Handbook of
Health Behavior Research II
Provider Determinants

Handbook of Health Behavior Research II
Provider Determinants

Edited by

David S. Gochman
University of Louisville
Louisville, Kentucky

Springer Science+Business Media, LLC

Library of Congress Cataloging-in-Publication Data

Handbook of health behavior research / edited by David S. Gochman.
p. cm.
Includes bibliographical references and indexes.
Contents: I. Personal and social determinants -- II. Provider determinants -- III. Demography, development, and diversity -- IV. Relevance for professionals and issues for the future.

ISBN 978-1-4899-1762-1
1. Health behavior. 2. Health behavior--Research. I. Gochman, David S.
[DNLM: 1. Health Behavior--handbooks. 2. Research--handbooks. W 49 H236 1997]
RA776.9.H363 1997
613--dc21
DNLM/DLC
for Library of Congress 97-14565
CIP

ISBN 978-1-4899-1762-1 ISBN 978-1-4899-1760-7 (eBook)
DOI 10.1007/978-1-4899-1760-7

Originally published by Plenum Press, New York in 1997
Softcover reprint of the hardcover 1st edition 1997

http://www.plenum.com

10 9 8 7 6 5 4 3 2 1

DEDICATION

Throughout my career I have been helped and encouraged by many persons. There are a few whose help was so special that my debt to them is enormous. It is in recognition of what I owe them that this *Handbook* is dedicated to Zelda S. Ackerman, O. J. Harvey, and D. Eldridge McBride, and to the memories of John H. Russel, William A. Scott, and John P. Kirscht. Mrs. Ackerman, my advisor in New York City's High School of Music and Art (now LaGuardia High School), facilitated my early entrance into academia. "Mac" McBride and John Russel, inspired and committed teachers, advisors, and counselors during my formative years at Shimer College, served as role models and continued as my friends over the decades. Bill Scott and O. J. Harvey were encouraging and supportive advisors during my graduate training at the University of Colorado. Bill taught me methodological rigor and innovation, and O. J. encouraged me to think in new and divergent ways. Both of them maintained high standards for their own performance, and demanded no less from me and others.

Jack Kirscht was a pioneer in health behavior research, a community activist, and a person of great wit, humor, and charm. In 1967 he convinced me to come to the University of Michigan's School of Public Health and to bring my research interests in cognitive development and structure to the area of health behavior. He was also a contributor to my 1988 book. Health behavior research lost a giant with his untimely death. He is very much missed by many as a friend and colleague and as a teacher and scholar.

Contributors

Cynthia L. Arfken, Center for Health Behavior Research and Diabetes Research and Training Center, Washington University, St. Louis, Missouri 63108

Zeev Ben-Sira, Late of School of Social Work, Hebrew University of Jerusalem, and Louis Gutmann Israel Institute of Applied Social Research, Jerusalem, Israel

Eric G. Benotsch, Department of Psychology, University of Iowa, Iowa City, Iowa 52242

Beth C. Bock, Miriam Hospital and Brown University School of Medicine, Providence, Rhode Island 02906

Daniel M. Cabrera, Department of Community Health Sciences, School of Public Health, University of California, Los Angeles, California 90095-1772

Victoria L. Champion, School of Nursing, Indiana University, Indianapolis, Indiana 46202-5117

Joan C. Chrisler, Department of Psychology, Connecticut College, New London, Connecticut 06320

Alan J. Christensen, Department of Psychology, University of Iowa, Iowa City, Iowa 52242

Noreen M. Clark, School of Public Health, University of Michigan, Ann Arbor, Michigan 48109-2029

Alexander Cohen, Consultant—Occupational Human Factors, 6752 East Farmacres Drive, Cincinnati, Ohio 45237

Michael J. Colligan, Education and Information Division, National Institute for Occupational Safety and Health, Cincinnati, Ohio 45226

Thomas L. Creer, Department of Psychology, Ohio University, Athens, Ohio 45701-2979

Wendy Demark-Wahnefried, Sarah Stedman Center for Nutritional Studies, Duke University Medical Center, Durham, North Carolina 27710

Colleen Di Iorio, Rollins School of Public Health, Emory University, Atlanta, Georgia 30322

M. Robin DiMatteo, Department of Psychology, University of California, Riverside, California 92521

Jennifer R. Egert, Department of Psychology, Social, and Health Sciences, Duke University, Durham, North Carolina 27710

Edwin B. Fisher, Jr., Center for Health Behavior and Diabetes Research and Training Center, Washington University, St. Louis, Missouri 63108

Russell E. Glasgow, Oregon Research Institute, 1715 Franklin Boulevard, Eugene, Oregon 97403

David S. Gochman, Kent School of Social Work, University of Louisville, Louisville, Kentucky 40292

Peggy Greco, Nemours Children's Clinic, 807 Nira Street, Jacksonville, Florida 32207

Frederic W. Hafferty, Department of Behavioral Sciences, University of Minnesota School of Medicine, Duluth, Minnesota 55812

Marie R. Haug, University Center on Aging and Health, Case Western Reserve University, Cleveland, Ohio 44106-7131

Joan M. Heins, Center for Health Behavior Research and Diabetes Research and Training Center, Washington University, St. Louis, Missouri 63108

Cheryl A. Houston, Center for Health Behavior Research and Diabetes Research and Training Center, Washington University, St. Louis, Missouri 63108

Donna B. Jeffe, Center for Health Behavior Research and Diabetes Research and Training Center, Washington University, St. Louis, Missouri 63108

Robin A. Kearns, Department of Geography, University of Auckland, Auckland, New Zealand

Deirdre Levstek, Department of Psychology, Ohio University, Athens, Ohio 45701-2979

Bess H. Marcus, Miriam Hospital and Brown University School of Medicine, Providence, Rhode Island 02906

Kevin D. McCaul, Department of Psychology, North Dakota State University, Fargo, North Dakota 58105

Anna Miller, School of Nursing, Ball State University, Muncie, Indiana 47306

Donald E. Morisky, Department of Community Health Sciences, School of Public Health, University of California, Los Angeles, California 90095-1772

C. Tracy Orleans, Fox Chase Cancer Center, 510 Township Line Road, Cheltenham, Pennsylvania 19012

Bernardine M. Pinto, Miriam Hospital and Brown University School of Medicine, Providence, Rhode Island 02906

Barbara K. Rimer, Duke Comprehensive Cancer Center, Duke University Medical Center, Durham, North Carolina 27710

Jeffrey C. Salloway, Department of Health Management and Policy, University of New Hampshire, Durham, New Hampshire 03824

Joseph L. Scarpaci, Department of Urban Affairs and Planning, Virginia Polytechnic Institute and State University, Blacksburg, Virginia 24061-0113

Timothy W. Smith, Department of Psychology, University of Utah, Salt Lake City, Utah 84112

Roslyn K. Sykes, Center for Health Behavior Research and Diabetes Research and Training Center, Washington University, St. Louis, Missouri 63108

James A. Trostle, Five College Medical Anthropology Program, Mount Holyoke College, South Hadley, Massachusetts 01075

Yvonne M. Vissing, Department of Sociology, Salem State College, Salem, Massachusetts 01970

Tim Wysocki, Nemours Children's Clinic, 807 Nira Street, Jacksonville, Florida 32207

Preface to All Volumes

THE STATE OF THE ART

The *primary* objective of this *Handbook* is to provide statements about health behavior research as a basic body of knowledge moving into the 21st century. It is expected that the *Handbook* will remain in use and current through 2005, at least. The *Handbook* presents a broad and representative selection of mid-1990s health behavior findings and concepts in a single work. While texts and books of readings are available in related areas, such as health psychology (e.g., DiMatteo, 1991; Stone et al., 1987), medical anthropology (e.g., McElroy & Townsend, 1989; Nichter, 1992), medical sociology (e.g., Cockerham, 1995; Helman, 1990; Wolinsky, 1988), behavioral health (e.g., Matarazzo, Weiss, Herd, Miller, & Weiss, 1984), behavioral risk factors (e.g., Hamburg, Elliott, & Parron, 1982), and changing health behaviors (Shumaker et al., 1990), none of these works was intended to address basic research-generated knowledge of health behavior, and none was intended to transcend individual disciplines. Accordingly, none of these works presents a broad and representative spectrum of basic health behavior research reflecting multidisciplinary activities. One work with a title identical to this one but for one word, the *Handbook of Health Behavior Change* (Shumaker et al., 1990), deals almost exclusively with applications. This *Handbook* thus presents the reader with the "state of the art" in health behavior research, something not found elsewhere.

In the context of this primary objective, it was not intended that the chapters be journal articles. Authors were encouraged to provide extensive coverage of their topics and to provide original findings to the degree that such findings were relevant. They were not encouraged to write research reports, and the reader should not expect the chapters to read as though they were journal articles.

HEALTH BEHAVIOR AS BASIC RESEARCH

Health behavior is not a long-established, traditional area of inquiry, comparable to chemistry or psychology, but a newly emerging interdisciplinary and multidisciplinary one. Health behavior is still establishing its identity as a domain of scientific research.

Although the earlier work (Gochman, 1988) that helped define it is now nearly a decade old, there are still relatively few institutional or organizational structures, i.e., departments and programs, that reflect the field, and few books and no journals are directed at it.

A *second* objective of the *Handbook* is to reaffirm the identity of health behavior and help secure its position as an important area of basic research, worthy of being studied in its own right. In the context of their discussion of the emergence of medical anthropology, Foster and Anderson (1978, pp. 2-3) stated: "When a sufficient number of researchers focus on the same, or related, topics, and as significant new data begin to appear, the stage is set for the emergence of a new discipline or subdiscipline. But some spark is essential to coalesce these emerging interests around a common focus; usually, it seems, an appropriate name supplies this spark." It is hoped that this *Handbook* will provide such a spark.

LEVELS OF ANALYSIS

Personal, Social, and Provider Determinants

A *third* objective, very much related to the first two, is to view health behavior research as transcending particular behaviors, specific illnesses or health problems or strategies for intervention, or single sets of determinants. One major way of achieving this objective is to look at health behavior in transaction with a range of personal, social systems: as an outcome or product, as well as a factor that affects these systems (in this context, the term *system* is often used interchangeably with *unit* or *entity*), rather than primarily as a set of risk factors or as targets for interventions directed at behavioral change. Volumes I and II of this *Handbook* thus deal largely with characteristics of the system of concern, and focus on specific health behaviors, or specific health problems or conditions, as ways of demonstrating the impact of these systems.

Volume I begins with conceptualizations of health and health behavior and then moves from smaller to larger systems, demonstrating how health behavior is determined by—and often in transaction with—personal, family, social, institutional and community, and cultural factors. These levels of analysis cannot be neatly differentiated, and at times the distinctions between them are arbitrary: Families, organizations, and institutions are all social systems. Moreover, although all individuals differ in their responses to and interpretations of family, social, and cultural norms, personalities and cognitive structures nonetheless reflect family, social, and cultural factors; additionally, families, social groupings, and organizations all reflect elements of the culture in which they exist. Furthermore, the categorizing and sequencing of sections and chapters in no way reflect an attempt to exclude material that deals with other levels of determinants; they serve primarily to facilitate focusing more on one of these determinants than on others. Volume I concludes with an integration that relates categories of health behaviors to characteristics of personal and social systems, identifies common themes, and suggests future research directions.

Since so much of health behavior is determined by providers—the health professionals and institutions that comprise the care delivery system—Volume II examines the way encounters with health providers determine health behaviors, and how health behaviors and the providers reciprocally affect one another. Volume II begins with an overview section on communication, continues with a section on interactional and structural determinants, i.e., professional characteristics, perceptions, power, and role relations, and organizational, locational, and environmental factors; and then presents major sections on the impact of provider characteristics on adherence to and acceptance of both disease-focused and lifestyle regimens.

Populations and Professional Applications

Volume III begins with an overview section on the demography of health behavior and continues with an examination of health behaviors in a range of populations selected on the basis either of the life-span continuum; of a health status risk due to an existing condition, a socially constructed label, or restrictive economic and environmental conditions; or of membership in defined communities. Volume IV examines the relevance of knowledge generated by health behavior research for the training and clinical (and other) practice activities of health professionals; for health services management and health policy; and for planned applications in school, family, community and workplace settings, and the media. Volume IV aims to position health behavior research in the 21st century through a discussion of the four major disciplines that inform health behavior research: health psychology, medical anthropology, medical geography, and medical sociology. Volume IV also presents a working draft of a taxonomy of health behavior and of a matrix framework for organizing health behavior knowledge.

Glossary and Index

Each of the volumes concludes with a glossary of health behavior concepts and definitions, and an index. Both of these reflect the contents of the entire *Handbook*.

A FRAMEWORK FOR ORGANIZING HEALTH BEHAVIOR KNOWLEDGE: A WORK IN PROGRESS

A Taxonomy for Health Behavior

Reviewing the contributed chapters in a volume with the editorial objective of integration led to the development of a "work in progress" taxonomy of health behaviors that became a primary organizing principle for the final chapter of each of the first three volumes. The taxonomy continued to evolve from Volume I to Volume III. The integration of Volume I would have been modified and organized slightly differently had it been written *after* those for Volumes II and III, but the fundamentals remained the same. Virtually all of the health behavior findings reported could be subsumed under one of six categories: health cognitions; care seeking; risk behaviors; lifestyle; responses to illness, including adherence; and preventive, protective, and safety behaviors.

A Matrix Framework

The working taxonomy appears in a different way in Volume IV. With one minor modification—the distinction between nonaddictive and addictive risk behaviors—it combines with the range of personal and social systems used as organizing principles in Volumes I and II, and in the integration chapters for Volumes I through III, to become part of a matrix framework for organizing health behavior knowledge. This framework is presented in Chapter 20 of Volume IV, entitled "Health Behavior Research, Cognate Disciplines, Future Identity, and an Organizing Matrix: An Integration of Perspectives."

DIVERSITY OF PERSPECTIVES

A *fourth* objective is to assure that the reader is exposed to varied perspectives in conceptual models, disciplines, populations, and methods, as well as to nonmedical frames of reference. The *Handbook* exposes the reader to a range of theories and models. The contributors bring expertise from their training or professional involvements in varied disciplines, including (in alphabetical order) anthropology, biology, communications, dentistry, education, engineering, ethics, geography, health management and policy, health promotion and health education, medicine, nursing, psychiatry, psychology, public health, social work, and sociology.

DIVERSITY OF READERS

A *fifth* objective is to assure the relevance of the *Handbook* for persons in a number of fields who are interested in issues related to research in health behavior. The potential readership includes researchers in the social and behavioral sciences who want to know more about health behavior in general, or particular aspects of it, or who want to develop their own health behavior research; students in courses that integrate social and behavioral science and health, in disciplines such as anthropology, psychology, and sociology, and in professional programs in dentistry, medicine (including psychiatry), nursing, public health, and social work; professionals who provide, plan, implement, and evaluate health services and programs: fitness and exercise physiologists; family planners; health educators and promoters; health managers; health planners; hospital administrators; nutritionists; pharmacists; physicians in community and family practice; physiatrists; public health dentists, nurses, physicians; rehabilitation therapists; social workers; and so forth.

THE PRACTICAL RELEVANCE OF HEALTH BEHAVIOR RESEARCH

The practical value of increasing knowledge and understanding of health behavior through rigorous, systematic research is implicit in the grave concern with health status in many contemporary societies. Solutions to an appreciable number of health problems require large-scale efforts at local, regional, and national levels to develop and enforce policies to control, minimize, and ultimately reduce air, land, and water pollution; the hazards of transportation; and the risks of the workplace environment. Many of these solutions transcend individual health behaviors. Solutions to other health problems, however, involve policies, programs, and processes that interact with the personal health behavior of individuals and the population at large, in their family, social, workplace, institutional, and community milieus.

As material in Volume IV demonstrates, attempts to change individual health behaviors, either through individual therapeutic interventions or through larger-scale health promotion or health education programs, have been less than impressive. Many attempts are purely programmatic, hastily conceived, and lacking in theoretical rationale or empirical foundation. A major reason for this is the lack of *basic* knowledge about the target behaviors, about the contexts in which they occur, and about the factors that determine and stabilize them. Basic research in health behavior, aside from being worthy of study in its own right, may very well increase the effectiveness of interventions and programs designed to bring about behavioral change.

DELIBERATE OMISSIONS

Notably absent from the *Handbook* are chapters devoted to topics such as "Type A" personality, psychosomatics, and stress. While these considerations may be linked to health status, and sometimes to health behavior, they have been omitted because they are more generally models for understanding the etiology of disease and illnesses. Furthermore, while "holism" has become a catchword among many who disavow the traditional medical model, the term has come to include charlatanism and cultism, as well as some impressive approaches to treatment. At present, it remains more a statement of faith suggesting future research alternatives than a body of well-thought-through, rigorously conducted research. Moreover, caution against a reverse "ethnocentrism" and overly romanticized views of non-high-technological medicine is cogently provided by Eisenberg and Kleinman (1981). In their words (Eisenberg & Kleinman, 1981, p. 10): "Healing ceremonies can be efficacious, but hardly substitute for antibiotics or surgery." Accordingly, there is no section on "holism" or "holistic medicine" or "holistic health" in the *Handbook*.

REFERENCES

Cockerham, W. C. (1995). *Medical sociology* (6th ed.). Englewood Cliffs, NJ: Simon & Schuster.

DiMatteo, M. R. (1991). *The psychology of health, illness, and medical care: An individual perspective*. Belmont, CA: Brooks/Cole.

Eisenberg, L., & Kleinman, A. (Eds.). (1981). *The relevance of social science for medicine*. Dordrecht, Netherlands: Reidel.

Foster, G. M., & Anderson, B. G. (1978). *Medical anthropology*. New York: Wiley.

Gochman, D. S. (Ed.). (1988). *Health behavior: Emerging research perspectives*. New York: Plenum Press.

Hamburg, D. A., Elliott, G. R., & Parron, D. L. (Eds.). (1982). *Health and behavior: Frontiers of research in the biobehavioral sciences*. Washington, DC: National Academy Press.

Helman, C. G. (1990). *Culture, health and illness* (2nd ed.). London: Wright/Butterworth.

Matarazzo, J. D., Weiss, S. M., Herd, J. A., Miller, N. E., & Weiss, S. M. (Eds.). (1984). *Behavioral health: A handbook of health enhancement and disease prevention*. New York: Wiley.

McElroy, A., & Townsend, P. K. (1989). *Medical anthropology in ecological perspective* (2nd ed.). Boulder, CO: Westview.

Nichter, M. (Ed.). (1992). *Anthropological approaches to the study of ethnomedicine*. Amsterdam, Netherlands: Gordon and Breach Science Publishers.

Shumaker, S.A., Schron, E. B., Ockene, J. K., Parker, C. T., Probstfield, J. L., & Wolle, J. M. (Eds.). (1990). *The handbook of health behavior change*. New York: Springer.

Stone, G. C., Weiss, S. M., Matarazzo, J. D., Miller, N. E., Rodin, J., Belar, C. D., Follick, M. J., & Singer, J. E. (Eds.). (1987). *Health psychology: A discipline and a profession*. Chicago: University of Chicago Press.

Wolinsky, F. D. (1988). *The sociology of health: Principles, practitioners, and issues* (2nd ed.). Belmont, CA: Wadsworth.

Preface to Volume II

PROVIDER DETERMINANTS OF HEALTH BEHAVIOR

Volume II focuses on health provider determinants of health behavior. In this context, the term *provider* broadly includes the professionals and institutions comprising the health care system—dentists, dieticians, exercise and fitness physiologists; health educators and health promotion specialists; health managers and planners; nurses, physiatrists, physicians, psychologists, psychiatrists, rehabilitation therapists; social workers and other health care professionals; and caregivers—together with the settings in which they encounter individuals—clinics, hospitals, program classrooms, professional offices, and so forth. The volume discusses aspects of the encounters between the individual—patient, client, or consumer—and the providers that affect health behavior. It is a complement to the coverage in Volume I of other determinants, one segment along a continuum of personal and social determinants.

The volume is organized into five sections. An overview focusing on critical dimensions of the information sharing and communication between the person or patient and professionals is followed by a section on interactional and structural determinants, including professional characteristics, roles, power, and locational issues. This section is followed by an overview of issues related to the ideology and political and economic context of adherence to or acceptance of regimens, a section on adherence to a range of disease-focused regimens, and a section on adherence to lifestyle regimens or programs. The volume concludes with an integration that relates categories of health behaviors to characteristics of health professionals and health institutions and of personal and social systems, identifies common themes, and suggests future research directions.

Acknowledgments

Many persons provided greatly valued assistance during the nearly four years from the time the *Handbook of Health Behavior Research* was conceptualized until its publication, and I owe all of them my thanks. The substantial help I received from some of them merits special recognition. Among the support staff at the Raymond A. Kent School, I especially wish to thank Shannon R. Daniels and Kelley E. Davis for their expeditious and careful photocopying of what must have seemed like tons of manuscripts, Jane Isert for her dedication in assuring that calls and mail from contributors and from the publisher reached me in a timely way, and Sally Montreuil-Palmarini for expediting mailings of material to contributors.

Among the highly professional and committed staff at the University of Louisville's Ekstrom Library, special thanks go to all of the reference librarians, and particularly to Carmen Embry (now at Barrier Islands Art Center) for some insightful content suggestions; Sharon Edge for her expediting access to materials; and S. Kay Womack (now at the University of Oklahoma) for her astute and knowledgeable guidance through computer and other literature searches, particularly in areas in which little had been written that was adequately indexed.

Thomas R. Lawson, Director of the Kent School, deserves recognition for his continued encouragement of my scholarly activities, his efforts in securing a sabbatical leave for me to assure the *Handbook*'s timely completion, and his generosity in providing necessary supplies and personnel resources.

A great debt is owed to all of the authors whose scholarly chapters grace the *Handbook*, and add immeasurably to its value, for the care they devoted to their work, and for their receptivity and constructive responses to the high density of editorial suggestions made throughout the *Handbook*'s progress. A number of authors and others also provided suggestions about potential contributors for several topics. Among those whose help in this quest was exceptional were M. Robin DiMatteo, Eugene B. Gallagher, Russell E. Glasgow, Michael R. Kauth, Jeffrey Kelley, James E. Maddux, Lillian C. Milanof, R. Prasaad Steiner, and David P. Willis.

Gene Gallagher, along with Zeev Ben-Sira (whose untimely death occurred prior to the final revision of his chapter), John G. Bruhn, Patricia J. Bush, Henry P. Cole, Reed Geertsen, Marie R. Haug, Richard R. Lau, Alexander Segall, and Ingrid Waldron had all contributed to the 1988 book. Their willingness to contribute anew to this one is most appreciated.

Finally, Richard Millikan merits special recognition for the excellence of his copyediting work, his ability to perceive issues that cross-cut the four volumes, and for his skill in helping me clarify my own thinking; and Eliot Werner, Executive Editor at Plenum Publishing Corporation, deserves special thanks for his vision and encouragement in the area of health behavior research, for his faith in the value of the *Handbook*, and for being laid back and calming in the face of my "overfunctioning" and obsessive-compulsivity.

Contents

I

OVERVIEW

INFORMATION SHARING AND COMMUNICATION

The processing of information between professional and patient is a critical component of communication. Hauser (1981) provided a review of empirical studies of information exchange, and Stiles, Putnam, and Jacob (1982) analyzed frameworks for conducting interviews. In an analysis of changes in physician interviewing styles, Armstrong (1984) pointed out that the old "medical gaze" that went hand in hand with the physician's aggressive interrogation of an essentially passive, inarticulate patient, followed by a physical examination, has evolved into a clinical perspective that allows greater amounts of input from the patient and a greater appreciation of the patient's view.

Nonetheless, despite such changes, information sharing and communication between physician and patient remain problematic. Wartman, Marlock, Malitz, and Palm (1981) cautioned that physicians' prescriptions of medication can be a substitute for meaningful communication with patients. The exploration by Boreham and Gibson (1978) of information-gathering and communication processes revealed that laypersons typically have been passive as information gatherers, despite changes in access to care, in the narrowing of the knowledge gap between professionals and clients, in the increasing chronicity—and thus increased needs for knowledge and information—of conditions that bring patients in for care, and the increasing degree to which poor communication is a source of patient dissatisfaction.

Observations of the verbal behavior of medical students and their patients showed the importance of provider communication initiatives. The frequency of patient questions and comments reflecting the content of the consultation and interaction was likely to increase when the providers themselves raised questions with the patient about the treatment (Robinson & Whitfield, 1987).

The Hayes-Bautista (1978) nontraditional conceptual paradigm for understanding the layperson–professional encounter is derived from a sociology of knowledge perspective. Hayes-Bautista pointed out that physicians and patients derive their knowledge and information from very different sources and that the attributes of their knowledge are different. Such differences lead to difficulties in effective communication.

Helman (1985) analyzed four components of the communication process: the patient's view of the origin, significance, and effects of a condition; the physician's view of these aspects; the physician's view of the patient's view; and the congruity of these three views. The physician is more likely to have a "disease" view, focusing on specific "objective" pathology; the patient is more likely to have an "illness" view, reflecting "subjective" feelings and experiences. Moreover, Helman observed, while physicians and patients might be in marked agreement on diagnosis and other components of the encounter, physicians showed limited knowledge of patients' explanatory beliefs. However, physicians' knowledge of patients' views was greater for patients who had completed college than for those who had not.

Although physicians recognize that their communications often require convergence toward the everyday language used by patients, and many perceive that their language actually does converge with that of patients, independent assessments by patients and nurses suggest that physician communication remains closer to medical language than to everyday speech (Bourhis, Roth, & MacQueen, 1989). A questionnaire study showing that patients and providers differed markedly in their understandings of a variety of terms revealed wider gaps in their understanding of psychological terms, such as "hysteria" and "neurosis," than of more straightforwardly medical terms (Hadlow & Pitts, 1991).

Heszen-Klemens and Lapinska (1984) observed how the behavior of Polish physicians affected the behavior of their patients. Using Bales's Interaction Process Analysis, they showed that patients' recall of instructions was greater when such instructions occurred more frequently in physicians' communications, when patients were allowed to act as partners in the encounter, when they asked more questions, and when physicians were friendlier. Recall worsened when the total amount of advice given by physicians (physician directiveness) increased.

An analysis by Stewart (1984) of patient-centered behaviors showed that when physicians asked patients for opinions and help, the result was increased patient satisfaction. Moreover, when physicians allowed patients to show negative feelings, patient satisfaction was also greater. Blanchard, Labrecque, Ruckdeschel, and Blanchard (1988) documented that large proportions of cancer patients want full disclosure of information, in contrast to physicians' assumptions that they should not reveal a cancer diagnosis to such patients.

The literature review by Mathews (1983) identifies a number of problem areas in the communication process and emphasizes the importance of shared knowledge, status, role, and ideology and of institutional restraints on sharing information. An analysis of provider communication styles by Campbell and associates (e.g., Campbell, Mauksch, Neikirk, & Hosokawa, 1990) suggested that such physician-patient interactions can be classified under four styles: curative, characterized by somatic diagnosis and treatment; patient education, characterized by providing information; caring, characterized by inclusion of psychosocial concerns and high levels of affiliation and control; and general, characterized by average levels of the other three.

Tuckett and Williams (1984) reviewed attempts to measure explanation and information giving and emphasized the need to improve and develop procedures to do so, particularly in relation to the "meaning" of the information sought and provided. Buijs, Sluijs, and Verhaak (1984) have developed a technique for assessing physicians' interview styles in relation to information gathering in the two distinct phases of the consultation process: diagnosis and prescribing. Physicians vary along the dimension of use of patient-centeredness and doctor-centeredness, depending on their use of patients' knowledge and experiences in relation to their own.

In the context of arguing for a role for counseling psychology in the training of physicians, Robins and Wolf (1988) present vignette-based data showing how physicians' linguistic responses to patients' confrontational statements have the potential to improve the communication process. A strategy of *asserting reciprocity*, in which the physician accepts the patient's point and offers to be of help in mutual problem solving, was suggested as a way of being both polite in a culturally acceptable way and facilitative of mutual understanding, in contrast to other more typical ways of responding that place patients in passive, compliant roles. Roter (1988), reporting on both a Bales Interaction Process Analysis and a meta-analysis, showed that a considerable degree of reciprocity existed in the physician-patient encounter.

DiMatteo's overview in Chapter 1 identifies

a number of issues inherent in communication between professionals and patients. These issues include patient needs for both support and information, changing interaction patterns and role relationships, professional characteristics, and adherence to regimens.

REFERENCES

Armstrong, D. (1984). The patient's view. *Social Science and Medicine*, *18*, 737-744.

Blanchard C. G., Labrecque M. S., Ruckdeschel, J. C., & Blanchard, E. B. (1988). Information and decision-making preferences of hospitalized adult cancer patients. *Social Science and Medicine*, *17*, 1139-1145.

Boreham, P., & Gibson, D. (1978). The informative process in private medical consultations: A preliminary investigation. *Social Science and Medicine*, *12*, 409-416.

Bourhis, R. Y., Roth, S., & MacQueen, G. (1989). Communication in the hospital setting: A survey of medical and everyday language use amongst patients, nurses and doctors. *Social Science and Medicine*, *28*, 339-346.

Buijs, R., Sluijs, E. M., & Verhaak, P. F. M. (1984). Byrne and Long: A classification for rating the interview style of doctors. *Social Science and Medicine*, *19*, 683-690.

Campbell, J. D., Mauksch, H. O., Neikirk, H. J., & Hosokawa, M. C. (1990). Collaborative practice and provider styles of delivering health care. *Social Science and Medicine*, *30*, 1359-1365.

Hadlow, J., & Pitts, M. (1991). The understanding of common health terms by doctors, nurses and patients. *Social Science and Medicine*, *32*, 193-196.

Hauser, S. T. (1981). Physician-patient relationships. In E. G. Mishler, L. R. Aramasingham, S. T. Hauser, S. D. Osherson, N. E. Waxler, & R. Liem (Eds.), *Social contexts of health, illness, and patient care* (pp. 104-140). Cambridge, England: Cambridge University Press.

Hayes-Bautista, D. E. (1978). Chicano patients and medical practitioners: A sociology of knowledges paradigm of lay-professional interaction. *Social Science and Medicine*, *12*, 83-90.

Helman, C. G. (1985). Communication in primary care: The role of patient and practitioner explanatory models. *Social Science and Medicine*, *20*, 923-931.

Heszen-Klemens, I., & Lapinska, E. (1984). Doctor-patient interaction, patients' health behavior and effects of treatment. *Social Science and Medicine*, *19*, 9-18.

Mathews, J. J. (1983). The communication process in clinical settings. *Social Science and Medicine*, *17*, 1371-1378.

Robins, L. S., & Wolf, F. M. (1988). Confrontation and politeness strategies in physician-patient interactions. *Social Science and Medicine*, *27*, 217-221.

Robinson, E. J., & Whitfield, M. J. (1987). Participation of patients during general practice consultations. *Psychology and Health*, *1*, 123-132.

Roter, D. L. (1988). Reciprocity in the medical encounter. In D. S. Gochman (Ed.), *Health behavior: Emerging research perspectives* (pp. 293-303). New York: Plenum Press.

Stewart, M. A. (1984). What is a successful doctor-patient interview? A study of interactions and outcomes. *Social Science and Medicine*, *19*, 167-175.

Stiles, W. B., Putnam, S. M., & Jacob, M. C. (1982). Verbal exchange structure of initial medical interviews. *Health Psychology*, *1*, 315-336.

Tuckett, D., & Williams, A. (1984). Approaches to the measurement of explanation and information-giving in medical consultations: A review of empirical studies. *Social Science and Medicine*, *18*, 571-580.

Wartman, S. A., Morlock, L. L., Malitz, F. E., & Palm, E. (1981). Do prescriptions adversely affect doctor-patient relationships? *American Journal of Public Health*, *71*, 1358-1361.

1

Health Behaviors and Care Decisions

An Overview of Professional–Patient Communication

M. Robin DiMatteo

The provision of high-quality health care for everyone in the United States remains an unattained goal because of limitations in financial resources. Evidence suggests, however, that reducing overall demand, particularly for high-cost, high-technology items, would make better use of these resources and thus increase the availability of medical services to all (Fries et al., 1993). This chapter will explore potential *behavioral* strategies for reducing overall demand and cost for medical services. These strategies involve interpersonal communication, adherence to recommendations for personal health behavior, and effective joint decision making on the part of medical practitioners and patients toward the goals of (1) reducing unnecessary, inappropriate medical treatment and (2) preventing chronic and acute illness and injury.

M. Robin DiMatteo • Department of Psychology, University of California, Riverside, California 92521.

Handbook of Health Behavior Research II: Provider Determinants, edited by David S. Gochman. Plenum Press, New York, 1997.

OVERVIEW

This chapter will examine health professional-patient communication as a central element in enhancing the effective and appropriate use of the opportunities presented by medical technology. Communication is essential to enhancing primary prevention (DiMatteo & DiNicola, 1982), to making effective medical decisions (DiMatteo, 1994a), to choosing appropriate treatments (Gambone, Reiter, & DiMatteo, 1994), to facilitating patients' coping with illness and avoidance of hopelessness (Kleinman, 1988), to enhancing the capacity to heal (Shapiro, 1960), and to assuming responsibility for chronic care (DiMatteo et al., 1993). The chapter will examine the growing evidence that patient satisfaction, communication of information, and practitioner concern for patients as individuals are valid and critically important indicators of the quality of medical care delivered to patients (Donabedian, 1980; Speedling & Rose, 1985) and predictors of health outcomes (Haug & Lavin, 1979; McBride et al., 1994; Speedling & Rose, 1985). Further, the chapter will consider challenges to medical "authority" that give rise to malpractice litigation, nonadherence to treatment, and patients' "doctor-shopping."

THE PROBLEM OF INAPPROPRIATE/ UNNECESSARY MEDICAL CARE

It is estimated that currently at least 20% of all health expenditures in the United States are for the delivery of medical care that is inappropriate and unnecessary (*Consumer Reports*, 1992). A medical intervention is considered inappropriate when the risk to the patient exceeds the potential benefit that might derive from the intervention (McGlynn, Kosecoff, & Brook, 1990). Considerable research shows that high-technology intervention (e.g., coronary artery bypass surgery) may not always be the best approach to a problem (e.g., heart disease) because much less expensive and much less risky long-term solutions (e.g., medication, dietary modification, smoking cessation, exercise, relaxation, and other lifestyle changes) may produce better overall outcomes. Researchers were first clued into the possibility that many routinely performed medical procedures might be unnecessary and inappropriate when they noted that despite massive regional variations in the frequency of administration of many medical procedures (among them cesarean section, tonsillectomy, and hysterectomy), health outcomes were similar (Fries et al., 1993; Leape et al., 1990; Wennberg, 1990; Wennberg et al., 1988). Variation due to physician habits and preferences suggested that some medical procedures may be done inappropriately, wasting health care dollars and exposing patients to unnecessary risk of morbidity and mortality.

Using a process for developing consensus among nationally recognized experts in a given field, researchers at the RAND Corporation (McGlynn et al., 1990) developed agreed-upon lists of the indications for various procedures and compared the medical records of thousands of patients with these criteria. Clear evidence of inappropriate overtreatment was found across the United States, including 14% of coronary artery bypass operations, 17% of coronary angiography procedures, 16% of tonsillectomies, 27% of tympanostomy tubes for recurrent otitis media, 50% of cesarean sections, 27% of hysterectomies, and 14% of laminectomies (Bernstein et al., 1993; Brook et al., 1990; Chassin, 1990; Gray, Hampton, Bernstein, Kosecoff, & Brook, 1990; Kleinman, Kosecoff, Dubois, & Brook, 1994).

Traditionally, physicians have made all the medical decisions that determine the course of a patient's care. Parsons (1951) has argued that physician and patient are separated by "the competence gap," which, because of the physician's superior knowledge, justifies physician maintenance of control. The proliferation of technological alternatives in medicine in recent years has further increased decision-making complexity and has taken emphasis off the patient as a person with unique outcome preferences (Lincoln, 1982; Lynn & DeGrazia, 1991). Research is beginning to confirm, however, that in order to apply medical technology most effectively, patient needs and preferences must be considered. Most medical conditions have behavioral components in which personal health behaviors and preferences figure in important ways (D. S. Brody, 1980; H. Brody, 1992).

Evidence is accumulating that an emphasis on communication can reduce the administration of unnecessary, inappropriate medical treatments that, partly because of patient preferences, are not the best choices for patients. The need to consider patient preferences is particularly salient in the realm of end-of-life decisions (Emanuel, Barry, Stoeckle, Ettelson, & Emanuel, 1991), but is also important in the choice of more conservative approaches to treatment. When given information and alternatives, patients select less invasive and less expensive treatment strategies than their physicians do (Wennberg, 1990). Further, better decisions are made when patients' values, expectations, and preferences are included in medical-care decisions.

COMMUNICATION: TWO FUNDAMENTAL ELEMENTS IN PATIENT CARE

The word "communicate" comes from the Latin *communis* ("common"); to communicate is to establish a commonness. In the words of DiMatteo and DiNicola (1982, p. 21): "In human social processes, communication involves the unrestricted exchange of meaning between people to establish a commonness of thought, attitude, feeling, and idea." Communication can be verbal, by means of words, or nonverbal, by means of signs.

It is important to remember that physician and patient may share a language and culture, but still fail to understand each other well. Illness and pain are subjective experiences dependent upon meaning and interpretation (Kleinman, 1988), and provider-patient communication is impeded by anxiety, emotional upset, differences in knowledge and social power, medical jargon, and time limits. As Barnlund (1976, p. 721) has noted, "The factors that complicate the process of shared meaning are nearly all present in doctor-patient encounters."

Two major elements of effective provider-patient communication affect health outcomes: (1) accurate transmittal of information from patient to practitioner and from practitioner to patient and (2) the practitioner's emotional support and understanding of the patient as a unique person and of his or her emotional needs and personal experience in medical care.

Regarding the first aspect, it should be noted that effective, accurate communication of information is far from standard in medical care as it is currently rendered. Research on the medical visit has involved recording (by standardized observation, audiotape, or videotape) and painstakingly analyzing thousands of medical-care visits.

Most research on provider-patient communication has been conducted on physicians as the providers. Although allied health professionals (nurses, technicians, health educators) can contribute significantly to patient education and behavior change, it is the case that they typically do so as extensions of physicians and by acting under physicians' direction. Health care delivery in the United States is currently dominated and controlled by physicians (Freidson, 1970; Starr, 1982), and changes in that delivery are likely to involve substantial physician input and regulation. For these reasons, this chapter focuses on physician-patient relationships, though much of what is reviewed and recommended is of course also relevant to other health professionals.

This research has demonstrated that physician-patient communication is often so poor that close to half of all patients leave their doctors' offices not knowing what they have been told and what they are supposed to do to take care of themselves (DiMatteo, 1991). Physicians regularly use medical terms that patients do not understand, and patients are unwilling or lack sufficient skill to articulate their questions (Christy, 1979; Roter, 1984). While 90% of patients place a high value on having as much information as possible from their physicians, and want to know about potential outcomes of and alternatives to treatment recommendations (Roter & Hall, 1992), such information is rarely provided to them (Faden, Becker, Lewis, Freeman, & Faden, 1981). In the course of medical visits that average 20 minutes, an average of less than 1 minute is spent giving patients any information at all (Waitzkin & Stoeckle, 1976). Observations of physician-patient interactions show that physicians actually discourage patients' voicing of concerns, expectations, and requests for information (Svarstad, 1976; West, 1984). Without information and the opportunity to participate in discussion during the medical care visit, the patient is, in effect, being told what to do (Wolf, 1988). Lack of sufficient explanation, poor patient understanding, and lack of consensus between physician and patient lead directly to therapeutic failure largely because of patients' failure to adhere to practitioners' recommendations (DiMatteo, 1994b).

Effective communication of information between medical providers and their patients has been identified as a positive influence on patient outcomes. Theoretically, benefits would be expected from patients' participating in their own care. Pickering (1979) has noted that in about 90% of medical conditions, either there is no indisputable, clear-cut treatment or the effectiveness of a treatment is unknown. Given that many clinical decisions are arbitrary and are influenced by physicians' habits and personal preferences (Eisenberg, 1979), it is reasonable to take patient preferences into account. Mutual exploration of alternatives toward the goal of agreement can help physician and patient form realistic expectations of various rational alternatives. Since patients tend to be more risk-averse than their physicians and to favor more conservative interventions that are less threatening to their quality of life (McNeil, Weichselbaum, & Pauker, 1978), it follows that patient involvement in the decision process is likely to lead to less invasive, less expensive interventions and, overall, an approach to solving the medical problem that is more satisfactory to the patient. As D. S. Brody (1980, p. 721) puts it: "Armed with a basic understanding of the nature of the problem, the patient is now capable of constructively challenging the foundations of the physician's reasoning. This interchange should lead to a more rational, thorough, open consideration of the various alternatives." Negotiation and constructive challenge lead physician and patient to examine their points of disagreement and prevent patients' expressions of dissatisfaction through noncompliance and malpractice litigation (Roter & Hall, 1992). Health professionals who communicate effectively with their patients will be able to determine and, if necessary, alter the two most important aspects of enhancing adherence: the patient's belief in the utility of the regimen (by finding an effective regimen that the patient can believe in) and existing barriers to patient adherence (by finding a regimen that the patient can follow) (DiMatteo et al., 1993). When patients cannot assert their preferences to their physicians, they often privately make plans for their own medical well-being, even to the point of making decisions not to adhere to medical regimens (Donovan & Blake, 1992; Hayes-Bautista, 1976). Noncompliance may be an active coping strategy to restore a lost sense of control (Rodin & Janis, 1979).

Empirical research has borne out these predictions, and the consensus of this research on outcomes is that patients benefit greatly from taking an active role in their medical-care choices (R. M. Kaplan, 1991). Starfield and colleagues (Starfield et al., 1979) showed that patients experienced greater improvement when physician and patient agreed on their expectations for follow-up. In other research, patients have been given information, have been trained in the skills necessary to request information during the medical visit, or have been taught to negotiate solutions with their physicians and take responsibility for decisions about their own care (Greenfield, Kaplan, & Ware, 1985). The structure of the medical interaction has been arranged to force joint decision making (such as by having the patient and physician coauthor the patient's medical record) (Fischbach, Sionelo-Bayog, Needle, & Delbanco, 1980). These interventions have helped patients to become much more active, ask more questions, and express greater satisfaction with their care (Roter, 1983; Roter & Hall, 1992). As a result of these interventions, patients have also experienced much greater alleviation of their symptoms and better control of their chronic conditions, greater improvement in their overall medical condition, less distress and concern about their illnesses, and better response to surgery and invasive diagnostic procedures (Egbert, Battit, Welch, & Bartlett, 1964; Johnson & Leventhal, 1974; S. H. Kaplan, Greenfield, & Ware, 1989). Patients who are involved in choices about their care also feel a greater sense of control over their health and their lives, demonstrate better adherence to the treatment that they have helped to decide upon, and have more positive expectations for their health (Speedling & Rose, 1985). Patients who participate in and share responsibility for their health decisions are less likely to blame their physicians if something goes wrong (Wagener & Taylor, 1986). Further, as Fisher (1983) has found, when patients question their physicians' decisions and ask about possible alternatives (e.g., medical management instead of surgery), their physicians typically change treatment decisions and are less likely to treat problems surgically.

The cost of failing to collaborate is high for both patients and health professionals. When they avoid discussion and its inevitable ***but manageable*** conflicts, providers and patients create relationships in which their expectations are never discussed. Kleinman and colleagues have demonstrated that the failure to elicit patients' desires and expectations about care actually can have devastating effects on therapeutic success (Kleinman, Eisenberg, & Good, 1978). When patients are not informed and involved, they give less adequate histories (Waitzkin & Stoeckle, 1972) and tend to delay in reporting important symptoms (Hackett, Cassem, & Raker, 1973).

The second aspect of provider-patient communication that is of importance involves empathy and the understanding of patients' feelings. This aspect of care has traditionally been a source of discomfort for physicians, and warnings are sounded regularly against what is termed "emotional involvement" in patients' lives (Marvel, 1993). As H. Brody (1992, p. 264) notes, however, "The cemetery is filled not with the corpses of patients who died because their overinvolved physicians became irrational and ineffective but rather with those of sufferers whose physicians attended to their diseases but failed to heal because of the multiple characterological barriers that cause physicians not to get close enough." If the physician attends only to disease and ignores suffering, he or she may cure but still fails to heal (Cassell, 1985). To quote H. Brody (1992, p. 259) again: "To be compassionate in response to the suffering of the patient is ... one of the most powerful things a physician can do."

The interpersonal behavior of physicians during office visits has been found to be associated with patients' satisfaction with medical care, their recall of medical information provided, and their subsequent adherence to prescribed regimens (Hall, Roter, & Katz, 1988). Patient satisfaction with medical treatment is greater if patients trust their providers (DiMatteo & DiNicola, 1982). Emotional support of patients appears to enhance positive expectations for healing, including placebo effects (Roter & Hall, 1992). The patients of physicians who are more sensitive to and emotionally expressive with nonverbal communication are more satisfied and more adherent to recommendations for treatment (DiMatteo, Hays, & Prince, 1986; DiMatteo, Linn, Chang, & Cope, 1985). Research demonstrates that physicians who make patients feel rushed or ignored, devalue their views, fail to respect and listen to them, and fail to understand their perspectives are more likely to be sued for medical malpractice (Hickson et al., 1994; Levinson, 1994). Importantly, there is empirical evidence that the interpersonal sensitivity of physicians is positively correlated with technical skills as a physician (DiMatteo & DiNicola, 1981); technical skill does not appear to be sacrificed in the development of the capacity to respond to patients' feelings.

BARRIERS TO EFFECTIVE PROVIDER–PATIENT COMMUNICATION

Despite considerable evidence that effective physician-patient communication provides many advantages to the therapeutic relationship, the practice of medicine today involves limitations in and physician control of information exchange. As Beisecker (1990, p. 104) says, "Even though they feel they have a right to challenge a doctor's authority, few patients ever do." A quarter century of research shows that patients want as much information about their medical care as they can obtain (Roter & Hall, 1992), but that they tend to be behaviorally passive in medical encounters. Patients tend to ask few questions, and they provide little information beyond what is directly asked for by their physicians (Beisecker, 1990).

Many factors influence effective communication in medical care. Certain sociodemographic characteristics are related to reduced communication, among them patients' lower income and education (Barnlund, 1976) and greater age (Putnam, Stiles, Jacob, & James, 1985). Female patients communicate more with physicians and ask more questions than do males, although male physicians tend to give shorter and less technical answers to female patients than to male patients (Wallen, Waitzkin, & Stoeckle, 1979). In comparison with male physicians, female physicians have been found to conduct longer and more talkative visits with their patients, to create a more positive interpersonal climate, and to be better listeners (Hall, Irish, Roter, Erhlich, & Miller, 1994).

Patients' attitudes also affect their willingness to ask questions and challenge physician authority. Patients with a more consumerist approach to medical care are more likely to seek information and to be assertive in the medical visit (Haug & Lavin, 1983), although only if the visit is long enough for meaningful discussion to take place (at least 19 minutes) (Beisecker & Beisecker, 1990).

Research on medical jargon suggests that a significant element in the misunderstanding between providers and patients involves the use by providers of technical terms that patients do not understand. Studies show that physicians often vastly overestimate the number and complexity of technical terms that their patients can understand, and that despite their confusion, patients typically do not ask for clarification (Barnlund, 1976).

Patients' ability to participate in their own health care depends upon having information, but studies suggest that physicians typically do not volunteer information (Roter, 1977; Waitzkin, 1985; West, 1984). Research also shows that physicians often react negatively to their patients' assertiveness (Beisecker, 1990) and may actively discourage patients' information seeking by ignoring questions, giving ambiguous responses, or changing the topic (West, 1984).

Physicians also tend to control and limit the amount of information they elicit from patients by asking them serial, closed-ended questions. Sankar (1986) has noted that patient provision of more information than the physician requests is seen as problematic by many physicians, and in some cases as rendering the problem more complex than the physician is prepared to handle. Many physicians fear that allowing patients to tell their own stories will require a large time investment (Kleinman, 1988), but research suggests that in most cases the time required does not exceed 2½ minutes (Beckman, Frankel, & Darnley, 1985). Interestingly, when a patient, by interjecting and volunteering details, does provide more information than the physician has solicited, physician and patient are more likely to arrive at a common definition of the patient's problem (Rost, Carter, & Inui, 1989).

From the practitioner's point of view, several factors contribute to poor communication with patients. First, many physicians harbor the misconception that patients do not want to know much about their medical care (Beisecker, 1990; Beisecker & Beisecker, 1990). Second, the pressures of professional practice limit the time available for communication with patients (Beisecker & Beisecker, 1990; DiMatteo & DiNicola, 1982). As Waitzkin (1985) has noted, however, physicians make choices in this regard. Waitzkin found that the more time physicians spent talking with patients, the fewer patients they had time to see and the less money they earned. Third, medical practice in the United States tends to be technology-driven. Testing, despite its limitations in reliability, is invoked for diagnosis much more than is the taking of a detailed medical history, which requires considerable skill at talking with patients (Putnam et al., 1985). Fourth, medicine in the United States tends to focus on intermediate outcomes (such as alteration in tissue) that may have little to do with the outcomes that affect a patient's quality of life (Eddy, 1990; Starr, 1982). Physicians' inattention to patients' quality of life tends to limit discussion with them of their overall well-being. Fifth, medical education in the United States does not prepare physicians for effective communication in practice. Communication skills actually diminish rather than improve over the course of medical training (Helfer, 1970).

From the patient's point of view, there are also certain factors that impede provider-patient communication. First, in terms of social power in the interaction, patients are at a decided disadvantage wearing a paper robe and sitting on an examining table with feet dangling. Second, unlike normal social discourse, in the medical visit the physician directs the conversation by asking questions and limiting the patient's responses (Waitzkin, 1991). Third, a patient's attempts at being assertive and actively asking questions are roundly discouraged and often met with the physician's anger and anxiety (Roter, 1977; West, 1984). In one analysis of medical interactions, patient assertiveness was met with attempts by the physician to regain control by asserting superiority and by questioning the patient's intelligence, stability, and normality (Beisecker, 1986). Fourth, physician-patient interactions are typically conducted in a manner that is relatively efficient, if not in fact rushed, with the physician controlling the amount of time it will take (Fisher, 1983). Patients tend to be deferent in response to this control, partly because of the physician's social power. Many patients believe, too, that urgency conveyed in the interaction has to do with patient care emergencies (taking care of other, sicker patients and saving lives) and are reluctant to take up time with their questions (DiMatteo, 1993). Of course, office-based medical practice presents few if any true clinical emergencies. Physician urgency is more about economics and the exigencies of reimbursement (Waitzkin, 1985). Fifth, anxiety, illness, and pain may pose particular challenges to the management of an already difficult social interaction. Sixth, there are several broader societal factors that affect physician-patient communication. One such factor is that the "competence gap" (Parsons, 1951) between physician and patient is broadened by the tremendous societal limitations in the availability of information about health and medical care. Patients have limited knowledge and technical skills with which to access and evaluate this information, and control of personal medical information such as copies of test results (which may be available to the patient only through the physician) limits patients' use of information about their personal medical cases (Fisher, 1984). Finally, the medical meeting is a "micropolitical" encounter in which content of the communication and the control of information reinforces social status and power relationships that parallel those in the broader society, in which physicians maintain social dominance (Waitzkin, 1991).

MODELS OF PATIENTS' INVOLVEMENT IN THEIR OWN CARE

Social theory of the physician-patient relationship has been guided by a series of models that have evolved through increasing levels of patient autonomy. Parsons (1951) argued that the social contract requires patients to submit to the "authority" of the physician, the basis of which lies in the physician's gatekeeping control of "the sick role." The sick role involves a status that grants the patient exemption from normal social responsibilities in exchange for seeking technically competent medical help and complying fully with medical recommendations. Because physicians control the legitimacy of patients' claims to the sick role, they have the right to tell patients what to do. According to Parson's theory, the social contract further allows patients to relax into complete trust in their physicians; because physician and patient have a "fiduciary relationship," the physician can be trusted to do what is in the patient's best interest.

The validity of these theoretical assumptions comes into question for several reasons. First, more recent views of American medicine suggest that its practitioners and organizations uniformly operate from strong motives for financial profit (Starr, 1982; Stevens, 1989). It follows, then, that providers of medical services have at least some goals that are different from those of their patients (Gambone & Reiter, 1991). Second, given the difficulties of communication, it is unlikely that any physician will know enough about any given patient's values and beliefs about what constitutes personal quality of life to make unilateral decisions that are truly in the patient's best interest. Given these limitations in the authority-based model, other models have been developed to guide research into optimal physician-patient relationships.

Theorists have noted for many years that patients can and should be active participants in their medical care. The Szasz and Hollender (1956) "mutual participation" model of therapeutic interaction places the patient and physician in a joint, cooperative venture, with their mutual goal being the patient's well-being. The "active patient orientation" approach (Schulman, 1979) likewise has patients involved and personally responsible for taking care of their health. These theorists have built their picture of the doctor-patient relationship on the importance of mutuality, arguing that physician and patient basically have the same goals and if a patient is involved and interested, the means to achieve those goals can be agreed upon. At the opposite extreme of theoretical positions is the approach of the consumer movement, which argues for patient autonomy (sole decision-making power) as essential to combat physician paternalism (Haug & Lavin, 1983).

Most current models of communication in the medical visit acknowledge, to some degree, the inevitability and the *value* of conflict in the physician-patient relationship (Katz, 1984). These models require active patient involvement in the negotiation of expectations and goals and the means for achieving them, as in the contractual model of Veatch (1972). Freidson (1961, 1970) likewise has argued that conflict is necessary in the therapeutic relationship and that the encounter is, and should be, a process of negotiation between physician and patient. Relatedly, Lazare and colleagues have supported the negotiated approach to patienthood (Lazare, Eisenthal, Frank, & Stoeckle, 1978), and models of shared decision making (e.g., Speedling & Rose, 1985) have supported the value of involving patients by incorporating their preferences into the decision-making process.

These models support, to varying degrees, the importance of "bargaining" and "negotiation" between practitioner and patient. The purpose of the negotiation, of course, is not just to have the patient accept the physician's definition of the problem and preferred solution. Rather, the goal is to have the physician accept the possibility that the patient has a different definition of the problem, different goals, and a different idea of what methods are acceptable for achieving those goals. D. S. Brody (1980, p.720) states it thus: "The extent to which there is true mutual participation will depend largely on physicians' flexibility in considering alternative courses of action." D. S. Brody points out that the best decision will be reached if the physician develops an empathic attitude in which the patient's internal frame of reference is understood and the situation is viewed through the patient's, not the physician's, value system. Likewise, the best approach to decision making and the resolution of conflict does not involve the patient's telling the physician what to do. D. S. Brody has argued that questioning or challenging the physician's every move is not productive and—like looking over the shoulder of a plumber who is trying to fix the sink—is a detriment to getting the job done. It is necessary that the physician make some decisions (such as which of several similar medications to choose once physician and patient have decided that the *type* of medication under consideration is the appropriate therapy). In a model in which decisions are truly shared, every decision made by the physician will be made in the context of considerable knowledge of the patient's personal values, expectations, and goals for treatment (H. Brody, 1992).

BUILDING A MODEL OF PRACTITIONER–PATIENT COMMUNICATION

An effective practitioner-patient relationship requires that they jointly recognize and examine disparate goals and collaboratively evaluate the means to achieve those goals. The patient's definition of what constitutes personal quality of life and related personal goals (such as avoiding surgery or maintaining fertility) and personal evaluations of risk and benefit must prevail in the evaluation of possible courses of action. The process of negotiation between practitioner and patient involves developing courses of action that are consistent with the patient's values and goals and that also satisfy the physician's values and goals (whether they are for some parameter in the patient's physiological condition or for the management of the physician's practice-related parameters such as time and income). It must be recognized that the most effective interaction will occur if physician and patient each fully understands the goals and preferences of the other (DiMatteo, Reiter, & Gambone, 1994).

Effective physician-patient communication also involves the recognition that each individual brings unique expertise to the encounter. The physician's expertise involves medical knowledge and clinical experience; the patient's involves knowing the role that the problem plays in quality of life and life goals, the effects of many variables on symptom character and control, and the patient's own ability to follow a proposed treatment regimen (DiMatteo & DiNicola, 1982).

The process of resolving conflict brings physician and patient closer to mutually acceptable solutions (Taylor, 1979). If physician and patient have such disparate views that conflict cannot be resolved, it is better to know sooner rather than later in their relationship. Patients who offer little resistance to prescription during a medical encounter may be adapting to a social situation that they feel unable to control or resist (Rodin & Janis, 1979), and the physician is likely to interpret their apparent passive acceptance as a sign of commitment instead of as a warning sign of noncompliance (DiMatteo, 1994b). When the physician is unaware of the patient's perspective, continuity of conflict, not resolution, is inevitable. Thus, it has been suggested that physicians should *stir up* conflict by exploring patients' assessments and feelings about all proposed actions (Speedling & Rose, 1985) and that they should actually lead therapeutic conversations to legitimate expressions of differences and conflicts, making clear that the encounter is one in which differences can be resolved through negotiation (Lazare et al., 1978).

How much do patients want to be involved in their care? Research shows, perhaps not surprisingly, that few patients want to make *all* their medical decisions on their own. The proportion who want to participate in their medical decisions varies from study to study, depending upon the age and education level of the respondents and the manner in which they are asked. In addition, as illness severity increases, preferences for information and decision-making involvement tend to decrease, even among physician-patients (Ende, Kazis, Ash, & Moskowitz, 1989; Ende, Kazis, & Moskowitz, 1990) (although these studies are based on hypothetical scenarios, not on actual clinical situations). Blanchard, Lebrecque, Ruckdeschel, and Blanchard (1988) found that 92% of cancer patients wanted to receive all the information available, but only 69% preferred to participate in medical decisions. Of those who wanted all the information, 24.9% preferred the physician to make the therapeutic decisions. Casselith, Zupkis, Sutton-Smith, and March (1980) found that many cancer patients preferred a participatory role and that those who were involved in their treatment decisions were more hopeful than those who were not. Patients who preferred to participate in treatment decisions were younger and better educated than those who did not: 87% of those 20-39 years of age preferred to participate, versus 62% of those 40-59 and 51% of those 60 and older. Those who wanted all information in the three age groups constituted 96%, 79%, and 80%, respectively. Strull, Lo, and Charles (1984) studied patients who were on average in their late 50s and early 60s. In their study, 55% of patients preferred "quite a lot" or "very extensive" discussion about their hypertensive therapy. Physicians in the study tended significantly to underestimate patients' preferences for "discussion about therapy" (which can reasonably be interpreted to mean participation). More highly educated patients preferred greater amounts of discussion. When asked who should make the decision about medicine for treatment of high blood pressure, 53% preferred to be involved.

Methodological Issues

The studies that have examined patient preferences for involvement have yielded equivocal and sometimes confusing results for several reasons. First, these studies have varied considerably in the measures they have used. For example, some studies have asked patients about their desire to make medical decisions; others have asked about patients' wishes to participate through detailed discussions with their physicians. Second, variations in preferences have not been systematically tracked as a function of patients' demographic characteristics. Results vary from study to study partly because of variations among subjects. Third, research on patients' decision-making preferences is seriously in need of strong theoretical underpinning and hypotheses regarding the meaning of patients' preferences. For example, a patient's decision not to take sole responsibility for making therapeutic treatment choices is not the same as passing the sole decision-making responsibility to the physician (Clarke, 1986). Patients' preferences to discuss treatment with their physicians likely involve their expectations that their physicians will fully understand and take into account their values, preferences, and goals when making medical decisions. Fourth, factors beyond those that have been studied explicitly may be operating in patients' stated preferences for involvement in medical choices. For example, there is often a significant social gap between patients and their typically higher-status physicians. In response to feelings of intimidation, patients may remain unassertive about their desire for involvement (D. S. Brody, 1980).

It is important to keep in mind that the debate over whether patients should be involved in decision making about their care is typically confined to practicing physicians and researchers seeking to find common ground for practitioners and patients to cooperate. Medical ethicists, on the other hand, are resoundingly clear about this issue. They hold that there exists an *ethical imperative* that physician and patient have reciprocal responsibility to share decision making (Pellegrino, 1976). It is even argued that some decisions are uniquely the patient's to make (Clarke, 1986).

In all forms of approach to decision making, there needs to be an emphasis on the patient's quality of life and a recognition that the patient will always know more about himself or herself than the physician ever will. As Lynn and DeGrazia (1991, p. 325) point out, quality of life choices are personal and should be made by the patient because the patient has to live with the results: "What matters to the patient, and what should matter to the practitioner, is the patient's future possibilities. More specifically, what is important is the character of the alternative futures that the patient could have and choosing among them so as to achieve the best future possible, with the ranking of outcomes determined by the patient's preferences." Physician and patient must explore together and discuss the chances of achieving the goals that they have jointly decided upon and consider the chances of achieving the entire goal picture—life as the patient would like to live it (Eddy, 1990).

Practical Methodologies

If physician-patient collaboration in decision making is to accomplish the goals examined above, it needs to be based upon an exceptionally good mechanism for facilitating open, unimpeded communication between physician and patient. H. Brody (1992) has suggested that one way to achieve such communication is through the "conversation model." In this model, the patient continually makes known to the physician his or her values, preferences, and constraints. The physician engages in a process of "transparency," "thinking out loud" about possible courses of action, the recommended interventions, and their possible implications, using language that is accessible to the patient. Each decision involves a choice about an immediate course of action and the "alternative futures" that are likely to follow from each choice. Transparency and the conversation model require a significant shift in the traditional medical therapeutic relationship and an acceptance that discussion, at least initially, takes some time and may be best accomplished with continuity of care.

Transparency and conversation can be facilitated by a methodology for focusing physician-patient discussion on various essential elements of care. As a structured approach, PREPARED™ is a system designed to enhance provider-patient communication and patient self-efficacy and satisfaction (Gambone & Reiter, 1991; DiMatteo et al., 1994). This system involves a checklist or agenda, which helps to make the provider-patient meeting more focused and save time. Following the PREPARED™ protocol, provider and patient discuss the recommended procedure (P), the reason for the recommendation (R), the patient's and provider's outcome expectations (E), the probability of achieving those expectations (P), and reasonable treatment alternatives (A), risks (R), and expenses (including direct and indirect costs) (E), before making a decision (D). Including patients in the decision-making process using PREPARED™ has been shown to contribute to an overall reduction in the utilization of hysterectomy (Gambone & Reiter, 1991) and hysterectomy for chronic pelvic pain (Reiter, Gambone, & Johnson, 1991). Recent data suggest that in hypothetical decision-making situations, consumers have increased self-efficacy after being trained to use PREPARED™.

RESOLVING THE DIFFERING PERSPECTIVES OF PHYSICIAN AND PATIENT

Research on medical decision making points to the need for continued, detailed theoretical development and empirical examination of several elements of physician-patient communication. The role of these elements in facilitating more appropriate health care choices and increased patient responsibility for health actions is gradually gaining support, and further examination of them promises to improve physician-patient communication considerably.

Discussion of the Patient's Problem

Research in the general population shows that at any given time, 75-90% of people experience symptoms that could be considered clinically relevant (though not necessarily requiring treatment), but only one third of them at some point seek medical help for the symptoms (Kellner, 1986; Pennebaker, 1982). A patient's problem may or may not have a diagnosis, and a diagnosis may or may not be a problem to the patient. Patients' decisions to attend to medical problems depend upon several social-psychological factors such as the focus of their attention, the salience of the symptoms, their bodily awareness, their threshold for discomfort, their childhood training and experiences, their cultural background, the circumstances of their lives at the time, and the meaning of the symptoms (DiMatteo, 1991). Given that illness and pain are essentially subjective phenomena, the physician who detects an abnormality must take care to consider fully what harm the problem is causing or is likely to cause in the future (see Gambone et al., 1994). If the patient experiences no symptoms or perceives no interference in the activities of living, and the problem is unlikely to threaten the patient's future health or span of life, it is possible that correction of the problem would constitute unnecessary medical treatment. If, on the other hand, the problem is likely to threaten life and future health (such as a malignant growth or a habit of cigarette smoking), effective physician-patient communication toward patient acceptance of the potential value of the regimen is essential for the patient to make a sustainable commitment to all elements of treatment or health behavior change (DiMatteo et al., 1993).

It is necessary that complete information be communicated to the patient so that the patient can exercise the ultimate right to decide whether and how the problem is to be treated (Pellegrino, 1976). In practice, resolution of the patient's perspective with that of the physician will require effective communication and negotiation about the patient's life plan.

Discussion of the Physician's and the Patient's Goals and Preferences

Typically, patients and physicians have rather broad and sometimes very different goals for the medical encounter (H. Brody, 1992). Physicians perform diagnostic and other procedures to achieve several goals, which may include ruling out diagnoses (even the most esoteric ones); arresting, attenuating, or managing disease processes; avoiding malpractice litigation; conforming to their training and local practice standards; having an exciting and interesting career; managing time in a busy practice; and optimizing income. Patients also seek and conform to the recommendations of medical care to achieve several goals, which may include: living longer, being more active and feeling better, maintaining personal dignity and autonomy, relieving their anxiety or their boredom, and obtaining exemption from work and other requisite activities. Even when the physician's and the patient's goals coincide, the patient's goals are likely to be somewhat more complex and involve more psychosocial elements than the physician expects will be the case (Kleinman, 1988). While both may agree, for example, that pain should be relieved, the patient may also wish to remain alert and cognitively functional at work, as well as emotionally responsive at home. The physician's goal (to control the patient's pain) may be achieved quite easily with certain medications, but these medications may negate the patient's more complex goals. Negotiation of physician and patient expectations for treatment is essential if the goals of both parties are to be realized.

Since the typical provider-patient interaction fails to take into account the inevitable differences in character and complexity of the practitioner's and the patient's preferences and goals, it comes as little surprise that patient noncompliance rates prevail at upward of 40% for simple regimens and 70-80% for complex lifestyle changes (Brownell, Marlatt, Lichtenstein, & Wilson, 1986; Epstein & Cluss, 1982). Without meticulous attention in their communicative interchange to honest exploration and assertive presentation of their respective preferences, physician and patient will not fully understand each other's perspectives. Practitioner and patient need precise examination of what constitutes quality of life for the patient; they need detailed discussion and mutual understanding of their values and preferences. Further, full consideration of the patient's complex goals involves careful analysis of the means to various ends and the effect these means and ends are likely to have on those complex goals.

Assumptions by a patient that a well-liked and even personally similar physician will automatically know and adhere to the patient's unarticulated preferences are likely to result in misunderstanding and poor choices. As an example of the problem with such assumptions, consider the actual case of a married couple who typically spent a good deal of time talking with each other and who knew each other's general values quite well. In a discussion of their personal preferences for life-sustaining treatment under varied circumstances, each tried to predict whether the other would want necessary, but temporary, life-sustaining intervention if rendered quadriplegic after an accident. Both guessed wrong, possibly because both assumed their personal preferences would be the same—which they were not. If spouses do not know each other's personal preferences for health care intervention without specifically discussing them, how likely are physicians and patients to have such knowledge without detailed discussion?

Risks of Health-Related Action and Inaction

Risk is defined in the 1980 edition of the *Oxford American Dictionary* as "exposure to the possibility of meeting danger or suffering harm or loss." Every action involves risk and must be considered in the context of the expected benefits of acting. Medical care, of course, carries certain risks, such as those of bad memories, indignity, pain (short- or long-term), disability, and even death. Risk tends to be salient to physicians and patients for very different reasons. The physician fears bad reputation and malpractice litigation if harm befalls the patient; the patient is the one who has to live with harm and its consequences.

The examination and understanding of risk is a fundamental element in medical care. In most realms of health care, choices are available among several alternative approaches to management (such as among different medications or between immediate surgery and "watchful waiting"). Each course of action (or inaction) carries a risk of harm. Research as far back as that on the health belief model (Becker, 1974; Rosenstock, 1988) has shown that patients form and act on their own opinions about the risk/benefit ratio. Although they might be wrong, emphasizing one over the other, they nevertheless typically choose to act on the basis of their beliefs. Recent research on patient adherence to treatment regimens suggests that in the realms of both prevention and treatment of cancer, patients formulate assessments of the costs (including risks) versus the benefits and expected efficacy of health promotion or medical care action and *decide* whether or not they *intend* to adhere to treatment. Intention is one of the two direct and highly significant predictors of actual behavior (presence or absence of practical barriers to behaving being the other [DiMatteo et al., 1993]). Effective communication includes confrontation and examination of the risks and benefits of various courses of action and must be undertaken before patients' own active, but possibly ill-informed, decision-making processes lead to poor outcomes.

Risk and Informed Consent

The requirement that patients be formally apprised of the risks of certain medical treatment became incorporated into medical practice in 1957 with the introduction of the legal mandate for informed consent (H. Brody, 1992). The procedure for informed consent represents the only mechanism by which information about risk is typically communicated to patients in medical practice in the United States today. H. Brody (1992) has noted that physicians tend to see informed consent as a legal practice, not as part of medical care. The actual execution of informed consent in medical practice almost negates its purpose, for several reasons: (1) Information about risk is typically given to patients only in high-consequence situations, such as surgery, where risks are appreciable in size and scope. Procedures with somewhat less severe, but still important, potential consequences (such as pain and disability) typically do not prompt any communication of risk information. (2) Information about risk is almost always given *after* a decision has been made about whether and how to treat the problem. (3) The process of "obtaining" informed consent usually involves obtaining the patient's signature on a legalistic document under enormous social and normative pressure (e.g., the morning of surgery). (4) Information that risk *exists* is provided, but the exact probability of a bad outcome such as bleeding, infection, or death is typically not presented. Since patients vary tremendously in their assessments of risk, this information is essential for truly informed consent (Lynn & DeGrazia, 1991). Some patients may perceive a 1% chance of an untoward outcome as quite high; others may perceive it as quite low. (5) The impact of potential negative outcomes tends almost never to be spelled out. Discussion of, for example, the likely consequences of infection or bleeding and the effect that these consequences might have on life as the patient wishes to live it are typically not part of the informed consent discussion.

Methodological Issues

Research on informed consent as it is carried out in practice suggests that there is often minimal provision of clear information about risks and that physicians and patients demonstrate very limited congruence in their understanding of the risks of agreed-upon medical procedures (Wu & Pearlman, 1988). Further, several studies have shown that patients are much more risk-averse than are their physicians and, when given complete information, choose much more conservative treatments than do their physicians (O'Meara, McNutt, Evans, Moore, & Downs, 1994; McNeil et al., 1978). This research strongly suggests that decision making in medical care should involve shared responsibility for negotiating *all aspects* of a choice, including the type and amount of risk that the physician and patient are willing to take. Risk should never be a separate issue tagged on after the decision is made. Rather, it is an integral part of the analysis of all the possible options and how they fit into the patient's life goals (Kassirer, 1983).

Two primary arguments seem to be levied against providing patients with risk information. First, when the case is made against patients' rights to all risk information, the admonition against disclosing remote risks (such as a 1 in 40,000 chance of mortality associated with a given diagnostic procedure) is almost always called into play. In a model of true physician–patient collaboration, disclosure of remote risk should depend upon patient preference (H. Brody, 1992). To some patients, remote risk is irrelevant; to others, it figures into decisions in important ways. Further, even very remote risk may be quite relevant when the necessity of an intervention is in question.

Second, the way in which information about risk is "framed" can have a large effect on how it is perceived, such as patients accepting a procedure with a 90% chance of surviving but rejecting one with a 10% chance of dying (e.g., Tversky & Kahneman, 1981). Both physicians and patients are susceptible to framing effects. If patients are to make the best decisions for their own lives, they should be given all relevant risk information to talk over with people who have other points of view (such as a skeptical family member and a physician who provides a truly independent second opinion [Hughes, 1993]).

Consideration of Alternative Treatments

When providers make recommendations to their patients for courses of health action, these recommendations typically involve a single course of action (Wu & Pearlman, 1988). Wu and Pearlman (1988) found that in over 100 observations of procedures, ranging from injecting and giving oral medication to performing invasive diagnostic procedures, physicians' communicated information about alternatives only 12% of the time. When interviewed, physicians and patients demonstrated congruence in their understanding of the alternatives only 25% of the time. Further, Fisher (1983) found that when patients asked questions about possible alternatives to surgery, their physicians changed treatment decisions. When patients repeatedly asked if the proposed treatment was necessary or indicated that they did not want surgery unless absolutely necessary, their physicians chose other methods of treatment.

FUTURE RESEARCH QUESTIONS

Several research questions have been posed throughout this chapter, and a few more suggest themselves: First, there needs to be an exploration of the effects of the timing of information transmittal in the health care interaction and an examination of the methods and timing of conflict resolution. Second, the role of information and conflict arousal and resolution on malpractice litigation needs to be explored. To what precise extent does patients' involvement in their medical-care decisions reduce the tendency to blame the physician in the event of a less than optimal outcome? Third, the question of how best to present information to patients and involve them in their health care decisions, particularly to enhance their commitment to the most appropriate decisions for them, needs to be explored. Decision analysis, for the most part, is a difficult methodology for both patients and physicians (Lincoln, 1982). Further research is needed on how the process of shared decision making might be improved for both patients and physicians, to enhance its appropriateness and effectiveness in improving the patient's life.

CONCLUSION

This chapter has examined the role of health professional-patient communication in enhancing patients' responsibility for their personal health care decisions and the effective and appropriate use of the opportunities presented by medical technology. It has been argued that effective communication is essential to the enhancement of patients' quality of life by ensuring that patients' goals remain at the forefront of medical intervention. Barriers to effective provider-patient communication in the medical encounter have been analyzed, and essential elements of effective therapeutic communication have been proposed.

The primary message of this analysis has been that regardless of the prevailing model of communication, patients are, and always have been, in charge of their own fate. When patients appear to be deferent to medical authority, they covertly regulate their health actions, such as by hidden noncompliance. Optimal health care decisions require collaborative decision making by providers and patients regarding the necessity of recommended health care action, patients' goals and preferences, and attendant risks and alternative courses of action.

This chapter has focused on one primary point: The best course of action in medical care is not always the one with the least risk of harm to the patient. Neither is it necessarily the one with a dramatic technical intervention. It is, as Eddy (1990) has noted the one that will lead to the outcome that the patient finds most desirable. The goal of shared power and decision making in the practitioner-patient relationship "is to use both powers—physician's and patient's—in tandem to produce, as efficiently as possible, the best and most skilled application of medical knowledge to the patient's problems to secure an outcome that best aids the patient in living out his life plan" (H. Brody, 1992, p. 112).

ACKNOWLEDGMENT. This work was supported by Intramural and Field Research Grants from the University of California, Riverside.

REFERENCES

Barnlund, D. C. (1976). The mystification of meaning: Doctor-patient encounters. *Journal of Medical Education, 51*, 716-725.

Becker, M. H. (1974). The health belief model and sick role behavior. *Health Education Monographs, 2*, 409-419.

Beckman, H. B., Frankel, R. M., & Darnley, J. (1985). Soliciting the patient's complete agenda: A relationship to the distribution of concerns. *Clinical Research, 33*, 714A.

Beisecker, A. E. (1986). *Taking charge: Attempts to control the doctor-patient interaction*. Paper presented at the Second James Madison University Medical Communication Conferences, Harrisonburg, VA.

Beisecker, A. E. (1990). Patient power in doctor-patient communication: What do we know? *Health Communication, 2*(2), 105-122.

Beisecker, A. E., & Beisecker, T. D. (1990). Patient information-seeking behaviors when communicating with doctors. *Medical Care, 28*(1), 19-28.

Bernstein, S. J., McGlynn, E. A., Siu, A. L., Roth, C. P., Sherwood, M. J., Keesey, J. W., Kosecoff, J., Hicks, N. R., & Brook, R. H. (1993). The appropriateness of hysterectomy: A comparison of care in seven health plans. Health Maintenance Organization Quality of Care Consortium. *Journal of the American Medical Association, 269*(18), 2398-2402.

Blanchard, C. G., Labrecque, M. S., Ruckdeschel, J. C., & Blanchard, E. B. (1988). Information and decision-making preferences of hospitalized adult cancer patients. *Social Science and Medicine, 27*(11), 1139-1145.

Brody, D. S. (1980). The patient's role in clinical decision-making. *Annals of Internal Medicine, 93*, 718-722.

Brody, H. (1992). *The healer's power*. New Haven, CT: Yale University Press.

Brook, R. H., Park, R. E., Chassin, M. R., Kosecoff, J., Keesey, J., & Solomon, D. H. (1990). Carotid endarterectomy for elderly patients: Predicting complication. *Annals of Internal Medicine, 113*(10), 747-753.

Brownell, K. D., Marlatt, G. A., Lichtenstein, E., & Wilson, G. T. (1986). Understanding and preventing relapse. *American Psychologist, 41*, 765-782.

Cassell, E. J. (1985). *Talking with patients: Vol. 1. The theory of doctor-patient communication*. Cambridge, MA: MIT Press.

Cassileth, B. R., Zupkis, R. V., Sutton-Smith, K., & March, V. (1980). Information and participation preferences among cancer patients. *Annals of Internal Medicine, 92*, 832-836.

Chassin, M. R. (1990). Practice guidelines: Best hope for quality improvement in the 1990s. *Journal of Occupational Medicine, 32*(12), 1199-1206.

Christy, N. P. (1979). English is our second language. *New England Journal of Medicine, 300*(17), 979-981.

Clarke, D. B. (1986). Helping patients make health care decisions. *Euthanasia Review, 1*(2), 85-96.

Consumer Reports (1992). Wasted health care dollars. 7(57), 435-449.

DiMatteo, M. R. (1991). *The psychology of health, illness, and medical care: An individual perspective*. Pacific Grove, CA: Brooks/Cole.

DiMatteo, M. R. (1993). Expectations in the physician-patient relationship: Implications for patient adherence to medical treatment recommendations. In P. D. Blanck (Ed.), *Interpersonal expectations* (pp. 296-315). New York: Cambridge University Press.

DiMatteo, M. R. (1994a). The physician-patient relationship: Effects on the quality of health care. *Clinical Obstetrics and Gynecology, 37*(1), 149-162.

DiMatteo, M. R. (1994b). Enhancing patient adherence to medical recommendations. *Journal of the American Medical Association, 271*(1), 79, 83.

DiMatteo, M. R., & DiNicola, D. D. (1981). Sources of assessment of physician performance: A study of comparative reliability and patterns of intercorrelations. *Medical Care, 19*, 829-842.

DiMatteo, M. R., & DiNicola, D. D. (1982). *Achieving patient compliance: The psychology of the medical practitioner's role*. New York: Pergamon Press.

DiMatteo, M. R., Hays, R. D., Gritz, E. R., Bastani, R., Crane, L., Elashoff, R, Ganz, P., Heber, D., McCarthy, W., & Marcus, A. (1993). Patient adherence to cancer control regimens: Scale development and initial validation. *Psychological Assessment, 5*(1), 102-112.

DiMatteo, M. R., Hays, R. D., & Prince, L. M. (1986). Relationships of physicians' nonverbal communication skill to patient satisfaction, appointment noncompliance, and physician workload. *Health Psychology, 5*(6), 581-594.

DiMatteo, M. R., Linn, L. S., Chang, B. L., & Cope, D. W. (1985). Affect and neutrality in physician behavior. *Journal of Behavioral Medicine, 8*(4), 397-409.

DiMatteo, M. R., Reiter, R. C., & Gambone, J. C. (1994). Enhancing medication adherence through communication and informed collaborative choice. *Health Communication, 6*(4), 253-265.

Donabedian, A. (1980). *Explorations in quality assessment and monitoring: Vol. 1.* Ann Arbor, MI: Health Administration Press.

Donovan, J. L., & Blake, D. R. (1992). Patient non-compliance: Deviance or reasoned decision-making? *Social Science and Medicine, 34*(5), 507-513.

Eddy, D. (1990). Anatomy of a decision. *Journal of the American Medical Association, 263*(3), 441-443.

Egbert, L. D., Battit, G. E., Welch, C. E., & Bartlett, M. K. (1964). Reduction of postoperative pain by encouragement and instruction of patients. *New England Journal of Medicine, 270*, 825-827.

Eisenberg, J. M. (1979). Sociologic influences on decision-making by clinicians. *Annals of Internal Medicine, 90*, 957-964.

Emanuel, L. L., Barry, M. J., Stoeckle, J. D., Ettelson, L. M., & Emanuel, E. J. (1991). Advance directives for medical care: A case for greater use. *New England Journal of Medicine, 324*, 889-895.

Ende, J., Kazis, L., Ash, A., & Moskowitz, M. A. (1989). Measuring patients' desire for autonomy: Decision making and information-seeking preferences among medical patients. *Journal of General Internal Medicine, 2*, 23-30.

Ende, J., Kazis, L., & Moskowitz, M. A. (1990). Preferences for autonomy when patients are physicians. *Journal of General Internal Medicine, 5*, 506-509.

Epstein, L. H., & Cluss, P. A. (1982). A behavioral medicine perspective on adherence to long-term medical regimens. *Journal of Consulting and Clinical Psychology, 50*(6), 950-971.

Faden, R., Becker, C., Lewis, C., Freeman, J., & Faden, A. (1981). Disclosure of information to patients in medical care. *Medical Care, 19*, 718-733.

Fischbach, R. L., Sionelo-Bayog, A., Needle, A., & Delbanco, T. (1980). The patient and practitioner as authors of the medical record. *Patient Counseling and Health Education, 1*, 1-5.

Fisher, S. (1983). Doctor talk/patient talk: How treatment decisions are negotiated in doctor/patient communication. In S. Fisher & A. Todd (Eds.), *The social organization of doctor-patient communication* (pp. 135-157). Washington, DC: Center for Applied Linguistics.

Fisher, S. (1984). Doctor-patient communication: A social and micro-political performance. *Sociology of Health and Illness, 6*(1), 1-29.

Fried, C. (1974). *Medical experimentation, personal integrity, and social policy*. New York: American Elsevier.

Freidson, E. (1961). *Patients' view of medical practice*. New York: Russell Sage Foundation.

Freidson, E. (1970). *Professional dominance*. Chicago: Aldine.

Fries, J. F, Koop, C. E., Beadle, C. E., Cooper, P. P., England, M. J., Greaves, R. F, Sokolov, J. J., Wright, D., & the Health Project Consortium. (1993). Reducing health care costs by reducing the need and demand for medical services. *New England Journal of Medicine, 329*(5), 321-325.

Gambòne, J. C., & Reiter, R. C. (1991). Quality improvement in health care. *Current Problems in Obstetrics, Gynecology, and Fertility, 14*, 151-175.

Gambone, J. C., Reiter, R. C., & DiMatteo, M. R. (1994). *The PREPARED provider: A guide for improved patient communication*. Beaverton, OR: Mosbyl Great Performance.

Gray, D., Hampton, J. R., Bernstein, S. J., Kosecoff, J., & Brook, R. H. (1990). Audit of coronary angiography and bypass surgery. *Lancet, 335*(8701), 1317-1320.

Greenfield, S., Kaplan, S., & Ware, J. E., Jr. (1985). Expanding patient involvement in care: Effects on patient outcomes. *Annals of Internal Medicine, 102*, 520-528.

Hackett, T. P., Cassem, N. H., & Raker, J. W. (1973). Patient delay in cancer. *New England Journal of Medicine, 289*, 14-20.

Hall, J. A., Irish , J. T., Roter, D. L., Erlich, C. M., & Miller, L. H. (1994). Gender in medical encounters: An analysis of physician and patient communication in a primary care setting. *Health Psychology, 13*, 384-392.

Hall, J. A., Roter, D. L., & Katz, N. R. (1988). Meta-analysis of correlates of provider behavior in medical encounters. *Medical Care, 25*, 399-412.

Haug, M. R., & Lavin, B. (1979). Public challenge of physician authority. *Medical Care, 17*, 844-858.

Haug, M. R., & Lavin, B. (1983). *Consumerism in medicine: Challenging physician authority*. Beverly Hills, CA: Sage.

Hayes-Bautista, D. E. (1976). Modifying the treatment: Patient compliance, patient control and medical care. *Social Science and Medicine, 10*, 233-238.

Helfer, R. E. (1970). An objective comparison of the pediatric interviewing skills of freshman and senior medical students. *Pediatrics, 45*, 623-627.

Hickson, G. B., Clayton, E. W., Entman, S. S., Miller, C. S., Githens, P. B., Whetton-Goldstein, K., & Sloan, F. A. (1994). Obstetricians' prior malpractice experience and patients' satisfaction with care. *Journal of the American Medical Association, 272*(20), 1583-1587.

Hughes, K. K. (1993). Decision making by patients with breast cancer: The role of information in treatment selection. *Oncology Nursing Forum, 20*(4), 623-628.

Johnson, J. E., & Leventhal, H. (1974). Effects of accurate expectations and behavioral instructions on reactions during a noxious medical examination. *Journal of Personality and Social Psychology, 29*, 710-718.

Kaplan, R. M. (1991). Health-related quality of life in patient decision making. *Journal of Social Issues, 47*(4), 69-90.

Kaplan, S. H., Greenfield, S., & Ware, J. E., Jr. (1989). Assessing the effects of physician-patient interactions on the outcomes of chronic disease. *Medical Care, 27*(3), S110-S127.

Kassirer, J. P. (1983). Adding insult to injury: Usurping patients' prerogatives. *New England Journal of Medicine, 308*, 847-853.

Katz, J. (1984). *The silent world of doctor and patient*. New York: Free Press.

Kellner, R. (1986). *Somatization and hypochondriasis*. New York: Praeger.

Kleinman, A. (1988). *The illness narratives: Suffering, healing, and the human condition*. New York: Basic Books.

Kleinman, A., Eisenberg, L., Good, B. (1978). Culture, illness and care: Clinical lessons from anthropologic and cross-cultural research. *Annals of Internal Medicine, 88*, 251-258.

Kleinman, L. C., Kosecoff, J., Dubois, R. W., & Brook, R. H. (1944). The medical appropriateness of tympanostomy tubes proposed for children younger than 16 years in the United States. *Journal of the American Medical Association, 271*(16), 1250-1255.

Lazare, A., Eisenthal, S., Frank, A., & Stoeckle, J. (1978). Studies on a negotiated approach to patienthood. In E. B. Gallagher (Ed.), *The doctor-patient relationship in a changing health scene* (pp. 119-139). NIH Publication No. 78-189. Washington, DC: U.S. Department of Health, Education, and Welfare.

Leape, L. L., Park, R. E., Solomon, D. H., Chassin, M. R., Kosecoff, J., & Brook, R. H. (1990). Does inappropriate use explain small-area variations in the use of health care services? *Journal of the American Medical Association, 263*(5), 669-672.

Levinson, W. (1994). Physician-patient communication: A key to malpractice prevention. *Journal of the American Medical Association, 272*(20), 1619-1620.

Lincoln, T. L. (1982). *Medical decision-making for patients as individuals*. Paper presented at the 148th American Association for the Advancement of Science, National Meeting, Washington, DC, January 8.

Lynn, J., & DeGrazia, D. (1991). An outcomes model of medical decision making. *Theoretical Medicine, 12*, 325-343.

Marvel, M. K. (1993). Involvement with the psychosocial concerns of patients: Observations of practicing family physicians on a university faculty. *Archives of Family Medicine, 2*(6), 629-633.

McBride, C. A., Shugars, D. A., DiMatteo, M. R., Lepper, H. S., O'Neil, E. H., & Damush, T. M. (1994). The physician's role: Views of the public and the profession on seven aspects of patient care. *Archives of Family Medicine, 3*, 948-953.

McGlynn, E. A., Kosecoff, J., & Brook, R. H. (1990). Format and conduct of consensus development conferences: Multi-nation comparison. *International Journal of Technology Assessment in Health Care, 6*(3), 450-469.

McNeil, B. J., Weichselbaum, R., & Pauker, S. G. (1978). Fallacy of the five-year survival in lung cancer. *New England Journal of Medicine, 299*, 1397-1401.

National Center for Health Statistics. (1992). *Health United States, 1991*. DHHS Publication No. [PHS] 92-1232. Hyattsville, MD: Public Health Service.

O'Meara, J. J., McNutt, R. A., Evans, A. T., Moore, S. W., & Downs, S. M. (1994). A decision analysis of streptokinase plus heparin as compared with heparin alone for deep-vein thrombosis. *New England Journal of Medicine, 330*(15), 1864-1869.

Parsons, T. (1951). *The social system*. New York: Free Press.

Pellegrino, E. D. (1976). Medical ethics, education, and the physician's image. *Journal of the American Medical Association*, *235*, 1043-1044.

Pennebaker, J. W. (1982). *The psychology of physical complaints*. New York: Springer-Verlag.

Pickering, G. (1979). Therapeutics: Art or science? *Journal of the American Medical Association*, *242*, 649-653.

Putnam, S. M., Stiles, W. B., Jacob, M. C., & James, S. A. (1985). Patient exposition and physician explanation in initial medical interviews and outcome of clinic visits. *Medical Care*, *23*, 74-83.

Reiter, R. C., Gambone, J. C., & Johnson, S. R. (1991). Availability of a multidisciplinary pelvic pain clinic and frequency of hysterectomy for pelvic pain. *Journal of Psychosomatic Obstetrics and Gynecology*, *12*, 109-112.

Rodin, J., & Janis, I. L. (1979). The social power of health-care practitioners as agents of change. *Journal of Social Issues*, *35*, 60-81.

Rosenstock, I. M. (1988). Enhancing patient compliance with health recommendations. *Journal of Pediatric Health Care*, *2*(2), 67-72.

Rost, K., Carter, W., & Inui, T. (1989). Introduction of information during the initial medical visit: Consequences for patient follow-through with physician recommendations for medication. *Social Science and Medicine*, *28*, 315-321.

Roter, D. L. (1977). Patient participation in the patient-provider interaction: The effects of patient question asking on the quality of interaction, satisfaction, and compliance. *Health Education Monographs*, *5*, 281-315.

Roter, D. L. (1983). Physician/patient communication: Transmission of information and patient effects. *Maryland State Medical Journal*, *32*, 260-265.

Roter, D. L. (1984). Patient question asking in physician-patient interaction. *Health Psychology*, *3*(5), 395-410.

Roter, D. L., & Hall, J. A. (1992). *Doctors talking with patients/patients talking with doctors*. Westport, CT: Auburn House.

Sankar, A. (1986). Out of the clinic into the home: Control and patient-physician communication. *Social Science and Medicine*, *22*, 973-982.

Schulman, B. A. (1979). Active patient orientation and outcomes in hypertensive treatment. *Medical Care*, *17*(3), 267-280.

Shapiro, A. (1960). A contribution to a history of the placebo effect. *Behavioral Science*, *5*, 109-135.

Speedling, E. J., & Rose, D. N. (1985). Building an effective doctor-patient relationship: From patient satisfaction to patient participation. *Social Science and Medicine*, *21*(2), 115-120.

Starfield, B., Steinwachs, D., Morris, I., Bause, G., Siebert, S., & Westin, C. (1979). Patient-doctor agreement about problems needing follow-up visit. *Journal of the American Medical Association*, *242*, 344-346.

Starr, P. (1982). *The social transformation of American medicine*. New York: Basic Books.

Stevens, R. (1989). *In sickness and in wealth: American hospitals in the twentieth century*. New York: Basic Books.

Strull, W. M., Lo, B., & Charles, G. (1984). Do patients want to participate in medical decision making? *Journal of the American Medical Association*, *252*(21), 2990-2294.

Svarstad, B. (1976). Physician-patient communication and patient conformity with medical advice. In D. Mechanic (Ed.), *The growth of bureaucratic medicine* (pp. 220-238). New York: Wiley.

Szasz, T. S., & Hollender, M. H. (1956). A contribution to the philosophy of medicine: The basic models of the doctor-patient relationship. *Archives of Internal Medicine*, *97*, 585-592.

Taylor, S. E. (1979). Hospital patient behavior: Reactance, helplessness, or control? *Journal of Social Issues*, *35*, 156-184.

Tversky, A., & Kahneman, D. (1981). The framing of decisions and the psychology of choice. *Science*, 211(30), 453-458.

Veatch, R. M. (1972). Models for ethical medicine in a revolutionary age: What physician-patient roles foster the most ethical relationship? *Hastings Center Report*, *2*, 5-7.

Wagener, J. J., & Taylor, S. E. (1986). What else could I have done? Patients' responses to failed treatment decisions. *Health Psychology*, *5*, 481-496.

Waitzkin, H. (1985). Information giving in medical care. *Journal of Health and Social Behavior*, *26*, 81-101.

Waitzkin, H. (1991). *The politics of medical encounters*. New Haven, CT: Yale University Press.

Waitzkin, H., & Stoeckle, J. D. (1972). The communication of information about illness: Clinical, sociological, and methodological considerations. *Advances in Psychosomatic Medicine*, *8*, 180-215.

Waitzkin, H., & Stoeckle, J. D. (1976). Information control and the micropolitics of health care: Summary of an ongoing research project. *Social Science and Medicine*, *10*, 263-276.

Wallen, J., Waitzkin, H., & Stoeckle, J. D. (1979). Physician stereotypes about female health and illness: A study of patient's sex and the information process during medical interviews. *Women & Health*, *4*, 135-146.

Wennberg, J. E. (1990). Outcomes research, cost containment, and the fear of health care rationing. *New England Journal of Medicine*, *323*, 1202-1204.

Wennberg, J. E., Mulley, A. G., Jr., Hanley, D., Timothy, R. P., Fowler, F. J., Jr., Roos, N. P., Barry, M. J., McPherson, K., Greenberg, E. R., Soule, D., Bubolz, T., Fisher, E., & Malenka, D. (1988). An assessment of prostatectomy for benign urinary tract obstruction: Geographic variations and the evaluation of medical care outcomes. *Journal of the American Medical Association*, *259*, 3027-3030.

West, C. (1984). *Routine complications: Troubles with talk between doctors and patients*. Bloomington: Indiana University Press.

Wolf, S. M. (1988). Conflict between doctor and patient. *Law, Medicine, and Health Care*, *16*(3-4), 197-203.

Wu, W. C., & Pearlman, R. A. (1988). Consent in medical decision making: The role of communication. *Journal of General Internal Medicine*, *3*, 9-14.

II

INTERACTIONAL AND STRUCTURAL DETERMINANTS

In addition to issues of communication, encounters between individuals and institutions within the health care system are mediated by interactional determinants, such as perceptions, roles, and power relationships, and by structural determinants, such as the organizational and locational dimensions of the physical institutions themselves.

INTERACTIONAL DETERMINANTS

Perceptions

Perceptions include beliefs, expectations, evaluations, and other cognitive elements discussed in Volume I, particularly in Chapters 1-7. Patients and clients enter the encounter with their own personal—often idiosyncratic—perceptions of their conditions, of medical and other health professionals, and of the institutions in which care is sought or provided. Lederer (1952) provides a dramatic and much-referred-to picture of the sick person's perspective that identifies the constricted view of the world and the concreteness, anxiety, need for reassurance, egocentricity, and ambivalence toward the physician that characterize the experience of feeling sick. Professionals enter these encounters with *their* perceptions of patients in general, of particular patients, of the patient's condition, of themselves and other professionals, and of the institutions in which they conduct their work.

Anderson and Helm (1979) noted the inevitably differential appraisals within the professional-layperson encounter. The initial "realities" of the encounter are different for each. At the outset, the patient perceives his or her condition in an immediate, personal, subjective manner and is often in a state of crisis. The physician, in contrast, perceives the patient as typifying an instance of some condition. For the patient, the encounter is exceptional, evoking anxiety and concern for expenses. For the physician, the encounter is routine (Anderson & Helm, 1979, p. 263). The encounter often culminates in what Anderson and Helm term a "negotiated reality." Helman (1990) further emphasized the differences in these two realities. For physicians, the basic premises of the encounter reflect scientific rationality; an emphasis on objective, numerical assessment and on physiochemical data; and beliefs that diseases are entities. Increasing reliance on tests and laboratory procedures can result in the physician's being less inclined to listen carefully to the patient and to take a history. For patients, the basic premises are that the disease or illness is something that they have, rather than something in an organ; that the illness is a personalized, subjective experience (Helman, 1990, chap. 5).

Research related to such perceptions can be

grouped under the following headings: client perceptions of professionals, professional perceptions of clients, marginalization, incongruities in perceptions, and perceptions of satisfaction.

Client Perceptions of Professionals

Among the earliest reports of client perceptions of professionals is the seminal study by Freidson (1961, chap. 3) of patients enrolled in New York City's Health Insurance Plan (HIP) and patients of private practitioners. Freidson showed that patients were slightly more likely to perceive the private practitioners as taking greater personal interest in them, but to perceive the HIP physicians as providing more competent care.

In a population of London dental patients, Liddell and May (1984) found that patients perceived their regular dentists more favorably, e.g., as more competent, more likeable, and more careful, and less indifferent, less mercenary, and less unsympathetic, than they perceived dentists in general. Moreover, these perceptions were related to the patients' age and gender, as well as to prior frightening dental experiences. Strauss observed (1976) that black patients have different perceptions of dentists and of dental treatment than do white patients, that they are more likely to expect to have an extraction, that they expect the dental treatment to be painful, and that they are less likely to express criticism of the professional.

In a different vein, Rosen (1977) found that women who were experiencing unwanted conceptions, who had a regular physician, and who chose to terminate the pregnancy did not perceive their primary care physicians as a source of advice in relation to their pregnancy. However, Adamson and Watts (1976) found that maternity patients perceived maternity nurse practitioners to be especially helpful in providing information and support and more helpful than physicians in several ways, e.g., showing concern and reassurance and providing information and explanations.

Finally, in the context of examining "doctor-shopping" behavior, Kasteler, Kane, Olsen, and Thetford (1976) observed that patients have begun to perceive their physicians as "commodities," rather than as "gods." This shift in perception is related to the increase in consumerism in health care.

Professional Perceptions of Clients

Professionals often demonstrate stereotyping in their perceptions of patients. McCranie, Horowitz, and Martin (1978) report on the degree of gender-based stereotyping in medical diagnosis; misdiagnosis has a high potential for inappropriate and unsatisfactory encounters between female clients and male medical practitioners. These researchers' vignette-based study failed to show a differential psychiatric diagnosis based on gender, but they acknowledge the problem of generalizing from such simulations to real encounters. On the other hand, Verbrugge (1984) was able to demonstrate that while men and women are equally likely to receive a psychiatric primary diagnosis, women are more likely to receive a secondary psychiatric diagnosis; that some differences exist in the kinds of services that are made available to men and to women, if not in the amounts of such services; that nonpsychiatrists are less equitable in their treatment of the genders than are psychiatrists; and that distressed women receive more care.

The issue of stereotyping also arises in the examination by Frazier, Jenny, Bagramian, Robinson, and Proshek (1977) of the incongruence between dentists' views of patients' beliefs and values and the patients' actual beliefs and values. Data revealed that practitioners' inferences are influenced by patients' socioeconomic status. McKinlay (1975) reported that physicians, particularly older ones, underestimated patients' grasp of the meanings of a range of medical terms. Moreover, the physicians continued to use these terms, even though they believed (mistakenly) that patients would not understand them.

Gerbert (1984), using videotaped simulations demonstrating three combinations of patient likability and competence, observed that these patient characteristics had an effect on case management. For example, recommendations for psychological referral were less likely to be made for likeable patients, and likeable-competent patients were more often encouraged to maintain close contact with the physician's office. Hall, Epstein, DeCiantis, and McNeil (1993) provide evidence that physicians' liking for their patients may itself be a reflection of patient satisfaction and health status and is influenced by gender: Physicians tended to like male patients more than females.

Gender issues also emerge in a study of the differential communication patterns of male and female physicians. For example, female physicians conduct longer visits, communicate more positively, smile more, and ask more questions than male physicians (Hall, Irish, Roter, Ehrlich, & Miller, 1994).

Niemeyer (1991) has documented how provider expectations, operating through social labeling and stereotyping, can have an impact on some aspects of patient behavior. Within the context of workers' compensation, Niemeyer emphasizes, the narrow biomedical model prevents physicians from understanding the psychological and social components of patients whose recoveries from trauma are delayed. Consequently, they "blame" the patient for not recovering, attributing the lack of progress to "malingering" or to a desire for the secondary gain of illness. They then respond to such patients in negative ways, which further exacerbates the patients' distress and encourages additional illness behavior.

Westbrook, Nordholm, and McGee (1984) demonstrated that Australian and Swedish nonphysician health professionals (physiotherapists, occupational therapists, nurses) showed differences in their perceptions of patients that reflected their cultural differences in beliefs about responsibility for health. Australians viewed patients more favorably, as more likely to need counseling, as more dependent, and as more poorly adjusted than did the Swedes. The Australians, moreover, were more likely to speak with patients about feelings.

In their factor analysis of physicians' views of patients, Ford, Liske, Ort, and Denton (1967) demonstrated a consensus that effective practice depends on patients' being cooperative with treatment, well-adjusted, responsive to treatment, expressive of appreciation, and believers in their physicians' skills. The literature review by Hill (1978) of how different helping professions view their clients revealed a general pessimism about clients, particularly in relation to treatability, manageability, and likability.

The technology of measuring professional perceptions is slowly emerging. Ashworth, Williamson, and Montano (1984) have developed and begun the validation of a self-report instrument measuring physicians' perceptions about psychosocial aspects of care, including perceptions of the physician's role, perceptions about what patients want and don't want, and perceptions about physicians' reactions to patients as persons.

Marginalization

Provider perceptions often involve marginalization or stigmatization of groups of patients. Ghodse (1978, 1979) observed that emergency room physicians and nurses in London accident and emergency departments varied in their perceptions of drug-overdose patients depending on patient characteristics. Patients who overdosed accidentally on prescription medication were perceived more favorably than those who took an overdose in a suicide attempt or those who were drug-dependent. Moreover, the recommendations for further treatment reflected these differential perceptions.

Similarly, Roth (1986) identified instances of moral evaluation of clients in emergency room settings, demonstrating that professional staff were not morally neutral in how they perceive patients and that there was consensus that some categories of patients, e.g., drunks, are less deserving of emergency room care and others, e.g., unusual cases, are more deserving.

Leiderman and Grisso (1985) identified the

"gomer" (*G*et *O*ut of *M*y *E*mergency *R*oom, *G*rand *O*ld *M*an of the *E*mergency *R*oom) phenomenon and showed that ambiguity of diagnosis and impairment of both adult social role functioning and mental status were more likely to lead to a patient's being perceived and labeled as a gomer, with ensuing problems of patient management and failure to respond to treatment. Gomers were no more likely to be seriously ill initially than comparable controls, but they remained in the hospital longer and experienced mental deterioration to a greater degree.

A similarly marginalizing view is found in the concept of the "nudnik" (Maoz, Antonovsky, Ziv, Avraham-Shiloh, & Durst, 1985), a bothersome patient whose problems are apparently discounted as being nonsomatic and emotional. Furthermore, in a study of nurses in public and community health agencies, Keith and Castles (1975) showed how environmental and workplace characteristics contribute to professionals' fears and rejections of patients and to the emergence of stereotyping by professionals.

Incongruent Perceptions

Since shared or overlapping perceptions are presumed to facilitate satisfactory and productive encounters, the degree to which patient and professional perceptions are incongruent may impede appropriate interactions and consequently may have a negative or unanticipated effect on health behavior and ultimately upon health status. Innes (1977) identified factors in the training of physicians that lead to failures of the physician to perceive the patient appropriately, i.e., to perceive the patient as a product of situational as well as dispositional factors, and failures to be sensitive to patient feelings and emotional states. Innes further observes that such failures lead to inadequate communication, which in turn fails to satisfy patient needs and generates failure to comply with aspects of treatment.

Kahn, Anderson, and Perkoff (1973) observed that laypersons' perceptions of the worsening of conditions and their subsequent use of emergency rooms for treatment were incongruent with the perceptions of physicians. On the basis of a latent structure analysis of the "normative conflict" between physicians and patients, Sawyer (1980) concluded that despite evidence that physicians know that incongruity exists between their own and their patients' perspectives and norms, physicians continue to ignore patients' perceptions and assume that a "normative" consensus exists.

In her observations of patients in rehabilitation programs, Hill (1978) demonstrated that their perceptions of themselves and of their physicians were often determined by the policies of the rehabilitation unit in relation to authority and by patients' participation in their own care. She reasons that the policies and perceptions of the care unit may be incongruent with, and detrimental to, the entire rehabilitation process.

Complementing the individual and health professional perceptions that mediate communication are interactional characteristics such as perceptions of satisfaction, and role and power relationships.

Perceptions of Satisfaction

Patients' perceptions of satisfaction—their positive evaluations or assessments of care—have been a major focus of health behavior research. Satisfaction is complexly determined. It involves trust and patients' characteristics and needs, as well as their perceptions of physicians' technical and interpersonal skills together with their perceptions of whether or not they are responding appropriately to treatment.

Caterinicchio (1979) used path analysis to develop a model for predicting the degree of trust in patient-practitioner interactions on the basis of continuity, frequency, and success of treatment, as well as for predicting the relationships between perceived trust, anxiety, tolerance of pain, and perceived health outcomes. The findings demonstrated that trust, once established, continues even in the face of subsequent negative experiences.

Kasteler et al. (1976) demonstrated that the degree to which patients have confidence or trust in their physician's competence, the degree to which they are impressed with the physician's personal characteristics, and the convenience of location and office hours are all important determinants of "doctor-shopping," the degree to which individuals will change physicians and systematically seek out new ones.

Ross (e.g., Ross & Duff, 1982; Ross, Mirowsky, & Duff, 1982) has analyzed how patients' satisfaction leads them to return to the physician and relates both their satisfaction and their inclination to return to the interaction between the characteristics of the patient and of the practice setting, e.g., continuity of care, small or large setting. In addition, Mirowsky and Ross (1983) have shown that the relationship between satisfaction and use of pediatric services resembles a self-regulatory system: Although increased levels of satisfaction lead to increased use of services, at some point increased use eventually results in diminished satisfaction, which then leads to a reduction in use.

Hall, Roter, and Rand (1981) have developed ingenious techniques to filter out the expressive qualities of speech from the verbal content. In a study of the qualities of oral communication between patients and physicians, they observed, paradoxically, that patients' contentment was positively related to physicians' showing anger toward them, the anger being interpreted as reflecting a firm but fair attitude. Analysis of oral communication indicate that vocal qualities such as empathy, calmness, and dominance become especially important in the interpretation of verbal messages (Harrigan, Gramata, Lucic, & Margolis, 1989). Buller and Buller (1987) observed that patients' satisfaction with care was positively related to the degree of "affiliativeness" in their physicians' communications and negatively related to the degree of "control" in such communications.

Locker and Dunt (1978) systematically reviewed problems in the conceptualization and measurement of satisfaction. Zyzanski, Hulka, and Cassel (1974) have devised a psychometrically sound and widely used scale to measure satisfaction with medical care in general, but it does not deal with care provided by individual physicians or health professionals.

In chapter 2, on professionals' characteristics, Ben-Sira integrates a number of issues relevant to perceptions and interactions. Ben-Sira elaborates on the relationship between patient affective needs, perceptions of physician affective behavior, and patient satisfaction, and discusses professional perceptions and behaviors that lessen the likelihood that the patient will be satisfied.

Power and Control

A power/authority differential is characteristic of most encounters between laypersons and professionals. Professionals have greater power and authority by virtue of their training, knowledge, and skill. In exchange for their services to community and society, professionals are accorded a preferred and special status, which reinforces and augments this power and authority. Often, the power of the health professional is invoked to influence the behavior of individual patients, particularly in relation to compliance with a specified regimen. Issues related to power can thus be considered in terms of the general power and authority of the professional and in terms of patient compliance.

Professional Power and Authority

The professional power and authority of the physician can be observed in a number of ways. Stimson and Webb (1975), for example, demonstrated how physicians can control aspects of the encounter with patients by establishing clinic hours and appointment schedules and thus limiting their availability to patients. Patients, on their part, seek to counter this power by seeking additional information from other physicians they may be seeing or from pharmacists who fill their prescriptions.

The relationship between power and information exchange and communication was examined by the Australian obstetrical case study of Shapiro et al (1983) showing that women seldom received the information they sought or needed, those in public clinics apparently needing more and receiving disproportionately less than those in private care. These findings are interpreted as indicating that physicians maintain their power by selectively managing discussions to avoid providing information. Examples of the power of physicians to stigmatize and label (or, conversely, to destigmatize), for example, are provided by Volinn's (1983) analysis of professional reactions to alcoholism and leprosy.

Gerson (1976) viewed illness and the physician-patient encounter in terms of a political process, involving conflict between the patient's needs and the physician's control over work, as well as allocation of scarce resources. The analysis by Ermann (1976) of the shift from decision making by independent health care professionals, who were presumed to be controlled by their clients, toward decisions made by physicians who are employees of hospitals and other large health care organizations raises questions about what types of social institutions can provide appropriate countervailing power to serve as social controls in the health care area.

Waitzkin and Britt (1989) note that communication in many medical encounters veers away from discussion of the very important personal and social problems arising from family life, gender roles, life cycle, or occupational or employment stresses or insecurity that may be factors in risk and other self-destructive behavior. Instead, communication focuses on narrowly defined medical issues, thereby discounting concerns that are often of great importance to the patient. Interestingly (but not surprisingly), this pattern is found not only in the United States, but also in the former Soviet Union, eastern Europe, and China (although not in Cuba) (Waitzkin & Britt, 1989). Waitzkin and Britt interpret the narrow focus of communication within the encounter as a means of discouraging discussion of "macro" issues involving politics and economics and thus discouraging attempts to change social conditions. Such communication is seen to reinforce the oppression and domination of the existing power and political structure, including the power of physicians.

Different degrees of professional power might be inferred from differential prestige rankings observed in the health care delivery system. Factors such as gender and ethnicity were observed to affect the prestige rankings of 19 different health care occupations, ranging from physicians, dentists, and nurses to inhalation therapists and other members of allied health professions; such differences can influence the differential power of these occupations within the overall health care system (Aguirre, Wolinsky, Niederauer, Keith, & Fann, 1989).

In Chapter 3, Haug elaborates on the changing power and authority of medicine and its implications for health behavior.

Role Relations

Szasz and Hollender (1956/1975) described three basic models of physician-patient role relationships: activity-passivity, guidance-cooperation, and mutual participation. Each model specifies a different view of the hierarchy or symmetry in the relationship and allows for the satisfaction of different physician needs. For example, in the activity-passivity model, physicians can presumably gratify their needs for mastery and express their feelings of superiority. The study of pregnant women by Danziger (1978) showed the differential interactional outcomes depending on whether the model accepted by the physician was congruent or incongruent with that accepted by the patient.

In a study of physicians in a health maintenance organization, Barr and Steinberg (1985) identified two independent role dimensions, colleague dependency and client dependency, and observed that there was no unitary conception of the physician role, but rather that some saw themselves as bureaucrats, while others saw themselves as unhampered by nonmedical restraints. They did see themselves as moderately colleague-dependent, although few participated in organizational decision making.

Drew, Stoeckle, and Billings (1983) analyzed the giving of gifts to physicians in relation to physician-patient roles. They suggested that the gift-giving process contains elements of needs for reciprocity as well as elements of attempts to change the status and power imbalance of the relationship.

Shelp (1984) argues, moreover, that courage should be an important component of the physician's role, particularly in relation to the risks of medical uncertainty, in contexts in which there is no cure. Such courage on the part of the physician is presumed to elicit similar courage on the part of the patient facing pain and death. In relation to uncertainty, especially in the context of biomedical innovations leading to prenatal detection of inherited diseases, Sorenson (1974) showed that the traditional role relationship between physicians and patients was changing. The increased uncertainty was bringing about greater patient participation and less authoritativeness on the part of the physician.

Todd and Still's (1984) observations of four general practitioners working with terminally ill patients suggest the appropriateness of physicians expanding their narrowly defined traditional role as *medical* practitioner to include the role of *counselor*, since their task was no longer one of treating or curing medically, but of helping the patient cope with the inevitability of dying. Another role-related observation is found in the typology of Bucks, Williams, Whitfield, and Routh (1990), which suggests the existence of five types of general practitioner attitudes: egalitarian, traditional-speculative, traditional-careful, doctor-centered, and balanced-patient-centered.

In Chapter 4, Salloway, Hafferty, and Vissing examine changes in professional roles, emphasizing their increasing differentiation and the implications of role changes for client and patient behaviors.

STRUCTURAL DETERMINANTS

The structural characteristics of institutions in which health care is sought, i.e., the milieu in which the encounter between the patient and the professional occurs, have both organizational (or social) dimensions and environmental dimensions. The organizational dimensions broadly include goals and values; policies related to authority, decision-making, division of labor, and personnel; and managerial styles; as well as how these affect employee morale and productivity (e.g., Etzioni, 1964). The environmental dimensions broadly include such aspects as location; building height; room size and shape; arrangements of space, color, and texture; acoustics; and ventilation and lighting.

The linkages between institutional characteristics and the health behaviors of clients, patients, or consumers, the satisfaction of whose needs is presumably a goal or value of health care institutions, and the morale of whom is a concern of workplace institutions, have seldom been systematically examined. Gish (1984), for example, has proposed a framework for identifying health care institutions in terms of whether they are resource-oriented, disease-oriented, political decision makers, or organized sellers and purchases of health care, and has analyzed how these institutional aspects exhibit different values related to health care from country to country, particularly in regard to whether health is considered to be a social objective or a market commodity. This promising conceptual model, however, has not yet been subject to much empirical testing in relation to health behavior. The limited extant research can be discussed under three headings: organizational characteristics, environmental characteristics, and system barriers.

Organizational Characteristics

Two important organizational characteristics that have been related to health behavior are policies and organization of tasks.

Policies

In early research on institutional policies, Berkanovic, Reeder, Marcus, and Schwartz (1975), for example,examined the differential effects of prepayment and nonprepaid, fee-for-service policies in relation to the financing of care and found that prepayment did not lead to significantly greater difficulty in obtaining appointments or in seeing a physician without an appointment. Under the nonprepaid arrangements, however, patients were somewhat more dubious about their physician's ability.

The analysis by Wolinsky (1976) of attitudinal data related to health maintenance organizations (HMOs) indicated that the HMO policy of heavily emphasizing prevention, together with the HMOs' appeal to persons who were already more interested in prevention, would account for some of the apparent dissatisfaction with HMOs: Potential users are already likely to be involved in preventive care. Thus, when these persons joined an HMO, they would experience a "ceiling effect" in that they could not increase such utilization by very much. Luft (1978), on the other hand, concluded from examination of the literature on HMO services that the greater use of preventive services by HMO enrollees was attributable to their being covered for it financially, rather than to the HMOs' preventive ideology, since persons who were covered for preventive services under third-party fee-for-payment reimbursement policies did not differ from HMO enrollees in use of such services.

Hospitals themselves have norms, or unwritten policies, about things such as duration of stay. That they do is confirmed in a study conducted in the Netherlands (and thus not constricted by United States DRG regulations) that demonstrated far greater between-institutional than within-institutional variation in lengths of comparable hospitalization for comparable conditions (Westert, Nieboer, & Groenewegen, 1993).

Institutions also differ in degree of client participation in policy making. Glogow (1973), reviewing a variety of arguments both for and against increased community involvement and participation in developing and implementing policies for public health services, reasons strongly for increased openness in such policy formulation. The examination by Eardley et al. (1985) of attendance patterns at cervical screening clinics in Britain revealed that policies related to inviting the women but providing them with insufficient information, together with non-user-oriented policies such as requiring the woman to take the initiative in setting the appointment, had negative impacts on use of screening.

An enlightening analysis of how several organizational models interacted differentially with client consistencies and community institutions is found in the study by Dill (1994) of organizational responses to AIDS. Dill noted the appreciable effect that organizational environments have on the way in which an organization can respond to needs and crisis.

Task Organization

Hoping to find that staff/patient ratios and degree of bureaucratization of work routines were related to nurses' encouraging of postnatal maternal behavior, i.e., behaviors such as touching, smiling at, and otherwise reacting to their infants, Moss (1984) observed few clear-cut effects attributable to formal properties of hospitals' organization. Moss found that the greatest amount of maternal affectionate behavior occurred in a setting in which there was fairly well differentiated task organization and in which mothers had moderate control over their own activities, rather than in a setting in which tasks were loosely organized and mothers had greater degrees of control. Moss introduces intervening factors, such as strict task organization leading to nurses having more time at their disposal to work with mothers, and the differential impact of lack of structure on women of different social classes, to account for the absence of straightforward organizational effects.

One critical component of task organization is "role discretion." Greenley and Schoenherr (1981) observed that "role discretion," the ability to make autonomous work decisions, is the single attribute that has an impact on client satisfaction. Greenley and Davidson (1988) provided a further examination of the effects of role discretion, together with an analysis of other institutional characteristics, such as claimed and de facto "domains" and availability of resources, on care-seeking behavior and on patient satisfaction.

Finally, the role of "queues," referring to the manner in which persons waiting to receive a service must wait upon those providing it (e.g., Finlay, Mutran, Zeitler, & Randall, 1990), is examined in relation to how medical residents organize their work. Rather than perform in a way that would minimize queues, make the system appear to function more efficiently, and thus generate organizational rewards for themselves, or reduce their loads by referring patients elsewhere, the residents demonstrated a strong commitment to patient care by taking the time needed with patients and by providing thorough examinations when necessary, even though this practice increased patient waiting time (Finlay et al., 1990).

Environmental Characteristics

Three environmental characteristics that have been specifically related to health behavior are size, location, and space.

Size

Ross and Duff (1982) examined a variety of organizational factors in relation to experiences and satisfaction with patient care and observed that clients who had good experiences with quality care within a large, bureaucratic multispecialty prepaid clinic were more likely to make appropriate, need-based return visits than were clients of smaller, fee-for-service practices. The size of the bureaucracy was apparently less of a barrier to care than the financial constraints of the fee-for-service arrangements. Size and impersonal treatment are not in themselves deterrents to care seeking.

Mishler (1981), reviewing research findings related to institutional size, noted that increased size had a negative impact on health, that patients in larger institutions tended to be less open and less free in expressing their feelings. Larger institutions apparently place less emphasis on understanding patients' personal problems. While Mishler observed reflected health status rather than health behavior, the findings point to some important directions for health behavior research: the effects of size on patient–physician interactions and on patient acceptance of regimens.

Location

Bohland (1984) analyzed use of emergency rooms for primary care in an urban Oklahoma county and found that geographic proximity of the site was as important a determinant of its use as patients' socioeconomic status. Davis and Kunitz (1978) reported that while the Navajo have distinctively different morbidity rates than does the larger United States population, reflecting both their poverty and their not yet completed transition from a population primarily at risk for acute infectious diseases to one primarily at risk for chronic diseases, the frequency with which they use hospital health services is attributable more to the proximity and thus to the accessibility of these services than to medical need. Moreover, although the data do not address the issue, the Navajo apparently use both traditional and scientific care.

Geographic differences in use of services have been observed. Chassin (1993) suggests that such differences are attributable not so much to inappropriate use of services in high-use areas or to uncertainty among physicians about appropriate procedures, as to geographic or locational differences in physician enthusiasm for selected high-technology procedures.

Space

In a dramatically written analysis of how public places are experienced, Hiss (1987a,b) calls attention to the important role that total perception of the environment plays in people's feelings of comfort and well-being as well as in their behavior. Hiss suggests that the scale of the physical environment, its opportunities for viewing, its richness and other characteristics must be considered in plans for buildings and neighborhoods.

Armstrong (1985) has provided a cogent analysis of the implications of changes in the physical context of British primary care, from practice conducted within the physician's own living quarters, through practice conducted within a separate part of the physician's home, to practice in clinics. The changes in the physical spatial arrangements were perceived to be causally associated with changes in the characteristics of the physician-patient encounter, as well as in the meanings of medical practice and community health.

Eyles (1990), reviewing the spatial configurations of health care from a geographer's perspective, suggests that spatial and locational factors have important implications for health behaviors, particularly for utilization. A complementary analysis of spatial and locational issues is found in the discussion by Moon (1990) of how spatial allocations and distributions should be integrated with health policy. Whitehead, Fusillo, and Kaplan (1988) integrated concepts of size, space, and other environmental characteristics and argued for consumer participation in the design of the physical environment of health care settings. The innovative study by Ornstein (1992) of perceptions of a reception area showed that factors such as selection and arrangement of furnishings, plants, and artwork convey messages about the considerateness of the organization. Such research has implications for the design of waiting rooms and clinical offices to maximize their positive messages and their appeal to patients and their families.

In Chapter 5, Scarpaci and Kearn expand on spatial and locational issues and introduce the critical concept of "sense of place."

System Barriers

Finally, a few studies have considered system barriers in the context of structural determinants. In their analysis of social, cultural, and demographic factors in utilization of health services, Berkanovic and Reeder (1974) extrapolate from available evidence and suggest that professional prejudices about clients' race, moral status, or responsibility for illness may serve as barriers to utilization of services. Furthermore, Rundall and Wheeler (1979) demonstrated that not having a regular source of care, problems in transportation to care sites, and long waiting times were all system barriers to utilization of preventive services.

REFERENCES

Adamson, T. E., & Watts P. A. (1976). Patients' perceptions of maternity nurse practitioners. *Public Health Reports, 66,* 585-586.

Aguirre, B. E., Wolinsky, F. D., Niederauer, J., Keith, V., & Fann, L-J. (1989). Occupational prestige in the health care delivery system. *Journal of Health and Social Behavior, 30,* 315-329.

Anderson, W. T., & Helm, D. T. (1979). The physician-patient encounter: A process of reality negotiation. In E. G. Jaco (Ed.), *Patients, physicians and illness* (3rd ed.) (pp. 259-271). New York: Free Press.

Armstrong, D. (1985). Space and time in British general practice. *Social Science and Medicine, 20,* 659-666.

Ashworth, C. D., Williamson, P., & Montano, D. (1984). A scale to measure physician beliefs about psychosocial aspects of patient care. *Social Science and Medicine, 19,* 1235-1238.

Barr, J., & Steinberg, M. K. (1985). A physician role typology: Colleague and client dependence in an HMO. *Social Science and Medicine, 20,* 253-261.

Berkanovic, E., & Reeder, L. G. (1974). Can money buy the appropriate use of services? Some notes on the meaning of utilization data. *Journal of Health and Social Behavior, 15,* 93-99.

Berkanovic, E., Reeder, L. G., Marcus, A. C., & Schwartz, S.

(1975). The effects of prepayment on access to medical care: The PACC experience. *Milbank Memorial Fund Quarterly: Health and Society, 53,* 241-253.

Bohland, J. (1984). Neighborhood variations in the use of hospital emergency rooms for primary care. *Social Science and Medicine, 19,* 1217-1226.

Bucks, R. S., Williams, A., Whitfield, M. J., & Routh, D. A. (1990). Towards a typology of general practitioners' attitudes to general practice. *Social Science and Medicine, 30,* 537-547.

Buller, M. K., & Buller, D. B. (1987). Physicians' communication style and patient satisfaction. *Journal of Health and Social Behavior, 28,* 375-388.

Caterinicchio, R. P. (1979). Testing plausible path models of interpersonal trust in patient-physician treatment relationships. *Social Science and Medicine, 13A,* 81-99.

Chassin, M. R. (1993). Explaining geographic variations: The enthusiasm hypothesis. *Medical Care, 31,* YS37-YS44.

Danziger, S. K. (1978). The uses of expertise in doctor-patient encounters during pregnancy. *Social Science and Medicine, 12,* 359-367.

Davis, S., & Kunitz, S. J. (1978). Hospitalization utilization and elective surgery on the Navajo Indian reservation. *Social Science and Medicine, 12B,* 263-272.

Dill, A. (1994). Institutional environments and organizational responses to AIDS. *Journal of Health and Social Behavior, 35,* 349-369.

Drew, J., Stoeckle, J. D., & Billings, J. A. (1983). Tips, status and sacrifice: Gift giving in the doctor-patient relationship. *Social Science and Medicine, 17,* 399-404.

Eardley, A., Elkind, A. K., Spencer, B., Hobbs, P., Pendleton, L. L., & Haran, D. (1985). Attendance for cervical screening—Whose problem? *Social Science and Medicine, 20,* 955-962.

Ermann, M. D. (1976). The social control of organizations in the health care area. *Milbank Memorial Fund Quarterly: Health and Society, 54,* 167-183.

Etzioni, A. (1964). *Modern organizations.* Englewood Cliffs, NJ: Prentice-Hall.

Eyles, J. (1990). How significant are the spatial configurations of health care systems? *Social Science and Medicine, 30,* 157-164.

Finlay, W., Mutran, E. J., Zeitler, R. R., & Randall, C. S. (1990). Queues and care: How medical residents organize their work in a busy clinic. *Journal of Health and Social Behavior, 31,* 292-305.

Ford, A. B., Liske, R. E., Ort, R. S., & Denton, J. C. (1967). *The doctor's perspective: Physicians view their patients and practice.* Cleveland: Press of Case Western Reserve University.

Frazier, P. J., Jenny, J., Bagramian, R. A., Robinson, E., & Proshek, J. M. (1977). Provider expectations and consumer perceptions of the importance and value of dental care. *American Journal of Public Health, 67,* 37-43.

Freidson, E. (1961). *Patients' views of medical practice.* New York: Russell Sage Foundation.

Gerbert, B. (1984). Perceived likability and competence of simulated patients: Influence on physicians' management plans. *Social Science and Medicine, 18,* 1053-1059.

Gerson, E. M. (1976). The social character of illness: Deviance or politics. *Social Science and Medicine, 10,* 219-224.

Ghodse, A. H. (1978). The attitudes of casualty staff and ambulance personnel towards patients who take drug overdoses. *Social Science and Medicine, 12,* 341-346.

Ghodse, A. H. (1979). Recommendations by accident and emergency staff about drug-overdose patients. *Social Science and Medicine, 13A,* 169-173.

Gish, O. (1984). Values in health care. *Social Science and Medicine, 19,* 333-339.

Glogow, E. (1973). Community participation and sharing in control of public health services. *Health Services Reports, 88,* 442-448.

Greenley, J. R., & Davidson, R. E. (1988). Organizational influences on patient health behaviors. In D. S. Gochman (Ed.), *Health behavior: Emerging research perspectives* (pp. 215-229). New York: Plenum Press.

Greenley, J. R., & Schoenherr, R. A. (1981). Organization effects on client satisfaction with humaneness of service. *Journal of Health and Social Behavior, 22,* 2-18.

Hall, J. A., Epstein, A. M., DeCiantis, M. L., & McNeil, B. J. (1993). Physicians' liking for their patients: More evidence for the role of affect in medical care. *Health Psychology, 12,* 140-146.

Hall, J. A., Irish, J. T., Roter, D. L., Ehrlich, C. M., & Miler, L. H. (1994). Gender in medical encounters: An analysis of physician and patient communication in a primary care setting. *Health Psychology, 13,* 384-392.

Hall, J. A., Roter, D. L., & Rand, C. S. (1981). Communication of affect between patient and physician. *Journal of Health and Social Behavior, 22,* 18-30.

Harrigan, J. A., Gramata, J. F., Lucic, K. S., & Margolis, C. (1989). It's how you say it: Physicians' vocal behavior. *Social Science and Medicine, 28,* 87-92.

Helman, C. G. (1990). *Culture, health and illness* (2nd ed.). London: Wright/Butterworth.

Hill, C. E. (1978). Differential perceptions of the rehabilitation process: A comparison of client and personnel incongruity in two categories of chronic illness. *Social Science and Medicine, 12,* 57-63.

Hiss, T. (1987a). Experiencing places—I. *The New Yorker,* June 22, 45-68.

Hiss, T. (1987b). Experiencing places—II. *The New Yorker,* June 29, 73-86.

Innes, J. M. (1977). Does the professional know what the client wants? *Social Science and Medicine, 11,* 635-638.

Kahn, L., Anderson, M., & Perkoff, G. T. (1973). Patients' perceptions and uses of a pediatric emergency room. *Social Science and Medicine, 7,* 155-160.

Kasteler, J., Kane, R. L., Olsen, D. M., & Thetford, C. (1976). Issues underlying prevalence of "doctor-shopping" behavior. *Journal of Health and Social Behavior, 17,* 328-339.

Keith, P. M., & Castles, M. M. (1975). Fear and rejection of patients by health practitioners. *Social Science and Medicine, 9*, 501-505.

Lederer, H. D. (1952). How the sick view their world. *Journal of Social Issues, 8*, 4-15.

Leiderman, D. B., & Grisso, J-A. (1985). The gomer phenomenon. *Journal of Health and Social Behavior, 26*, 222-232.

Liddell, A., & May, B. (1984). Patients' perceptions of dentists' positive and negative attributes. *Social Science and Medicine, 19*, 839-842.

Locker, D., & Dunt, D. (1978). Theoretical and methodological issues in sociological studies of consumer satisfaction with medical care. *Social Science and Medicine, 12*, 283-292.

Luft, H. S. (1978). Why do HMOs seem to provide more health maintenance services? *Milbank Memorial Fund Quarterly: Health and Society, 56*(2), 140-168.

Maoz, B., Antonovsky, H., Ziv, P., Avraham-Shiloh, L., & Durst, N. (1985). The family doctor and his "nudnik (bothersome) patients": An exploratory study. *Israeli Journal of Psychiatry and Related Sciences, 22*, 95-104.

McCranie, E. W., Horowitz, A. J., & Martin, R. M. (1978). Alleged sex-role stereotyping in the assessment of women's physical complaints: A study of general practitioners. *Social Science and Medicine, 12*, 111-116.

McKinlay, J. B. (1975). Who is really ignorant—physician or patient? *Journal of Health and Social Behavior, 16*, 3-11.

Mirowsky, J., & Ross, C. E. (1983). Patient satisfaction and visiting the doctor: A self-regulating system. *Social Science and Medicine, 17*, 1353-1361.

Mishler, E. G. (1981). Social contexts of health care. In E. G. Mishler, L. R. Amarasingham, S. D. Osherson, S. T. Hauser, N. E. Waxler, & R. Liem (Eds.), *Social contexts of health, illness, and patient care* (pp. 79-103). Cambridge, England: Cambridge University Press.

Moon, G. (1990). Conceptions of space and community in British health policy. *Social Science and Medicine, 30*, 165-171.

Moss, N. (1984). Hospital units as social context: Effects on maternal behavior. *Social Science and Medicine, 19*, 515-522.

Niemeyer, L. O. (1991). Social labeling, stereotyping, and observer bias in workers' compensation: The impact of provider-patient interaction on outcome. *Journal of Occupational Rehabilitation, 1*(4), 251-269.

Ornstein, S. (1992). First impressions of the symbolic meanings connoted by reception area design. *Environment and Behavior, 24*(1), 85-110.

Rosen, R. H. (1977). The patient's view of the role of the primary care physician in abortion. *American Journal of Public Health, 67*, 863-865.

Ross, C. E., & Duff, R. S. (1982). Returning to the doctor: The effect of client characteristics, type of practice, and experience with care. *Journal of Health and Social Behavior, 23*, 119-131.

Ross, C. E., Mirowsky, J., & Duff, R. S. (1982). Physician status characteristics and client satisfaction in two types of practice. *Journal of Health and Social Behavior, 23*, 317-329.

Roth, J. A. (1986). Some contingencies of the moral evaluation and control of clientele: The case of the hospital emergency service. In P. Conrad & R. Kern (Eds.), *The sociology of health and illness: Critical perspectives* (2nd ed.) (pp. 327-333). New York: St. Martin's Press.

Rundall, T. G., & Wheeler, J. R. C. (1979). The effect of income on use of preventive care: An evaluation of alternative explanations. *Journal of Health and Social Behavior, 20*, 397-406.

Sawyer, D. (1980). Normative conflict and physician use: A latent structure approach. *Journal of Health and Social Behavior, 21*, 156-169.

Shapiro, M. C., Najman, J. M., Chang, A., Keeping, J. D., Morrison, J., & Western, J. S. (1983). Information control and the exercise of power in the obstetrical encounter. *Social Science and Medicine, 17*, 139-146.

Shelp, E. E. (1984). Courage: A neglected virtue in the patient-physician relationship. *Social Science and Medicine, 18*, 351-360.

Sorenson, J. R. (1974). Biomedical innovation, uncertainty, and doctor-patient interaction. *Journal of Health and Social Behavior, 15*, 366-374.

Stimson, G., & Webb, B. (1975). *Going to see the doctor: The consultation process in general practice*. London: Routledge & Kegan Paul.

Strauss, R. P. (1976). Sociocultural influences upon preventive health behavior and attitudes toward dentistry. *American Journal of Public Health, 66*, 375-377.

Szasz, T. S., & Hollender, M. H. (1956/1975). A contribution to the philosophy of medicine: The basic models of the doctor-patient relationship. In T. Million (Ed.), *Medical behavioral science* (pp. 432-440). Philadelphia: Saunders. (Reprinted from *Archives of Internal Medicine*, 1956, *97*, 585-592.)

Todd, C. J., & Still, A. W. (1984). Communication between general practitioners and patients dying at home. *Social Science and Medicine, 18*, 667-672.

Verbrugge, L. M. (1984). How physicians treat mentally distressed men and women. *Social Science and Medicine, 18*, 1-9.

Volinn, I. J. (1983). Health professionals as stigmatizers and destigmatizers of diseases: Alcoholism and leprosy as examples. *Social Science and Medicine, 17*, 385-393.

Waitzkin, H., & Britt, T. (1989). Changing the structure of medical discourse: Implications of cross-national comparisons. *Journal of Health and Social Behavior, 30*, 436-449.

Westbrook, M. T., Nordholm, L. A., & McGee, J. E. (1984). Cultural differences in reactions to patient behaviour: A comparison of Swedish and Australian health professionals. *Social Science and Medicine, 19*, 939-947.

Westert, G. P., Nieboer, A. P., & Groenewegen, P. P. (1993). Variation in duration of hospital stay between hospitals and between doctors within hospitals. *Social Science and Medicine*, *37*, 833-839.

Whitehead, B. A., Fusillo, A. E., & Kaplan, S. (1988). The design of physical environments and health behavior. In D. S. Gochman (Ed.), *Health behavior: Emerging research perspectives* (pp. 231-241). New York: Plenum Press.

Wolinsky, F. D. (1976). Health service utilization and attitudes toward health maintenance organizations: A theoretical and methodological discussion. *Journal of Health and Social Behavior*, *17*, 221-236.

Zyzanski, S. J., Hulka, B. S., & Cassel, J. C. (1974). Scale for the measurement of "satisfaction" with medical care: Modifications in content, format and scoring. *Medical Care*, *12*, 611-620.

2

Professionals' Characteristics and Health Behavior

Zeev Ben-Sira

INTRODUCTION

This chapter addresses the trends in interprofessional relations among three health professions—medicine (with the focus on primary care), nursing, and social work—and their effect on health behavior in relation to the role of stress in the onset, severity, and outcome of disease. It begins with a brief review of approaches to the stress-health relationship, underscoring the importance to the treatment process of coping with patients' emotional problems. The trends toward medical specialization and the dehumanizing potential of such specialization are then reviewed with a specific focus on the reluctance of general practitioners to demonstrate affective behavior. Affective behavior refers to acts aimed at establishing a physician-patient relationship such that the physician accepts the patient as a human being who may have anxiety-arousing problems frequently over and above the identifiable somatic disturbance—problems that can hardly be alleviated by mere technical-medical procedures.

Following the analysis of medical practice, some characteristics of the nursing profession are examined. Questions are raised concerning whether nurses can compensate or should be expected to compensate, for physicians' reluctance to demonstrate affective behavior, and issues in interprofessional confrontation are presented. Finally, some characteristics of social work in health care are examined, and parallel questions are raised about social workers' capacity to cope with the psychosocial aspects of health care.

The chapter concludes with suggestions regarding the effect of professional progress and interprofessional confrontation on health care and promotion.

Zeev Ben-Sira • Late of School of Social Work, Hebrew University of Jerusalem, and Louis Gutmann Israel Institute of Applied Social Research, Jerusalem, Israel.

Zeev Ben-Sira passed away before he was able to complete the revision and final review of this chapter. Recognizing his terminal illness, he entrusted its completion to the editor, who may not have done justice to the final product.

—DSG

Handbook of Health Behavior Research II: Provider Determinants, edited by David S. Gochman. Plenum Press, New York, 1997.

THE STRESS–DISEASE RELATIONSHIP: A DAMAGING CYCLE

Accumulating evidence suggests that stress contributes to the onset of, seriousness of, and recovery from disease (e.g., Antonovsky, 1979; Ben-Sira, 1991; Monat and Lazarus, 1991, p. 9; Pearlin, 1991). Evidence also suggests that disease itself can be a stressor (Ben-Sira, 1982a,b, 1988a). A person's subjective appraisal of the meaning and severity of an "objective" somatic episode can play an important role in that episode's becoming a stressor. Evidence further suggests that subjective appraisal of health is a central intervening factor between physician-diagnosed somatic episodes and the experience of stress. Subjective appraisal of health, in turn, is contingent on physician-diagnosed somatic episodes and on control of individual and environmental resources (Ben-Sira, 1991, pp. 147–148).

Occurrence of a somatic disturbance, then, has the potential of setting into motion a *damaging cycle* by causing persons to make detrimental appraisals of their own health. This detrimental appraisal can precipitate stress. Stress in turn can aggravate the risk of a further deterioration of the person's health. For persons in the disadvantaged strata of society (i.e., those with fewer resources at their disposal, the detrimental effect of somatic disturbances on their perceived health and consequent stress can be more perilous than for others.

THE BIOPSYCHOSOCIAL APPROACH AND ADVANCES IN MEDICINE

Evidence suggests that moderating the subjective detrimental appraisal is a critical requisite for minimizing the effect of the damaging cycle (Ben-Sira, 1991). Since the relative availability of treatment resources contributes to the appraisal of health, the need to ameliorate the subjective detrimental appraisal will increase as these resources decrease.

Evidence also suggests that the distress due to the subjectively assessed meaning and severity of a somatic disturbance, rather than the disturbance itself, will stimulate medical help-seeking. Patients evidently aspire to realize two goals by turning to a physician. Although the overt goal in help-seeking is to solve the health problem, the latent goal—alleviation of the anxiety underlying the subjective assessment of the severity of the medical problem—is often the decisive goal (Ben-Sira, 1976, 1980, 1982c).

The Need for Physicians to Manifest Affective Behavior

Since health problems are conventionally viewed as exclusively medical (cf. Illich, 1986), physicians are likely to be regarded as the only competent helping agents (Ben-Sira, 1988a). In view of patients' inability to judge the quality and effectiveness of the "instrumental" (medical, technical) intervention, and medicine's frequent inability to provide an immediate solution to the problem, evidence suggests that patients tend to base their judgment on the physicians' "affective" (humane, person-oriented) behavior (Ben-Sira, 1976,1980, 1982a, 1988a). Data suggest that the physician's affective behavior may function to enhance confidence and consequently to moderate stress not only by being emotionally supportive but also by providing "lay-intelligible clues." These clues are likely to serve as a basis for a patient's assessment of the effectiveness and quality of the intervention and of the physician's competence (Ben-Sira, 1982b, 1987a, 1990b). Such affective behavior, then, can halt the damaging cycle by improving patients' assessment of their health and consequently fulfilling a stress-mode-rating function.

Evidence (Ben-Sira, 1987a) further suggests that a physician's affective behavior can enhance a patient's lasting generalized confidence in the medical profession's efficacy in solving health problems over and above that particular encounter with the physician. Confidence, in turn, may fulfill a health-promoting function by reinforcing a belief in the surmountability of health problems, by reducing the health-hazardous consequences of stress, and by decreasing the frequency of physician visits that themselves can have distressing consequences (Ben-Sira, 1988a).

The Need for a Biopsychosocial Approach

The concept of a biopsychosocial approach developed by Engel (1977) refers to the integrated application of biomedical, psychological, and social factors in the understanding and treatment of health problems. This approach advocates viewing patients' and their families' psychosocial problems as an inherent component of medical intervention.

Family practice is the medical speciality that professes a biopsychosocial approach (Henao, 1985; Pattison & Anderson, 1978, p. 85). Israeli evidence, however, does not reveal a significant difference in demonstration of affective behavior between certified specialists in family practice and general practitioners (GPs). GPs even showed a somewhat higher inclination to incorporate affective behavior in their treatment. On the other hand, private fee-for-service primary care practitioners showed a greater likelihood of demonstrating affective behavior than did salaried physicians (Ben-Sira, 1985). Since physicians are aware of the role of their affective behavior in patients' assessment of the quality of the medical intervention and of physician proficiency (Ben-Sira, 1986a), it was suggested that physicians' inclination to demonstrate affective behavior is greatly motivated by the desire to attract a clientele (Ben-David, 1958; Ben-Sira, 1985).

Affective Behavior and Patient Participation

An explanation of the concepts of "affective behavior" and "patient participation in medical decision making" (cf. Haug, 1994) is in order at this point.

Affective behavior has been defined operationally as (1) attributing therapeutic importance to and (2) engaging in (a) warm, open relations with the patient, (b) attentiveness to problems even if unrelated to disease, (c) gathering information about personal and family problems, (d) gathering information about social relations, and (e) explaining the rationale of diagnosis and treatment (Ben-Sira, 1988a, p. 94).

Such behavior broadens the channels of interaction by bridging the status gap. Physicians do so by demonstrating sincere interest in patients' pressing personal problems (even if not directly related to their medical problems), tolerating patients' expectations, and minimizing professional "esotericity" by explaining in lay-intelligible terms the rationale of the diagnosis and treatment (Ben-Sira, 1988a, p. 93). The importance of physicians' affective behavior, then, is its potential to ameliorate the hazardous consequences of patients' negative assessment of the somatic disturbance (Ben-Sira, 1982c, 1986a).

Patient participation refers to the patient's sharing with the physician the responsibility for the intervention (Haug, 1994). The aim of this sharing is both to counteract professional dominance (Freidson, 1986) and to counterbalance the waning, and possibly even the further depreciation, of the physician's professional authority (Burnham, 1982; Haug, 1976, 1994; Haug & Lavin, 1981; Haug & Sussman, 1969; Starr, 1978).

The goal of *affective behavior*, contrary to the goals of patient participation, is to reinforce the patient's confidence in the physician's competence and professional authority. Sick individuals, who have reached the point at which professional help is indispensable, need the support of a competent and trustworthy physician with the best available knowledge-based professional authority to cope with their problems. Physicians' capacity to reinforce confidence lies in their sincere attentiveness to all of the patients' problems, their explanations of the rationale for their decisions, and their supportive behavior. It aims at bridging the status gap without depreciating the physicians' professional authority (Ben-Sira, 1987a, 1988a,b, 1990a).

One may question whether patient participation carries the risk of exacerbating the patient's anxiety, entailing as it does both the requirement that the patient share the responsibility for the consequences of the intervention and the explicit aim of diminishing the physician's professional authority (Johnston, 1994). Margalith (1993) suggests that *literal* patient participation in decision making where patients could choose between two possible types of a minor surgical intervention did not alleviate their anxiety. On the other hand, a feeling that they had received adequate information about their condition as well as about both the nature and the possible consequences of the intervention *without* participating in the decision regarding the intervention did alleviate their anxiety.

The conclusion derived from the data was that patients derive emotional homeostasis from a perception of having had the nature of their disorder and their treatment explained intelligibly and of having been addressed as human beings by a competent professional—a professional who has the authority and proficiency to carry out the needed intervention. Margalith concludes that physicians' "affective" behavior, rather than patients' involvement in the decision-making process, enhances patients' well-being.

Potential Negative Consequences of Affective Behavior

Physicians may perceive affective behavior as depriving them of authority by exposing the inadequacies and limitations of medicine. Indeed, as a protective mechanism, they may refrain from affective behavior in order to maintain or even widen the status gap. An inclination to refrain from affective behavior may particularly characterize salaried primary care practitioners (PCPs), whose knowledge base, by definition, is generalistic rather than biomedically specialized (Ben-Sira, 1985, 1986b), and who may therefore be more defensive.

The reluctance of salaried PCPs to demonstrate affective behavior is explained also by the nature of their practice. Evidence suggests that PCPs can rarely derive professional satisfaction from their routine interventions and that they have a rather low status in the eyes of both the professional community and patients. Demonstration of authoritarian rather than affective behavior apparently fulfills a status-compensating function (Ben-Sira, 1986b, 1988a,b, 1990a,b).

The greater likelihood that private fee-for-service practitioners will demonstrate affective behavior is explained by their perceiving that behavior as a means of attracting a clientele; hence, affective behavior has a "rewarding" property (Ben-David, 1958; Ben-Sira, 1988b, 1990a).

Utilization Patterns

The reluctance of PCPs to demonstrate affective behavior is likely to initiate a *damaging cycle* involving both dissatisfied, overutilizing patients and frustrated salaried physicians. Data from a comprehensive study among Israeli PCPs and ex-patients (Ben-Sira, 1988a) highlight the effects of a damaging cycle. The cycle began with the physicians' reluctance to demonstrate affective behavior. The patients were consequently dissatisfied with solutions that required repeated physician visits, and the physicians, in turn, felt overwhelmed by redundant visits that prevented them from carrying out "good" medical practice.

The data suggest that about one third of the patients treated by PCPs maintain that they have not received an adequate solution of their problem and will have to make repeated visits for the same problem (Ben-Sira, 1988a, pp. 19–20). Satisfaction with the treatment, the feeling that the medical problem has been adequately solved and hence will not require a return visit, and a consequent decrease in physician visits are all contingent on physicians' affective behavior (pp. 61–65). The data suggest a relationship in which patients' satisfaction with physicians' affective behavior increases their satisfaction with physicians' instrumental (biomedical) behavior, which in turn leads to patients perceiving their problem as being solved. The perceived solution of the problem explains their positive appraisal of their health, and subsequently their enhanced emotional homeostasis (pp. 22-25). A decrease in their satisfaction increases the likelihood that they will turn to private fee-for-service practitioners (pp. 77-79). The data suggest that private fee-for-service practitioners are attributed with far higher professional competence and inclination to demonstrate humane concern than are salaried physicians (pp. 80-81)—these attributions being explained by their greater likelihood of demonstrating affective behavior (pp. 74-75).

The data further underscore the role of individual resources in both help-seeking patterns and emotional homeostasis. A decrease in socioeconomic status (SES) is related to a decrease in satisfaction with medical care and to an increase in both the need for recurrent visits and the number of visits per year accounted for by dissatisfaction with the physician's intervention and consequent failure to alleviate the patient's stress (Ben-Sira, 1988a, pp. 33-42).

Salaried PCPs define nearly one third of patients' presenting complaints as redundant, compared to private fee-for-service PCPs, who describe only 14% as such (Ben-Sira, 1988a, p. 105). Salaried family practitioners tend to view the volume of redundant visits to be somewhat greater than do GPs (33% versus 29%) (p. 111). Salaried PCPs complain more than private practitioners of being "flooded" by too many patients. Family practitioners tend to voice such complaints more often than GPs (p. 121). The feeling of being flooded by the volume of visits is contingent on the likelihood that visits will be defined as redundant (p. 135). The data corroborate earlier evidence suggesting that private fee-for-service practitioners are more likely than salaried ones to demonstrate affective behavior (p. 103), and family practitioners are less inclined than GPs to demonstrate such behavior (p. 109).

The data suggest that salaried GPs achieve crucial gratification by adhering to the perceived expectations of the professional community and even more so to those of the employing agency. The weight of these expectations in shaping salaried physicians' behavior is more decisive than the perceived expectations of patients (Ben-Sira, 1988a, p. 121). The professional community is perceived as primarily rewarding biomedical excellence; the employing agency, as primarily rewarding adherence to administrative procedures and assistance in promoting the agency's political goals. Physicians perceive these agencies as expecting less affective behavior from them than do patients (p. 119).

The data suggest, then, the mutually distressing potential of the *damaging cycle* for both patients and physicians. Moreover, the overutilization inherent in this cycle can propagate such adverse health consequences as unnecessary diagnoses, "overtreatment," and overmedication (Illich, 1986). Salaried physicians may maintain that being flooded by "redundant" complaints hinders them from engaging in "good medicine" for those who are really in need. Thus, physicians may feel not merely unrewarded but even "punished" by being confronted by redundant cases. Physicians argue that the visits they most frequently defined as redundant were demands for sick certificates without justification, demands for medications without medical justification, and "trivial complaints" not requiring a physician's advice (Ben-Sira, 1988a, p. 104).

Israel has universal unlimited provision of free health care to all sectors of the Israeli population. With decreasing SES, however, come decreases in individuals' feeling of having received an adequate solution to their health problem, increases in their need for recurrent visits, increases in the frequency of their physician visits (Ben-Sira, 1988a, p. 37), and aggravated stress (p. 34). Aggravated stress is more of an impetus among those of lower SES than among those of higher SES to present emotional problems to physicians—problems that PCPs are likely to define as redundant (p. 104).

The data thus suggest that persons with fewer resources—and thus with greater needs for medical support—face a higher risk that their pleas for help will be labeled as redundant.

Primary Care Practitioners' Stereotyping of Patients: A Protective Mechanism

Affective behavior may also be regarded as undermining professionals' ability to render responsible medical assistance: PCPs often have to make decisions in the face of a high degree of uncertainty. Obtaining accurate and relevant information from the patient constitutes an important input for reaching such decisions. Affective behavior may be perceived as counterproductive, since it encourages the patient to convey "irrelevant," unnecessary, or inaccurate information together with redundant complaints. Responses and information that conflict with physicians' cultural framework and professional viewpoint are likely to be interpreted as challenges to professional authority (Gerbert, 1984; Roth, 1986; Zola, 1966). Curtailed authority, in turn, may be perceived as jeopardizing their ability to render care according to their professional judgment, possibly leading to being accused of professional incompetence and irresponsibility (Allen, 1994; Ben-Sira, 1986b, 1988a, 1990b). Such fears can become acute when physicians are confronted with pressures from patients who insist that they respond to "redundant" complaints and unjustified demands.

PCPs are likely to seek ways of protecting themselves against the distress of "authority-challenging" patients by distancing themselves from commitment to patient problems—commitment that carries the risk of being accused of failure to discharge their professional responsibility. Under such circumstances, physicians may attempt to attribute the responsibility for possible failure to the patient.

Detecting "authority-challenging" patients who interfere with the physician's practice of "good medicine" may serve as a protective mechanism, "saving" the physician from investing time, effort, and interest in such frustrating patients. Thus, physicians may look for "clues" in patients' external appearance that may facilitate classification, and hence stereotyping, of patients according to their anticipated behavior. On the basis of their experience, physicians may believe themselves capable of recognizing types of patients as soon as they enter the office.

Stereotyping, then, refers to the physician's use of clues indicating that the patient is likely to challenge the physician's authority as a basis for categorizing the patient as ***bad*** or ***undesirable*** (Papper, 1970). This stereotyping protects physicians against both frustrations and accusations of failure in discharging their professional responsibility.

Secondary analysis of a comprehensive interview study carried out by the author among a sample of Israel primary care practitioners was aimed at elucidating the factors that may predispose physicians to stereotype patients (Ben-Sira, 1993). The data suggest that the inclination to stereotype patients as "bad" or "undesirable" is contingent on *patient-related* predictors that in turn are conditioned by *physician-related* predictors.

As to patient-related predictors, the data suggest that PCPs' inclination to stereotype patients is contingent on their suspicion that the patient entering the office is likely to (1) present redundant complaints, (2) give unsatisfactory information, and (3) display unsatisfactory compliance. The propensity to anticipate such patient behavior, in turn, is contingent on the physician's own cognizance of professional weakness ("physician-related predictors") involving (1) limitations in the physician's professional experience ("experience mainly with trivial cases"), (2) inadequate professional progress, and (3) inadequate professional confidence.

Primary Care and Stress Alleviation: The Israeli Experience

In the wake of the growing specialization of medicine, it seems reasonable to view primary medical care as the most appropriate medium for rendering comprehensive, humane, stress-alleviating medical care. Comprehensive humane medical care would seem to be particularly attainable in a health care system, such as Israel's, that provides universal unlimited coverage for the entire population. A system like this would seem to be particularly beneficial for socioeconomically disadvantaged patients who more than others are in need of alleviation of their health-related emotional problems.

Evidence suggests, however, that the pressures inherent in the system are likely to impede the provision of such care and even to motivate PCPs to search for mechanisms to protect themselves against authority-depriving patient behavior—mechanisms that counter the inclination to demonstrate affective behavior toward patients. Israeli data suggest that in a prepaid system in which unlimited medical care is provided by salaried practitioners, the trend toward "challenging physician authority, [and] patients ... asserting their right to be autonomous actors in a medical encounter" (Haug, 1994, p. 4) advocated by proponents of patient participation in medical decisions can lead to counterproductive outcomes.

One may also question whether the trend toward patient participation may bring about the entrenchment of private physicians in the defense of their authority. Could the trend toward "question[ing] the legitimacy of the physicians' dominance" (Haug, 1994, p. 3) lead to defensive responses similar to the aforediscussed inclination to stereotype patients?

NURSING AND BIOPSYCHOSOCIAL PRACTICE

In view of physicians' reluctance to view "affective" behavior as an inherent component of medical treatment, are nurses to be regarded as the proficient providers of this component of medical intervention?

According to Benner and Wrubel (1989), nurses occupy an intermediary role between patients and physicians in coping with patients' emotional problems. There is reason, however, to question whether that role might not relieve physicians from the necessity of incorporating affective behavior as an inherent and indispensable component of medical intervention. Affective behavior serves as both a basis for a patient's appraisal of the quality and effectiveness of the physician's intervention and a mechanism for bridging the status gap (Ben-Sira, 1982b). Thus, compensation by other professionals for a lack of affective behavior on the physician's part seems inconceivable.

Nurses envision collaborative practice involving physicians and nurses as a bridge over the gap between the need for and the provision of biopsychosocial health care. Attainment of this kind of health care implies, according to Smoyak (1986), a *shared* responsibility whereby each professional can make a discrete input, on the basis of "equality in the making of decisions about the needs and problems of patients. Contributions from nurses about the care required may be largely socio-cultural and contributions from the physicians may be largely physiological, but each would be valued equally" (p. 83). Steel (1986, p. 5) envisions that "one of the major benefits of collaboration by doctors and nurses in patient care is the expectation that care will be coordinated, collaboratively planned, incorporate each other's areas of expertise, and be delivered in a planned fashion."

Doctor-nurse collaboration, in which each profession can provide its discrete knowledge-based input, has the potential of contributing to patients' well-being by integrating affective and instrumental components in the medical intervention. Lysaught (1986) concludes on the basis of empirical evidence that "when physicians and nurses worked in fully collaborative care patterns, there emerged a form of complementary role enactment ... [in which] physicians and nurses not only functioned in some overlapping ways, but also worked quite differently in discrete areas, such that the patient ... benefited significantly ... [in terms of] hastened return to work, better compliance with treatment regimens, decreased rates of readmission, and higher levels of satisfaction with the practitioners and the care delivered" (pp. 17-18).

Lamb and Stempel (1994) underscore the contribution of nurse practitioners in improving individuals' health through appropriate case-management procedures. They conclude that "several small descriptive studies indicate that individuals who work with nurse case managers spend fewer days in the hospital and intensive care units, have fewer hospital admissions and use the emergency room less frequently."

In the field of primary care, it has been noted that an HMO study suggested that the most satisfied patients had nurse practitioners who were more involved in their care and had greater influence over treatment decisions. Patients tended to be more satisfied when both the primary physician and the nurse practitioner were known to them.

Yedidia (1986) recounts evidence on the role of nurse practitioners in primary care in encouraging patients to verbalize their health concerns and consequently in eliciting an array of patient concerns and questions for which the physicians had no time.

The literature emphasizes the increasing status of nursing as a profession (Lysaught, 1986) that aspires to institute a distinctive professional knowledge base and to establish an autonomous professional territory and status (Lambertson, 1971). These aspirations bring about intrusions into territories that traditionally were physicians' exclusive domain and counteract nurses' subordinate position vis-à-vis physicians (Steel, 1986)—developments that can bring about interprofessional conflicts (Steel, 1986; Yedidia, 1986). Questions may be raised regarding the extent to which these developments come at the expense of meeting patients' biopsychosocial needs and eventually affecting patients' health behavior.

SOCIAL WORK AND BIOPSYCHOSOCIAL PRACTICE

The mandate of social work is to improve the quality of life from a psychosocial standpoint by "promoting or restoring a mutually beneficial interaction between individuals and society" (Second Meeting, 1981). In the words of Neugeboren (1985), "The maximum benefit for the client may be achieved by modifying both person and situation.... It is impossible to separate the individual from the situation, as there is a continuous interaction between the two" (p. 9).

The psychosocial outlook of social work equips social workers to deal concomitantly with the individual and the social problems of afflicted persons and their families. Social work, then, has the proficiency to provide the needed social care to afflicted persons by integrating coping with the pressures inherent in disease and those coming from their social environment. Such an integrative approach, which characterizes the "generic" nature (M. Sheppard, 1991) of social work, has the potential of alleviating patients' stress and consequently contributing to recovery.

The role of social work in health care has long been recognized as an established specialty (cf. Ben-Sira, 1987b; Carlton, 1984; R. J. Estes, 1984; Falck, 1984; Schlesinger, 1985). M. Sheppard (1991) quotes a report by the British Department of Health defining the role of social work in health care as "the assessment of social factors contributing to diagnosis; providing advice on social factors affecting discharge from hospital; and provision, if necessary, of long term after care support. Additionally in the primary health setting the role advocated include[s] therapeutic work with individuals, families or groups; mobilizing practical resources and liaison with outside agencies; educating the team on social factors in health care" (M. Sheppard, 1991, pp. 6–7).

Social workers are the most appropriate agents for coping with the psychosocial components of health care in relation "to assisting persons in need to identify and to cope emotionally and instrumentally with unmet demands (i.e., stressors) that may have affected the onset and severity of disease or are a consequence of it. Coping emotionally means moderating the subjectively perceived threat of these demands, thus reducing their homeostasis-disturbing impact. Coping instrumentally means changing environmental stressors (e.g., improving economic conditions) ... [by] a well grounded identification of unmet needs and the provision of competent, hypothesized-to-be-effective assistance, [based on] the social worker's informed decisions reached by a process of knowledge-based judgments" (Ben-Sira, 1987b, p. 81).

Since interventions in the psychosocial domain must take the patient's medical condition into account, collaboration with medical professionals is inevitable. Yet to legitimize their influence on health-care decisions, and to reach autonomously professional decisions in the psychosocial domain, the collaboration must be on an equal-status basis, with an explicit recognition of the social worker's professional authority in the psychosocial domain (Connery, 1953; H. E. Estes, 1981, pp. 3-6; Falck, 1984, pp. 9-10). Evidence suggests, however, that collaboration on an equal-status basis "is more the exception than the rule" (Pollin & McKinney-Cashion, 1984, p. 284).

Social Worker–Nurse Collaboration

The legitimization of equal-status collaboration is particularly critical in the social worker–nurse relationship, since nurses, due to their combined medical and psychosocial knowledge base, are likely to view themselves as the most proficient and competent to render the needed assistance.

Patients, who invariably conceive of a somatic disturbance as a medical problem, are likely to view nurses more than social workers as the competent agents for providing the needed assistance (Ben-Sira, 1987b). Cousins (1983), on the basis of his experience as a patient, maintains that in the wake of the growing depersonalization imposed by medical technology, the nurses' "knowledge ... dissolved much of the forbidding and arcane nature of the technology.... The information a nurse is frequently able to give a patient pertaining to complicated procedures and the mysterious indicators in the diagnostic technology [is essential]" (p. 181).

Failure to recognize social workers' professional expertise for interventions in the psychosocial domain of health care and to create the conditions for collaboration on an equal-status basis is likely to deprive both health professionals and patients of valuable inputs for promoting the efficacy of treatment.

CONCLUSION

Professional Progress and Health: Cui Bono?

Despite the increasing recognition of the contributory role of stress in the onset and severity of, and recovery from, a disease (Cohen & Cordoba, 1982; Cooper, 1983, 1984; Lundberg, Thorell, & Lind, 1975; Norbeck and Peterson-Tilden, 1983), physicians are reluctant to incorporate coping with patients' emotional state as an inherent component of medical intervention. Physicians may regard emotional support as both peripheral to the core of medicine and a time-consuming luxury at the expense of devoting their time and expertise to treating the "real" medical problems (Ben-Sira, 1985, 1986b, 1988a,b, 1990b; Johnston, 1994). Evidently, the reluctance to incorporate affective behavior in the medical intervention stems not only from its "peripheral" nature but also from its possible authority-depriving potential (Ben-Sira, 1986b, 1988a).

Nurses' drive toward professionalization (Philips, 1994; Smith, 1994) has brought about intrusion into areas that physicians regard as exclusively their territory, such as "comprehensive health assessment ... based upon history, physical examination, and appropriate diagnostic and screening procedures ... manag[ing] the health problems of individuals through clinical interventions ... possess[ing] the necessary expertise to unite cure and care functions within the domain of primary care" (Yedidia, 1986, p. 89). One may question whether nurses' drive toward specialization and professionalization comes at the expense of providing high-quality nursing assistance to physicians by carrying out their directives, shifting this kind of activity to less qualified practical nurses and physician aides.

The aspiration to enlarge professional knowledge bases often leads to encroachment into other professional territories and interprofessional confrontations. These confrontations, though overtly legitimized by the goal of improving care and cure, latently focus on questions of status and authority.

Professional Progress and Satisfaction of Health Needs

The crucial question, however, is the extent to which professional progress and the effort of enlarging professional territories come at the expense of satisfying afflicted persons' needs. Though the underlying overt rationale for progress and enlargement of professional territories is doubtless the improvement of care and cure, such change carries the latent danger that coping with patients' psychosocial needs will be neglected as an inherent component of medical intervention.

Israeli data (Ben-Sira, 1988b) suggest that perceptions of the professional community's norms and expectations are decisive in determining the focus of professional behavior, dwarfing the importance of meeting those patient needs that are perceived as peripheral to the biomedical mainstream.

On the other hand, however, the accumulating evidence regarding the importance of physicians' affective behavior can hardly be disregarded. To what extent can nurses compensate for physicians' neglect of that behavior? Considering the crucial role that affective behavior plays in providing "lay-intelligible" clues and patients' expectations that such behavior will be manifested by the physicians who bear the ultimate responsibility for treatment, compensation may be hardly feasible. Doubtless, nurses can serve as emotional support agents, yet emotional support is only one aspect of affective behavior.

Moreover, scrutiny of the literature on nursing as a profession may reveal that much of their aspiration focuses on their professional expansion in the biomedical field.

Under these circumstances, it stands to reason that from the patients' perspective, a significant part of their health needs are likely to remain unresolved. It may be recalled that when patients seek medical help, they indeed seek to satisfy two goals—the overt goal of solution of their health problem and the latent goal of alleviating their anxiety (Ben-Sira, 1976). Failure to satisfy the latter goal is likely to have health-hazardous consequences, as is particularly evident in light of the growing understanding of the stress-health relationship.

FUTURE RESEARCH ISSUES

The preceding analysis highlights the need for probing the issues underlying the rather pessimistic outlook that characterizes the current situation. First, it seems necessary to investigate the specific factors that underlie physicians' disinclination to demonstrate affective behavior. Research in this field will have to elucidate the role of factors such as status, rewards, specialization, and power drive in determining physicians' orientation.

Another issue that seems necessary to resolve is the role of social worker-physician collaboration in shaping physicians' orientation.

These are current research objectives to be pursued by doctoral students tutored by the author.

REFERENCES

Allen, J. (1994). From both sides of the stethoscope: The physician. *Los Angeles Times*, May 10, E3.

Antonovsky, A. (1979). *Health, stress and coping*. San Francisco: Jossey-Bass.

Ben-David, J. (1958). The professional role of the physician in bureaucratized medicine. *Human Relations*, *11*, 261-266.

Benner, P., & Wrubel, J. (1989). *The primacy of caring: Stress and coping in health and illness*. Menlo Park, CA: Addison-Wesley.

Ben-Sira, Z. (1976). The function of the professional's affective behavior in client satisfaction: A revised approach to interaction theory. *Journal of Health and Social Behavior, 12*, 3-11.

Ben-Sira, Z. (1980). Affective and instrumental components in the physician-patient relationship: An additional dimension in interaction theory. *Journal of Health and Social Behavior, 21*, 170-180.

Ben-Sira, Z. (1982a). Life change and health: An additional perspective on the structure of coping. *Stress, 3*, 18-28.

Ben-Sira, Z. (1982b). Stress potential and esotericity of health problems: The significance of the physician's affective behavior. *Medical Care, 20*, 414-424.

Ben-Sira, Z. (1982c). Lay evaluation of medical treatment and competence: Development of a model of the function of the physician's affective behavior. *Social Science and Medicine, 17*, 1013-1018.

Ben-Sira, Z. (1985). Primary medical care and coping with stress and disease: The inclination of primary care practitioners to demonstrate affective behavior. *Social Science and Medicine, 21*, 485-498.

Ben-Sira, Z. (1986a). The stress-resolving component in primary medical care. *Stress Medicine, 2*, 339-348.

Ben-Sira, Z. (1986b). The plight of primary medical care: The problematics of committedness to practice. *Social Science and Medicine, 22*, 699-712.

Ben-Sira, Z. (1987a). The stress bounding capacity of the physician's affective behavior: An additional dimension of health promotion. In J. H. Humphrey (Ed.), *Human stress: Current selected research*. Vol. II (pp. 15-36). New York: AMS Press.

Ben-Sira, Z. (1987b). Social work in health care: Needs, challenges and implications for structuring practice. *Social Work in Health Care, 13*, 79-100.

Ben-Sira, Z. (1988a). *Politics and primary medical care: Dehumanization and overutilization*. Aldershot, England: Gower.

Ben-Sira, Z. (1988b). Affective behavior and perceptions of health professionals. In D. S. Gochman (Ed.), *Health behavior: Emerging research perspectives* (pp. 305-317). New York: Plenum Press.

Ben-Sira, Z. (1990a). Universal entitlement for health care and its implications on the doctor-patient relationship. In G. L. Albrecht (Ed.), *Advances in medical sociology* (pp. 99-128). Greenwich, CT: JAI Press.

Ben-Sira, Z. (1990b). Primary care physicians and the patients' stress: Professional centered vs. patient centered orientation. In J. H. Humphrey (Ed.), *Human stress: Current selected research*, Vol. IV (pp. 1-10). New York: AMS Press.

Ben-Sira, Z. (1991). *Regression, stress, and readjustment in aging*. New York: Praeger.

Ben-Sira, Z. (1993). *Physicians' predisposition to stereotype patients: A stress-buffering mechanism* Paper presented at the Interim Conference of the Sociology of Mental Health Working Group of the ISA. Rome, Italy, June.

Ben-Sira, Z. (1994). *Immigration, integration and readjustment*. Jerusalem: Louis Guttman Israel Institute of Applied Social Research.

Ben-Sira, Z., & Duchin, R. (1981). *Ambulatory medical service in Israel: Utilization patterns and image*. Jerusalem: Louis Guttman Israel Institute of Applied Social Research.

Burnham, J. C. (1982). American medicine's golden age: What happened to it? *Science, 215*, 1474-1479.

Carlton, T. O. (1984). *Clinical social work in health settings*. New York: Springer.

Cohen, J., & Cordoba, C. (Eds.). (1982). *Psychological factors in cancer*. New York: Raven Press.

Connery, M. (1953). The client of effective teamwork. *Journal of Psychiatric Social Work, 22*, 59-60.

Cooper, C. L. (1983). *Stress research: Issues for the eighties*. New York: Wiley.

Cooper, C. L. (Ed.). (1984). *Psychosocial stress and cancer*. New York: Wiley.

Cousins, N. (1983). *The healing heart*. New York: Norton.

Engel, G. L. (1977). The need for a new medical model: A challenge for bio-medicine. *Science, 196*, 129-136.

Estes, H. E. (1981). The team context. In M. R. Haug (Ed.), *Elderly patients and their doctors* (pp. 132-136). New York: Springer.

Estes, R. J. (1984). Social workers in health care. In R. J. Estes (Ed.), *Health care and the social services* (pp. 3-22). St. Louis, MO: Green.

Falck, H. S. (1984). Social work in health settings. In A. Lurie & G. Rosenberg (Eds.), *Social work administration in health care* (pp. 7-15). New York: Haworth.

Freidson, E. (1986). The medical profession in transition. In L. H. Aiken & D. Mechanic (Eds.), *Applications of social science to clinical medicine and health policy* (pp. 63-79). New Brunswick, NJ: Rutgers University Press.

Gerbert, B. (1984). Perceived liability and competence of simulated patients: Influence on physicians' management plans. *Social Science and Medicine, 12*, 341-346.

Haug, M. R. (1976). Erosion of professional authority: A cross-cultural inquiry in the case of the physician. *Milbank Memorial Fund Quarterly: Health and Society, 54*, 83-105.

Haug, M. R. (1994). Elderly patients, caregivers, and physicians: Theory and research on health care triads. *Journal of Health and Social Behavior, 35*, 1-12.

Haug, M. R., & Lavin, B. (1981). Practitioner or patient—Who is in charge? *Journal of Health and Social Behavior, 22*, 212-229.

Haug, M. R., & Sussman, M. B. (1969). Professional authority and the revolt of the client. *Social Problems, 17*, 153-161.

Henao, S. (1985). A system's approach to family medicine. In S. Henao (Ed.), *Principles of family medicine* (pp. 24-40). New York: Brunner/Mazel.

Illich, I. (1986). The epidemics of modern medicine. In N. Black, D. Bosswell, A. Gray, S. Murphy, & J. Popay (Eds.), *Health and disease* (pp. 24-40). Philadelphia: Open University Press.

Johnston, B. D. (1994). The bureaucrat will see you now. *Los Angeles Times*, February 7, B7.

Lamb, G. S., & Stempel, J. E. (1994). Nurse case management from the clients' view: Growing as insider expert. *Nursing Outlook*, *42*, 7-13.

Lambertson, E. C. (1971). Not quite M.D., more than P.A. *Hospitals*, *45*, 70-71.

Lundberg, U., Thorell, T., & Lind, E. (1975). Life changes and myocardial infarction: Individual differences in life change scaling. *Journal of Psychosomatic Research*, *19*, 27-32.

Lysaught, J. P. (1986). Retrospect and prospect in joint practice. In J. Steel (Ed.), *Issues in collaborative practice* (pp. 15-33). Orlando, FL: Grune & Stratton.

Margalith, I. (1993). *Disclosure of information, participation in clinical decision-making, and patient well-being: The case of patients with ureteral calculi*. Unpublished doctoral dissertation [in Hebrew, English abstract]. Jerusalem: Hebrew University.

Monat, A., & Lazarus, R. S. (1991). Introduction: Stress and coping—current issues and controversies. In A. Monat & R. S. Lazarus (Eds.), *Stress and coping* (3rd ed.) (pp. 1-15). New York: Columbia University Press.

Neugeboren, B. (1985). *Organization, policy, and practice in the human services*. New York: Longman.

Norbeck, J. S., & Peterson-Tilden, V. (1983). Life stress, social support and emotional disequilibrium in complications of pregnancy: A prospective multivariate study. *Journal of Health and Social Behavior*, *24*, 30-46.

Papper, S. (1970). The undesirable patient. *Journal of Chronic Disease*, *22*, 777.

Pattison, E. M., & Anderson, R. C. (1978). Family health care. *Public Health Reviews*, 7, 83-134.

Pearlin, L. I. (1991). The study of coping: An overview of problems and directions. In J. Eckenrode (Ed.), *The social context of coping* (pp. 261-276). New York: Plenum Press.

Philips, J. R. (1994). A vision of nursing research priorities. *Nursing Science Quarterly*, 7, 52.

Pollin, I. S., & McKinney-Cashion, M. (1984). Community based social work with the chronically ill. In R. J. Estes (Ed.), *Health care and the social services*. St. Louis, MO: Green.

Roth, J. A. (1986). Some contingencies of the moral evaluation and control of clientele: The case of the hospital emergency service. In P. Conrad & R. Kern (Eds.), *The sociology of health and illness: Critical perspectives* (2nd ed.) (pp. 327-333). New York: St. Martin's Press.

Schlesinger, E. G. (1985). *Health care and social work practice*. St. Louis, MO: Times Mirror/Mosby.

Second Meeting on Conceptual Frameworks. (1981). Working statements on the purpose of social work. *Social Work*, *26*, 6.

Sheppard, M. (1991). *Mental health work in the community: Theory and practice in social work and community psychiatric nursing*. London: Falmer.

Smith, M. C. (1994). Beyond the threshold: Nursing practice in the next millennium. *Nursing Science Quarterly*, 7, 6-7.

Smoyak, S. A. (1986). Problems in interprofessional relations. In J. Steel (Ed.), *Issues in collaborative practice* (pp. 77-85). Orlando, FL: Grune & Stratton.

Starr, P. (1978). Medicine and the waning of professional sovereignty. *Daedalus*, *197*, 175-193.

Steel, J. E. (1986). An overview. In J. Steel (Ed.), *Issues in collaborative practice* (pp. 3-14). Orlando, FL: Grune & Stratton.

Yedidia, M. (1986). Nurse practitioner-physician collaboration in primary care: Survival of an innovation. In J. Steel (Ed.), *Issues in collaborative practice* (pp. 87-104). Orlando, FL: Grune & Stratton.

Zola, I. K. (1966). Culture and symptoms: An analysis of patients' presenting complaints. *American Sociological Review*, *31*, 615-630.

3

Physician Power and Patients' Health Behavior

Marie R. Haug

INTRODUCTION

As the end of the 20th century approaches, few would argue that the relationship between physicians and patients in Western industrialized countries is the same as it was a generation ago. The media remind the public that physicians can make dreadful mistakes and can be sued successfully for seven-figure damages; that some physicians are impaired by alcohol, drug abuse, or old age; and that they can charge exorbitant or unwarranted fees—in short, that physicians are all too human. The patient who believed and trusted the doctor's every word and considered it a duty to comply with "doctor's orders" is gradually becoming obsolete, as people achieve more years of education and grow more medically sophisticated.

To these threats to physician authority must be added the dangers to physician autonomy that arise from their work locations in bureaucratic structures. As noted in an earlier review (Haug & Lavin, 1983, p. 10):

> ... while authority concerns power over others, autonomy is the power not to be compelled by others. Physicians have enjoyed both types: the right to give patients "doctor's orders" that will be accepted, and the right not to have anyone else, whether bureaucratic boss or fellow physician, interfere with their work.

Various types of managed care systems in countries throughout the industrial world constrain physicians from performing, ordering, and billing for procedures that are too expensive and may not be necessary. Identifying and understanding these relatively recent developments calls for a review of the roots of physician power and the sources of the challenges to that power.

THEORIES OF PROFESSIONAL POWER

Power is the ability to compel behavior in another, regardless of the other's own desires. It may take the form of raw force, which is rarely if ever a factor in professional-client or professional-colleague relationships. In these contexts, the compelling force is authority, the right to rule that is accepted by others as valid and legitimate.

Marie R. Haug • University Center on Aging and Health, Case Western Reserve University, Cleveland, Ohio 44106-7131.

Handbook of Health Behavior Research II: Provider Determinants, edited by David S. Gochman. Plenum Press, New York, 1997.

Weber (1961) proposed three sources of such legitimated power: traditional, charismatic, and legal-rational. Each is relevant to the power of the physician with respect to patients and coprofessionals.

Traditional authority flows from past history and custom. In Britain, the practice of medicine was long identified with the aristocratic elite; only gentlemen with university degrees from Oxford or Cambridge were admitted to the Royal College of Physicians when it was founded in 1518 (Elliot, 1972; Haug, 1975). In the United States, the Flexner report in 1910 shut off poor boys' pathway to medicine. It was the sons of wealthy prestigious families who had the wherewithal for medical training, particularly abroad, who came to dominate medicine (Kunitz, 1974). A history of upper-class position clothed physicians in the authority of status.

Charismatic authority was based on the extraordinary mystical quality of the priest and medicine man in earlier times. The image of the kindly, dedicated family physician who carried the same mystique is rapidly fading among the public (Belkin, 1993; Shorter, 1985). Similarly, in bureaucratic settings, the charisma of the leading surgeon or world-famous physician may be losing some of its force among colleagues and coworkers.

More generally applicable to all physicians is legal-rational authority. Licensure laws and regulations of various kinds prohibit the practice of medicine by anyone not properly credentialed. The power of the state backs the authority of physicians over patients by giving them the sole legal right to act as doctors. However, the state not only grants but also limits professional power. The temptation to provide excessive service to enhance income (Ohsfeldt, 1993) may be tempered in the United States by such state-provided constraints as Medicare rules with respect to the elderly and disabled. In other countries, the autonomy of the physician in making medical decisions may be contained by limits imposed by national medical care insurance systems (Hafferty & McKinlay, 1993).

One source of power and authority that Weber did not capture is monopolized knowledge. Larson (1977) considered professional knowledge to be a form of property, a resource used to maintain power and eliminate competition by limiting access to training and thus to credentials. Parsons (1951) identified unshared knowledge as justifying the right of physicians to exercise control over their patients. His concept of the "sick role" long dominated sociological thinking on physician-patient relationships. In this model of physician-patient interaction, sick persons are excused from normal duties, provided they try to get well by seeking care from a physician and complying with the regimen prescribed. Because of the "competence gap" between patients and doctors (Parsons, 1975), the knowledgeable practitioners must have full authority over the ignorant patients in order that the latter can be cured and resume their presickness roles and obligations.

The sick-role concept has been criticized from two distinct but related directions, which may be characterized as the conflict model and the negotiating model. Those who espouse a conflict model of society criticize the sick role as assuming equivalence of purpose and values between physicians and patients. The potential for conflict inheres in any medical interaction (Freidson, 1970). Patients' perspectives and expectations often differ from those of the practitioner, on cultural or class grounds, and these differences moderate patients' acceptance of treatment recommendations and compliance with regimen (Mechanic, 1982). In the conflict situation, physicians may use the tactic of information control to maintain their power, while patients attempt to limit that power by information seeking.

A consumerism perspective on the part of the patient also challenges the sick role model: "It focuses on purchasers' (patient's) rights and seller's (physician's) obligations, rather than on physician's rights (to direct) and patient obligations (to follow directions) ..." (Haug & Lavin, 1981, p. 213). Just as consumers negotiate the terms of purchase of any commodity, patients can negotiate the terms under which they will buy the physician's advice, including both diagnosis and treatment plans. The negotiating model of physician-patient interactions defines how the conflict between the parties can be amicably resolved, by entering into a partnership for solving the patient's problems (Bursztajn, Feinbloom, Hamm, & Brodsky, 1990). For this approach to work, however, the patient needs to secure health information, make rational choices, and be ready to play an active role in determining the terms of care (Pratt, 1978).

Esoteric knowledge is also an advantage for physicians in bureaucratic settings. Freidson (1986) reiterated the position taken in his earlier seminal works on the dominance of the physician in the medical arena (Freidson, 1970). His chief interest then was on the power of the physician over other occupations in the medical division of labor, involving both the authority to give orders to nurses, paraprofessionals, and others and the autonomy to be free from taking orders from administrators or even from some peers. Later, Freidson (1986) focused on the position of the physician in relation to administrative and supervisory personnel who often now control access to the tools and services needed to carry out medical work, clearly a threat to autonomy. On both flanks, physician power is being eroded. Witness the increasingly successful battle of nurse-midwives to practice without physician oversight and the growing "corporatization" of medical care under the rule of conglomerates that hedge physician clinical freedom (Salmon, 1984) even to the point that some predict physicians will become "proletarianized" (McKinlay & Arches, 1985).

At the same time, the negotiating or partnership model implicitly empowers patients to act as equals in any interaction with a health provider. By challenging physician authority, patients are asserting their right to be autonomous actors in a medical encounter. Indeed, as physicians' autonomy is being assailed by coworkers and administrators, their authority is being undermined by autonomy demands of their patients. Some limited material on the attitudes and reported experiences of the public is useful in showing that characteristics of patients have an effect on the balance of power between the giver and the receiver of care (Bursztajn et al., 1990). Still fewer data are available on physician characteristics that might tip that balance (Roter & Hall, 1992). Many studies seem to assume that physicians are homogeneous in all respects, when in fact their differences in age, gender, specialty, or beliefs can have a marked effect on the nature of the physician-patient relationship.

FACTORS IN PATIENT POWER

Age

The age cohort of the patient is a critical variable in determining events in a medical encounter. The old-old cohort, those currently 85 and over, were born before technological and scientific developments produced dramatic changes in medical care. Buffeted by two major depressions, many could afford to use a physician's services only in desperate emergencies, when such help was seen as lifesaving. Also, older persons are more likely to have little education and to have been trained to accept the authority of persons higher on society's status ladder (Haug & Lavin, 1983). Compare these attributes to those of persons now in their 20s and early 30s, who have heard about both medical miracles and medical mistakes, who are likely to have had at least a high school or perhaps some college education, and who appear to have little respect for authority (Haug, 1993).

Thus, a patient's age could well influence whether the patient acts out the sick role or attempts to take a more egalitarian negotiating approach to the doctor. Although earlier studies did not directly determine whether respondents had actually attempted to negotiate an acceptable diagnosis or treatment with their attending physician, respondents did show, by claiming they were willing to challenge, or had actually challenged, medical authority, that they did not accept the sick-role model, with its requirement of unquestioning acceptance of the physician's advice (Haug, 1979). Older patients may also be at a disadvantage in the power game because of the stereotypical attitudes of their practitioners. One study has shown that old people are less able than younger ones to get the doctor to listen to their problems and attend to their concerns. Overriding the wishes of the patient in this way is evaluated as a subtle form of ageism and "reflects a liability in power dynamics" (Greene, Adelman, Charon, & Hoffman, 1986, p. 121).

Gender and Race

Gender and race characteristics could also be expected to affect the nature of the encounter. Because blacks, given the paucity of practitioners of their own race, are usually constrained to deal with white physicians, they may be more reserved and less forthcoming in interacting with them (Santos, Hubbard, & McIntosh, 1983). Women make more physician visits than men (Verbrugge, 1985), and familiarity might foster a less submissive role despite the conventional wisdom that women are generally unaggressive. Indeed, female gender has been related to challenging attitudes and behaviors in one research endeavor (Haug & Lavin, 1979).

Education and Knowledge

Bridging the competence gap would empower the patient. Accordingly, patients with higher education and better health knowledge should have the confidence to question what the physician suggests. And indeed this expectation has been borne out, with respect to both attitudes and reported behavior. Those with more education and knowledge of health matters are consistently more challenging of physician authority (Haug & Lavin, 1983; Shorter, 1985). One aspect of this knowledge concerns patients' access to their own medical records. In applauding the passage of a New York State law mandating that patients be given such records, the sponsor of the legislation explicitly noted the relationship between knowledge and power. He commented that the law "says patients have a much larger role in making decisions about their treatment, that patients are equal to doctors and no longer subservient to their decisions" (Sullivan, 1986). The role of the media in educating the public on health matters should not be underestimated. With the growing interest in health, TV specials on new discoveries, both technological and biomedical, are not uncommon and are available to members of all classes. "Doctor books" and how-to manuals have proliferated in recent years, but are perhaps more appealing to the middle class than to other groups.

Health Status

Szasz and Hollender (1956) were among the first to point out that the nature of the patient–physician relationship could vary depending on the health condition of the patient, with an adult–adult, egalitarian interaction most common when the patient was not in dire physical straits. In this respect, a curious reversal in effect between attitudes and behaviors was found in two studies. Persons who considered their health to be excellent, or did not have a disabling chronic condition, were more likely to declare their willingness to challenge a physician's authority, but those who assessed their health as poor or had a chronic condition that interfered with normal activity were more likely to have translated attitude into action, claiming to have openly disagreed with their physician in the past (Haug & Lavin, 1983). It was as though patients who were not well believed that they had not been satisfactorily treated, perhaps because they had not been "cured," and had at some point confronted the physician with this presumed failure. This speculation is reinforced by the fact that in one study, in which a question was asked about prior experiences with medicine, those who claimed that they had been the victims of medical error were more likely to report challenging behavior (Haug & Lavin, 1979). Similarly, those who admitted that they often did not comply with their medical regimens were also the most likely to be challengers (Haug & Lavin, 1983). Clearly, those dissatisfied with the treatment plans or outcomes of care were inclined to refuse to accept the physician's authority.

FACTORS IN PHYSICIAN POWER

Age

Physician characteristics can either enhance or erode their power in relationships with patients. Unfortunately, the tendency to treat all physicians as undifferentiated actors has resulted in very little empirical data, forcing much of the following discussion to be speculative. For example, the effect of age on physician power vis-à-vis patients is not known. Older doctors may carry an aura of the wisdom of years, which enhances their authority, or they may be considered out-of-date, which diminishes it. Newly minted doctors can be evaluated either as greenhorns or as being up on the latest medical breakthroughs, with opposite effects on their authority. There is some limited evidence on the effects of age on physician attitudes concerning older patients. Younger doctors are likely to be more ageist in their attitudes than are their older colleagues (although the elderly can be ageist too). Doctors under 65 are likely to be less egalitarian, less patient, less attentive, and less respectful with older patients, and less willing to raise psychosocial issues with them (Adelman, Greene, Charon, & Friedmann, 1990). Younger doctors may not take the time to provide information to the elderly or to be as supportive to older patients when they bring up issues (Adelman, Greene, & Charon, 1991). Older patients are given less time for a consultation (Clark, Potter, & McKinlay, 1991). Stereotyping the aged also affects doctors' communication styles. They use simplified language and take on a patronizing air, blaming older patients, but not younger, for forgetfulness (Ryan & Cole, 1990).

Gender

A few clues exist on the effects of provider gender. An analysis of actual interactions of patients with male and female physicians revealed that male physicians tend to interrupt their patients while they are talking more than patients interrupt them. With women, the opposite is true. Patients interrupt female physicians more than the latter interrupt them (West, 1984). Assuming that the act of interruption is an expression of dominance, these findings suggest the lesser power and authority of women. Such a conclusion also resonates with the stereotype of women as less aggressive and assertive than men, two behaviors that can express power. Women physicians tended to take a more power-sharing, egalitarian approach than their male colleagues (Weisman & Teitelbaum, 1985). Also, female physicians talk more than men, and give more attention to the history segment of a consultation, which is critical in uncovering the patient's point of view about the meanings of his or her symptoms. This attentiveness in turn is likely to produce medical recommendations that are more attuned to the patient's cultural beliefs and consequently are more effective. Also, women physicians have generally been found to be more egalitarian in treating their patients, spending more time in medical visits, and providing more information and positive support (Roter, Lipkin, & Korsgaard, 1991).

Race

The effect of the practitioner's race on power relations with patients is rarely studied. Given that black physicians are in the minority in the United States, cross-race interactions are more likely to involve white physicians and black patients. Such a mix would superimpose racial dominance on professional authority and exacerbate the power imbalance.

Practice Style

Another factor in the equation is what might be called the physician's practice style. Those who are willing and able to take the time to explore fully with the patient the various options for care and treatment, along with their rationale and possible effectiveness, at the same time respecting the patient's values and concerns, are acting in ways that diminish their power. As Waitzkin and Stoeckle (1976) have claimed, mystification and withholding of information are the major techniques used to maintain the professional's authority. Demystification tends to equalize the participants' power.

Medicine is not an exact science. There is a great deal of uncertainty as to both correct diagnosis and effective treatment (Fox, 1957). Physicians whose style is to share this uncertainty openly with their patients may generate trust, but simultaneously are revealing that their claim to authority is not absolute. Indeed, it has been suggested that failure to be open is a sign of lack of confidence: "Many doctors are authoritarian because ... they are afraid to be found out as wrong ... not as good as they should be" (Haug, 1976b, p. 30). Uncertainty becomes most obvious in treating chronic conditions, like renal failure, or incurable diseases, like AIDS. Physicians do not have a cure and therefore cannot easily claim authority.

The attitude of the provider toward time is another element of practice style. Fee-for-service doctors must fit many patients into a limited number of hours, in part for economic reasons. Those who handle an assembly line of patients in different cubicles give short shrift to patients who ask a lot of questions and who want to be part of decision making concerning their care because such patients interfere with the flow. Patients have little time to exercise power in these circumstances. Indeed, in one study, practitioners who saw 50 or more patients a day were less likely to accommodate to patient challenge than those who saw fewer than 30 (Haug & Lavin, 1983).

Practice style is also linked to specialty. Surgery probably offers the most clear-cut case of an authority-based practice style (Cassell, 1987). The process of securing informed consent may be marked by persuasion rather than real information giving, and is often pro forma (Miller, 1986). The major interaction between physician and patient occurs when the latter is unconscious. In the course of a surgical procedure, the physician makes decisions to excise or not to excise without consultation with the patient. In that context, the physician's power appears to be absolute, but that is not necessarily so. The practitioner is still constrained by payment regulation in the patient's insurance program, of which the surgeon is usually well aware (Clark, Potter, & McKinlay, 1991).

Social Status

One final factor should not be overlooked. Physicians' social status is almost universally higher than that of all patients except the most prestigious and economically well-off. Although technically patients "employ" doctors and should have higher status as "employers" (Wiemann, Gravell, & Wiemann, 1990), this is rarely the case. In fact, only upper-class patients are given more time and fuller explanations than the average (Pendleton & Bochner, 1980). Thus, class differences reinforce physician power over patients.

PHYSICIAN AUTONOMY

Factors in the organizational setting of care have an effect on physician autonomy, the physician's power not to be compelled by others. In a competitive fee-for-service system, it is conceivable that a practitioner would bow to patients' wishes in order to keep their business. If the predictions of a coming doctor glut prove true, such behavior could become common. On the other hand, "demanding," not at all submissive, patients have been identified in prepaid group plans, such as health maintenance organizations (HMOs), because they feel free to invoke organizational rules to get their way (Freidson, 1973). Yet one research project found that HMO-based physicians were more likely to accept patient challenge, although this could be because they tended to be younger (Haug & Lavin, 1983). Furthermore, the power relationship may shift depending on the locale of care. Patients seen in a hospital are less able to challenge their physician's demands than are patients in a physician's office (Goss, 1981). Physicians may also be at a relative disadvantage in dealing with those patients seen in their own homes, their own familiar turf (Zola, 1986).

The societal context of care is beginning to receive scrutiny as the effects of global issues in a number of areas suggest the need to examine physician autonomy and authority cross-culturally. The role of the state in financing and consequently regulating various aspects of medical practice (Frank & Duran-Arenas, 1993) is having a profound effect on physician autonomy throughout the world. In the United States, attempts to control rising health care costs, as examplified by increasing charges to governmental funds for services to the aged (Medicare) or the poor (Medicaid), have produced a web of regulations and payment limitations. For example, diagnostic related groups (DRGs) set limits on hospital charges according to illness, but health care managers and doctors shift care outside of hospitals to preserve their incomes (Light, 1993). Insurance companies set limits on what care doctors can provide and expect to be paid. Similarly, large medical care groups like HMOs determine what procedures are covered and what non-HMO specialists can be used. The autonomy of physicians has been constrained by direct limitations, not on what they can do, but on what they can be paid for doing, by institutional sources. Light (1993, p. 78) calls this the "countervailing power of institutional buyers," which has set limits but not completely negated physician autonomy. Organized physician and political organizations enter the fray to curtail the attempted dominance of the institutional buyers, in a seesaw battle that will likely continue for some time to come.

The same type of situation can be observed in other countries. In Great Britain, the National Health Service has increasingly come under state scrutiny, often in terms of local authorities' power to establish rules limiting payments (Larkin, 1993). In that country, as in others, physicians have organized to preserve their clinical autonomy from the regulations imposed by government funding rules and insurance companies' payment regulations. A struggle for control between doctors and the state can also be documented in Australia (Willis, 1993) and New Zealand (Fougere, 1993), as well as other locales with publicly financed sickness services and physician organizations that seek to preserve their power and income (Hafferty & McKinlay, 1993).

PATIENT CONSUMERISM

Outlines of the new role of the patient as active consumer instead of passive recipient of care began to sharpen in the late 1960s in the United States. It was a time of revolt against traditional authority, among students, antiwar activists, and feminists (Haug & Sussman, 1969). Reeder (1972) was among the first specifically to identify patients as consumers in a changing physician-patient relationship. The general ferment of the times was fed with respect to the medical arena by the dawning realization that physicians could make dreadful mistakes. One of the most dramatic of these errors was the use of the sedative thalidomide for pregnant women, with the result that their babies were born with flipperlike appendages instead of arms or legs. These and other mistakes in treatment sparked a surge of widely publicized malpractice suits, some of which produced large damage awards (Charles, 1993; Ritchey, 1993). With widespread doubts about practitioners' advice, it is small wonder that estimated rates of noncompliance run high: Perhaps 60% of patients do not follow their doctor's advice, and 50% do not take prescribed medications as they have been instructed (Becker, 1985). Generally, noncompliance is likely to result from physician withholding of information or restricted responsiveness (Hauser, 1981), as well as high costs or unexpected side effects of a prescribed regimen.

Still another factor has diminished patients'

acceptance of physician authority. Outright fraud in doctors' billing is increasingly being uncovered, a symptom of the basic contradiction between concern for patients' quality of life and practitioners' economic interests (Jesilow, Pontell, & Geis, 1993). The public is also aware of physicians' conflicts of interest when recommending tests and treatments in facilities they wholly or partly own (Rodwin, 1993), thus fattening their bank accounts at the possible expense of patients' well-being or comfort. In fact, evidence of the public's diminishing confidence in physicians can be found in the widespread recommendation that patients should seek independent second opinions rather than rely exclusively on one practitioner's advice.

How do physicians respond to these developments? Many recognize that patient attitudes toward them are changing. In one study, 58% of practicing physicians surveyed believed that patients were more challenging than in the past (Haug & Lavin, 1983). In an earlier study, a similar perception was expressed as well by practitioners in Great Britain and the U.S.S.R. (Haug, 1976a). Leaders in academic medicine have drawn the same conclusion: that the traditional conceptions of professional authority are being challenged by a more educated and more egalitarian society (Pellegrino, 1977). Stoeckle at Harvard Medical School is among those who argue that these changes in patients' expectations require a more negotiating approach to arriving at a diagnosis and treatment plan (e.g., Becker, 1985; Cockerham, 1992; Lazare, Eisenthal, Frank, & Stoeckle, 1978). In fact, it has been found that a physician's assuming an authoritarian stance may diminish the likelihood of patient compliance (Svarstad, 1986). Telling patients about the probable risks and benefits of treatments or procedures, and letting them decide what course to follow, is another option recommended by some physicians (Bursztajn et al., 1990).

A study of medical students and their teachers showed that some academic physicians share these views about patient autonomy and are apparently passing on some of their opinions to their students (Lavin, Haug, Belgrave, & Breslau, 1987). Between the time they first entered medical school and six years later, when they had completed their first year of residence, over 40% of 124 students studied had changed their views and accorded less authority to physicians and more autonomy to patients than earlier. The greatest change occurred among those who originally had given little weight to patient rights or had believed that physicians should have authority in dealing with patients. At least in the academic setting studied, the faculty was adapting to changes in the physician-patient relationship and apparently transmitting these perspectives to the student body. How these attitudes will be maintained in the "real world" of practice is uncertain, however, and a potential topic for further study.

FUTURE OF POWER RELATIONS

What, then, is the future of physician power and patient autonomy? Will the sick-role, authority-based model go into decline and the negotiating model dominate? Will the autonomy of physicians be maintained in increasingly bureaucratized health systems? Although it is always dangerous to extrapolate current trends into the future, some tentative predictions are in order. Consumerism on the part of patients is not likely to decline, but whether it will be more dominant is problematic. There are likely to continue to be people more comfortable with a dependent patient role (Bursztajn et al., 1990). Increasing levels of public education will not catch up with constantly expanding medical knowledge. Yet many common acute illnesses are self-limiting, or easily treated with self-care. People are more and more learning to handle their chronic conditions, monitoring their health states on a day-to-day basis. There is now a plethora of books on self-treatment for various ailments, along with academic analysis of self-care movements (Defriese, Woomert, Guild, Steckler, & Konrad, 1989).

The popularity of all forms of health self-care, from attention to diet and exercise to self-treatment for symptoms without resort to professional attention, is likely to continue. There is no evidence that lay medicine produces more ill effects than the iatrogenic problems resulting from faulty procedures and misdiagnoses of medical professionals (Light, 1983). Self-care has existed for many centuries and in many parts of the world. Its impact on the future power balance in the physician-patient relationship will probably be minimal. Such effects as it may have are likely to be in the direction of the patient. Unhappy experiences in dealing with a physician may well encourage patients to practice self-care rather than submit to an unpleasant interaction (Haug, 1986).

Along with the changes brought by increasing patient self-care is the bureaucratization of medicine, as it comes to be more and more a corporate enterprise, with a profit-making ethos (Salmon, 1984; Starr, 1982). As physicians' authority is being challenged by demands for patient autonomy, their autonomy is being hedged by bureaucratic rules (Dougherty, 1990; Relman, 1991). This change manifests itself most dramatically in care for the elderly in hospitals, where reimbursable lengths of stay are determined by Medicare through DRGs. The extension of such regulations to ambulatory care is already on the horizon. In large group practices, in which profit-making is also a consideration, the control may take the form of allotting only so much time to any patient visit, regardless of the complaint.

The intrusion of economic constraints into clinical practice is not new, but the changes now taking place are more far-reaching and more invasive than in the past (Luft, 1986). But what about their implications for physician-patient relationships? One can only speculate that limiting the physician's autonomy will of necessity reduce the range of available options in dealing with patient concerns; even if the physician wishes to follow the negotiating model, there will be fewer areas in which choices can freely be made. The potential exists for an encounter in which conflicts are resolved by physician fiat or by patient rejection.

Both patient power and physician autonomy are affected by rising public recognition that medicine is not an exact science, but is faced with uncertainty at many levels. The work of Bursztajn et al. (1990) is aimed at dealing with these uncertainties in patient care, an issue first addressed decades ago by Davis (1960) in the case of polio patients and by Fox (1957) with respect to physician training. The effect of uncertainty on clinical decision making has been addressed by Gerrity, Earp, and Devellis (1990) and by Gerrity, Earp, Devellis, and Light (1992), in two of the rare studies of the concept of uncertainty in actual clinical practice. A major theme that underlies these studies is physicians' fear of failure, with its implications for their self-image as powerful, all-knowing practitioners.

The resolution of this uncertainty can be linked to a major societal development that holds the potential for a revolution in medical care: technology. It is hardly necessary to document the extent and force of these changes, which allow studies of the living brain in full color through positron emission tomography (PET) scans, permit heart transplants with cadaver or artificial hearts, provide kidney dialysis, and offer birth control with a pill. Computers have been programmed to take medical or psychiatric histories. Data have been stored, and updated as new discoveries are reported, to allow the split-second calculation of the most likely diagnosis and preferred treatment, given an input of a constellation of symptoms. What was at one time mere speculation, that persons who know how to access computers could be their own doctors (Haug, 1977), is apparently coming to pass. The so-called "information superhighway" will allow those with computer skills and access, whose numbers are increasing rapidly, to seek medical advice with respect to both diagnosis and treatment. As pointed out by Cowley (1994), the public, by using the Internet, is quietly reinventing the health care system in this country. Three major computer encyclopedia programs, available for purchase for use on the Internet, offer evaluation of symptoms, explain care procedures, suggest diagnosis, and outline possible treatment (Bates, 1994).

In other uses, physicians can provide patients, puzzled by care options, with interactive videos that can outline the benefits and risks of various treatments and procedures, so that they can make decisions away from the stress and time pressures of a doctor visit (Kolata, 1994). The other side of the technological revolution gives more mystique, and perhaps power, to doctors, with the invention of new techniques for cochlear implants, bone replacements, and brain surgery (Bowers & Volz, 1994). More innovations, such as extended gene therapy, are likely to provide new evidence of physician power, particularly for those unfamiliar with the bureaucratic constraints that physicians must accommodate.

The effect of such developments on physician-patient relationships was explicitly considered in two early analyses. Reiser (1978) rejected the notion that turning over technical tasks to a computer would free physicians to give more attention to patients' social and psychological concerns. He believes that the practitioner will become even more technologically oriented by attachment to "the machine at the bedside" and will be even less open to nonbiological issues. Bursztajn, Hamm, and Gutheil (1984, p. 180) are concerned that the two models of medical decision making—paternalism and patient autonomy—may degenerate into the misuse of technology: "The use of technological aids (and technological mystification) to bolster the physician's authority is a commonly noted phenomenon. But ... greater patient involvement in decisions may also be expressed as a clamor for technological placebos." The authors sound this cautionary note even though they favor involving the patient in the process of decision making, as providing a context of mutual support in openly sharing the inevitable uncertainty of medical diagnosis and treatment potential. If mutual trust can be established through joint decision making, technology will be less likely to be used "as an escape from uncertainty" (p. 190). Moreover, trust arising from good interpersonal skills can help physicians avoid the trauma of malpractice suits (Hickson et al., 1994).

What, then, is the forecast? Undoubtedly, physician autonomy will decline, and perhaps prestige as well (Freidson, 1985), whereas patient autonomy will show some staying power. What is unlikely is that the age of paternalism will return in full flower (Beisecker & Beisecker, 1993). Physician-patient relationships will not revert to the old form for everyone. The most likely outcome has been stated in an earlier paper relative to paternalism versus patient autonomy: The "two competing models [will] apply differentially depending on the characteristics of the actors, their orientation to power and dependence, and the circumstances under which they meet" (Haug & Lavin, 1981, p. 222).

A GLANCE AT METHODOLOGICAL ISSUES

Effective research methods for studying the issues raised in this chapter are not easy to come by. Surveys asking about past experiences and past or current attitudes, although widely used, are problematic, whether conducted by face-to-face or telephone interviews. Respondents, both patients and physicians, may forget, misstate, or slip into socially acceptable covers for the realities of their behavior in an actual medical encounter. Observing that actual behavior has drawbacks on its own. This method imposes the ethical obligation to secure the consent of both parties and, of course, requires the presence of an observer, often with tape recorder or TV camera, during the interaction. Such a presence inevitably changes the participants' behavior to some degree, particularly at the beginning of an interaction sequence. Coding the communication patterns that result forces them into categories that may be only marginally effective in identifying the meaning of what goes on.

What all these caveats suggest is the utility of multiple methods in studying physician-patient power relations. A given single technique may be necessary, but will not be sufficient, to grasp all the nuances underlying the meanings and future implications of the communication clues for attitudes and behaviors of the participants. Existing methods and mathematical techniques may be elegant when assessed singly, but their claims should be presented modestly, with honest recognition that they can only partially represent actuality, in either belief or action.

UNANSWERED QUESTIONS

A rich agenda of research questions has been suggested by the present state of knowledge on power in physician-patient relationships. There is a need to know whether the egalitarian, negotiating pattern of interactions actually occurs during therapeutic encounters or whether the relationship reverts to the pattern of the physician in charge. In cases where the egalitarian interactions break down, there is also a need to know what the barriers are and what facilitates mutual decision making between physician and patient, including the characteristics of both parties. Although there are some data on patient characteristics that foster autonomy in dealing with physicians, they concern attitudes and reported behaviors, rather than actual interaction. The data on physician characteristics are even more limited, and again have little relevance to the effect of physician characteristics in real-life medical encounters. Studies of communication and language patterns during physician visits do not differentiate by type of practitioner. Clearly, what is needed are studies that compare characteristics of actors and settings in the two types of interaction model, the sick-role model and the negotiating model.

The effects of cultural and societal contexts are also unknown. Do people with symptoms in Brazil, China, Morocco, Finland engage in the sick role, or do they succeed in relating to health care professionals in a give-and-take way? Nobody really knows. Moreover, one can only speculate on the effects of rapidly expanding computer technology. If computers can beat humans in chess games, and if preschoolers can become computer-literate, how can physicians monopolize medical knowledge (Haug, 1988)? The potentials for technology in health care and illness treatment can hardly be imagined.

Nor is there knowledge of the health outcomes of the two types of interaction. Whether a particular mode affects compliance is not the issue, since that word implies following a physician's prescriptions, and indeed compliance may not be relevant to health outcome. One of the most difficult measurement problems is finding an appropriate indicator for the outcome of care. Preventing mortality is a poor one for most illnesses, few of which are life-threatening. Termination of morbidity may be a better measure, but it often occurs regardless of treatment, although it could be delayed by inappropriate care. Patient and/or practitioner satisfaction with the interaction may be interesting to know, but whether it is a valid measure of health outcome is quite another question.

The overarching research question restates the forecast proposed by Haug and Lavin (1981) as a subject for inquiry: Do the competing models apply differentially, depending on the characteristics of the actors, their orientations to power and dependence, and the circumstances under which they meet? And one must add another: What difference does it make for patient health outcomes?

REFERENCES

Adelman, R. D., Greene, M. G., and Charon, R. (1991). Issues in physician-elderly patient interaction. *Ageing and Society*, *11*, 127-148.

Adelman, R. D., Greene, M. G., Charon, R., & Friedmann, E. (1990). Issues in the physician-geriatric patient relationship. In H. Giles, N. Coupland, J. M. Wiemann (Eds.), *Communication, health and the elderly* (pp. 126-134). London: Manchester University Press.

Bates, B. (1994). Diagnosing yourself via computers. *Cleveland Plain Dealer*, September 20, 8-E.

Becker, M. H. (1985). Patient adherence to prescribed therapies. *Medical Care, 23*, 539-555.

Beisecker, A. E., & Beisecker, T. D. (1993). Using metaphors to characterize doctor-patient relationships: Paternalism versus consumerism. *Health Communication, 5*, 41-58.

Belkin, L. (1993). Public-image progress is bad for doctors. *Cleveland Plain Dealer*, June 27, i and 6-G.

Bowers, R., & Volz, J. (1994). Medicine's future. *Cleveland Plain Dealer*, October 25, 7-E.

Bursztajn, H. J., Feinbloom, R. I., Hamm, R. M., & Brodsky, A. (1990). *Medical choices, medical chances*. London: Delacorte Press.

Bursztajn, H. J., Hamm, R. M., & Gutheil, T. J. (1984). The technological target: Involving the patients in clinical choices. In S. J. Reiser & M. Anbar (Eds.), *The machine at the bedside* (pp. 177-191). London: Cambridge University Press.

Cassell, J. (1987). On control, certitude, and the "paranoia of surgeons." *Culture, Medicine and Psychiatry, 11*(2), 229-249.

Charles, S. C. (1993). The doctor-patient relationship and medical malpractice litigation. *Bulletin of the Menninger Clinic, 57*(2), 195-207.

Clark, J. A., Potter, D. A., & McKinlay, J. B. (1991). Bringing social structure back into clinical decision making. *Social Science and Medicine, 32*(8), 835-866.

Cockerham, W. C. (1992). *Medical sociology* (5th ed.). Englewood Cliffs, NJ: Prentice-Hall.

Cowley, G. (1994). The rise of cyberdoc. *Newsweek*, September 26, 54-55.

Davis, F. (1960). Uncertainty in medical prognosis: Clinical and functional. *American Journal of Sociology, 66*, 41-47.

DeFriese, G. H., Woomert, A., Guild, P. A., Steckler, A. B., & Konrad, T. R. (1989). From activated patient to pacified activist: A study of the self-care movement in the United States. *Social Science and Medicine, 29*(2), 195-204.

Dougherty, C. J. (1990). The costs of commercial medicine. *Theoretical Medicine, 11*(4), 275-286.

Elliott, P. (1972). *The sociology of professions*. London: Macmillan.

Fougere, G. (1993). Struggling for control: The state and the medical profession in New Zealand. In F. W. Hafferty & J. B. McKinlay (Eds.), *The changing medical profession: An international perspective* (pp. 115-123). New York: Oxford University Press.

Fox, R. (1957). Training for uncertainty. In R. K. Merton, G. Reader, & P. L. Kendall (Eds.), *The student physician* (pp. 207-241). Cambridge, MA: Harvard University Press.

Freidson, E. (1970). *Professional dominance*. New York: Atherton Press.

Freidson, E. (1973). Prepaid group practice and the new demanding patient. *Milbank Memorial Fund Quarterly: Health and Society, 51*, 473-488.

Freidson, E. (1985). The reorganization of the medical profession. *Medical Care Review, 42*, 11-35.

Freidson, E. (1986). *Professional powers*. Chicago: University of Chicago Press.

Frenk, J., & Duran-Arenas, L. (1993). The medical profession and the state. In F. W. Hafferty & J. B. McKinlay (Eds.), *The changing medical profession: An international perspective* (pp. 25-42). New York: Oxford University Press.

Gerrity, M. S., Earp, J. A. L., & Devellis, R. F. (1990). Physicians' reactions to uncertainty in patient care: A new measure and new insights. *Medical Care, 28*, 724-736.

Gerrity, M. S., Earp, J. A. L., Devellis, R. F., & Light, D. W. (1992). Uncertainty and professional work: Perceptions of physicians in clinical practice. *American Journal of Sociology, 97*(4), 1022-1051.

Goss, M. E. W. (1981). Situational effects in medical care of the elderly: Office, hospital and nursing home. In M. R. Haug (Ed.), *Elderly patients and their doctors* (pp. 147-156). New York: Springer.

Greene, M. G., Adelman, R., Charon, R., & Hoffman, S. (1986). Ageism in the medical encounter: An exploratory study of the doctor-elderly patient relationship. *Language and Communication, 6*, 113-124.

Hafferty, F. W., & McKinlay, J. B. (Eds.). (1993). *The changing medical profession: An international perspective*. New York: Oxford University Press.

Haug, M. R. (1975). The deprofessionalization of everyone. *Sociological Focus, 8*, 197-213.

Haug, M. R. (1976a). The erosion of professional authority: A cross-cultural inquiry in the case of the physician. *Milbank Memorial Fund Quarterly: Health and Society, 54*, 83-106.

Haug, M. R. (1976b). Issues in general practitioner authority in the national health services. *Sociological Review Monograph, 22*, 23-42.

Haug, M. R. (1977). Commuter technology and the obsolescence of the concept of profession. In M. R. Haug & J. Dofney (Eds.), *Work and technology* (pp. 215-228). Beverly Hills, CA: Sage.

Haug, M. R. (1979). Doctor patient relationships and the older patient. *Journal of Gerontology, 34*, 852-860.

Haug, M. R. (1986). Doctor-patient relationships and their impacts on self care of the elderly. In B. Holstein, K. Dean, T. Hickey, & L. Coppard (Eds.), *Self care and health behavior in old age*. Copenhagen: Croom Helm.

Haug, M. R. (1988). A re-examination of the hypothesis of physician deprofessionalization. *Milbank Memorial Fund Quarterly: Health and Society, 66* (Suppl. 2), 48-55.

Haug, M. R. (1993). The role of patient education in doctor-patient relationships. In J. M. Clair & R. M. Allman (Eds.), *Sociomedical perspectives on patient care* (pp. 198-210). Lexington: University Press of Kentucky.

Haug, M. R., & Lavin, B. (1979). Public challenge of physician authority. *Medical Care, 17*, 844-858.

Haug, M. R., & Lavin, B. (1981). Practitioner or patient—

Who's in charge? *Journal of Health and Social Behavior, 22*, 212-229.
Haug, M. R., & Lavin, B. (1983). *Consumerism in medicine: Challenging physician authority*. Beverly Hills, CA: Sage.
Haug, M. R., & Sussman, M. B. (1969). Professional autonomy and the revolt of the client. *Social Problems, 17*, 153-161.
Hauser, S. T. (1981). Physician-patient relationships. In E. G. Mishler, L. R. Amarasingham, S. T., Hauser, R., Leim, S. D., Osherson, & N. E. Waxler (Eds.), *Social contexts of health, illness and patient care* (pp. 104-140). London: Cambridge University Press.
Hickson, G. B., Clayton, E. W., Entman, S. S., Miller, C. S., Githens, P. B., Whetten-Goldstein, K., & Sloan, F. A. (1994). Obstetricians' prior malpractice experience and patients' satisfaction with care. *Journal of the American Medical Association, 20*, 1583-1587.
Jesilow, P., Pontell, H. N., & Geis, G. (1993). *Prescription for profit: How doctors defraud Medicaid*. Berkeley: University of California Press.
Kolata, G. (1994). Their treatment, their lives, their decisions. *The New York Times Magazine*, April 24.
Kunitz, S. T. (1974). Professionalism and social control in the progressive era: The case of the Flexner report. *Social Problems, 22*, 16-27.
Larkin, G. V. (1993). Continuity in change: Medical dominance in the United Kingdom. In F. W. Hafferty & J. B. McKinlay (Eds.), *The changing medical profession: An international perspective* (pp. 81-90). New York: Oxford University Press.
Larson, M. S. (1977). *The rise of professionalism*. Berkeley: University of California Press.
Lavin, B., Haug, M. R., Belgrave, L. L., & Breslau, B. (1987). Change in student physicians' views on authority relationships with patients. *Journal of Health and Social Behavior, 28*, 256-272.
Lazare, A., Eisenthal, S., Frank, A ., & Stoeckle, J. D. (1978). Studies on a negotiated approach to patienthood. In E. B. Gallagher (Ed.), *The doctor-patient relationship in the changing health scene* (pp. 119-139). Washington, DC: U.S. Government Printing Office.
Light, D. W. (1983). Lay medicine and the medical profession: An international perspective. In P. Herder-Dorneich & A. Schuller (Eds.), *Spontanität oder Ordnung: Laienmedizin gegen professionelle Systeme* (pp. 95-110). Stuttgart: Verlag W. Lohlhammer.
Light, D. W. (1993). Countervailing power: The changing character of the medical profession in the United States. In F. W. Hafferty & J. B. McKinlay (Eds.), *The changing medical profession: An international perspective* (pp. 69-80). New York: Oxford University Press.
Luft, H. S. (1986). Economic incentives and constraints in clinical practice. In L. H. Aiken & D. Mechanic (Eds.), *Applications of social science to clinical medicine and health policy* (pp. 500-519). New Brunswick, NJ: Rutgers University Press.
McKinlay, J. B., & Arches, J. (1985). Towards the proletarianization of physicians. *International Journal of Health Services, 15*, 161-195.
Mechanic, D. (1982). The epidemiology of illness behavior and its relationship to physical and psychological distress. In D. Mechanic (Ed.), *Symptoms, illness behavior and help seeking* (pp. 1-24). New Brunswick, NJ: Rutgers University Press.
Miller, B. L. (1986). *Autonomy and decision-making: The institution and the patient*. Paper presented at the Aging and Health symposium on decision-making in long term care, Cleveland, Ohio.
Ohsfeldt, R. L. (1993). Contractual arrangements, financial incentives, and physician-patient relationships. In J. M. Clair and R. M. Allman (Eds.), *Sociomedical perspectives on patient care* (pp. 96-113). Lexington: University Press of Kentucky.
Parsons, T. (1951). *The social system*. New York: Free Press.
Parsons, T. (1975). The sick role and the role of the physician reconsidered. *Milbank Memorial Fund Quarterly: Health and Society, 53*, 257-278.
Pellegrino, E. D. (1977). Medicine and human values. *Yale Alumni Magazine and Journal, 41*, 10-11.
Pendleton, D. A., & Bochner, S. (1980). The communication of medical information in general practice consultations as a function of patients' social class. *Social Science and Medicine, 14A*, 669-673.
Pratt, L. V. (1978). Reshaping the consumer's posture in health care. In E. B. Gallagher (Ed.), *The doctor-patient relationship in the changing health scene* (pp. 197-214). Washington, DC: U.S. Government Printing Office.
Reeder, L. G. (1972). The patient-client as consumer: Some observations on the changing professional-client relationship. *Journal of Health and Social Behavior, 13*, 402-416.
Reiser, S. J (1978). *Medicine and the reign of technology*. London: Cambridge University Press.
Relman, A. S. (1991). Shattuck lecture—The health care industry: Where is it taking us? *New England Journal of Medicine, 325*(12), 854-859.
Ritchey, F. J. (1993). Fear of malpractice litigation, the risk management industry, and the clinical encounter. In J. M. Clair & R. M. Allman (Eds.), *Sociomedical perspectives on patient care* (pp. 114-138). Lexington: University Press of Kentucky.
Rodwin, M. A. (1993). *Medicine, money and morals: Physicians' conflicts of interest*. New York: Oxford University Press.
Roter, D. L., & Hall, J. A. (1992). *Doctors talking with patients/patients talking with doctors*. Westport, CT: Auburn House.
Roter, D. L., Lipkin, M., Jr., and Korsgaard, A. (1991). Sex differences in patients' and physicians' communication during primary care medical visits. *Medical Care, 29*(11), 1083-1093.
Ryan, E. B., & Cole, R. L. (1990). Evaluative perceptions of

interpersonal communication with the elders. In N. Giles, N. Coupland, & J. M. Wiemann (Eds.), *Communication, health and the elderly* (pp. 173-188). London: Manchester University Press.

Salmon, W. (1984). Organizing medical care for profit. In J. B. McKinlay (Ed.), *Issues in the political economy of health care*. New York: Tavistock.

Santos, J. F., Hubbard, R. W., & McIntosh, J. L. (1983). Mental health and the minority elderly. In L. D. Breslau & M. R. Haug (Eds.), *Depression and aging: Causes, care and consequences* (pp. 51-70). New York: Springer.

Shorter, E. (1985). *Bedside manners: The troubled history of doctors and patients*. New York: Simon & Shuster.

Starr, P. (1982). *The social transformation of American medicine*. New York: Basic Books.

Sullivan, R. (1986). New York patients to have access to their medical records. *The New York Times*, Sept. 14, 30.

Svarstad, B. L. (1986). Patient-practitioner relationships and compliance with prescribed medical regimens. In L. Aiken & D. Mechanic (Eds.), *Applications of social science to clinical medicine and health policy* (pp. 438-459). New Brunswick, NJ: Rutgers University Press.

Szasz, T., & Hollender, M. H. (1956). A contribution to the philosophy of medicine: The basic models of the doctor-patient relationship. *AMA Archives of Internal Medicine*, *97*, 585-592.

Verbrugge, L. M. (1985). Gender and health: An update on hypotheses and evidence. *Journal of Health and Social Behavior*, *26*(3), 156-182.

Vissing, Y. M., Kallen, D. J., & Johnson, G. (1988). *Health care communication between parent, child, and physician in primary pediatric settings*. Paper presented at the Popular Culture Association meeting, New Orleans, March 23-26.

Wagenfeld, M. O., Vissing, Y. M., Markle, G. E., & Peterson, J. C. (1979). Notes from the cancer underground: Health attitudes and practices of participants in the laetrile underground. *Social Science and Medicine*, *13A*(4) 483-485.

Waitzkin, H., & Stoeckle, J. D. (1976). Information control and the micro-politics of health care: Summary of an ongoing research project. *Social Science and Medicine*, *10*, 263-276.

Weber, M. (1961). Legitimate order and types of authority. In T. Parsons, E. Shils, & D. Naegele (Eds.), *Theories of society: Vol. I* (pp. 229-235). New York: Free Press.

Weisman, C. S., & Teitelbaum, M. A. (1985). Physician gender and the physician-patient relationship: Recent evidence and relevant questions. *Social Science and Medicine*, *20*, 1119-1127.

Wells, K. B., Ware, J. E., & Lewis, C. E. (1984). Physician attitude in counseling patients about smoking. *Medical Care*, *22*, 360-365.

West, C. (1984). *Routine complications: Troubles with talk between doctors and patients*. Bloomington: Indiana University Press.

Wiemann, J. M., Gravell, R., & Wiemann, M. C. (1990). Communication with the elderly: Implications for health care and social support. In N. Giles, N. Coupland, & J. M. Wiemann (Eds.), *Communication, health and the elderly* (pp. 229-242). London: Manchester University Press.

Willis, E. (1993). The medical profession in Australia. In F. W. Hafferty & J. B. McKinlay (Eds.), *The changing medical profession: An international perspective* (pp. 104-114). New York: Oxford University Press.

Wolinsky, F. D. (1988). *The sociology of health: Principles, practitioners, and issues* (2nd ed.). Belmont, CA: Wadsworth.

Zola, I. K. (1986). Reasons for non-compliances and failure of the elderly to seek care. In R. W. Moskowitz & M. R. Haug (Eds.), *Arthritis and elderly* (pp. 72-84). New York: Springer.

4

Professional Roles and Health Behavior

Jeffrey C. Salloway, Frederic W. Hafferty, and Yvonne M. Vissing

INTRODUCTION

In the rapidly changing field of health care, professionals are inundated with a host of structural issues that affect how they perceive their roles, how they are perceived by the patient, and how they interact with patients. These structural issues include political, economic, organizational, scientific, and technological forces that promote change in even the most routine delivery of health care. In order for health care professionals to interact with patients in ways that both enhance communication and improve well-being, it is useful for professionals to have a clear understanding of how traditional roles of health care providers have changed and what these changes mean in routine interaction with patients. This chapter will explore the changing nature of roles for health care providers, the social forces that cause these role changes, and what the role alterations mean for routine provider-patient interactions.

Physician-patient relationships are dynamic in nature; the interaction within the dyad is fluid and symbiotic, while role relationships between doctors and patients as aggregate groups are always evolving (Katz, 1984). The traditional relationship between health care providers and patients has been transformed from a strict paternalistic model into one more closely resembling a partnership. While secondary prevention and tertiary prevention in the treatment of illness are still major components of the health care delivery system, it is argued in this chapter that prevention at the level of primary care in which health rather than disease is the focus, has become a more publicly valued and desirable behavior. This shift from disease focus has resulted from complex structural causes and certainly has affected the role of health care providers in a variety of critical ways. First, as the focus of the field has shifted from pathology to disease pre-

Jeffrey C. Salloway • Department of Health Management and Policy, University of New Hampshire, Durham, New Hampshire 03824. **Frederic W. Hafferty** • Department of Behavioral Sciences, University of Minnesota School of Medicine, Duluth, Minnesota 55812. **Yvonne M. Vissing** • Department of Sociology, Salem State College, Salem, Massachusetts 01970.

Handbook of Health Behavior Research II: Provider Determinants, edited by David S. Gochman. Plenum Press, New York, 1997.

vention and health promotion (Hellstrom, 1995; Pelletier, 1978), the required skills and thus the provider roles have changed. Second, the health care provider is no longer regarded as the sole determinant of the patient's health care (Fitzpatrick, Hinton, Newman, Scrambler, & Thompson, 1984; Levin, Katz, & Holst, 1979). Third, new health care professional roles and norms have been created to address technological and economic changes in the field (Twaddle & Hessler, 1987). Finally, as professional roles and norms have changed, so have patient expectations and roles. All of these forces have created new, and sometimes challenging, norms, roles, expectations, and interactions for the provider (Fisher, 1986; Pilisuk & Parks, 1986).

While professional training and socialization may prepare health care workers for accepting these new professional roles, patients may retain traditional views about how health care providers "ought" to behave. As a result, patients often have different expectations than the health care provider holds, or demand behaviors that have become inappropriate for the provider. When this discontinuity of role expectation occurs, both providers and patient are likely to be frustrated with the interaction (Emanuel & Emanuel, 1992). This frustration can lead patients to "doctor-shop" or to compromise the quality of medical care as they search for interactions that meet their role expectations of how health care providers "ought" to be treating them (Suchman, 1965).

CONCEPTUAL FRAMEWORK

The patient visiting a physician arrives with an image of the provider's role and the way it should be performed. This image reflects the societal definition of the physician's role along with subcultural expectations as well as the conceptions formed by the patient from prior experiences. It is within this frame of reference that the patient attempts to evaluate the professional's qualifications and capabilities. In turn, the extent to which the provider can meet these expectations plays an important part in the patient's conformity to the prescribed treatment, the likelihood of return visits, and even the therapeutic effect gained through the influence of the provider's authority (Mechanic, 1978).

The work of Parsons (1951, 1975) is central to understanding the history of health care provider roles. As he analyzed the interface of society and medicine during the 1950s and '60s, Parsons noted several critical features of the physician's or health provider's role. First, he noted that caring for the sick is a functionally specialized, full-time professional activity, achieved through the development of a standard of technical proficiency. Second, the provider is expected to maintain a stance of affective neutrality, to approach the patient in objective and scientifically justified terms. Third, the ideology of the profession emphasizes the welfare of the patient, which the provider is to put above any personal interests. Thus, the health care provider has historically been expected to be the self-sacrificing expert who will always do what is best for the patient (Mechanic, 1978).

There is a widespread consensus within both the academic community and the medical community that there exists a professional role obligation for health care providers to impart not only technical services but also values to instill normative behaviors. But while the provision of technical services is one thing, the effect of interventions on patient attitudes and behaviors is quite another. Bloom (1963) noted that the interaction between patients and providers takes place within a sociocultural context that has a significant influence on the total interaction. For instance, in the days when doctors delivered several generations of babies to the same family, set the kids' broken bones, and knew the intricacies of their patients' lives in a longitudinal frame, the doctor-patient relationship was much different from that in the 1990s, when a doctor and a patient who have never seen each other before meet for six minutes and do not meet again for six months.

While their relationship is a specific instance of the interaction between two major categories of roles as provider and patient, each role player carries into the encounter two very special reference groups. For the provider, particular sets of values—which lead to specific norms and behaviors—serve as a dominating force in shaping the view of interaction with the patient. For the patient, the family, with its heritages and customs, provides a major framework for understanding interaction with the provider. In addition, both provider and patient are influenced by the many subcultures and other reference groups with which they have contact (Kurtz and Chalfant, 1984). Therefore, the doctor-patient relationship is subject not just to individual influences, but to professional, familial, and cultural ones as well.

While the provider-patient interaction occurs within an overarching sociocultural context, health care professionals' roles are highly influenced by their health subculture. These professional role players take their behavioral imperatives from the values of their health subculture and their role positions from within health care organizations. One of the professionals' role obligations, then, is to pass on the values and role expectations of the health subculture to their patients in an effort to create health care behaviors that are consistent with the values of the health care system. Within this theoretical framework, it is thus necessary to deal with issues of norms and values that define the role structure of professionals and socialization of patients into the value systems promoted by these professionals.

Cultural values and norms regarding health care contain implicit and explicit directives for action (professional and patient roles) that are to occur within health care organizations. Each player (provider or patient) has a role that includes prescriptions and proscriptions (do's and don'ts), prohibitions (taboos), and preferences (value hierarchies that dictate the order in which to implement prescriptions and proscriptions). For example, a physician learns that smoking tobacco is undesirable for patients (value) and that patients should not smoke (norm). It is the physician's role to encourage patients to quit smoking (prescription), but not to shout at them when they bring the subject up (proscription)—and not to threaten them with violence for smoking (prohibition). Given that real life is imminently complicated, if the patient is alcoholic and a smoker, it may be the physician's preference to deal with the threat of alcoholism first and attack the smoking later.

TRADITIONAL ROLE OF HEALTH CARE PROFESSIONALS

The traditional role of the health care provider has reflected a fascinating balance between a powerful authority figure who defines illness and a service provider who is compelled to address even minute requests in order to keep patients committed to the professional health care delivery system model. Physicians are society's authority on what "illness really is" (Freidson, 1970, p. 206) They decide who is sick and what should be done about it. In essence, physicians are the gatekeepers to most professional health resources, since these resources (such as prescription drugs and hospitals) cannot be used without their permission. Thus, Freidson argues that the behavior of health care providers constitutes the embodiment of certain dominant values in society (Cockerham, 1986, p. 113). The traditional values underlying the foundation of health care delivery prescribe specific normative behaviors for both patient and health care provider. In this model, a group of scientific experts identifies a set of ideal health care behaviors. This information is taught to health care providers during their socialization into their respective professions. In turn, these health care providers, working in health care delivery systems, are to transmit this information and in the process affect patient health. It is Balint's view of the health care profession that "every doctor has a vague, but unshakably firm idea of how a patient ought to behave when ill. It is as if the doctor had the knowledge of what was right and wrong for the patient to expect and to endure, and further, as if he had the ... duty to convert to his faith all the ignorant and unbelieving among his patients" (Balint, 1957, p. 216).

Providers must make patients feel that the medical model, in general, and medical expertise, in particular, warrant patient belief, compliance, and commitment. In this respect, their authority is supposedly used to improve the patient's well-being. But their authority also has the effect of keeping patients committed to the allopathic, patriarchal system of health care delivery. Health care providers have a vested interest in maintaining the support of their clientele for both personal and altruistically professional reasons. Sheff (1966) points out that since the overt role of the health care provider is to work for the good of the patient, providers have tended to feel it was better to impute illness to their patients than to deny it and risk overlooking or missing it. Patients come to health care providers with concerns that something may be wrong, and these concerns—real or imagined—must be addressed by the provider in some way (Tessler, Mechanic, & Dimond, 1976). Providers and patients engage in what W. T. Anderson and Helm (1979) call "reality negotiation," in which competing definitions of the situation are reviewed. They allege that the provider has the upper hand in deciding which definition is acceptable, because the provider has "the setting, language, latent status, stereotypical categorization of illness, tendency toward type 2 error (finding illness even if it is not there), and organizational clout—all supporting his or her definition of reality over the patient's" (Anderson & Helm, 1979, p. 269). Thus, "while the physician's job is to make decisions, including the decision not to do anything, the fact seems to be that the everyday practitioner feels impelled to do something, if only to satisfy patients who urge him to do something when they are in distress" (Freidson, 1970, p. 258).

Hall (1948) points out that this behavior is a natural part of the provider role, because in any medical practice, it is important to acquire a clientele, retain it, and improve its composition to one that may be more comfortable to the middle-class values held by many practitioners (Cockerham, 1986). In providing care, Hall alleges, the practitioner needs to play the role of a promoter, interacting with patients so as to secure their approval of the services provided. This role requisite, however, has led to allegations of overprescribing medication (Begley, 1994; Levy, 1992) and unnecessary surgery (Leape, 1992; Nickerson, Colton, Peterson, Bloom, & Hauck, 1976).

SOCIAL FORCES CHANGE PROVIDER ROLES

What caused the rise of new roles for health care providers? Certainly, structural forces amid political, economic, organizational, scientific, and technological institutions all drive changes in the institution of health care delivery. These forces need to be explored further, since they lay the foundation for many changes in the provider–patient role relationship.

First, rising costs of health care became the greatest single source of inflation in the United States economy (K. Anderson, 1991). Health care costs increased 400% over a 15-year period (Lewin, 1990). As a result, there were increased public demands for government intervention (Hollingsworth, 1981).

Second, the establishment of medical legislation and regulation, such as Medicare, Medicaid, professional standards review organizations (PSROs), diagnostic related groups (DRGs), and managed care through health maintenance organizations (HMOs) or other systems, have all resulted in a different financial reimbursement system, which has forced changes in health care delivery organizations and structures. In turn, the role of health care professionals has changed dramatically as they have been forced to alter their relationship with patients to meet organizationally imposed constraints on the delivery and utilization of health services and technologies (Emanuel and Brett, 1993). The central theme in these changes is that the physician is no longer in control of the health care that is provided. Health care organizations have now assumed this function, and thus organizations—not a particular health care provider—have the responsibility for the quality of care provided and its fiscal reimbursement. But as managed care systems become more prevalent, the doctor-patient relationship is faced with an unavoidable conflict as patient needs begin to exceed the available level of payment. More specifically, the physician and patient have been joined in the examining room by corporate interests, which have turned the traditional doctor-patient dyad into a triad of countervailing needs. Managed care has forced patient role changes especially in the direction of increased preventive and healthy behaviors and increased personal responsibility and partnership with health care providers (Advertisement, 1994).

Third, these changes have occurred simultaneously and in conjunction with the corporatization of American medicine (Starr, 1982). With health care delivery having become big business, the health care delivery field has transformed the charity and humanity of healing the sick into a lucrative financial investment for large-scale corporate enterprises.

Fourth, there has been a cultural shift in health care values, which has directly influenced social norms about health care. Reasons for the changes in health norms and values are discussed below.

Shifting Values and Behaviors

Professional and public norms for appropriate health care behavior shift when confronted with people who hold different cultural values regarding health, when scientific inconsistencies are faced, or as new behaviors emerge.

Time and values change standards in health care protocols and roles, as seen in public attitudes toward smoking (Flynn, Worden, & Secker-Walker, 1992; Popham, Poller, & Bal, 1993). Cardiac and asthmatic patients, who were once told to get plenty of rest, are now admonished to get exercise. In this respect, as "appropriate" health roles change, yesterday's complaint patient can become tomorrow's deviant.

Scientific inconsistencies also force shifts in values and behavior. For instance, what is the public to believe when it reads that there is no scientific evidence that women who do breast self-exams every month are less likely to die of breast cancer than women who do not conduct this exam? The writer goes on to say that physicians have long touted the importance of self-exams, but have done so essentially in good faith, in the absence of scientific data (Painter, 1995). Even the standard of when women should have mammograms has changed to a less rigorous one (Conkling, 1995). Similarly, when parents learn in the media that the latest scientific data indicate that athletic participation may not reduce unhealthy behavior among adolescents, the scientific validity of all exercise may be questioned (Skolnick, 1993).

When the traditional medical model failed to "cure" diseases for which nontraditional healers claimed success, alternative remedies gained attention. Patients may be convinced of the health benefits of a vegetarian diet, use of nutritional supplements, or other nontraditional remedies (Vissing & Burke, 1984; Wagenfeld, Vissing, Markle, & Peterson, 1979). By the end of the 1980s, a number of American adults equal to one in three were making more than 425 million visits annually to providers of unconventional therapy. This number is larger than the number of visits to all United States primary care physicians, and over $13.7 billion a year is spent on unorthodox remedies (Eisenberg, 1994). Even reimbursement programs may deem services such as acupuncture, herbalism, and homeopathy as legitimate and cost-effective (Cowley, King, Hager, & Hager, 1995).

A Growing Behavioral Component in the Scientific Literature

The scientific literature has grown to contain a series of latent behavioral imperatives in its findings. Etiological agents for many chronic diseases are thought to include a sedentary lifestyle, high-fat diet, smoking, high alcohol consumption, exposure to pathogenic agents, low dietary fiber, and other undesirable components and behaviors. Thus, the prevention of ailments is increasingly linked to changing the health behaviors of people at risk.

Life Expectancy Changes

Increases in life expectancy and epidemiology have resulted in the development of new health values. Demographers anticipate that people will live longer (Olshansky & Carnes [1944] project that by the year 2020, 52.4% of females will live beyond age 85), but with similar rates of morbidity and incapacity that result from chronic diseases (L. Verbrugge & Patrick, 1995; M. Verbrugge, Lepkowski, & Imanaka, 1989).

Promoting Health versus Extending Life

Rather than valuing behaviors that simply extend life, a health-oriented value system has become concerned with promoting behaviors that preserve a high-quality lifestyle, with its features of high physical mobility, positive mood, independent living, social connectedness, and freedom from debilitating symptoms.

Social Forces Influencing Provider Roles

The shift in medicine away from the treatment of acute diseases toward preventive health services to offset the effects of chronic disorders has dramatically changed the ways that providers and patients interact (Reeder, 1972). Where once treatment of acute and infectious conditions relied on short-term, biotechnical interventions such as quarantine, alcohol rubs to reduce fevers, and use of antibiotic drugs, the chronic and degenerative diseases of the late 20th century require different treatment approaches. Biomedical prescriptions have come to include a variety of behavioral components. For instance, bed rest for cardiovascular disease has been replaced by active, exercise-oriented cardiac rehabilitation; diabetes may control their disease by diet rather than medication. The socialization of health care providers into their respective professions has begun to rectify the traditional schizophrenic approach in which the physician promotes health only by identifying and managing illness.

Consumerism

As consumerism has developed, "the social role of the physician and the overall physician–patient relationship can hardly escape modification. In general, this modification has taken the form of physician and patient interacting on a more equal footing in terms of decision making and responsibility for outcome" (Cockerham, 1986, p. 179). Though health care advice is ostensibly based in scientific rigor, the American public has become increasingly confused and skeptical regarding that advice (Becker, 1993).

As a result of these trends, the health care field has developed a variety of new roles—roles that affect how patients perceive providers and what they expect.

CHANGING HEALTH CARE PROVIDER ROLES AND THEIR EFFECT

The model for providing health care to a patient has changed since the 1950s, when Parsons (1951) described normative role relationships. Blinded by medicine's claim of expert knowledge and professional authority, patients expected physicians to act paternally, placing patients' interests ahead of their own in a form of fiduciary responsibility. Parsons described and endorsed this unbalanced power relationship, in which the primacy of physicians was secured because of their expertise and professionalism.

Early modifications of the Parsonian model, such as the one advanced by Szasz and Hollender (1956), attempted to directly relate the patient's physiological symptoms with a three-tiered model of (1) activity–passivity, (2) guidance–cooperation, and (3) mutual participation But even with the recognition that conditions of chronic illness might require a more egalitarian relationship between the patient and the physician, models of the physician's role remained paternalistic and authoritarian for much of the 1950s and 1960s (see Wolinsky, 1988).

In many respects, it has taken changes in the larger social structure that governs health care delivery to usher in radical changes in the provider-patient relationship. How, then, has the provider role changed?

Role Differentiation among Health Care Providers

Structural changes have resulted in more and differentiated types of health care providers. While Marcus Welby may have been the one-stop, full-service physician who could deal with everything from surgery to psychotherapy and nutrition, modern health care professionals have been differentiated into highly specialized subprofessionals. A patient may utilize dozens of different types of health care providers in order to manage aspects of a single health care disorder. Physicians and nurses—and all their subspecialties—work alongside a host of technicians, medical records librarians, computer analysts, occupational therapists, physical therapists, nutritionists, social workers, psychiatrists, and the like. As a result, health care providers are more likely to operate in a team model than ever before.

This shift raises interesting questions for the role of the physician in health-related behaviors. As responsibility for behavior change becomes delegated across a broader spectrum of health professions, physicians become marginalized both as producers of relevant knowledge and as deliverers of that knowledge to patients. Shedding the role of behavioral change agent in some ways reduces the professional power of the physician and makes that role increasingly a technical exercise with diminished human contact.

Nowhere is the increase in a profession's internal differentiation more evident than in nursing (Garner, Smith, & Piland, 1990). Formerly, nursing distinctions were few, including categories of licensed practical nurse, nurse's aide, operating room nurse, and floor nurse. By the 1990s, the range included ophthalmologic nursing, nephrology nursing, oncology nursing, cardiovascular nursing, perinatal and women's health nursing, psychiatric nursing, post-operative nursing, postanesthesia nursing, and so on. Professional organizations range from the American Holistic Nurses Association to the American Association of Neuroscience Nurses.

Role specialization in medicine is hardly a new phenomenon. Claims heralding the death of the generalist appeared as early as the beginning of the 20th century (Konold, 1962; Shryock, 1967), barely a half century after the founding of the American Medical Association in 1847. Trends supporting a specialty-oriented and procedure-based medicine were continuing in the 1990s. Despite a policy emphasis on primary care in both the 1970s and the 1990s, the trend toward specialization and thus internal differentiation has continued to accelerate. For example, by 1995, the American Board of Medical Specialties (ABMS) had recognized 70 subspecialty areas, 40 of them having been approved since 1980 and 13 since 1990 (Martini, 1992). Although subspecialty incomes show signs of weakening (Mika, 1994; Page, 1994), and while medical school graduates are beginning to show an increased interest in generalist residency programs (Kassebaum & Szenas, 1994), subspecialty medicine remains well entrenched within allopathic medicine.

Health Professional as Health Educator

The evolving role of the physician places much more emphasis on the notion of the physician as information bearer, interpretive agent, and general educator (Clarke, 1991; Machowsky, 1993; Mitchinson, 1995). This emphasis on the physician as facilitator and the importance of reciprocity in the physician-patient relationship has largely replaced the former paternalistic model (Emanuel & Emanuel, 1992). How such changes in the provider role will affect patient behavior can be determined only over time; it appears, however, that improved provider-patient interactions typically result in increased patient compliance and satisfaction (Hoppe, Farquhar, Stoffelmayr, Henry, & Helfer, 1988).

Health professionals (including but not limited to physicians) most often direct their health education activities in one of two ways: at the community level to address broad-based educational concerns or in the clinical health setting for individual-level education.

Community Health Educator. One need only glance at popular American culture to ascertain the widespread acceptance of the provider as educator and health advocate. Community health educators are expected to work with large numbers of people in nonclinical settings. They teach the risks of disease, the importance of healthy behaviors, or resource referral. Often, community health educators have a public health focus and can serve small groups of individuals, student groups, or entire segments of society. While community health educators are frequently identified with smoking cessation programs, hypertension screening programs, and the like, they may also deal with large-scale public information and policy development. Representatives of health care professions, such as the American Medical Association, American Hospital Association, and countless others, routinely testify before Congressional committees, are quoted as reliable new sources, and issue position statements on ideal health care behaviors and systems for delivering care. Health care providers write advice columns in newspapers, endorse commercial products, and appear on television and distribute video cassettes to disseminate information about what they perceive to be optimal health behaviors. Embedded in all of these activities is the normative expectation that health care providers have the knowledge and authority to determine what constitutes health care and can affect their patients' behavior.

But the increase in public exposure has also been accompanied by a crisis of credibility as important health announcements of today are retracted tomorrow (Price, 1989; Shibata, Mack, Paganini-Hill, Ross, & Henderson, 1994; Thompson, 1994). For instance, the public is confused about whether milk is healthful (Hellmich, 1992), whether one should use butter or margarine (Bass, 1995; Deveny, 1993; Mashberg, 1994), or whether women should conduct breast self-exams every month (Painter, 1995). It may come as no surprise that there has been an increase in "health habit complacency" (Marwick & Gunby, 1993).

Clinical Health Educator. The clinical health educator works in clinical settings and takes responsibility for educating patients and families about diagnoses and their management. This role is directed specifically at treatment or adherence behaviors and, to a somewhat lesser extent, preventative and other health behaviors. Often, the clinical health educator works closely with a particular service and has substantive expertise. Examples include the diabetes educator or the ostomy management specialist. Because of the heavy clinical knowledge base required for these roles, the roles require training in both substantive and behavior management areas.

Health Professional as Health Advocate

Professionalism has traditionally implied that the professional-client relationship is governed by a system of ethics and advocacy in which providers are prepared to advance the interests of the patient before the interests of any other entity, including their own. A system of ethics implies that the professional has internalized a normative system with regard to practice and that that normative system is the sole guide to the relationship. Advocacy, as part of the system of ethics, implies that the professional will use great discretion to address the particular needs of individual patients and to respond in the face of uncertainty and ambiguity.

A system guided by ethics and principles of advocacy works well for the management of health-related behaviors. The professional is expected to recommend treatment behaviors and health behaviors that are best for the patient regardless of cost or time consumed. However, changes in health care delivery toward managed care also bring with them the potential for erosion of ethics and advocacy in the health professional-patient encounter.

Health Professional as Partner in Patient Health

As patient roles have changed, patients may expect providers to take more time with them and interact with them as equals in the partnership process in search of better health. Studies indicate that cues used by patients to estimate a provider's competence may not reflect the provider's technical abilities and knowledge. Rather, cues usually reflect the provider's apparent interest in the patient, willingness to give time to hear the patient's complaint, and similar concerns. The provider's willingness to socialize with the patient may be seen as an index of interest; one's confidence and authority may be perceived as indications of expertise, and rapid arrival at a diagnosis and a treatment plan may be viewed as evidence of competence. While patients vary widely in their sophistication and knowledge, the compatibility of patient expectation and provider performance has important implications for the success of the relationship (Goffman, 1974; Mechanic, 1978).

More Professionals, Increased Role Ambiguity

While new occupational groups are charged with more specific health-related behaviors, they also are confronted with new sources of role conflict and role ambiguity. It appears almost ironic that as organized medicine has moved to proclaim a new era of the generalist, ancillary providers, flush with their new certifications and specialty aspirations, are staking out vigorous claims over technologies and services—all buttressed by a national mania for controlling health care expenditures. Ancillary providers generally cost less than physicians and, with backup provided by more expert providers, are often as effective (Abrams, 1993; Garfield, 1970).

While clear roles provide structured expectations and guidelines for behavior, ambiguous situations now regularly occur in doctor-patient interactions. Sometimes, it is difficult for health care providers to know exactly which role to play, as in the following exchange: The doctor asks a patient, "Do you smoke?" The patient answers, "Yes, but I switched to a low-tar, low-nicotine cigarette and I smoke fewer cigarettes." How should the doctor respond? The physician may experience role ambiguity in seeking to choose the "correct" response. Should the provider applaud the patient's efforts at change, and meld praise with the admonition that such behavior is good—but not good enough? Or should the patient be admonished for still smoking? "Correct" choices for provider behavior are unclear.

Another example of role ambiguity occurs when the provider is "caught" between being a selfless motivator for patient health and being a savvy economic entrepreneur. Working with a smoking patient will require time for patient education about the risks of smoking, identifying the availability of smoking cessation programs, or counseling the patient about a decision to use a nicotine patch. These actions, while laudable, are frequently not reimbursable and are time-consuming. Providers may view these low-yield encounters as stealing important time away from other patients who need and who will benefit from their more technical medical expertise. Thus, while the role prescriptions for different elements of the single role, there lie potential role strains that are difficult to resolve and still keep the whole role intact.

Increased Competition and Changing Roles

As more health care providers enter the delivery system, and as technical and service roles intersect, it is harder for a patient to decide when to seek the services of other providers. It is also difficult for a professional to refer the patient to other providers when it is possible for that professional to supply the rudimentary core of services that others provide. The assignment of responsibility for health-related behavior in the currently evolving delivery system is done with neither precision nor clarity. For instance, nurses have traditionally claimed expertise in assisting in their adaptation to illness, its complications, and its avoidance (Clarke, 1991; Mitchinson, 1995). Nutritionists now take an active role in passing on their expertise about the management of food-related behaviors (Haughton, Shaw, 1992). Occupational therapists, pharmacists, physical therapists, and a host of other role players also claim legitimate expertise in the management of health-related behavior. Their roles often overlap, compete, and occasionally conflict.

Viewing competition in the health care delivery system from another vantage point, patients are not immune from issues of competition. Providers who have heavy caseloads can be selective about patients they choose to see, and they can be "too busy" for potentially problematic patients. This situation can lead to inadequate serving of some patients by health care providers. Some patients who have difficult health problems or compliance problems may be rejected as "bad" patients (Cato 6, 1982; Konner, 1987; Leiderman & Grisso, 1985; Mizrahi, 1986; Wells, Ware, & Lewis, 1984). Only when a patient accepts the provider's diagnosis and treatment regimen will the physician consider the encounter a successful one (Kurtz & Chalfant, 1984).

Role Differentiation

The transfer of role responsibilities from physicians to nonphysicians is not without contention or possible risk. As long argued by allopathic medicine, alternative providers and allied health professionals often receive less training, and the training they do receive is less predicated on scientific principles than that received by physicians. Among other things, this relative paucity of training renders alternative providers less able to exercise discretionary decision making, and therefore less able to act independently, especially in situations involving clinical uncertainty. It follows, therefore, that patients may be at a greater risk—particularly at the point of initial contact with the health care system—if these points are staffed by providers other than the most highly skilled professionals.

For this and other reasons, a national program of medical effectiveness research was undertaken (Raskin & Maklan, 1991), particularly with the creation of the Agency for Health Care Policy and Research and its Medical Treatment Effectiveness Program (MEDTEP). These forces and the rationales that are being developed are revolutionizing the practice of medicine (Hafferty & Light, 1995). As of late 1995, the future of the Agency for Health Care Policy and Research was in doubt, making it impossible to gauge the long-range impact of medical effectiveness research on health behavior and professional roles.

Role Changes and Communication Shifts

When several generations of a family saw the same physician, a familiarity naturally evolved in the doctor-patient interaction. Providers would automatically have in mind certain information concerning the patient, and patients felt comfortable telling intimate details that one might normally never tell a stranger. But as role differentiation has proliferated in the heath care field, patients may find themselves providing the same information over and over, or refusing to mention more sensitive facts.

Changes in communication and relationships also evolve when patients expect a traditional role relationship but are met with one that emphasizes personal responsibility. Minor changes in the expected interaction patterns of one partner can drastically influence the behavior of the other; for instance, when the patient expects a "magic bullet" to cure diabetes and the provider insists upon a diet and exercise regime, the patient may be dissatisfied with the provider.

As Haug and Lavin (1981, 1983) note, provider power and authority can be wielded in a variety of ways to produce differential patient outcomes. No longer is the doctor's word sacred, as is evident from the growing recourse to second medical opinions. Communication between patients and providers may be comfortable when both operate with expectations of a paternalistic relationship; successful interactions may also occur when both the provider and the patient expect partnership-egalitarian exchanges. However, role strain and conflict result when the patient and the physician hold differing expectations about how the other is to behave in the clinical setting (Vissing, Kallen, & Johnson, 1988).

'Onstage' versus 'Offstage' Interactions: Professional Role Strain

Patients may expect providers to give them medical advice when they pay for it in the office (onstage). However, they may not welcome the provider's attempts to point out the need to modify behavior when patient and provider encounter one another at a social gathering (offstage). Providers may ask whether, as professionals, they can ever legitimately step out of the health care professional role (Goffman, 1974). Strains on the offstage patient and provider interaction may be complicated further if the patient sees the provider smoking, overweight, not wearing a seatbelt, consuming "forbidden" foods, and so on (Nelson et al., 1994).

On occasion, the health care professional may also have legitimate reason to resent the patient who aggressively seeks extensive—not to mention unremunerative—advice in a social setting.

All of this is predicated on the question of whether society views the physician role as being setting-specific or involving broader responsibilities. But even if the physician role is accorded a master status (Dotter & Roebuck, 1988), and thus extended beyond the structural boundaries of the medical workplace (e.g., clinic or hospital setting), patients may still view some forms of interaction as appropriate only in certain settings. Thus, in the office, the physician can be preemptive, but at a party, health issues can be raised only by the patient. In other words, the physician may always be on call, but the patient cannot be put on the carpet.

Difficulties in Practicing the Professional Role

Health care providers themselves may not practice what they preach (McBride, Plane, Underbakke, Hill, and Wiebe, 1995), and what one provider believes to be of importance another provider may not (Holcomb et al., 1985). But health care providers may be expected to embody personally those behaviors that they seek to instill in their patients. The Pew Health Professional Commission (Langfitt, 1991) asserts that the education and training of health professionals is out of step with the evolving health needs of the American people. In assessing attitudes and skills that health professionals should possess in order to meet the health needs of the public, their report alleged that the traditional physician role must change to include increased emphasis on preventive health skills and consumer satisfaction, and a willingness to engage in formal review (physician report cards). The commission called for physicians to institute a "bottom-up" approach employing skills, attitudes, and values that would help patients to become healthy.

RESEARCH ON PROFESSIONAL ROLES

Inquiries into the physician-patient relationship, including its impact on health, treatment decisions and outcomes, and patient compliance and satisfaction, remain a ubiquitous part of medical research. The range of topics covered under this banner is extensive and includes themes such as physician attitudes and reactions toward patients (Bush, Cherkin, Barlow, 1993;

Fried, Stein, O'Sullivan, Brock, & Novak, 1993; Hahn, Thompson, Willis, Stern, & Budner, 1994; Packer, Prendergast, Wasylenski, Toner, & Ali, 1994), patient attitudes and reactions toward physicians (Daaleman & Nease, 1994; Frederikson & Bull, 1995; Greco, Brownlea, & McGovern, 1995; Stump, Dexter, Tierney, & Wolinsky, 1995), physician-patient communication and its impact on clinical decision making (Frederikson & Bull, 1995; Roberts, Cox, Reintgen, Baile, & Gibertini, 1994), concurrence between patients' and physicians' assessments (Punamaki & Kokko, 1995), medication noncompliance (McLane, Zyzanski, & Flocke, 1995), the influence of gender on the physician's practice style (Bertakis, Helms, Callahan, Azari, & Robbins, 1995), and issues such as physician counseling and smoking cessation (McIlvain, Susman, Davis, & Gilbert, 1995; Ockene et al., 1994), patient preferences for test result disclosure (Schreiber, Leonard, & Rieniets, 1995), and the importance of physician recommendations in patients' decision to donate preoperative autologous blood (Ferguson, Strauss, & Toy, 1994).

Methodological approaches extend from descriptively oriented case studies, retrospective and cross-sectional surveys, participant observation and related field work, and the analysis of historical and archival documents (e.g., Braslow, 1995) to prospective observations and clinical trials employing randomization and blinding strategies (e.g., Smith et al., 1995; SUPPORT Principal Investigators, 1995).

Project scope can vary from a study of a particular clinic, hospital, or training program to large, multisite, million-dollar studies designed to comparatively and causally assess how training interventions, shifts in organizational policies, or work structure can affect patient outcomes and patient satisfaction. Perhaps surprisingly—perhaps not—efforts to document improvements in provider-patient interactions have remained frustratingly elusive (see SUPPORT Principal Investigators, 1995).

With the growth of managed care, attempts to measure patient satisfaction, along with corollary topics like cost containment, clinical outcomes, provider practice styles, and the relationship of culture to patient satisfaction (Baider, Ever-Hadani, & De-Nour, 1995), have come to dominate studies of physician-patient relations. As of November 24, 1995, the MEDLINE data base listed 4093 citations attached to the key word "patient satisfaction," with over 2500 of these articles published after 1992.

But while these and other aspects of the physician-patient relationship remain the legitimate object of both scientific study and concern, it is important to realize that virtually all empirically based inquiries into provider-patient interactions focus on rather restricted questions about particular interactive styles and strategies, about the divulging of certain types of information, or about participant perceptions—all important issues but not issues at the level of roles per se. The notion of social roles is more of a macrolevel concept, something that is concerned with broad aspects of social exchange. It is concerned with values and normative expectations and it is influenced by institutional and organizational contingencies, but it transcends these elements as well. It is something more amenable to commentary than analysis and, given the pace of change, more evolutionary than intervention-specific.

As health care moves into the 21st century, the broad picture of professional roles and health behavior will continue to be shaped by managed care systems and corporate ownership of medical work settings. Studies will be conducted, but more than in the past, they will be company-specific, unpublished, and deal with topics of "customer" satisfaction, employee productivity, and system efficiency. Findings will be considered as proprietary and as having organization-specific utility rather than any broader "scientific" relevance or applicability. Workers will be trained to adapt to a changing work environment rather than to perform particular tasks. Work itself will be structured around the introduction of practice guidelines, organizational deskilling (the transference of work functions once controlled exclusively by physicians or nurses down the occupational hierarchy), cross-training (preparing workers for multiple and changing job responsibilities), and organizational certification, with who does what increasingly set by employers as opposed to the traditional "right" of specialty organizations and associations to establish who is and is not qualified to perform particular tasks (Hafferty & McKinlay, 1995; Hafferty & Raskin, 1994). Even the problems identified as needing study will be set more by the major funding sources—corporate and federal (e.g., efficiency and productivity for the former, "policy relevant" for the latter)—than by any notion of theoretical or conceptual relevance. The voices of the public and of researchers increasingly will become more distant from each other and more irrelevant to the debate.

CONCLUSIONS

The roles of health care providers have evolved from providing treatment (in which professionals prescribe behaviors that are specific to the amelioration of illness, the reduction of symptoms, and the prevention of complications) to advocating for health behaviors. Unlike treatment behaviors, health behaviors are directed at risk reduction, and place the burden of responsibility for good health squarely upon the patient's shoulders.

This emphasis on individual responsibility has two important implications. First, there is no health professional mediating between the knowledge experts and the client, who is not (yet) a patient. Self-care, a health fad of the 1970s, has become part of the mainstream health care delivery system (Shye, Javetz, & Shuval, 1991) and accounts for billions of dollars spent yearly on over-the-counter drugs and a variety of health supplements. Second, the client is reasonably free to choose from among those practices defined as desirable whether they be offered by allopathic physicians, chiropractic physicians, naturopaths, dieticians, herbalists, health food faddists, or old wives whose tales seem believable or whose knowledge claims have gained a certain cultural credibility. In short, a greater amount of health-relevant information is now available.

This wide availability creates a reasonably open market for ideas in which no single profession is able to control the quantity and content of information about health behaviors and how they are to be practiced. A person already practicing health behavior who becomes a patient is far more likely to behave autonomously, having already demonstrated a degree of self-directedness in matters of health. This implies a very different relationship between practitioner and patient—one in which the provider has become "deprofessionalized" or egalitarianized (Graham, 1994; Haug & Lavin, 1981, 1983).

How well will patients adhere to the new mandate for health and healthful behaviors? Patients routinely fail to follow the directives of health professionals; hypertensives refuse to limit sodium intake, diabetics eat illegal foods, smokers continue to light up, overweight people neglect to lose weight and exercise, patients fail to keep follow-up appointments or finish antibiotic prescriptions, and the like. But as the economic reimbursement screws are tightened, as access to health care becomes more difficult, and as the relationship between lifestyle choices and chronic disease becomes better understood, patients may find that they engage in more preventive behavior out of necessity. Time will prove whether or not they will.

Accompanying the shift in health roles has been the development of a new norm of personal responsibility in health that ranges from the Congressional thrust for health care reform to the kitchens of America. Health has become a new form of morality that includes fitness, a variety of abstentions, slenderness, and dietary regulations (Fiatarone, Marks, & Ryan, 1990). However, the notion of health as a new morality has raised concern among sociologists (Becker, 1993; Kronenfeld, 1988), ethicists (Caplan, 1993), and others (Morreim, 1994) who fear that patient blame will become the modus operandi for responding to health care problems. For example, "If only you had eaten properly and exercised regularly, you would never have this cardiovascular condition." This new morality in health fails to consider the wide variability in health beliefs and practices (Shye, et al., 1991; Retchin, Wells, Valleron, & Albrecht, 1992). Additionally, experts fear that identification of the social and environmental causes of health problems will recede, along with governmental- and corporate-level responsibility, and that issues of quality health care will be reassigned to individuals rather than to the health care system.

The role implications of such a move are substantial if health care providers are asked to shift from a traditional role of nonjudgmental patient advocate to corporate agents who will monitor and direct access to the health care system based on their evaluation of patient culpability. Social science is in search of new models, but none has emerged that captures the essence of the new role structure. The role structure is in flux, and is yet to be determined.

REFERENCES

Abrams, H. S. (1993). Harvard community health plan's mental health redesign project: A managerial and clinical partnership. *Psychiatry Quarterly, 64*(1), 13-31.

Advertisement. (1994). Access Health. *Wall Street Journal*, April 6, A17.

Anderson, K. (1991). Medical cost inflation outstrips all industry. *USA Today*, May 16, A13.

Anderson, W. T., & Helm, D. T. (1979). The physician-patient encounter: A process of reality negotiation. In E. G. Jaco (Ed.), *Patients, physicians and illness* (3rd ed.) (pp. 259-271). New York: Free Press.

Baider, L., Ever-Hadani, P., & De-Nour, A. 1995. The impact of culture on perceptions of patient-physician satisfaction. *Israel Journal of Medical Sciences, 31*(2-3), 179-185.

Balint, M. (1957). *The doctor, his patient, and the illness*. New York: International Universities Press.

Bass, F. (1995). Butter or margarine? Don't worry, doctors say, they both can kill you. *Houston Post*, March 10, A20.

Becker, M. H. (1993). A medical sociologist looks at health behavior. *Journal of Health and Social Behavior, 34*(1), 1-6.

Begley, S. (1994). The end of antibiotics. *Time*, March 28, 46-52.

Bertakis, K. D., Helms, L. J., Callahan, E. J., Azari, R., & Robbins, J. A. (1995). The influence of gender on physician practice style. *Medical Care, 33*(4), 407-416.

Bloom, S. (1963). *The doctor and his patient*. New York: Russell Sage Foundation.

Braslow, J. (1995). Effect of therapeutic innovation on perception of diseases and the doctor-patient relationship: A history of general paralysis of the insane and malaria fever therapy. *American Journal of Psychiatry, 152*(5), 660-665.

Bush, T., Cherkin, D., & Barlow, W. (1993). The impact of physician attitudes on patient satisfaction with care for low back pain. *Archives of Family Medicine, 1993*(3), 301-305.

Caplan, A. (1993). Dangers in the rhetoric of personal responsibility toward health care. *Atlanta Constitution*, July 15, A:13.

Cato 6. (1982). Dirtball. *Journal of the American Medical Association, 247*, 3059-3060.

Clarke, A. C. (1991). Nurses as role models and health educators. *Journal of Advanced Nursing, 16*(10), 1178-1184.

Cockerham, W. (1986). *Medical sociology*. Englewood Cliffs, NJ: Prentice-Hall.

Conkling, W. (1995). The great mammogram controversy: National Cancer Institute guidelines. *American Health, 14*(April), 10-13.

Cowley, G., King, P., Hager, M., & Hager, D. (1995). Going mainstream. *Newsweek*, June 26, 56-57.

Daaleman, T. P., & Nease, D. E., Jr. (1994). Patient attitudes regarding physician inquiry into spiritual and religious issues. *Journal of Family Practice, 39*(6), 564-568.

Deveny, K. (1993). Marketscan: Health doubts cut into margarine sales. *Wall Street Journal*, June 24, B1.

Dotter, D. L., & Roebuck, J. B. (1988). The labeling approach re-examined: Interactionism and the components of deviance. *Deviant Behavior, 9*(1), 19-32.

Eisenberg, J. M. (1994). If trickle-down physician workforce policy failed, is the choice now between the market and government regulation? *Inquiry, 31*,(3), 241-249.

Emanuel, E. J., & Brett, A. S . (1993). Managed competition and the patient-physician relationship. *New England Journal of Medicine, 329*(12), 879-882.

Emanuel, E. J., & Emanuel, L. L. (1992). Four models of the physician-patient relationship. *Journal of the American Medical Association, 267*(16), 2221-2226.

Ferguson, K. J., Strauss, R. G., & Toy, P. T. (1994). Physician recommendation as the key factor in patients' decisions to participate in preoperative autologous blood donation programs: Preoperative autologous blood donation study group. *American Journal of Surgery, 168*(1), 2-5.

Fiatarone, M. A., Marks, E. C., & Ryan, N. D. (1990). High intensity strength training in nonagenarians: Effects on skeletal muscle. *Journal of the American Medical Association, 263*, 3029-3034.

Fisher, S. (1986). *In the patient's best interest: Women and the politics of medical decisions*. New Brunswick, NJ: Rutgers University Press.

Fitzpatrick, R., Hinton, J., Newman, S., Scrambler, G., & Thompson, J. (1984). *The experience of illness*. New York: Tavistock Publications.

Flynn, B., Worden, J., & Secker-Walker, R. (1992). Prevention of cigarette smoking through mass media intervention and school programs. *American Journal of Public Health, 82*, 827-834.

Frederikson, L., & Bull, P. (1995). Evaluation of a patient education leaflet designed to improve communication in medical consultations. *Patient Education Counselor, 25* (1), 51-57.

Freidson, E. (1970). *Profession of medicine: A study of the sociology of applied knowledge*. New York: Harper & Row.

Fried, T., Stein, M., O'Sullivan, P., Brock, D., & Novak, D. (1993). Limits of patient autonomy: Physician attitudes and practices regarding life-sustaining treatments and euthanasia. *Archives of Internal Medicine, 153*(6), 722-728.

Garfield, S. R. (1970). The delivery of medical care. *Scientific American, 222*, 15-23.

Garner, J. F., Smith, H. L., & Piland, N. F. (1990). *Strategic nursing management: Power and responsibility in a new era*. Rockville, MD: Aspen Publishers.

Goffman, E. (1974). *Frame analysis*. New York: Harper & Row.

Graham, J. (1994). Self-care: A new trend in changing industry. *Denver Post*, June 12, G:1.

Greco, M., Brownlea, A., & McGovern, J. (1995). Utilising patient feedback in the RACGP training program: An exploratory study. *Australian Family Physician, 24*(6), 1077-1081.

Hafferty, F. W., & Light, D. W. (1995). Professional dynamics and the changing nature of medical work. *Journal of Health and Social Behavior* (extra issue), 132-153.

Hafferty, F. W., & McKinlay, J. B. (1995). *The transformation of American medicine revisited; What's in store for American medicine*. Paper presented at the 90th Annual Meeting of the American Sociological Association, Washington, DC, August 19-23.

Hafferty, F. W., & Raskin, I. (1994). *Medical effectiveness research and the future of medicine as a profession*. Paper presented at the 89th Annual Meeting of the American Sociological Association, Los Angeles, August 5-9.

Hahn, S., Thompson, K., Wills, T., Stern, V., & Budner, N. (1994). The difficult doctor-patient relationship: Somatization, personality and psychopathology. *Journal of Clinical Epidemiology, 47*(6), 647-657.

Hall, O. (1948). The informal organization of the medical profession. *Canadian Journal of Economics and Political Sciences, 12*, 30-44.

Haug, M. R., & Lavin, B. (1981). Practitioner or patient: Who's in charge? *Journal of Health and Social Behavior, 22*, 212-229.

Haug, M. R., & Lavin, B. (1983). *Consumerism in medicine: Challenging physician authority*. Beverly Hills, CA: Sage.

Haughton, B., & Shaw, J. (1992). Functional roles of today's public health nutritionist. *Journal of the American Dietetic Association, 92*(10), 1218-1222.

Hellmich, N. (1992). Nutritional do's and don'ts can spoil an appetite. *USA Today*, October 8, D1.

Hellstrom, O. (1995). Health promotion and clinical dialogue. *Patient Education Counselor, 25*(3), 247-256.

Holcomb, J. D., Mullen, P. D., Fasser, C. E., Smith, Q., Martin, J. B., Parks, L. A., & Wente, S. M. (1985). Health behaviors and beliefs in four allied health professions regarding health promotion and disease prevention. *Journal of Allied Health, 14*(4), 373-385.

Hollingsworth, J. A. (1981). Inequalities in levels of health in England and Wales. *Journal of Health and Social Behavior, 22*, 268-283.

Hoppe, R., Farquhar, L., Stoffelmayr, B., Henry, R., & Helfer, M. (1988). A course component to teach interviewing skills in informing and motivating patients. *Journal of Medical Education, 63*, 176-181.

Kassebaum, D. G., & Szenas, P. L. (1994). Graduates' interest in generalist specialties rises for a second year. *Academic Physician and Scientist* (November), 2-3.

Katz, J. (1984). *The silent world of doctor and patient*. New York: Free Press.

Konner, M. (1987). *Becoming a doctor: A journey of initiation in medical school*. New York: Penguin Books.

Konold, D. E. (1962). *A history of American medical ethics 1847-1912*. Madison: State Historical Society of Wisconsin.

Kronenfeld, J. J. (1988). Models of preventive health behavior, health behavior change, and roles for sociologists. *Research in the Sociology of Health Care*, 7, 303-328.

Kurtz, R. A., & Chalfant, H. P. (1984). *The sociology of medicine and illness*. Boston: Allyn and Bacon.

Langfitt, T. W. (1991). *Healthy American: Practitioners for 2005. A report of the Pew Health Professions Commission*. Durham, NC: Pew Health Professions Commission, Duke University Medical Center.

Leape, L. L. (1992). Unnecessary surgery. *Annual Review of Public Health, 13*, 363-383.

Leiderman, D. B., & Grisso, J.-A. (1985). The gomer phenomenon. *Journal of Health and Social Behavior, 26*, 222-232.

Levin, L., Katz, A., & Holst, E. (1979). *Self care: Lay initiatives in health*. New York: Prodist.

Levy, S. B. (1992). *The antibiotic paradox: How miracle drugs are destroying the miracle*. New York: Plenum Press.

Lewin, M. (1990). IFC report. New York: Families USA Foundation.

Machowsky, S. L. (1993). The role of the health educator. *Insight, 18*(2), 14-15.

Martini, C. J. M. (1992). Graduate medical education in the changing environment of medicine. *Journal of the American Medical Association, 268*(9), 1097-1105.

Marwick, C., & Gunby, P. (1993). Survey suggests rise in health habit complacency. *Journal of the American Medical Association, 269*(16), 2061-2062.

Mashberg, T. (1994). Distress at the dairy case. *Boston Globe*, May 17, 20.
McBride, P., Plane, M. B., Underbakke, G., Hill, R., & Wiebe, D. (1995). Medical student's health habits: Do future physicians have healthy lifestyles? *Wisconsin Medical Journal*, *94*(1), 45-46.
McIlvain, H., Susman, J. L., Davis, C., & Gilbert, C. (1995). Physician counseling for smoking cessation: Is the glass half empty? *Journal of Family Practice*, *40*(2), 148-152.
McLane, C., Zyzanski, S., & Flocke, S. (1995). Factors associated with medication noncompliance in rural elderly hypertensive patients. *American Journal of Hypertension*, *8*(2), 206-209.
Mechanic, D. (1978). *Medical sociology*. New York: Free Press.
Mika, M. (1994). Higher pay for primary care. *American Medical News*, *37*(37), 1, 7.
Mitchinson, S. 1995. A review of the health promotion and health beliefs of traditional and project 2000 student nurses. *Journal of Advanced Nursing*, *21*(2), 356-363.
Mizrahi, T. (1986). *Getting rid of patients: Contradictions in the socialization of physicians*. New Brunswick, NJ: Rutgers University Press.
Morreim, E. H. (1994). Redefining quality by reassigning responsibility. *American Journal of Law and Medicine*, *20*, 1-2, 79-104.
Nelson, D. E. Giovino, G. A., Emont, S. L., Brackbill, R., Cameron, L. L., Peddicord, J., & Mowery, P. D. (1994). Trends in cigarette smoking among US physicians and nurses. *Journal of the American Medical Association*, *271*(16), 1273-1275.
Nickerson, R., Colton,T., Peterson, O., Bloom, B., & Hauck, W. (1976). Doctors who perform operations: A study of in-hospital surgery in four diverse geographic areas. *New England Journal of Medicine*, *295*, 921-926.
Ockene, J., Kristeller, J., Pbert, L., Hebert, J., Luippold, R., et al. (1994). The physician-delivered smoking intervention project: Can short-term interventions produce long-term effects for a general outpatient population? *Health Psychology*, *13*(3), 378-281.
Olshansky, S., & Carnes, B. (1994). Demographic perspectives on human senescence. *Population and Development Review*, *20*(March), 57-80.
Packer, S., Prendergast, P., Wasylenski, D., Toner, B., & Ali, A. (1994). Psychiatric residents' attitudes toward patients with chronic mental illness. *Hospital and Community Psychiatry*, *45*(11), 1117-1121.
Page, L. (1994). Early signs of a shakeout: Specialists face the future. *American Medical News*, *37*(37), 1, 7-8.
Painter, K. (1985). Breast self-exams: Wise precaution or waste of time? *USA Today*, June 12, D1-2.
Parsons, T. (1951). *The social system*. New York: Free Press.
Parsons, T. (1975). The sick role and the role of the physician reconsidered. *Milbank Memorial Fund Quarterly: Health and Society*, *53*(3), 257-278.
Pelletier, K. (1978). *Mind as healer, mind as slayer: A holistic approach to preventing stress disorders*. London: G. Allen & Unwin.
Pilisuk, M., & Parks, S. (1986). *The healing web: Social networks and human survival*. Hanover, NH: University Press of New England.
Popham, W., Poller, L., & Bal, D. (1993). Do anti-smoking media campaigns help smokers quit? *Public Health Reports*, *108*(July-August), 510-513.
Price, J. (1989). Reduced cancer risk is a perk of heavy coffee drinking. *Washington Times*, November 20, A7.
Punamaki, R. L., & Kokko, S. J. (1995). Content and predictors of consultation experiences among Finnish primary care patients. *Social Science and Medicine*, *40*(2), 231-243.
Raskin, I. E., & Maklan, C. W. (1991). Medical treatment effectiveness research: A view from inside the Agency for Health Care Policy and Research. *Evaluation and the Health Professions* (June), 161-186.
Reeder, L. G. (1972). The patient-client as a consumer: Some observations on the changing professional client relationship. *Journal of Health and Social Behavior*, *13*(December), 406-412.
Retchin, S. M., Wells, J. A., Valleron, A. J., & Albrecht, G. L. (1992). Health behavior changes in the United States, the United Kingdom, and France. *Journal of General Internal Medicine*, *7*(6), 615-622.
Roberts, C. S., Cox, C. E ., Reintgen, D. S., Baile, W. F., & Gibertini, M. (1994). Influence of physician communication on newly diagnosed breast patients' psychologic adjustment and decision-making. *Cancer*, *74*(Suppl.), 336-341.
Schreiber, M., Leonard, M., & Rieniets, C. (1995). Disclosure of imaging findings to patients directly by radiologists: Survey of patients' preferences. *American Journal of Roentgenology*, *165*(2), 467-469.
Scheff, T. (1966). *Being mentally ill*. Chicago: Aldine.
Shibata, A., Mack, T. M., Paganini-Hill, A., Ross, R. K., & Henderson, B. E. (1994). A prospective study of pancreatic cancer in the elderly. *International Journal of Cancer*, *58*(1), 46-49.
Shryock, R. H. (1967). *Medical licensing in America, 1650-1965*. Baltimore: Johns Hopkins University Press.
Shye, D., Javetz, R., & Shuval, J. T. (1991). Lay self-care in health: The views and perspectives of Israeli lay people. *Social Science and Medicine*, *33*(3), 297-308.
Skolnick, A. A. (1993). Studies raise doubts about benefit of athletics in reducing unhealthy behavior among adolescents. *Journal of the American Medical Association*, *270*(7), 798, 800.
Smith, R., & Hoppe, R. (1991). The patient story: Integrating the patient- and physician-centered approaches to interviewing. *Annals of Internal Medicine*, *115*(6), 470-477.
Smith, R., Lyles, J., Mettler, J., Marshall, A., Egeren, L. V., et al. (1995). A strategy for improving patient satisfaction by the intensive training of residents in psychosocial medicine: A

controlled, randomized study. *Academic Medicine, 70*(8), 729-732.

Starr, P. E. (1982). *The social transformation of American medicine: The rise of a sovereign profession and the making of a vast industry*. New York: Basic Books.

Stump, T. E., Dexter, P. R., Tierney, W. M., & Wolinsky, F. D. (1995). Measuring patient satisfaction with physicians among older and diseased adults in a primary care municipal outpatient setting. *Medical Care, 33*(9), 958-972.

Suchman, E. (1965). Social patterns of illness and medical care. *Journal of Health and Human Behavior,6*, 2-16.

SUPPORT Principal Investigators. (1995). A controlled trial to improve care for seriously ill hospitalized patients: The Study to Understand Prognoses and Preferences for Outcomes and Risks of Treatments (SUPPORT). *Journal of the American Medical Association, 274*(20), 1591-1598.

Szasz, T., & Hollender, M. (1956). A contribution to the philosophy of medicine: The basic models of the doctor-patient relationship. *Journal of the American Medical Association, 97*, 585-588.

Tessler, R., Mechanic, D., & Dimond, M. (1976). The effect of psychological distress on physician utilization. *Journal of Health and Social Behavior, 17*, 353-364.

Thompson, W. G. (1994). Coffee: Brew or bane. *American Journal of Medical Science, 308*(1), 49-57.

Twaddle, A., & Hessler, R. (1987). *A sociology of health*. New York: Macmillan.

Verbrugge, L., & Patrick, D. (1995). Seven chronic conditions: Their impact on U.S. adults' activity levels and use of medical services. *American Journal of Public Health*, (February), *5*, 173-182.

Verbrugge, M., Lepkowski, J., & Imanaka, Y. (1989). Comorbidity and its impact on disability. *Milbank Memorial Fund Quarterly: Health and Society, 67*(3-4), 450-485.

Vissing, Y. M., & Burke, M. A. (1984). Nursing professionals and the art of visualization. *Journal of Psychosocial Medicine and Mental Health, 22*(1), 29-34.

5

Locational Attributes of Health Behavior

Joseph L. Scarpaci and Robin A. Kearns

The traditional conceptualization of space and place as determinants of health behavior has focused on the institutional and facility attributes of health care delivery. Institutional features include the financial (public versus private) and practitioner-specific (nurse, physician, midwife) characteristics of service delivery. Facility aspects of a health care setting refer to the physical dimensions of the medical or health care encounter between patient and provider. Embedded in conceptualizing the facility are aspects of location, space, and place. Practitioners' offices, hospitals, emergency rooms, free-standing ambulatory-care settings, patients' homes, and worksites are just a few of these facilities. Locational attributes of a facility refer to its proximity, centrality, and convenience.

Since the early 1990s, the literature surrounding the conceptualization of the physical environment of health care has been broadened by a more theoretically informed discussion of place and space. Place and space are differing yardsticks by which the world is described and analyzed. The former term is anchored in human experience, whereas the latter has its roots in more abstract thinking (Kearns & Joseph, 1993). Generally speaking, different scholarship goals have directed investigations of these concepts with respect to health behavior. Research that has viewed space and location in geometric terms arises from the positivist tradition that holds explanation as the goal, whereas humanistic interpretations of place seek to understand rather than explain. In so doing, humanistic work often focuses on experience (which includes feelings and perceptions) as well as behavior (which compromises specific actions, and associated decision making). The sense of place concept, for instance, pays attention to what goes on within a particular health care facility rather than simply to where that facility rests within the larger spatial distribution of health services.

Drawing largely on debates within medical geography and on research examples from the United States, Chile, and New Zealand, this chap-

Joseph L. Scarpaci • Department of Urban Affairs and Planning, Virginia Polytechnic Institute and State University, Blacksburg, Virginia 24061-0113. **Robin A. Kearns** • Department of Geography, University of Auckland, Auckland, New Zealand.

Handbook of Health Behavior Research II: Provider Determinants, edited by David S. Gochman. Plenum Press, New York, 1997.

ter outlines the salient points of the nexus between place and health. It begins with the more traditional aspects of the physical environments of health care delivery. Next, it turns to a discussion of place and space. It concludes by showing how a continuous engagement of the structure-agency question and other aspects of social theory will provide a richer epistemology in which to investigate the locational attributes of health settings and the health behaviors associated with these attributes. The term *setting* is used throughout this chapter to refer to conventional "bricks-and-mortar" notions of place as well as the psychosocial implications that such places inherently bring to provider-patient encounters.

LOCATIONAL ATTRIBUTES, QUALITY OF CARE, AND HEALTH CARE CONSUMPTION

Accessibility to and quality of health care services are important factors in the utilization of health services, and the physical setting of a medical encounter brings these two concepts together in unique ways. The place of care has inherent attributes that either attract patients or deter them from seeking services. In general, measures of the quality of care have been provider-determined, because the objective procedures of assessing "good" care are easier to document than the subjective view held by the patient. Provider assessments of quality often center upon the "application of the science and technology of medicine, and of the other health sciences, to the management of a personal health problem" (Donabedian, 1980, p. 4). The medical profession throughout most of this century has therefore established standards of quality (Caper, 1988; Starr, 1982). Peer review—the assessment of medical care by colleagues in the same specialty—forms a central part of assessing quality of care (Donabedian, 1985). Technical components of care that may or may not be germane to the physical setting, but certainly relate to its quality, include diagnosis accuracy, appropriateness of drug prescription, and postoperative infection rates (Weitzman, 1990). Again, quality pertains to studies of health behavior and physical settings because of the axiom that better-quality care is more likely to increase service use than lower-quality care.

Quality of care is a central gauge of hospital performance, and finding robust, readily available quality-of-care measures remains a challenge. Cleverley and Harvey (1992) uncovered evidence that quality is tied to several measures of financial performance. Examining eight low-quality hospitals, they noted that the facilities had fewer staff hours per adjusted discharge and lower investment in capitals assets than the median measures for hospitals matched by bed size and region. However, Levitt (1994) built on their approach by examining the relationship between quality of care and investment in property, plant, and equipment (PPE) in hospitals. His data consisted of peer review organization (PRO) and generic quality screen (GQS) reviews and confirmed failures over a five-year period for Massachusetts hospitals. The principal findings showed that PPE in Massachusetts hospitals is correlated with GQS confirmed failure rates. Thus, investment in PPE—a key feature of the physical environment of Western medicine—predicts certain dimensions of quality of care in hospitals. Levitt (1994, p. 726) concludes that while this finding is useful, his methodology "misses important dimensions of quality ... [of] patient satisfaction."

In contrast to provider assessments of quality care, patients tend to emphasize the interpersonal aspects of quality. Here, the analytical lens shifts from technical competence to patient perception or, as Evans (1993) describes it, from "high tech" to "high touch." Unable to judge technical matters, patients concentrate on the concern and interest shown by providers (Donabedian, 1985). Patients are put off by physicians with heavy patient loads, inconsistent evaluations, brief office visits, and treatments that are delegated to so many providers that the patient lacks a sense of who is in charge (Allman, Yoels, & Clair, 1993). At the risk of overgeneralization, it would appear that smaller, aesthetically pleasing settings in which patients can spend enough time to explain their symptoms to a provider will be more attractive to patients than crowded, hurried, and busy facilities. In the United States medical marketplace, high-cost medical care characterizes the former, while public care points up the latter. Despite the increase in medical equipment—most of which tends to be place-specific (specialty treatment centers, hospitals)—patients continue to discern the difference between good technology and good care.

Theoretically, then, professionals stand to benefit if they can understand the kinds of settings in which patients are satisfied with their care. Patient satisfaction is likely to be strongly associated with compliance with physician orders. Compliance with a prescribed regimen, in turn, may lead to greater relief and improvement in health status. From an applied perspective, understanding how settings influence utilization and other health behaviors improves health planning and the allocation of scarce resources in a medical market with finite goods and services (Feldstein, 1981). As Americans become more expert as consumers, they acquire higher expectations about what kind of health care they want, where it should be delivered, and what constitutes good care (Kovner, 1990). These heightened expectations have implications for the institutional and facility aspects of health care.

INSTITUTIONAL AND FACILITY ASPECTS OF HEALTH CARE DELIVERY

Sources of geographic differences in health care delivery systems can be identified in a number of ways. Institutional and facility aspects of health care delivery vary according to the size and distribution of select populations, sex, age, marital status, and other features, as well as the population's relationship to physical structures in the health care ensemble. These features are ecological because they draw on the relationships between environments and people. Significantly, these environments include physical and social elements (Hawley, 1950).

Population characteristics and how people relate to their environment shape the organization of health services. In market-driven health care systems, highly specialized medical services tend to cluster in urban areas because such areas are the point of maximum access and contain a larger user population to sustain the financial solvency of specialty services. Metropolitan areas also afford agglomeration economies for providers and potential cost savings for consumers. If accessibility is thought of as a potential link, then it stands to reason that specialty medical services concentrate in high-density urban centers where that potential can be maximized. Clearly, the locational attributes of a health service (proximity, centrality, convenience) cannot solely determine the use of that medical service because of financial, cultural, or psychological barriers. In that regard, accessibility and utilization are highly related.

Perhaps the most basic tenet of the ecological dimensions of health care delivery is the distance-decay factor, which states that medical-care utilization is inversely related to proximity to providers or facilities. While the importance of distance seems axiomatic, it is often neglected in facility planning and health services research. Such an idea dates back to the work of Edward Jarvis, who examined the prevalence of lunacy in western Pennsylvania. He concluded that residents living closer to a mental hospital were more likely to be admitted to those facilities than were patients who lived farther away (Jarvis [noted in Meade, Florin, & Gesler, 1988]). Research subsequent to Jarvis's pioneering work has led to more refined distance-decay models and examinations of Jarvis's Law. A common equation in use is

$$f = k/d^b,$$

where f is the frequency of patient-provider contact, d equals distance, and k and b are parameters that must be determined for a given setting (Meade, et al., 1988). The latter parameters usually examine the rate of distance-decay, which in turn translates into the "steepness" of the curve that measures the drop-off rate of facility attendance. The axiom is that as distance increases, utilization wanes.

Market-driven health care in the United States often addresses physician location as a response to socioeconomic and geographic factors. The underlying assumption in this case is that providers (supply) will locate at a midpoint between the locale of the "tools of their trade" (hospitals where they have staff privileges, ancillary services for diagnostic and laboratory work), the profiles of the service areas (cultural amenities, quality of schools, leisure activities available), and the location of their clients (demand). Hospitals where physicians have staff privileges may also assist the physicians in acquiring office space adjacent to the hospitals. A host of correlation- and regression-based research on factors influencing physician location has used the state, county, and city as the unit of analysis. The aim of this research is to calibrate the relationship between the characteristics of the area and the distribution of medical doctors. Variants of the following model assess this relationship:

$$P = a \pm b_1X_1 \pm b_2X_2 \pm \ldots b_mX_m$$

where independent variables (X) are suspected to influence the supply of physicians (P). Partial regression coefficients (b) assess the elasticity of the dependent variables to changes in all independent variables. While this inferential model does not specifically address patient behavior, the assumption in a market setting is that one can understand a given environment indirectly by understanding physician behavior (Joseph & Phillips, 1984, p. 94).

Geographic and ecological theories of the distance-utilization relationship have surfaced in both national health care policy acts and empirical studies. The enactment of the Hospital Survey and Construction (Hill-Burton) Act of 1946 recognized the lack of hospital services in rural areas. For nearly four decades, federal outlays sought to remedy secondary care in rural settings. However, the "brick-and-mortar" approach to hospital utilization was unable to address the problem of physician retention in rural hospitals. Though funding has been discontinued, Hill-Burton produced a spate of research assessing the distribution and utilization of health services in geographically underserved areas. For example, Jehlik and McNamara (1952) documented the relationship of distance to differential utilization (e.g., to distinct health personnel and facilities). Their work underscored the importance of distance in explaining patterns of health care use among the American farm population. Ciocco and Altman (1954) observed a decline in the use of urban specialists in their western Pennsylvania study even though resources were evenly distributed. In its simplest form, then, the locations of health services and providers remain perhaps the most basic attributes of the health care environment, but also perhaps one of its least understood (Shannon & Dever, 1974).

Land use and population density are chief determinants of the utilization of health services (Twaddle & Hessler, 1977). Not only the distributions of rural and urban residents, but also the distribution of population over space and the modalities by which health services become used, are important in determining land-use patterns. Even in socialized medical settings that are not driven exclusively by market forces, expensive services used by relatively few people imply distortions in matters of equity and resource allocation. This distortion is evident, for example, in the concentration of medical specialties (neurosurgery) in a service area that can sustain the use of that service financially (market economies) or justify the diversion of state resources (socialist or centrally planned economies). Thus, the nature of specialization and the urban-rural profile of a target population cannot readily be separated. China, for instance, is highly rural and depends greatly on generalists and "barefoot doctors" who work in small population units where their services can be easily consumed (Roemer, 1985). In highly urban countries such as the United States and the United Kingdom, therapeutic and diagnostic procedures concentrate in cities to maximize accessibility to their highly urban populations.

One aspect of the salience of the environment in determining health behavior surfaces in the hierarchy of medical care services, regardless of whether the setting is rural and underdeveloped (Good, 1987; Stock, 1982), urban and underdeveloped (Scarpaci, 1988b), or advanced and industrial (Mayhew, 1986). The classic model of health care delivery based on population size and the level of medical-care specialty is embodied in Central Place Theory. The application of this theory, which is based on land-economics studies in north Germany in the 19th century, to health services research identifies three levels of services. High-order medical services are concentrated in large cities capable of drawing on a service population from a large geographic area. These services include specialized tertiary facilities and specialty services. Major metropolitan areas adopt these functions. A secondary, intermediate service refers to medium-order goods and services. In health care delivery, this translates as secondary care such as hospitals and clinics. Accordingly, a population threshold between large metropolis and small town sustains this service. At the lower end of Central Place Theory, one finds low-order goods and services. These services might include a primary care physician, some more common specialties (obstetrics-gynecology, pediatrics) and primary health care services. Low-order goods and services prevail among smaller towns and communities (Figure 1) because they cannot support a minimum (threshold) population for more sophisticated care. At the same time, though, large metropolitan areas also require low-order services and facilities for routine and nonspecialized care. A theoretical interpretation based merely on population size would predict potential help-seeking behaviors to cities for tertiary (high-order), secondary (medium-order), and primary care (low-order) services. This may also explain why large hospital chains rationalize their locations in line with economic principles of central places.

The organization of health services presents defining features that patients and providers often recognize when providing or consuming services, respectively. In the United States, medical-practice organizations have evolved in response to changing market and regulatory conditions. Two major trends have characterized the use of health services in the past three decades. One is the rise in ambulatory care. Outpatient visits to hospitals have increased dramatically since the 1960s. Nonfederal short-term hospitals had a 55% rise in outpatient visits from 1970 to 1980, while inpatient visits rose by just 24%. Increases in outpatient visits stemmed from a corporate structure in which diversification and ambulatory care, specialized management and marketing, an increasingly elderly population, and economies of scale combined with an expanded asset base among hospitals (Katz, Mitchell, & Markezin, 1982).

A second trend is the shift from general to specialized practice and from solo to corporate practice. Solo practice, traditionally portrayed as the (male) physician in his neighborhood, provided a wide array of services. It was not uncommon for the physician to work out of his home and make house calls. Representing small town America of the 19th century and the early part of the 20th century, solo practice has gradually become less common in United States medical care. Citizens of other industrial nations of western Europe and in Canada and Great Britain have access to a greater percentage of primary care physicians. Recent data show that about 50% of physicians in most western European nations and 72% of Canadian physicians work as primary care physicians. In comparison, the United States percentage is 29% and is declining (Koop, 1993). If primary care physicians are the most likely to work in solo or smaller group practices (Ernst & Yett, 1985), then this trend bodes poorly for the small, more "personalized" setting of health care delivery that characterized American medicine the first half of the 20th century. Indeed, only 14% of medical students graduating in 1992 began a career in primary care (Koop, 1993).

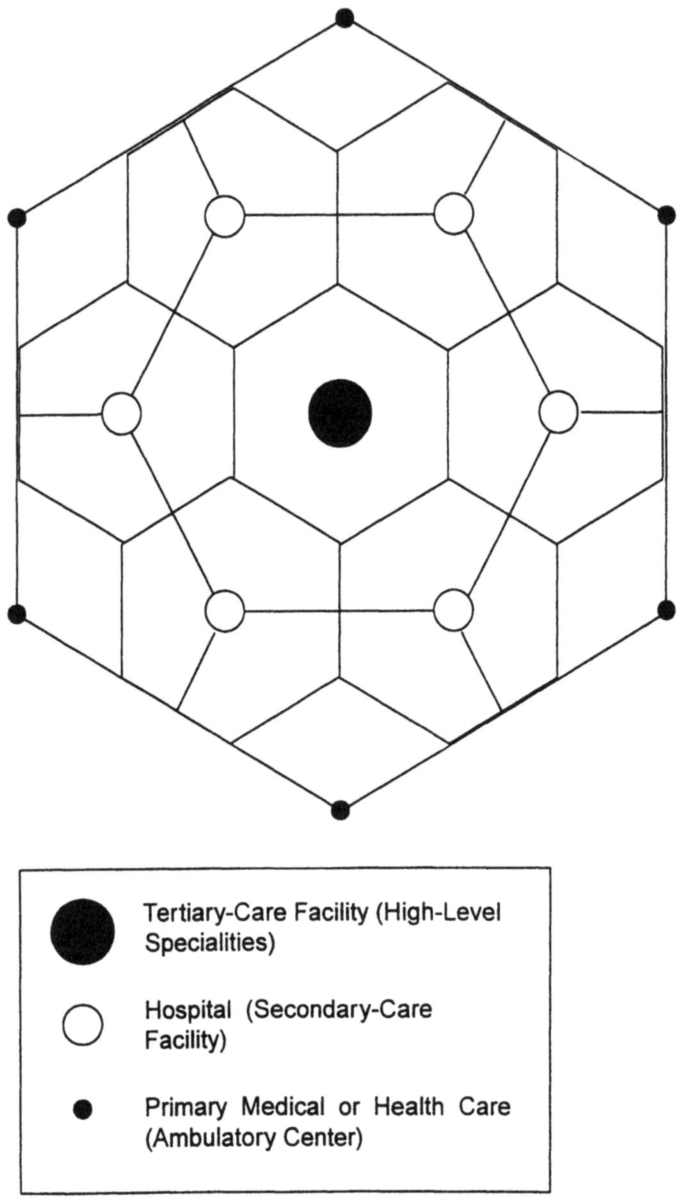

Figure 1. Central place theory and a hierarchy of health services.

Partnerships, group practices, and hospital practices are replacing primary care solo practitioners. These new forms represent economies of scale in providing medical services (sharing overhead, clerical, and billing staffs; insurance pooling) and in complementing the division of labor. This complementarity allows for the sharing or rotating of shifts in hospital practices as well as greater flexibility in staffing hours and taking in new patients and market share. The shift from solo to group practices is well illustrated by the rise in health maintenance organizations (HMOs). These medical practices tend to provide savings in the patient's overall medical costs because the incentive is to keep the patient healthy. They put strong emphasis on preventive health care such as annual medical examinations, routine well-baby checkups, and weight, stress, and exercise programs that are often affiliated with the HMO. To pool risks and keep costs down, consumers may also be forced to relinquish some aspects of choice such as drawing on a smaller pool of providers, more tightly controlled and limited hospitalizations, and generally more rigorous criteria about what gets done for a patient, who does it, and what the patient is entitled to receive from the bundle of services provided for by a set premium. Such a scenario contrasts with the non-HMO insured consumer, who may have greater choice of provider and of diagnostic and imaging facilities.

If a defining feature of the American health care system is the progressive shift to group practices, clearly, providers and patients must be gaining some benefits. Providers benefit from economies of scale, staffing flexibility, more ancillary services, and other amenities. Patients allegedly profit from group practices as well: location of multiple services under a single roof, easier access to referrals, and possibly a better understanding of medical costs (Table 1). Yet group practices are not trouble-free. Providers must contend with a loss of freedom, less individual decision making, ceilings on salary earnings, and other detriments. Patients must contend with less choice in providers, the possibility of higher personnel turnover, and maybe even less provider incentive for care. Table 1 makes it clear that while the trend toward group practices necessarily influences the physical setting of United States health care, there are both merits and detriments to those environments.

That the medical profession has become the main arbiter of technical skill and medical knowledge is widely accepted. The profession has consolidated its power, and its typical work setting enables it to provide distinctive medical experiences unavailable in nontypical settings. Rothman (1982), for instance, documents that a home delivery is a different birthing experience from one in a hospital. In good measure, maternity patients relinquish considerable decision-making ability to the physician, resulting in patients' inability to care for themselves and to make independent decisions. If the comfort of giving birth in the home is a growing trend, then the hospital industry's response would seem to be the rapid incorporation of "birthing centers" to emulate home environments.

The importance of locational attributes of a medical experience varies even when some physical aspects are held constant. For example, Fisher (1988, p. 142) has shown that hysterectomies are more likely to be recommended and performed in clinics staffed by residents than by attending staff and professors of medicine. Residents are also likely not to perform Pap smears in family practice clinics, even among potentially high-risk populations. Kisch and Reeder (1969) showed long ago that even in the same physical setting, patients in hospitals can identify with considerable reliability, providers whose care they deem as "better." Thus, controlling for the location of service delivery, patients discern which providers are better than others. Even though the physical environment influences the nature of the medical encounter in key ways, these examples also point to the risk of overly rigid geographic or facility determinism.

AMBULATORY CARE UTILIZATION BY PATIENTS IN THE UNITED STATES

If the settings of health care encounters have become more diverse in recent years, ambulatory care still remains the dominant setting. In 1991, there were approximately 670 million visits made to non-federally employed, office-based physicians. This number translates into 2.7 visits per person. Nearly half (48.9%) of all office visits were made by persons 25–64 years of age. The

Table 1. Some Advantages and Disadvantages of Group Practice[a]

Advantages	Disadvantages
From the perspective of the health services provider	
1. Availability of professional manager	1. Less individual freedom
2. Organizational responsibility for patient	2. May lead to excess use of specialist
3. Less physician administrative time	3. Fewer outside consultants
4. Shared capital expense	4. Possible reduced identity with patient and community
5. Shared financial risk	5. Group rather than individual decision making
6. Better coverage and shared on-call	6. Share all problems
7. More flexible working hours	7. Must work with others
8. More peer interaction	8. Less individual incentive and more security-oriented
9. Increased access to specialists	9. Income limitations
10. Broader array of ancillary services	10. Income-distribution arguments
11. Stable income for providers	
12. No direct financial concern with patient	
13. Lower initial investment	
14. More time for continuing education	
15. More flexible vacation time	
16. Generally excellent benefits	
17. Possible efficiencies of scale	
18. Use of nonphysician practitioners	
From the perspective of the group practice patient	
1. Care under one roof	1. Less freedom of choice of provider
2. Availability of specialists, lab, other facilities	2. Possible lessening of provider–patient relationships
3. Improved coverage and emergency care	3. Possible overuse of ancillary services
4. Medical and administrative records centrally located	4. Possible high provider turnover
5. Referrals simplified	5. Heavy patient loads, and waiting times may be increased
6. Peer interaction among providers	6. Less provider incentive for care
7. Better administration of group	7. More bureaucracy
8. Efficiency may be promoted in patient care	
9. Possibly better knowledge of medical care cost	

[a]From Williams (1980). Note that some advantages and disadvantages could be included under both the provider and the patient category.

elderly (>65) accounted for about a quarter (23.3%) of all visits, while females made 59.8% of all office visits. The largest proportion of office visits were to physicians specializing in family and general practice (24.6%). The proportion of office visits from referrals increased slightly between 1990 and 1991, from 5.5% to 6.2%.

There appears to be consistency in the kinds of physicians most Americans see, including follow-up visits to them. In 1991, for instance, most patients (83.3%) making an office visit had seen the same physician previously, and 6 out of 10 visits were follow-up visits for a previously treated medical episode. Because of the many ways of paying for visits, as well as the different types of copayments, no clear pattern emerges of the kind of financial profile that is most conducive to ambulatory visits. About one third (35.8%) of ambulatory visits were paid for by commercial insurance, and 23.6% were financed by out-of-pocket payments. Medicare coverage accounted for 21.2% of all ambulatory visits, while prepaid plans and HMOs accounted for 15.1% (CDCP, 1994, p. 2).

Patients' age, sex, race, and geographic location revealed different pattens of ambulatory care utilization. As noted earlier, women made most (59.8%) of all office visits in 1991, translating into an average of 3.1 visits for females versus 2.2 visits for males. Visits increased notably beyond age 24. White persons accounted for 87.8% of all visits, while African-Americans and Asian-Pacific Islanders registered 8.7% and 3.0%, respectively. White persons on average had a higher annual visitation rate (2.8 visits per person) than African-Americans (1.9 visits) in 1991, suggesting that demographically related structural barriers to care share equal footing with characteristics of the physical environment in shaping utilization behavior. Geographically, rates did not vary significantly among the Midwest, West, and Northeast. The South, however, registered an overall lower visit rate than the rest of the country, possibly due to financial accessibility.

The pattern of ambulatory utilization breaks down clearly by physician specialty. Of the 13 specialties for which there were data in 1991, the 4 leading specialties (general and family practice, internal medicine, pediatrics, and obstetrics and gynecology) accounted for nearly 60% of all ambulatory visits. The least utilized specialties (psychiatry, urological surgery, cardiovascular diseases, and neurology) registered just 18.8% of all ambulatory visits. The general breakdown of specialty utilization is in line with general patterns of utilization in recent years.

Ambulatory clinics are usually free-standing facilities not connected to the hospital with which they associate. They fill a gap left by the abdication of private doctors in caring for the poor or the uninsured, provide convenience for day surgery, and serve as a transfer point for patient referral. Since the early 1980s, free-standing ambulatory facilities (known as "doc-in-the boxes") serve a market niche directed at middle-income patients, or at least those patients with a credit card. Minor household or sports injuries can easily be handled in these free-standing facilities, and the costs are lower than those of outpatient treatments in hospital emergency rooms. As well, minor acute episodes such as colds, flus, and abrasions can readily be treated at these facilities when regular caregivers are unavailable or their offices are closed. Indeed, the suburban landscape of America shows an increase of these free-standing ambulatory care centers as they vie for locations comparable to those of other retailers in convenience and locational attributes.

The first free-standing ambulatory center opened in Phoenix, Arizona, in 1970. Indeed, the South and West of the United States have registered the greatest regional growth in these new facilities. Lowell-Smith (1993) contends that these regions represent a more lenient regulatory setting that allows providers to set up those (mainly) for-profit facilities, and are also home to a rapidly growing "sun belt" population (south, southeast, southwest, and west coast states) that lacks a regular provider because of the large numbers of newcomers from other regions. The sun belt is also the environment in which all types of for-profit health care facilities are increasing faster than the national rate, as is the percentage of the medically vulnerable (Bohland, 1990). In 1983, these centers performed about 400,000 minor surgical procedures on an outpatient basis, increasing fivefold (to 2,000,000) by 1989 (Henderson, 1989). By 1992, these ambulatory centers provided 17% of all outpatient surgery (Henderson, 1993). Unfortunately, more is known about the provider side of these centers than about the user profiles of patients attending them.

PATTERNS OF HOSPITAL UTILIZATION IN THE UNITED STATES

Hospitals and clinics are the modern shrines of the medical-care system, with their wondrous collection of diagnostic and imaging technology. As well-defined points in the landscape, they symbolize power, expertise, and a semiotic space in which patient and provider converge (Apter & Sawa 1984; Feinsilver, 1993). Access to hospitals and tertiary care clinics usually requires referral from a provider who is recognized by the facility, except in emergency settings. The great American dilemma stems from the 37 million uninsured persons who often appear in the emergency rooms of hospitals and clinics for nonemergency care or for care that could be provided in another ambulatory setting (Koop, 1993). The heavy loading of self-referral cases in central urban hospitals has had the long-standing stigma of producing "conflict arising from efforts to cull the 'illegitimate' patients" (Roth, 1971, p. 319). Clearly, determining who is "legitimate" and who is not, coupled with lengthy waits, makes nonemergency treatment in emergency rooms an unpleasant experience for the patient. Whether it is in regard to seeking medical care at a hospital or clinic by default (uninsured) or through a referral (insured), the following question raised in the late 1970s seems more germane than ever: "The hospital is symbolic of the Western cult of technology that preserves life, and that people have been willing to invest in it to the point of their own bankruptcy, we must raise the question: is it important?" (Twaddle & Hessler, 1977, pp. 234-235).

Hospitals certainly are important, since they are the major setting for secondary and tertiary care. Curiously, though, nonmedical factors have determined their use in the recent past more than have medical factors. The average length of stay (ALOS), for instance, has fallen in most kinds of hospitals (see below). Insurance plans and prospective payment criteria have curtailed the allowable length of reimbursable internment. Teaching hospitals generate costlier medical encounters and, traditionally, attract more interesting (rare) cases for the medical students' education, differing somewhat from the kinds of options available at nonteaching facilities. Nonmedical amenities, also part of a place's attributes, may play a role—about which little is known—in how the patient perceives the quality of medical care and in the psychological impact the patient's state of mind (as determined by such variables as physical design, cleanliness, judgment of food, staff treatment, room decor) has on medical outcomes.

The hospital's traditional linkages to the community at large, other than referrals made by medical staff, include two types of outpatient clinics: the emergency room and the ambulatory-care clinic. Emergency rooms aim to provide crisis management of highly acute and sudden-onset trauma. As noted, emergency rooms in many United States cities are increasingly being used for nonemergency routine care that could be provided in an ambulatory clinic or physician's office. Whether because of inconvenient primary care physician hours or a lack of insurance on the part of patients, emergency rooms provide a good amount of nonemergency care, and this care has cost implications. They do not serve as major referral points for consuming secondary or tertiary care, however, except when warranted; fiscal pressures tend to force emergency rooms to stabilize patients and discharge them as soon as clinically feasible.

Because the hospital is perhaps the most visible "symbol" in the United States health care landscape, it deserves description in this discussion of the physical environment of health care. Several patterns emerge in the utilization of hospitals over the past decades, reflecting structural changes in the United States health care delivery system. Since 1980, the number of beds, average daily census, occupancy rate, and ALOS have declined in United States community hospitals. These include state and local government hospitals, private for-profit hospitals, and private not-for-profit hospitals. The same trend is apparent in state and local government hospitals alone, except in the ALOS, which has risen from 7.3 days in 1980 to 7.8 days in 1991. One interpretation is that the rising cost of hospitalization is forcing more patients (and bad debt) into these public hospitals. In contrast, private for-profit community hospitals have had lower and more stable ALOSs than their public counterparts (6.5 days in 1980 and 6.3 days in 1991), reflecting perhaps the greater ability of the for-profit management to screen their patients. A similar though less striking pattern surfaces among nongovernmental not-for-profit community hospitals (e.g., Catholic hospitals).

The next two figures distinguish trends in utilization for selected years from 1950 through 1991 for investor-owned (for-profit) short-term general and other hospitals (Figure 2) and their nongovernmental nonprofit counterparts (Figure

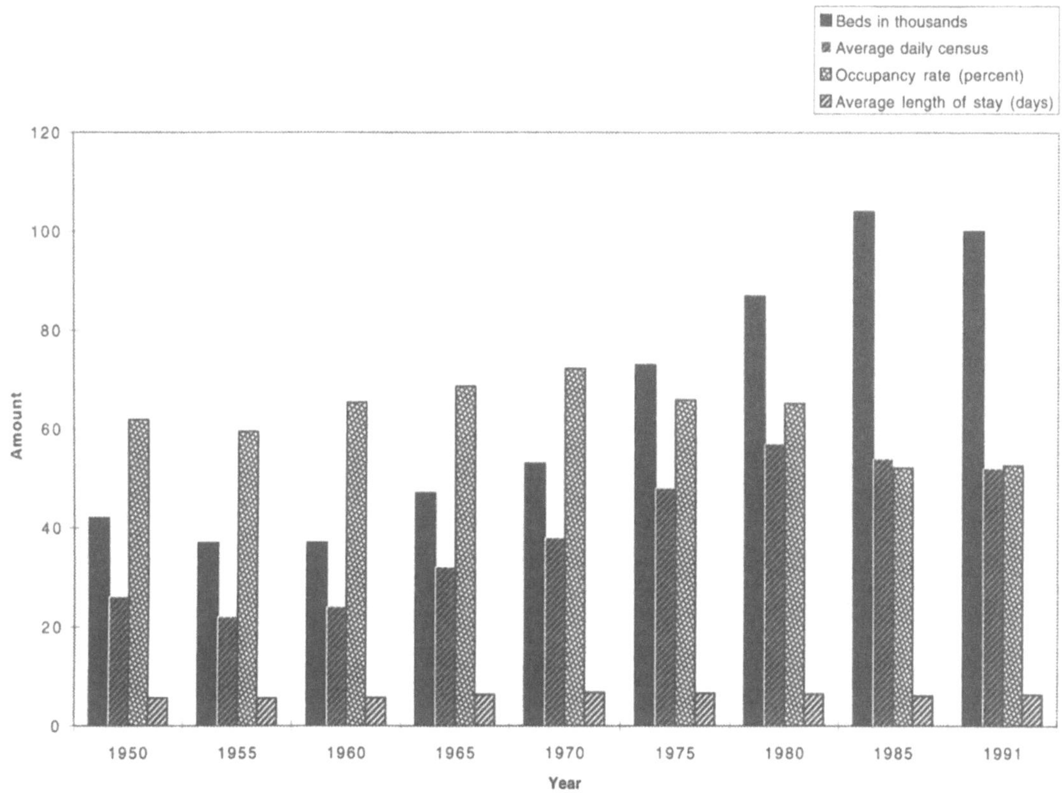

Figure 2. Trends in utilization for selected years from 1950 through 1991 for investor-owned (for-profit) short-term general and other special hospitals.

3). Between 1970 and 1985, the number of for-profit beds nearly doubled in the United States. After peaking in 1970, occupancy rates fell to just under 60% for for-profits in 1991 (Figure 2), while averaging 68.6% for nonprofits in 1991 (Figure 3). Thus, the nature of hospital ownership over the past few decades reveals that private, for-profit hospitals have historically had lower occupancy and ALOS rates. These supply-side features, however, say nothing about the motivations and help-seeking behaviors of the patients in these health care settings. Instead, they reflect the corporatization of health care in the United States as a defining feature in hospitalization (Bohland & Knox, 1989; Salmon, 1985).

The next section examines a case study of patient use and satisfaction with care from the demand side of the health care encounter. Such an examination raises questions about the ways in which patients react to the physical, social, and even political context of the health care environment.

HELP-SEEKING BEHAVIORS: PREDICTING USE OF AND SATISFACTION WITH CARE

Considerable international research has attempted to distill the essential features of environmental attributes of health care facilities in

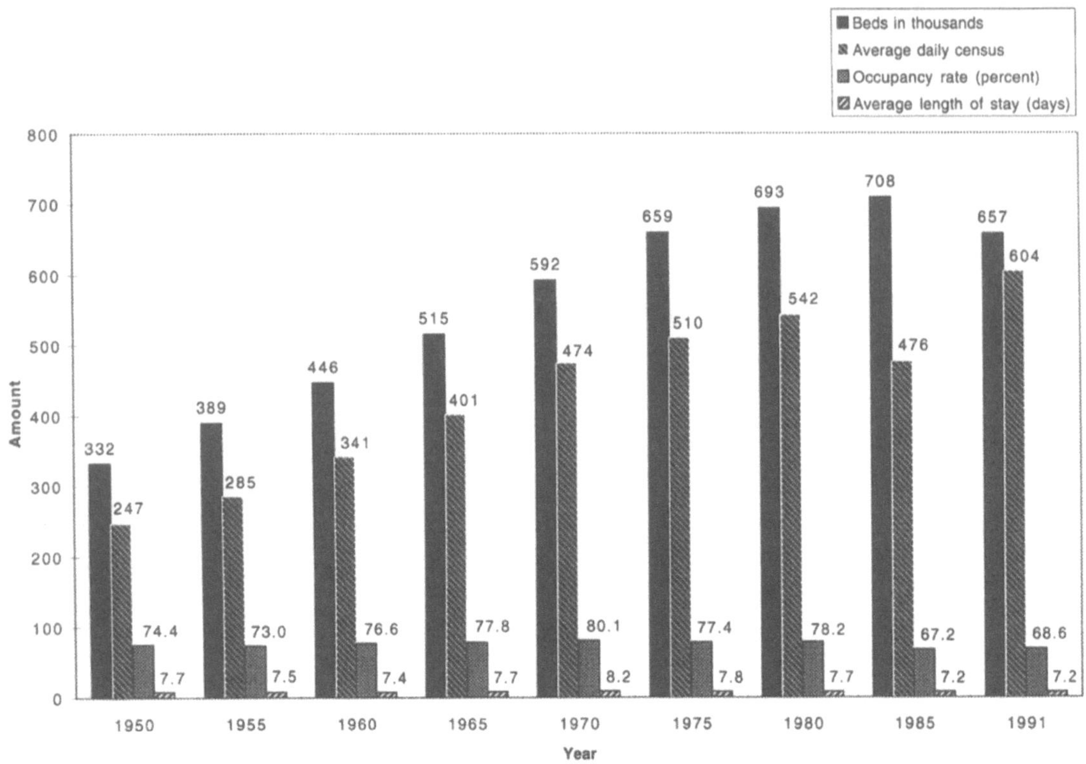

Figure 3. Trends in utilization for selected years from 1950 through 1991 for nongovernment not-for-profit short-term general and other special hospitals.

trying to predict use and satisfaction. Methodologically, the task is compounded by trying to hold constant the attributes of the patients while assessing their interaction with health care delivery setting. As noted, spatial variables are antecedents to seeking care. The Bice and White (1971) review of the World Health Organization's international study of medical care utilization found that the "use of physicians' services decreases ... with increasing distance to physicians. Regardless of income bracket, the use of physician services is distinctly greater among persons living near a physician than among other distance groups ..." (p. 254). Kohn and White (1976, p. 50) found in a similar international study that 77% of all patients lived within 15 minutes of an ambulatory care center.

While the distance factor seems well documented, the attributes of place and their allure to patients are less clear. Cultural differences in consumer beliefs and values about the composition of "good" care complicate any universal truth. The seminal study by Cartwright (1967) of general practitioners in England and Wales is insightful. Based on open-ended responses, Cartwright asked British patients to identify the attributes of physicians that they appreciated most. None of the respondents claimed that being physically touched by a physician was an important characteristic of their physician examination. By contrast, "touching" was often cited in a study of 140 low-income patients at a public health clinic in Santiago, Chile (Scarpaci, 1988a). Following Freidson (1961), it would appear that patients' definitions of physician competence is strongly tied to the kind of "personal interest" physicians display. "Personal interest" is culturally defined, however, as shown by the British and Chilean studies.

Methodological Issues

Highly accurate models have yet to be developed that predict the satisfaction of care and the frequency of utilization of care based on variables that assess the health care "environment" (both physical and cultural). Shortell (1980) showed that regression models of utilization in biomedical settings usually explain 15-25% of variance. Mechanic (1979) found that explained variance ranges between 16% and 25%. Wolinsky (1978) assembled 29 independent variables in trying to explain the utilization of services but could explain only between 9% and 12% of model variance and patient satisfaction levels. In the same study of low-income Chileans noted earlier, Scarpaci (1988a) found that only 26% of model variance in predicting patient satisfaction and 29% of model variance in predicting the quality of care were explained by multiple-regression models. That multivariate models of utilization and satisfaction explain relatively little variance may derive from specification or measurement error, calling into question the role of validity in variable conceptualization (Scarpaci, 1993). Moreover, there may be little variation in the dependent variable because of a "halo effect" in patient response; patients generally answer favorably so as not to appear rude and ungrateful.

Clearly, there is inherent difficulty in comparative medical care research and the assessment of qualitative aspects of medical care encounters. As Kohn and White (1976) pointed out some time ago, nonmaterial variables are difficult to conceptualize, let alone operationalize. However, these relatively low rates of explained variance point to the need to step back from formal measurement and, through alternative methodologies, attempt to understand (rather than explain) the locational attributes of health behavior. The following section presents insights into the links between place, space, and health that have been gained when the rigor of conventional survey research has been maintained.

PLACE, SPACE, AND HEALTH

It is the profession and practice of medicine, as expressed in the landscape through patterns of health care delivery, that has preoccupied this chapter. Social scientists are increasingly recognizing, however, that health and medicine involve different, and at times competing, discourses and belief structures. Indeed, a significant body of research has shown that in Western societies, the most enduring determinants of health status are social (Eyer, 1985). Employment status and income levels, for example, have been cited as critical determinants of health in the much-publicized Black Report in Britain (Townsend & Davidson, 1982). A decade after this controversial report was released, it was shown not only that the patterns of gradients in class affiliation and health status had persisted, but also that the disparities had widened (Davey Smith, Bartley, & Blane, 1990). These findings endorse a view that while the empirical reality of disease remains grounded in the realm of biomedical science, the experience of health and ill health is ultimately a socially constructed phenomenon.

This recognition of the social construction of health experience is a cue for social scientists to take seriously lay perceptions, experiences, and beliefs in terms of how they can shape the meaning of geographically specific medical care. As Eyles (1993) notes, the vantage point of the medical practitioner or health care provider should not be granted special privilege in the quest to understand health experience. This perspective can assist in understanding the locational attributes of health behavior. The intellectual formula for achieving such pluralism calls for an infusion of humanistic perspectives that aims to situate the determinants of health behavior somewhere between the conventional empirical approaches to health care utilization and the more phenomenological dimensions of health experience. This involves viewing the idea of place as not just location, but further as a relationship between social position (i.e., "place in the world") and a center of lived meaning (Eyer, 1985; Kearns, 1994).

A point of departure for a humanistic perspective on health care delivery is the recognition that health care settings can be more than simply locations within urban or rural space; rather they can be meaningful places that, because of their symbolism or nonmedical functions, can take on an "added value above and beyond places of health care per se. A key concept for appreciating these "extralocational" dimensions of health care facilities is sense of place, which, according to Tuan (1974), involves the meaning people attach to places that have a particular significance for them.

In traditional conceptualizations of place and space by geographers and other social scientists interested in the locational attributes of health behavior, "place" has been at last implicitly equated with location, and "space" has been represented in geometric terms. Nodes of health care delivery such as hospitals and clinics have therefore been studies as places of service delivery within urban or rural space and its more abstract representations (such as Central Place Theory discussed earlier). In this context, space has been viewed as simply a container for activities. Of course, the world is neither as simple nor as bland as these social scientific abstractions, so researchers have acknowledged the effects of tangible barriers to accessing health care facilities such as topographic features. Such barriers to physical accessibility are less common in urban environments, but other locales present barriers to effective accessibility, such as inefficient public transport networks, unacceptably high costs, or the language difficulties and class conflicts experienced by patients in attempts to consult a physician (Joseph & Phillips, 1984; Scarpaci, 1988b). This focus on potential accessibility (or utilization behavior) assumes, however, that service delivery sites are point-specific locations rather than experienced and meaning-laden places. In this section, work connecting space, place, and health will be explored and highlighted with examples from New Zealand research.

Earlier sections of this chapter have argued that the location of services as well as institutional and facility characteristics can influence the utilization behaviors of patients. Three further dimensions of location will be discussed from the perspective that health care facilities are more than simply sites of activity. These interrelated dimensions are symbolism, sense of place, and the nonmedical role of health care locations. They will be considered with respect to New Zealand health care examples: private accident and medical clinics, home as a birthing place, and isolated rural clinics. As Gesler (1991) points out, one can "read" places for their symbolic meaning. Symbols have discrete locations; indeed, they may be concrete in the literal sense in the case of monuments. Yet less obvious elements of the build environment such as hospitals can also have strongly symbolic properties that can be "read off" the landscape through the lens of local culture. Modern medical facilities symbolize authority and influence the context in which patient and provider meet (Apter & Sawa, 1984). A rural community hospital, for instance, may have been built through local efforts, and may be a site of significant local employment, serving not only as a medical center but also indirectly as a place of sociability and information exchange. Thus, a hospital can symbolize more than simply a local component of the regional health care system. Rather, it can become an integral part of the fabric of a community with threats of closures precipitating considerable mobilization and protest (Kearns & Joseph, 1993; Joseph & Kearns, in press).

In Western countries such as New Zealand, health sector reforms have involved the introduction of market-based ideology and the subsequent construction of health care as a product rather than a service. As health care users have been recast as "consumers" rather than "patients," so too has the symbolism of health care facilities changed. Greater prominence has been given to signs and advertising, with clinics themselves increasingly becoming embedded within landscapes of consumption, often juxtaposed with activities such as cafes and retail stores. Under the influence of "postmodern" architecture and the culture of consumption, newer for-profit health care facilities proclaim their location through "place advertisement" techniques. In other words, bold design, catchy slogans, and locations adjacent to shopping malls have significantly altered the sense of place experienced by users. In a patient survey, over one fifth of Auckland respondents at two such clinics rated aspects of the ambiance of the clinic as features they most liked (out-rating issues such as cost and quality of medical care). Thus, for these users, the *form* of the clinics appeared to rival their *function* in importance. From this perspective, the consumption of health care clearly involved more than just the purchase of services at selected sites from providers with certain qualities. Rather, it involved the generation of patterns of behavior by means of the design of service sites, the image of health care projected, and the advertising of the product consumed. Indeed, inasmuch as "consumers" report enjoying simply being in these new clinics, one can go as far as to say that the spaces of health care provision are consumed in the course of visiting the places of medical care (Barnett & Kearns, in press).

The idea of "sense of place" has been developed by so-called "humanistic" geographers to describe the consciousness that people have of places that have a special significance to them. Most obviously, this consciousness relates to home, where people feel "in-place" rather than "dis-placed" (Kearns, 1993). This perspective on place can provide a tool to interpret the recent revival of home as a locus of health behavior, evidenced in the home birthing as well as the home death (or hospice) movements. Earlier in the chapter, changing utilization patterns generated by maternity services in the United States were described. In New Zealand, the trend toward home birthing has been given impetus by the Nurses Amendment Act (1990), which legalized independent midwifery. By the mid-1990s, approximately 4% of births occurred at home. In a study exploring the perspectives of women choosing this option, three dimensions of the home location (compared to hospital) were identified by participants as important: the higher degree of *control* they could experience at home, the continuity they experienced from pregnancy to parenthood in both social support and place of care, and the sense of feeling in-place in their home environments (Abel & Kearns, 1992). Central to this analysis was a recognition that home is a place of paramount significance in women's lives, and not simply another maternity service location option within urban space. The women's narratives revealed that whereas they might have felt *dis-placed* in a hospital setting, they felt very much *in-place* (as well as in control) in their home environment. It is important to point out that this example is not presented to suggest that all women will feel similarly about the home location. Indeed, it is likely that the majority of women will continue to feel better placed seeking obstetric care in institutional settings.

Home has been described by Tuan (1974) as a broad, elastic concept, and indeed the firmer the links between people and place, the more a dwelling or local community can satisfy the basic human need for roots. Although the idea of place has been extensively investigated by geographers, there has been little examination of the ways in which the presence and use of health facilities can add to the experience of place itself. In a study of the significance of publicly funded community outpatient clinics in the Hokianga, a remote rural area populated predominantly by Maori in northern New Zealand, "clinic day" was shown to be more than simply an occasion for physician-patient interactions (Kearns, 1991). Rather, it was an opportunity for the broader "health" of the community itself to be enhanced through social interaction and information exchange in the waiting areas of the clinics. Through fieldwork that involved a standardized period of participant observation at each of the ten community clinics, it was established that the highest proportion of waiting area conversations (23% overall) involved community concerns. A wide range of issues were noted as being discussed (e.g., the condition of local roads, the problem of wandering dogs, progress toward fund raising for a community canoeing team). Significantly, the second most frequent conversation category (16%) was health concerns. Patients were observed to be discussing not their personal ailments, but—sometimes prompted by posters and pamphlets—general health issues such as what types of food should be featured at community events. Of particular interest is that some people who came and participated in clinic conversations in the waiting areas had no intention of consulting the visiting physician or nurse. Rather, they recognized the clinic as a location that generated a sociable context in which information could be exchanged.

This study indicates that one implication of bringing health services to the population served rather than expecting individuals and families to travel out of their area to seek care is that people feel more at ease to talk, both to the service providers and to others sharing the medical setting, to whom the clinic has become as familiar as the school or general store. The center of the Hokianga health system is a 32-bed hospital at Rawene, and here a survey was undertaken asking all those present at the hospital on a particular day (patients as well as medical and general staff) what they considered to be unique about the hospital. It was found that 68% of respondents cited place-centered perceptions (e.g., "the family atmosphere"), rather than health system characteristics (e.g., ease of admitting patients) (Kearns, 1991).

Each of these examples has pointed toward medical interactions being a necessary but not sufficient element in the experience of health care places. The experience of place involves dimensions such as "belonging" that are hard to quantify, yet are fundamental to human experience. Seeking an understanding of these dimensions through qualitative methodologies can therefore provide rich insights into the way locations of health care can have "added value" in terms of people's experience of place.

STRUCTURE, AGENCY, AND HELP-SEEKING BEHAVIOR

This section suggests a merger between a socioecological perspective in examining health behavior and health care settings and the ways in which patients experience place. This approach consists of methodologies that draw on the quantitative and empirically descriptive statistics of documenting a delivery system and the more qualitative and interpretive methods used to gauge how consumers experience different places discussed in the last section. To illustrate this, the discussion draws on the help-seeking behavior of a low-income population in Santiago, Chile.

In 1983, Chile was in its tenth year under military rule. During the previous decade, social expenditures, including those for health care, had been sharply curtailed, as the government aimed to introduce more privately financed delivery of medical care. This policy change departed markedly from a trend since the 1950s of increasing the size and scope of the welfare state in Chile (Scarpaci, 1990).

Three kinds of health services existed in 1983; public health clinics and hospitals run by the National Health Service System for the indigent or working poor, public and private facilities for middle-income users of the National Health Fund (partially subsidized care), and private facilities for the well-off. About 70% of the nation received medical care from the first category, the National Health Service System, from which the following study is taken.

Figure 4 represents a hypothetical accessibility surface based on a set of assumptions. An algorithm generated by a SYMAP graphics program mapped out peaks of relatively good accessibility and valleys of areas that are relatively deprived. Using data from 54 primary care clinics, a hypothetical accessibility surface was gener-

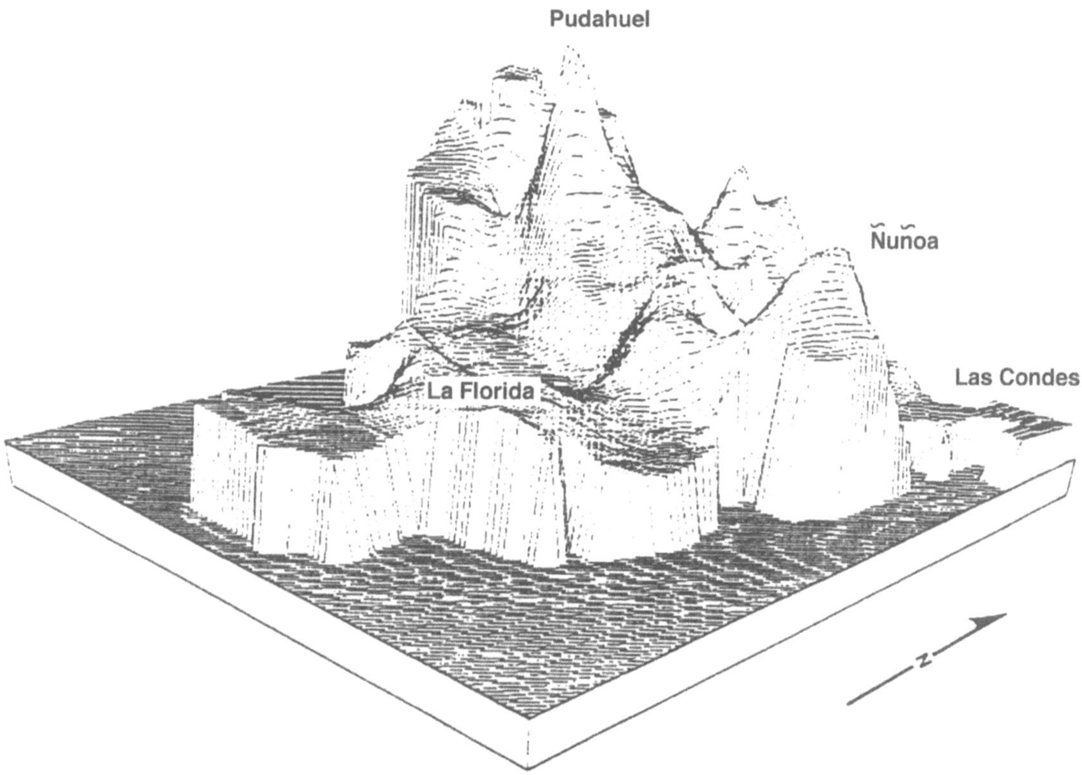

Figure 4. Accessibility surface of primary care in Santiago, Chile.

ated using interpolation for each clinic's service area across the contiguous metropolitan surface. The number of physician hours worked weekly at each facility represented the supply of medical care, while the aggregate demand was estimated based on the density of clinics in a particular area and the relative isolation or proximity of clinics to each other. Underlying this calculation is the notion that Euclidean space could be used as a surrogate for actual utilization because no topographic barriers exist in the valley of Santiago. Health care, moreover, is free. The calculation for the model generating the accessibility surface is:

$$A_i = \sum_{i=1}^{n=54} \frac{Sj}{Dij^k}$$

where *Ai* is the summary index of accessibility of clinics at point *i*, *Sj* is the size of the clinic at location *j* measured by the number of physician hours worked weekly, *Dij* is the distance between *i* and *j*, *k* is the distance-decay function denoting the falloff in attendance at a given facility, and *n* is the number of clinics (54).

The accessibility surface identifies disparity in the primary health care environment of Santiago, Chile (Figure 4). Municipalities to the south (such as La Florida) have clinics that are less accessible than most others. By contrast, municipalities on the western edge of the metropolis (Pudahuel) have relatively "better" accessibility to primary health care clinics. This better accessibility results from the greater supply of physician hours worked weekly and the greatly density of clinics in that part of the city. Under the assumptions of no topographic barriers and free access to medical facilities, the commuter-generated surface presents one dimension of the role of the physical environment. This top-down metropolitan planning approach does not measure, however, the perceptions and levels of satisfaction among users of these facilities.

The investigation of these low-income health care users next moved into predictors of patient use of and satisfaction with primary medical care. A survey of 140 frequent users of primary care provided the primary data for the regression trials. Variables from the questionnaire comprised one of two models: demographic and organizational. Demographic variables (age, life cycle, family size, gender) are fixed attributes of users and are not amenable to administrative intervention. These immutable features of the user population are helpful, however, in pointing out group needs. Organizational variables assess clinical procedures performed on patients, factors influencing their travel and waiting time, ecological conditions of patients' neighborhoods, and their spatial behavior while seeking primary care. The organizational model, unlike its demographic counterpart, is subject to administrative or policy intervention (Scarpaci, 1988a, p. 88; Shortell, 1980, p. 67).

A series of regression trials sought out the best general linear model in predicting the frequency of visits. Six variables explained 26.8% of the model variance; half of the variables were locational (travel time, waiting time, and interaction variable created by crossing travel time and linear distance from clinic to home) and half were demographic (time ill before coming to clinic, mother accompanying young child, and a life-cycle variable measuring the presence of children in the home). Intuitively, the model is appealing because it suggests that mothers with young children who live relatively close to the family make up a good share of the user population. As experienced patients, they are more familiar with the clinic procedures and methods for securing a turn in the lengthy queue, which often requires getting to the clinic before dawn to reserve a limited spot (telephone appointments were not accepted).

The same study examined a set of variables that would best predict patient satisfaction. This inquiry moved the discussion from the macroscale of health planning to the intricacies of patient perceptions about the medical encounter, place, and space. The dependent variable—a Likert-scale response measuring whether patients found the primary medical-care examination to be very good, good, fair, poor, or very poor—was best predicted by four independent variables that explained 29.6% of model variance. These independent variables measured whether or not patients disliked something about the clinic in an open-ended response, whether or not the physician touched them or displayed interest in them, the receipt of a free prescription drug or a referral to diagnostic procedures at the local hospital (usually a blood test or an X ray), and the presence of young children in the household. the findings show that patients differentiate between the place and space of health care provision (an average 4.2-hour queue, dirty facility and bathrooms, discourteous ancillary staff who schedule appointments) from the medical encounter (the care and concern displayed by the attending physician). When patients were asked why they had made their Likert-scale responses about care, the majority said "The physician touched me" or "The doctor examined me well and listened." Clearly, no physical examination can occur without physical contact between provider and patient. Follow-up questioning with the patients and the physicians revealed that the "touching" and "listening" responses underscored the different class backgrounds of the two groups and the physicians showed no disdain toward the patient. Normally, when patients perceive that physicians are standoffish, they contend that the physicians hurry through the examination, with disdain for them. In this instance, however, patients did not perceive that the college-educated physicians—with distinct language and dress that placed them in the upper-income neighborhood of Santiago (*barrio alto*)—were rushed during the average 20-minute examination. It is noteworthy that the urban poor at this clinic were using one of the as yet untouched public services that had not been privatized or greatly curtailed in the free-market privatizations that characterized the military government since 1973. Despite the dismantling of the Chilean welfare state, patients also replied that they attended that particular clinic because they felt a sense of affiliation with it and that it was a right (*un derecho*) of their citizenship, and not just because they lived in that service area. Once again, patients were able to tease out the medical encounter and the place and space of health care provision (Scarpaci, 1988a).

This example of the help-seeking behavior of the Santiago urban poor reveals the interplay between structure and human agency, a conceptualization often ignored in the study of the physical environments of health settings. Human agency in its starkest form refers to the capabilities of humans (Gregory, 1994). Cutler, Hindess, Hirst, and Hussain (1977) contend that human agency includes those entities that are capable of occupying the locus of decisions in a set of social relations that are determined by custom or law. By extension, one can see in the context of help-seeking behavior the comportment of patients who not only behave within the confines of the "sick role," but also are capable of assessing satisfaction within a physical, cultural, and political setting. The Chilean study found patients perceiving the quality of care at three levels: (1) the facility and its ancillary staff, (2) the medical encounter between patient and physician, and (3) the larger political economy of Chile in 1983. Levels (1) and (2) represent the structural factors in the human agency and structure equation. Methodologically, it is clear that a combination of techniques must be employed in order to assess the essence of the "meaning" of the health care and help-seeking behavior; closed- and open-ended responses, multiple regression, and the sociopolitical environment in which the patient lives all relate to outcomes of quality care and frequency of use.

If structure and agency are important conceptual categories in the study of the physical settings of health care behavior, then researchers must search for new, multidisciplinary ways of operationalizing and conceptualizing "setting," "location," and "quality care." Giddens (1984) has argued that although human agency has been defined in terms of patients' intentions, the crux of analyses should aim to integrate the physical and psychosocial locational attributes of health care settings. Doing so enables researchers to infuse studies of place ("bricks and mortar") with socially defined meaning. Extending this argument to the patient-environment setting, it must be recognized that patients' interactions with a health care delivery system are not all purposive. Patients may seek solace from providers as a means to allay some of the pressures of urban poverty. Symptomatic children may be likely to get better without medical intervention, but that is little comfort to a distraught parent. Lastly, patients no doubt tell physicians and social scientists things that are socially acceptable given the prescribed roles of "physician" and "researcher." In the end, multiple-regression left about 70% of the variance "unexplained" in predicting utilization ($r^2 = 0.268$) and satisfaction ($r^2 = 0.296$) (Scarpaci, 1988b).

Mechanic (1979, p. 387) asked rhetorically, "Why do major multivariate studies of physician utilization find trivial psychosocial and organizational effects?" The answer may lie in variable misspecification. It is clear, however, that multiple regression is just one response from a logical positivist perspective. Researchers may move closer to understanding the complex facets of patient and provider interaction, and the attendant effects of the physical environment, by conceptualizing their questions in the human agency and structure framework.

CONCLUSIONS

The locational attributes of the health care encounter are related in complex ways to how patients perceive the quality of care. Nonmedical amenities in the United States health care system shape help-seeking behavior in ways that may be better understood by corporate marketers than by social scientists. Researchers have a better grasp of the institutional and facility aspects of health care delivery and the geographic and administrative array of services than they do of the psychosocial factors that motivate patients. However, health services, from primary care to specialty tertiary services, consistently demonstrate a spatial pattern that stems from the population threshold required to sustain that economic activity. Indeed, the changing suburban landscape in America increasingly reveals new modes of delivery such as free-standing ambulatory care centers, which were rare as recently as the 1970s.

Changing modes of health care finance and the questioning of authority by consumers combine to give new meaning to today's health care setting. No longer is the physician an isolated agent who works out of a back office and whose supplies and tools are all contained in the "little black bag." Nevertheless, two out of three Americans still visit a general and family practice physician, and this remains the main setting for ambulatory visits. Ambulatory care also continues to show greater use among women, a pattern that has held steady for some time. Hospital utilization has become more varied because of the rise of for-profit investor-owned facilities and the decline of the community nonprofit hospital. As health care continues to consume an increasing share of the gross domestic product, these new types of for-profit settings appear to achieve the seemingly impossible task of containing cost and capturing market share.

If locational attributes of health care delivery shape the nature of the medical encounter, the examples presented in this chapter suggest a need to look for new methodologies and concepts to understand the role of concepts such as human agency and sense of place in research. To that end, the role of human agency in research on help-seeking behaviors has been decidedly absent. Logical positivist approaches, mainly through multivariate studies, fail to fully "explain" what best predicts patient use and satisfaction. Filling this void could easily constitute a research agenda for years to come.

REFERENCES

Abel, S., & Kearns, R. A. (1992). Birth places: A geographical perspective on planned home birth in New Zealand. *Social Science and Medicine*, *33*, 825-834.

Allman, R. M., Yoels, W. C., & Clair, J. M. (1993). Reconciling the agendas of physicians and patients. In J. M. Clair & R. M. Allman (Eds.), *Sociomedical perspectives on patient care* (pp. 29-46). Lexington: University Press of Kentucky.

Apter, D. W., & Sawa, N. (1984). *Against the state: Politics and social protest in Japan*. Cambridge, MA: Harvard University Press.

Barnett, J. R., & Kearns, R. A. (in press). Shopping around: Consumerism and the use of private accident and medical clinics in Auckland, New Zealand. *Environment and planning A.*

Bice, T. W., & White, K. L. (1971). Cross-national comparative research and the utilization of medical care. *Medical Care*, *9*, 253-271.

Bohland, J. (1990). State variations in the distribution of the medically vulnerable: The impact of health policy. In K. Kodras & J. P. Jones (Eds.), *Geographic dimensions of United States social policy* (pp. 134-153). London: Edward Arnold.

Bohland, J., & Knox, P. (1989). Growth of proprietary hospitals in the United States: A historical geographic perspective. In J. L. Scarpaci (Ed.), *Health services privatization in industrial societies* (pp. 26-64). New Brunswick, NJ: Rutgers University Press.

Caper, P. (1988). Defining quality in medical fare. *Health Affairs*, 7, 1.

Cartwright, A. (1967). *Patients and their doctors: A study of general practice*. New York: Atherton.

CDCP (Centers for Disease Control and Prevention). (1994). *Vital and health statistics: National ambulatory medical care survey: 1991 summary*. DHHS Publication No. (PHS) 94-1777. Washington, DC: U.S. Government Printing Office.

Ciocco, A., & Altman, I. (1954). *Medical service areas and distances traveled for physician care in western Pennsylvania*. PAS Monograph No. 19. Bethesda, MD: U.S. Public Health Service.

Cleverley, W. O., & Harvey, R. K. (1992). Is there a link between hospital profit and quality? *Healthcare Financial Management*, *9*, 72-80.

Cutler, A., Hindess, B., Hirst, P., & Hussain, A. (1977). *Marx's capital and capitalism today*. London: Routledge and Kegan Paul.

Davey Smith, G., Bartley, M., & Blane, D. (1990). The Black Report on socioeconomic inequalities in health ten years on. *British Medical Journal*, *301*, 373-377.

Donabedian, A. (1980). *Explorations in quality assessment and monitoring: Vol. 1. The definition of quality and approaches to its assessment*. Ann Arbor, MI: Health Administration Press.

Donabedian, A. (1985). *Explorations in quality assessment and monitoring: Vol. 3. The methods and findings of quality assessment and monitoring*. Ann Arbor, MI: Health Administration Press.

Ernst, R. L., & Yett, D. E. (1985). *Physician location and specialty choice*. Ann Arbor, MI: Health Administration Press.

Evans, H. H. (1993). High tech vs. "high touch": The impact of a medical technology on patient care. In J. M. Clair & R. M. Allman (Eds.), *Sociomedical perspectives on patient care* (pp. 82-95). Lexington: University Press of Kentucky.

Eyer, J. (1985). Capitalism, health and illness. In J. B. McKinlay (Ed.), *Issues in the political economy of health care* (pp. 23-59). New York: Tavistock.

Eyles, J. (1993). Feminist and interpretive method: How different? *The Canadian Geographer, 37*, 50-52.

Feinsilver, J. (1993). *Healing the masses: Cuban health politics at home and abroad*. Berkeley: University of California Press.

Feldstein, P. J. (1981). Economic success for hospitals depends on their adaptability. *Journal of the American Hospital Association, 55*(2), 77-79.

Fisher, S. (1988). *In the patient's best interest: Women and the politics of medical decisions*. New Brunswick, NJ: Rutgers University Press.

Freidson, E. (1961). *Patients' view of medical practice*. New York: Russell Sage Foundation.

Gesler, W. (1991). *The cultural geography of health care*. Pittsburgh: University of Pittsburgh Press.

Giddens, A. (1984). *The constitution of society*. Cambridge, MA: Polity Press.

Good, C. (1987). *Ethnomedical systems in Africa*. New York: Guilford Press.

Gregory, D. (1994). Human agency. In R. J. Johnston, D. Gregory, and D. M. Smith (Eds.), *The dictionary of human geography*. London: Blackwell.

Hawley, A. (1950). *Human ecology: A theoretical essay*. New York: Ronald Press.

Henderson, H. (1989). Surgery centers' success challenges hospitals. *Modern Healthcare, 19*, 78-80.

Henderson, H. (1993). Surgicenters cut further into market. *Modern Healthcare, 22*, 108-110.

Jehlick, P. J., & McNamara, R. L. (1952). The relation of distance to the differential use of certain health personnel and facilities and to the extent of bed illness. Rural Sociology, *17*, 261-265.

Joseph, A. E., & Kearns, R. A. (in press). Deinstitutionalization meets restructuring: The closure of a psychiatric hospital in New Zealand. *Health and Place*.

Joseph, A. E., & Phillips, D. R. (1984). *Accessibility and utilization: Geographical perspectives on health care delivery*. New York: Harper & Row.

Katz, G., Mitchell, A., & Markezin, E. (1982). *Ambulatory care and regionalization in multi-institutional health systems*. Rockville, MD, and London: Aspen.

Kearns, R. A. (1991). The place of health in the health of place: The case of the Hokianga special medical area. *Social Science and Medicine, 33*, 519-530.

Kearns, R. A. (1993). Place and health: Towards a reformed medical geography. *Professional Geographer, 46*, 111-115.

Kearns, R. A. (1994). Putting health and health care in place: An invitation accepted and declined. *Professional Geographer, 47*, 111-115.

Kearns, R. A., & Joseph, A. E. (1993). Space in its place: Developing the link in medical geography. *Social Science and Medicine, 37*, 711-717.

Kirsch, A.I., & Reeder, L. G. (1969). *Journal of Health and Social Behavior, 10*, 51-58.

Kohn, R., & White, K. (1976). *Health care: An international study*. New York: Oxford University Press.

Koop, C. E. (1993). Revitalizing primary care: A 10-point proposal. *Hospital Practice*, Oct. 15, 55-62.

Kovner, A. R. (1990). Futures. In A. R. Kovner (Ed.), *Health care delivery in the United States* (pp. 510-532). New York: Springer.

Leslie, C. M. (1980). Medical pluralism in world perspective. *Social Science and Medicine, 14B*, 191-195.

Lowell-Smith, E. (1993). Regional and intrametropolitan differences in the location of freestanding ambulatory surgery centers. *Professional Geographer, 45*, 398-407.

Mayhew, L. (1986). *Urban hospital location*. Boston: George Allen and Unwin.

Meade, M., Florin, J., & Gesler, W. (1988). *Medical geography*. New York and London: Guilford Press.

Mechanic, D. (1979). Correlates of physician utilization: Why do major multivariate studies of physician utilization find trivial psychosocial and organizational effects? *Journal of Health and Social Behavior, 20*, 387-396.

Roemer, M. (1985). *National strategies for health care organization: A world overview*. Ann Arbor, MI: Health Administration Press.

Roth, J. A. (1971). Utilization of the hospital emergency department. *Journal of Health and Social Behavior, 12*, 312-320.

Rothman, K. K. (1982). *In labor: Women and power in the birth place*. New York: W. W. Norton.

Salmon, W. (1985). Organizing medical care for profit. In J. B. McKinlay (Ed.), *Issues in the political economy of health care* (pp. 143-186). New York: Tavistock.

Scarpaci, J. L. (1988a). Help-seeking behavior, use, and satisfaction among frequent primary care users in Santiago de Chile. *Journal of Health and Social Behavior, 29*, 199-213.

Scarpaci, J. L. (1988b). *Primary medical care in Chile: Accessibility under military rule*. Pittsburgh: University of Pittsburgh Press.

Scarpaci, J. L. (1990). Medical care, welfare state and deindustrialization in the Southern Cone. *Environment and Planning D: Society and Space, 8*, 191-209.

Scarpaci, J. L. (1993). On the validity of language: Speaking, knowing and understanding in medical geography. *Social Science and Medicine*, *37*, 719-724.

Shannon, G., & Dever, G. E. (1974). *Health-care delivery: Spatial perspectives*. New York: McGraw-Hill.

Shortell, S. (1980). Factors associated with the utilization of health services. In S. J. Williams & P. R. Torrens (Eds.), *Introduction to health services*. New York: Wiley.

Starr, P. (1982). *The social transformation of American medicine*. New York: Basic Books.

Stock, R. (1982). Distance and the utilization of health facilities in rural Nigeria. *Social Science and Medicine*, *17*, 563-570.

Townsend, P., & Davidson, N. (1982). *Inequalities in health: The Black Report*. Harmondsworth, England: Penguin.

Tuan, Y.-F. (1974). Space and place: Humanistic perspective. *Progress in Human Geography*, *6*, 211-252.

Turshen, M. (1988). *The politics of public health*. New Brunswick, NJ: Rutgers University Press.

Twaddle, A. C., & Hessler, R. M. (1977). *A sociology of health*. St. Louis, MO: C. V. Mosby.

Weitzman, B. C. (1990). The quality of care: Assessment and assurance. In A. R. Kovner (Ed.), *Health care delivery in the United States* (pp. 353-380). New York: Springer.

Williams, S. J. (1980). Ambulatory and community health services. In S. J. Williams & P. R. Torrens (Eds.), *Introduction to health services* (p. 106). New York: Wiley.

Wolinksy, F. D. (1978). Assessing the effects of predisposing, enabling and illness-morbidity characteristics. *Journal of Health and Social Behavior*, *19*, 384-396.

III

ADHERENCE TO AND ACCEPTANCE OF REGIMENS

A. GENERAL PERSPECTIVES

An important corollary of the power issues discussed in Part II is what has traditionally been termed *compliance*, but is increasingly being referred to as *adherence* or *acceptance*. Whether and to what degree persons perform medically recommended or prescribed activities, and how they relate to and respond to medical regimens, are thought to be important factors in maintaining and improving health status, as well as critical areas of health behavior research. Yet there are reports (e.g., Stimson, 1974) indicating that persons demonstrate great variability in the degree to which they exhibit such acceptance of medical regimens and prescribed activities. There is no neutral word to refer to this behavior. Whatever term is used—be it "compliance," "obedience," or "adherence"—repeatedly emphasizes an assumed appropriate hierarchical authority structure, an implicit acceptance of the power and right of the professional to make demands, and an imperative for "submission" by the patient. For the purposes of this *Handbook*, the terms "adherence" or "acceptance" are preferable to "compliance." Whether one is preferable to the other is debatable. They are often used interchangeably and synonymously. Acceptance can be used freely as a substitute for adherence, but adherence is sometimes not a substitute for acceptance. For example, one can accept participation in a one-time lifestyle educational program, but it would not make sense to designate this as adherence.

As a rule, compliance research refrains from addressing physician failure to keep appointments, i.e., patients having to wait an hour or more beyond a scheduled appointment time, or with their inability to communicate clearly (e.g., McKinlay, 1975). It is implicit that compliance is normative and "good," that noncompliance is deviant and "bad," and that pressures must be exerted to induce normative, good, compliant behavior.

For convenience, and as a way of imposing some organization on a large number of subjects, the chapters on specific types of adherence are grouped arbitrarily into sections on "disease-focused" and "lifestyle" regimens.

TOWARD A RECONCEPTUALIZATION OF "COMPLIANCE"

Conrad (1985) reasons that an important issue in nonacceptance of medication is the meaning that the patient ascribes to the medication and the illness. Within the context of epilepsy, Conrad demonstrates that taking medication may be associated with the stigma of the condition and that not taking medication may represent attempts at self-regulation.

In a study of Chicano females, Hayes-Bautista (1976) concluded that compliance or noncompliance is an outcome of negotiations between the patient and the physician and that noncompliance—sometimes taking the form of decreasing or increasing the amount of medication taken—may reflect the patient's dissatisfaction with the treatment, as well as constitute a means whereby the patient can control the treatment process.

Kotarba and Seidel (1984) showed how some "pain-management" clinics perceive the chronic paint patient to be in need of social control and how seminars on the management of such patients seem to equate compliance with social control. Patients are discredited, their presentations are distorted, their stories are listened to cynically. From Kotarba and Seidel's analysis, one can see that the issues are social and behavioral, rather than medical; that compliance—or behaving properly—is a way of medicalizing a behavioral issue.

Stimson (1974) analyzed the legitimacy and "rationality" of the "view from the other side," the patient's views on medication, and showed how these views may often vary from the perspectives of the physician. Moreover, from the patient's perspective, not taking medication can be seen to be rational and appropriate. Furthermore, Stimson and Webb (1975, p. 11) pointed out that the patient's decision whether or not to accept medication is a result of reappraisal of the recommendation in light of additional consultation with others and of attempts to make sense out of what the patient knows about the condition and the medication.

Waissman (1985) provides insights into what might be termed the ultimate act of noncompliance: a "strike" in which patients of a French hemodialysis clinic refused to accept their treatment. In this context, they were showing—at great risk to themselves—their disapproval of some clinic management policies and were using noncompliance as a political tool, as a way of demonstrating their own social power.

The complexity of adherence, its multidimensionality, and its essentially "static" as opposed to changing or developmental nature are identified by Karoly (1993) as issues that need to be considered in any reconceptualization. Furthermore, since the level of adherence is dependent on the specificity of demands within a regimen, rather than intrapersonally consistent (e.g., Orme & Binik,1989), any reconceptualization of adherence would have to embrace its less than global nature.

Barofsky (1978) identified several alternative models of therapeutic relationships that could be substituted for the traditional model in which a powerful figure or institution requires compliant or conforming behavior. In such alternatives, coerciveness is increasingly replaced by self-management, and the relationship between the physician and the patient is that of a therapeutic alliance with the objective of increased self-care.

The analysis by Lipton and Hershaft (1985) of how dubious findings have been incorporated into medical practice on a large scale raises the question of the value to the patient of compliance with medical regimens and, with it, the value of the medical perspective. For many patients, nonacceptance of a regimen is an appropriate and healthy behavior!

In Chapter 6, on the history of compliance as a concept and as an area of empirical study, Trostle shows how extensively compliance is intertwined with economics and politics and how it reflects the powerful influences of physicians and pharmaceutical and nutrition companies. Trostle further demonstrates the medicalization of the purchase of consumer goods.

REFERENCES

Barofsky, I. (1978). Compliance, adherence and the therapeutic alliance: Steps in the development of self-care. *Social Science and Medicine*, *12*,369-376.

Conrad, P. (1985). The meaning of medications: Another look at compliance. *Social Science and Medicine*, *20*, 29-37.

Hayes-Bautista, D. E. (1976). Modifying the treatment: Patient compliance, patient control and medical care. *Social Science and Medicine*, *10*, 233-238.

Karoly, P. (1993). Enlarging the scope of the compliance construct: Toward developmental and motivational relevance. In N. A. Krasnegor, L. Epstein, S. B. Johnson, & S. J. Yaffe (Eds.), *Developmental aspects of health compliance behavior* (pp. 11-27). Hillsdale, NJ: Erlbaum.

Kotarba, J. A., & Seidel, J. V. (1984). Managing the problem pain patient: Compliance or social control. *Social Science and Medicine*, *19*, 1393-1400.

Lipton, J. P., & Hershaft, A. M. (1985). On the widespread acceptance of dubious medical findings. *Journal of Health and Social Behavior*, *26*, 336-351.

McKinlay, J. B. (1975). Who is really ignorant—physician or patient? *Journal of Health and Social Behavior*, *16*, 3-11.

Orme, C. M., & Binik, Y. M. (1989). Consistency of adherence across regimen demands. *Health Psychology*, *8* 27-43.

Stimson, G. V. (1974). Obeying doctor's orders: A view from the other side. *Social Science and Medicine*, *8*, 97-104.

Stimson, G., & Webb, B. (1975). *Going to see the doctor: The consultation process in general practice*. London: Routledge & Kegan Paul.

Waissman, R. (1985). A protest movement in a private clinic: An analysis of a patients' strike. *Social Science and Medicine*, *220*, 129-132.

6

The History and Meaning of Patient Compliance as an Ideology

James A. Trostle

INTRODUCTION

Patient compliance with regimens may be one of the most studied and least understood behavioral issues in medicine. Medical compliance was defined in the late 1970s as "the extent to which the patient's behavior (in terms of taking medications, following diets, or executing other lifestyle changes) coincides with medical or health advice" (Haynes, 1979). That definition continues to predominate almost two decades later. Virtually any North American medical journal published since the mid-1970s contains advertisements proclaiming that a particular product's simple dosage or low level of side effects will increase patient compliance. These proclamations are frequently used to advertise treatments for common chronic conditions such as arthritis, diabetes, and hypertension. Nevertheless, studies estimate that about half of the people who have chronic conditions like these are noncompliant with their medication regimens (Sackett & Snow, 1979).

This chapter discusses the reasons for therapeutic compliance having received such attention for two and a half decades. The chapter contends that the topic is better approached as an ideology supporting the authority of medical professionals than it is as a legitimate topic for behavioral research. The basic problem with most research on medical compliance is that it continues to be dominated by a series of ideological conceptions of the proper roles of patients and physicians. Though presented as a literature about improving medical services, the research literature about compliance is preeminently, although covertly, a literature about power and control. It is written largely by medical professionals about themselves and their clientele. It reveals the medical profession's worldview: The problem lies in patients' behavior or in doctor-patient interaction; the solution lies in patient education, behavioral reinforcements, and better doctor-patient communication. By reviewing 20th-century historical materials, the chapter will show that what physicians and other clinical professionals now call "compliance" is what they

James A. Trostle • Five College Medical Anthropology Program, Mount Holyoke College, South Hadley, Massachusetts 01075.

Handbook of Health Behavior Research II: Provider Determinants, edited by David S. Gochman. Plenum Press, New York, 1997.

once called "control." This approach shows more clearly the limitations of the compliance concept and the challenges it poses to research designed to understand and improve the appropriate use of medication. This historical perspective also shows that issues once seen as social, such as poor nutrition, lack of exercise, and alcohol abuse, have become medicalized and have fallen under the compliance rubric. Labeling failure to follow these nonmedical regimens as "noncompliance" (as though to do so were legitimately analogous to calling sin noncompliance with morality or crime noncompliance with law) suffers from the same ideological notions described in this chapter for medical noncompliance.

THE CLINICAL, ECONOMIC, AND ACADEMIC IMPORTANCE OF COMPLIANCE

To call compliance an ideology is not to derogate the clinical, economic, and academic reasons to study the use of medications. The irregular, diminished, or excessive consumption of medicine can impair health or extend illness. Some medications must be taken long after symptoms disappear, others are dangerous if taken in excess, many are ineffective unless a certain critical minimum level of medication is taken. Consumption that varies from professional expectations, and prescription that varies from accepted standards, can cause the therapeutic effectiveness of a medication to be misjudged both in individuals and in large-scale clinical trials.

Compliance is also important because it affects a large and profitable portion of the economy. The total value of shipments of pharmaceutical preparations in the United States in 1991 was $47.4 billion, or almost 1% of the nation's gross national product in that year (U.S. Department of Commerce, 1994). Pharmaceutical companies use compliance in their advertisements as a promotional strategy to increase market share and product sales. But compliance also serves other latent functions: Increased compliance is one among a set of positive attributes (also including low cost, few doses, few side effects, therapeutic efficacy) advertisers use to increase the visibility of their products and to enhance their company's positive image among physicians and the lay public.

Compliance continues to attract a great deal of attention in both clinical and social science journals: As of May 1995, more than 11,600 English-language research and review articles on the topic had been included in the *Index Medicus* and other bibliographic collections. A cumulative bibliography on the subject (Haynes, Sackett, & Taylor, 1979) listed only 22 articles in English published before 1960 and 850 published by 1978. Production of articles about compliance doubled about every five years between 1966 and 1985. The field even received its one journal in 1986, the *Journal of Compliance in Health Care*. This journal ceased publishing in 1989, and the rate of increase in compliance publishing appears to be slowing in the mid-1990s. Nonetheless, the absolute number of articles produced annually is still quite impressive: More than 700 articles on the topic were published in 1994 alone. Figure 1 dramatizes the growth and extent of research interest in this aspect of patient-doctor relationships.

COMPLIANCE AS AN IDEOLOGY

The purpose of this chapter is not to survey the compliance literature; that has been done often—even excessively—and well (DiMatteo & DiNicola, 1982; Eraker, Kirscht, & Becker, 1984; Haynes et al., 1979; Wright, 1993). Rather, its purpose is to argue that therapeutic "compliance" itself is a problematic concept with its own social history. Most of the many research articles on compliance have evaluated a range of possible determinants and measures, but few have asked why compliance itself has prompted such research enthusiasm or how it came to be so important. The present popularity of compliance can be better understood if it is analyzed as an *ideol-*

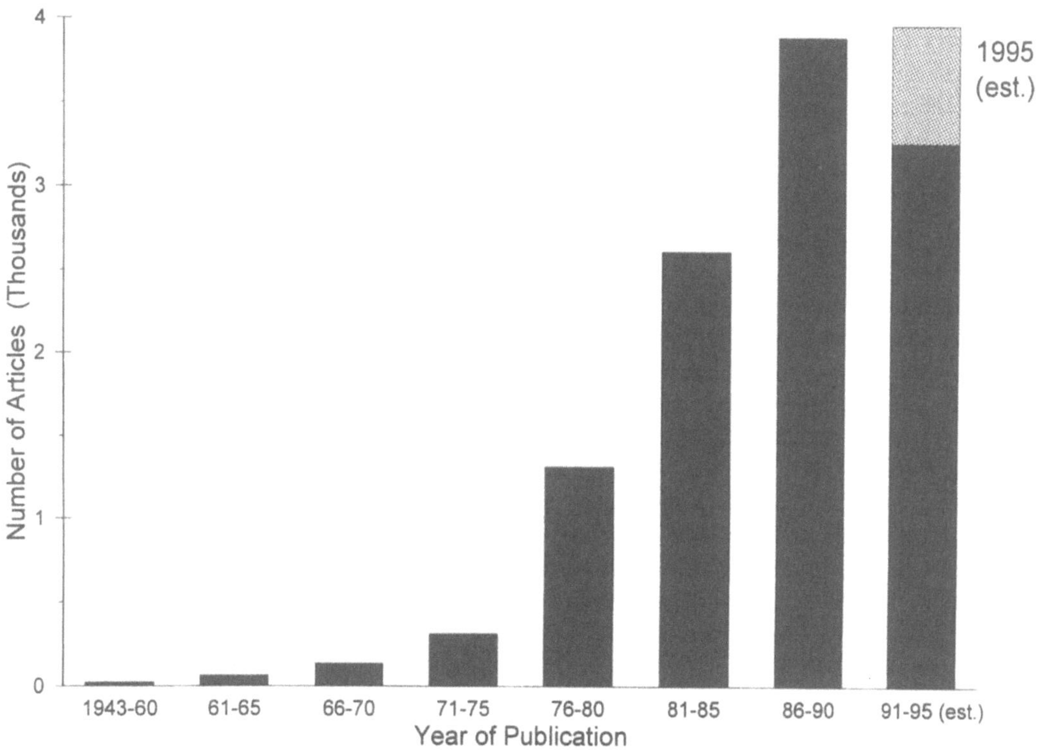

Figure 1. Compliance articles published by grouped year of publication. Adapted from Haynes (1979), Figure 1.1, and *Index Medicus* postings from 1978 to 1995.

ogy, i.e., a system of shared beliefs that legitimize particular behavioral norms and values at the same time that they claim and appear to be based in empirical truths. Ideologies help to transform power (potential influence) into authority (legitimate control). Compliance is an ideology that transforms physicians' theories about the proper behavior of patients into a series of research strategies, research results, and potentially coercive interventions that *appear* appropriate and that reinforce physicians' authority over health care. (Physicians are certainly not the only professionals involved in patient care, but they still largely determine the direction and intensity of medical interventions.) Looking at compliance as an ideology helps explain why research into the determinants of compliance has been largely inconclusive: This research has defined patient behavior in terms of professional expectations and has largely ignored health-related behavior that contradicts the profession's view of its own centrality to health care.

Social scientists might be expected to adopt an "outsider" perspective to facilitate investigating the differences between expert recommendations and lay responses. Unfortunately, those who write about compliance commonly adopt the worldview of the medical profession, a phenomenon labeled "management bias" by Roth (1962). When differences between expected and adopted behavior arise despite the best intentions and efforts of physicians and patients, research on the day-to-day use of medications certainly can contribute to improving health care and health status. But the future success of research under the rubric of compliance will be limited until the barriers posed by its present definition are recognized.

THE HISTORY OF COMPLIANCE AS AN IDEOLOGY

To date, there has been no historical work done on the topic of compliance, except for a few cursory paragraphs relying on what has become a standard set of anecdotes. Haynes (1979, p. 3), an editor of the first major compliance bibliography, stated facetiously that the "first recorded incident of human noncompliance in Judeo-Christian tradition" occurred when Eve ate the apple in the Garden of Eden. Compliance researchers commonly cite Hippocrates as their progenitor because he is reported to have said that "[the physician] should keep aware of the fact that patients often lie when they state that they have taken certain medicines" (Blackwell, 1992; Haynes, 1979; Lasagna, 1973). They also cite the renowned 19th-century clinician Sir William Osler, who wrote that "the desire to take medicine is perhaps the greatest feature which distinguishes man from animals" (quotation in Cushing, 1925 [cited in Becker & Maiman, 1980]). Though often repeated, these few anecdotes are inadequate, for the ideology of compliance does have a history.

The Origins of Compliance Research: Conventional Explanations

Most compliance researchers explained the growth of their literature by linking it to the development of antibiotics in the 1950s and the subsequent wide availability of these effective treatments. Authors such as Bissonette and Seller (1980), Haynes (1979), and Robins (1980) wrote that while noncompliance may have been occurring since the time of Hippocrates, only in the 1950s did physicians obtain many truly effective medications for the first time, and only then did it become as important for physicians to make sure that these medications were *consumed* by patients as it was to make sure the medications were properly chosen and prescribed.

This explanation mistakenly assumes that scientific measures of efficacy are the foundation of professional beliefs about clinical efficacy. The explanation is incomplete because it fails to acknowledge that most healers in any historical period (be they physicians, bone-setters, barbers, surgeons, or shamans) believe in and help to reinforce the curative powers of their treatments. Physicians in the 18th and 19th centuries relied on their so-called "heroic treatment," which consisted of bleeding, purging, mercurials, and blistering. Dissenting voices were raised, such as a remark by Oliver Wendell Holmes in 1860 that "I firmly believe that if the whole *materia medica* as now used could be sunk to the bottom of the sea, it would be all the better for mankind—and all the worse for the fishes" (quoted in Crout, 1980, p. 41). But by and large, 18th- and 19th-century physicians and healers also believed in the therapeutic effects of their actions, and they probably were just as concerned about compliance as any contemporary physician is. The efficacious treatments of one era become the outmoded therapies of the next. Even today, only a small proportion of clinical practices have been evaluated through careful experimental studies.

A history of medical compliance must therefore go beyond the efficacy of pharmaceuticals to explain the emerging popularity of the concept. It must refer to cultural beliefs in curative substances and the history of the profession of medicine. The history of compliance as an ideology can be uncovered by looking at legislation, medical journals, and advertisements that address and reveal the self-image of the medical profession. Such a history portrays the origins and growth of concerns about compliance: Rather than resulting solely from medical advances in the past three decades, contemporary concern for compliance is also a product of the growing monopoly of the medical profession over the past century.

The Origins of Compliance Research: An Alternative Explanation

The modern chronicles of compliance have missed a point made by Temkin (1964), a historian of medicine who pointed out that patients have had faith in drugs for longer than they have had faith in physicians. Most of the compliance literature suggests that the relationship between physician and patient is—and by inference should be—the most important factor determining the course of a person's health-related activities. Yet Temkin says that obtaining the medical *products* available primarily from physicians may be more important to patients than their relationships with physicians. Physicians are a historically and geographically bounded profession organized to provide health care, but the consumption of substances to cure illness has no such temporal or spatial boundaries. Labeling patients "noncompliant" because they follow their own ideas about their own care misses the point that this is what people have done since medicines were first used. Those who use the label mistakenly equate health care dominated by physicians—a specific outcome of a contemporary power distribution—with health management in general.

Much compliance research thus makes a crucial historical error. It places undue emphasis on one particular historical relationship between healers and the afflicted, the physician-patient relationship, and neglects the existence of more universal forms of obtaining care: self-management, and relying on family, friends, neighbors, and others. The very notion of compliance requires a dominant professional and a dependent layperson—someone to give advice, suggestions, or orders, and someone to carry them out. Yet even within North American and European societies, the structural dominance of the medical profession is not a timeless or universal phenomenon. United States physicians owe their dominance to 19th- and 20th-century legislative acts that helped to establish the "monopolizing" and "gatekeeping" functions of medicine: controlling who may practice the profession and where (licensing of practitioners and educational establishments, malpractice review), who may obtain and prescribe scarce valuable items like pharmaceuticals (controlled substance laws), what reasonable levels of payment are (Medicaid, Medicare), how much is known about costs and charges (restrictive advertising covenants), and a host of other structural constraints (Brown, 1979; Conrad, 1979; Duffy, 1984; Freidson, 1970, 1975; Klein, 1973; Starr, 1982; Stevens, 1971).

Rather than point to the efficacy of antibiotics to explain the growth of a concern for compliance with therapeutic regimens in the United States, one might point instead to this developing consolidation of the profession of medicine and to the growth and sales strategies of the pharmaceutical and proprietary drug industries. One example of this process comes from advertising in medical journals in the early 1900s, for example, which proudly proclaimed that companies were directing information to physicians rather than to patients. This practice reinforced physicians' beliefs that they were not only the most skilled but also the only proper source of health care for their patients. A selection of advertisements from campaigns for infant feeding materials shows the development of a new professional and industrial concern for controlling the behavior of the weak and the sick. These advertisements document that a concern for market control combined with a concern for therapeutic power evolved into a concern for patient compliance.

Nutritional Supplements and Infant Formula: Transforming Information Control into Patient Compliance

For much of the 19th century, physicians in the United States had little power: they were poorly trained, disorganized, and had little social prestige. During this time, patent medicine companies advertised their products directly to the general public. ("Patent" is a misnomer; their ingredients were copyrighted and thus private, rather than patented and public.) Up to the late 19th century, many miracle cures were touted as cheap alternatives to medical care. At the beginning of the 20th century, however, both organized medicine and the United States government began to legislate changes in the extent and kind of drug advertising directed at the public. The federal government began with the Pure Food and Drugs Act of 1906, setting initial standards for labeling drug ingredients and claims of efficacy, and in 1938 passed the Food, Drug, and Cosmetic Act with further restrictions and additional enforcement provisions. The American Medical Association (AMA) stopped accepting patent medicine advertisement in the *Journal of the American Medical Association* (*JAMA*) in 1905, and also began to rule on whether various products were acceptable for medical use. In 1924, it reserved the right to reject advertising for approved drugs from companies that derived earnings from other unapproved drugs. Though physicians and politicians both campaigned against misrepresentation of health products, they did so with somewhat different goals: The government meant to make consumer information more accurate, while the AMA wanted to make information accurate, as well as to control the amount of product information consumers received and thereby increase physician control over medicines and other health-related products (Apple, 1982, 1987; Starr, 1982).

Physicians in the early 20th century thus began to consolidate their control over the business of healing in the United States and to increase their influence over the health-related activities of their patients. (These efforts were paralleled by the growing public health movement in the United States, which argued for improving [and controlling] the collective health of the country by means of population interventions such as putting iodine into salt or, more recently, fluoridating water.) One early strategy in doctors' attempts to control patient behavior was to sell food products containing nutritional additives, thereby, at least ostensibly, circumventing patients' problems in taking nutritional supplements as suggested. This strategy was a means to resolve the problem now called noncompliance.

Some attempts to increase patient compliance were couched in terms of improving patient forgetfulness. This strategy was used in the following advertisement promoting evaporated milk with cod-liver oil extract printed in the 1934 *Journal of the American Medical Association* (102[4], 333):

> YOU FORGOT again MOTHER. Yes ... mothers *do* forget!
>
> How many mothers forget to give regularly the cod-liver oil you prescribe? Many doctors are now recommending DEAN'S so that the children under their care are assured a regular and definite supply of Vitamin "D". DEAN has put Vitamin "D", extracted from cod-liver oil (by the Zuckerman process), into evaporated milk. And you can't even taste it. Furthermore, DEAN'S is pure, selected, cow's milk from tuberculin-tested herds, unsweetened and evaporated to double richness. Developed especially for infant feeding, DEAN'S is also important in child and adult nutrition. We should like to send you Vitamin "D" Evaporated Milk Literature and a Standard Feeding Formula. May we?

Adding nutritional supplements to food products is a problematic strategy: On the positive side, the dietary supplement is consumed whenever the food product is consumed; no extra pills or syrups need to be taken. On the negative side, doctors can rely on a fixed proportion on the additive being consumed *only if the food product is consumed according to directions*. Moreover, the product provides the additive but does not require the continuing supervision of the physician. This was an economic hazard to the physician because it did not require return visits (Apple, 1982). Physicians gained control over return visits by emphasizing that these products could be misused by patients unless they were monitored. They emphasized the potential medical hazards to the patient and thereby avoided focusing on the economic hazard to their livelihood.

The potential problem was solved for infant formula preparations in a way that increased physician control over patient behavior and increased formula company revenues. The solution was simple and elegant: Formula companies took preparation directions and feeding schedules off containers of infant formulas and directed advertising at physicians rather than the lay public. Potential consumers could obtain the product only if they were under the care of a physician.

This change took place in a time of increasing government regulation, when infant formula companies decided to entrust physicians with control over their products. (This is called the "ethical push" route for advertising, while the "consumer pull" strategy is to advertise in the mass media directly to the public.) Physicians would be more respectable and profitable salesmen than the company sales force; as time passed, physician control over the distribution of certain health-related products began to appear natural and even necessary (see the recounting by Apple [1982] of the history of the formula-marketing decision). The sales strategy was expanded to vitamin supplements and became the model for subsequent marketing of prescription pharmaceuticals. The strategy was forthrightly articulated in the advertising section of *JAMA*, where one full-page advertisement in 1931 (*97*[8], 46) concluded with the following paragraphs:

> When the physician reads this class of exploiting advertisement which patronizingly refers to his endorsement of the most ridiculous claims, and later hears his patients knowingly repeating these to him, he cannot help asking himself these questions:
>
> (1) Should the layman receive his medical education, including his vitamin-mindedness, from the commercial house, or from his doctor?
>
> (2) Should the commercial house exploit vitamins in modern patent medicine style, or should the physician control their intelligent application?
>
> Mead Johnson & Company, for one, continue to feel that vitamin therapy, like infant feeding, should be in the hands of the medical profession, and consequently refuse to lend their aid to exploiting these valuable agents to the public. This house, for one, advertises its vitamin products exclusively to the medical profession and furnishes no directions to the public.

This deliberate company decision to advertise its marketing strategy was effective because it reflected and amplified a sentiment already common among United States physicians, namely, that the medical profession should maintain control over the distribution of infant formula. That sentiment was formalized in 1932, when the AMA passed a resolution requiring infant food companies that wanted AMA approval of their products to advertise those products only to physicians. This particular advertisement clearly goes beyond infant feeding, addressing vitamin therapy as well. But what is most interesting is that an ideology of physician control itself is being created and promoted here; an explicit announcement of support for physician control of patient behavior is used to sell products.

Another example of the ideology of physician control can be seen in a Mead Johnson & Company advertisement from 1931 (*JAMA*, *98*[2], 74). The full-page drawing shows a mother holding a baby, both of whom are looking at a physician behind his desk. The physician, dominant in the foreground though in profile, is looking at a large piece of paper in his hands, headed "Pediatric Case History." The mother cannot read what is written on the page in the doctor's hand, and she has a trusting and expectant expression on her face. The only text visible in the advertisement, superimposed on the case history, reads: "The Mead Johnson Policy of cooperating exclusively with physicians by refraining from suggesting or indicating the application of Mead's infant diet materials to the laity assures the patient's fullest cooperation with the physician." This is a telling portrayal of the marketing strategy of the producer, but it is also a snapshot of an image-making process. By controlling information, doctors gain power. By withholding information, they promote passivity and dependence.

Mead Johnson had the most visible "no laity advertising" strategy, used in its campaigns up until the mid-1940s for products ranging from infant formula to fish liver oil. But it was not the only company to extol this strategy. Similar claims were also made, for example, by the Corn

Products Sales Company for its Karo syrup for infant feeding (*New England Journal of Medicine*, [*NEJM*], *220*(2), x, 1939) and by the Nestlé corporation for its Lactogen infant formula (*NEJM*, *220*[5], ix, 1939). These advertisements demonstrate that: (1) a concern for controlling patient behavior antedated the development of antibiotics; (2) the United States medical profession's interest in maintaining control over patients' behavior and access to information was recognized and reinforced throughout the 1920s to the 1940s, before many effective medications became available; (3) professional self-interest was a significant factor in the movement to limit popular advertising of infant feeding products and of vitamins; and (4) the contemporary concern for "compliance" was openly articulated earlier in this century as a concern for patient "cooperation" and physician "control."

PHYSICIAN AUTHORITY AND THE STATUS OF COMPLIANCE

The concern for compliance is a cultural phenomenon intimately connected with the self-image of physicians and with their organized (and often successful) attempts to define the limits of their own discipline. Yet the respect and authority accorded physicians in the United States is of recent origin and has been diminished over the past decade (Haug & Lavin, 1983; McKinlay & Arches, 1985). Physicians have exercised their control over medical technology and pharmaceuticals only since the beginning of the 20th century. Now, at the end of that century, for-profit hospitals, health maintenance organizations (HMOs), and other types of medical groups are employing physicians as salaried workers; their growth is causing reductions in physicians' monopolistic power. Physician control over the technology of medical care is decreasing as pharmaceutical companies lobby for the right to advertise directly to consumers, the Food and Drug Administration moves drugs (such as cortisone) from prescription to nonprescription categories, and HMOs develop limited lists of approved medications. These changes reduce physicians' control over the technology of health care. Some would even argue that the preoccupation with compliance over the two decades preceding these changes was partly a consequence of the declining authority of the profession.

UNPACKING THE CONTEMPORARY IDEOLOGY OF COMPLIANCE

Contemporary research on medical compliance is burdened by the multiple meanings of the word "compliance." To pursue Haynes's witticism that noncompliance began in the Garden of Eden, if the term "noncompliance" can apply equally to a patient's nonconformity with medical advice and to a biblical figure's nonconformity with God's commandment, then what values does the term express? While Haynes was joking, the biblical example is not serendipitous: Haynes states that his definition of compliance was intended to be nonjudgmental. Some researchers urged that terms such as "nonadherence" or "defaulting" be substituted for "noncompliance" in an effort to escape the word's connotations of dominance and subservience (Barofsky, 1978; Kasl, 1975; Stimson, 1974; Stone, 1979). Others suggest terms such as "intelligent noncompliance" or "capricious compliance," the better to conceptualize those instances in which noncompliance makes sense or where compliance does not (Weintraub, 1976). Some have proposed replacing "noncompliance" with a label such as patient "self-regulation" (Schneider & Conrad, 1983) or "self-management" (Buchanan, 1982). This change would be made to emphasize that patients are ultimately responsible for their behavior and to counter the prevailing research emphasis that the physician needs to foster compliance. If unmodified, however, these terms overemphasize the patient's contribution to therapy and thus mirror the errors of relying on a physician-centered approach to compliance. An editor of the first compliance bibliography explicitly recognized that the term compliant "is troublesome to many people because it conjures up images of patient or client sin and serfdom" (Haynes, 1979, p. 2), but he stated that the editors knew of no acceptable alternative. Another editor of this volume called the various alternatives "technical jargon terms," thus implying that compliance is immune from such jargon.

Compliance is an ideology based in theories about the proper relationship between physicians and their clients. Yet its assumptions, definitions, and manifestations have been studied and reified as quantifiable categories of human behavior. Though compliance can be called a nonjudgmental concept, it rarely is used or studied as such. Much contemporary compliance research has manifested the theories about proper patient behavior seen in the following examples:

> Through instruction in health magazines, the *Reader's Digest*, and radio and television programmes, patients acquire that superficial knowledge which often emboldens them to question their doctor more closely than hitherto about their own complaints. Of course it is unlikely that a patient can have any real understanding about his illness, but the greater risk that he will obtain misguided information from less reliable sources has to be reckoned with. Greater profit, therefore, will be earned if the doctor affords time to talk to each patient with cardiac pain. (Evans, 1959, p. 252)

> Communication between doctor and patient ideally necessitates a certain degree of reciprocity. Each person has certain rights and obligations. When the doctor performs a service, the patient is obligated to reciprocate: first, by cooperating with the doctor in their interaction; and second, by complying with the medical recommendations once he leaves the doctor's office. (Davis, 1968, p. 284)

> In some instances, the patient, because his condition is not improving or is getting worse (due to his failure to follow the prescribed regimen) may start a malpractice action. On a less critical level, the patient, and his or her family and friends may decide to go elsewhere for their health care. In addition, a discontented patient is not likely to help a physician's reputation in the community. That is why it's important for the physician to understand the motivations for the patient's noncompliance. (Van Kamerik, 1978, p. 30 [from an article entitled "Why Don't Patients Do What You Tell Them?"])

> Whether your patient needs to be reassured or warned, he needs to be made aware of his responsibility for taking medication as directed. Just as he decided to seek treatment, so he must decide to take his drug correctly and follow other particulars of his therapeutic regimen. Most patients appreciate the idea of being active partners in their treatment. (Weibert & Dee, 1980, p. 9)

> Patient's perception of their own health ... may be more important than how well they understand their underlying illness, and there is evidence that intensive education programmes do not necessarily improve compliance. None the less, education of the patient is always to be encouraged, and if it does improve compliance then so much the better. (Aronson & Hardman, 1992, p. 1011)

These examples chart some of the changing rationales for physician concerns with compliance. Writing in the late 1950s, Evans (1959) portrayed patients as ignorant and prone to act on misguided information. He championed patient education as a strategy to prevent "improper" consults rather than to prevent illness. This view reflects the paternal role the profession adopted at the time. By the late 1960s, many physicians had replaced their role as stewards with a role as "therapeutic partners," but this partnership was a limited one. Davis (1968) articulated the doctor-patient relationship as a contract, but whereas most professional contracts stipulate that fees are to be exchanged for services, Davis suggested that patients reciprocate their doctor's services by cooperating with the doctor's agenda during the clinical interaction and complying with the doctor's recommendations afterward. Writing in the late 1970s, in the era of defensive medicine, Van Kamerik (1978) was more blunt: Physicians' self-interest should cause them to give effective treatments, try to understand noncompliers, and avoid malpractice suits or a damaged public image. A little later, Weibert and Dee (1980) portrayed a more subtle variant of the contractual model of doctor-patient relationships: Having freely and of his own volition sought treatment, the patient is thus responsible for internalizing the doctor's orders and following the regimen. Writing in the next decade, Aronson and Hardman (1992) adopted a more limited vision of their own power and suggested that education may not in fact be sufficient to increase compliance.

All these excerpts except the most recent one (Aronson & Hardman, 1992) assume that the professional consultation signals an end to the patient's decision making about caring for the complaint. Evans was motivated to protect the patient from other nonprofessional influences, while Van Kamerik wanted to protect the physician from legal action. Davis and Weibert and Dee presented more egalitarian models of how physicians and patients should interact, yet they both left no conceptual room for patients to disagree with or reject doctors' advice. Even Aronson and Hardman, who are willing to accord perception as much power as understanding, still suggest that patient education by physicians is always to be encouraged.

These ideological assumptions about patient-doctor relationships can be summarized as follows: Physicians are the proper ultimate authority over the actions of their patients; in exchange for a physician's services, a patient owes fees, cooperation, and compliance; noncompliance is usually the patient's fault; and physicians offer therapeutic partnerships to patients, not vice versa.

A small group of researchers have consistently argued for another vision of compliance. Even as the ideological assumptions described above were being expressed in the clinical literature, some social scientists were presenting alternative visions of medication usage that paid more attention to the patient's perspective (e.g., Conrad, 1985; Garrity, 1981; Hayes-Bautista, 1976; Stimson, 1974; Zola, 1981) or to the need for more social theory in the design of compliance research (Leventhal, 1985; Leventhal, Zimmerman, & Gutmann, 1984).

This alternative vision of compliance stressing the patient's perspective, the rationality of noncompliance, and the range of behaviors potentially linked to compliance has increased its visibility somewhat over the past decade. For example, studies concentrating on the patient perspective were reviewed by Morris and Schulz (1993), and Nichter and Vuckovic (1994) discussed a research agenda for anthropological studies of pharmaceutical practice. Vandereycken and Meermann (1988) used a psychological interaction approach to discuss the importance of doctor, patient, and family in noncompliance. Richardson, Simons-Morton, and Annegers (1993) did a detailed study of patients' perceived barriers to compliance. These are a few of the more recent studies that have avoided a focus on the noncompliant patient as a guilty party.

Some other compliance research has looked at medication usage as a behavioral rather than an ideological category. For example, Horwitz and Horwitz (1993) reviewed evidence suggesting that since compliance with placebo treatments also seems to improve health outcomes, compliance itself may have nonspecific therapeutic effects. They suggested that this possibility be discussed with patients, and they urged designers of randomized clinical drug trials to pay attention to possible "adherence effects" on health outcomes (Horwitz & Horwitz, 1993, p. 1866).

Other research has focused on more accurate measures of compliance over time. For example, Cramer, Scheyer, and Mattson (1990) experimented with a pill container that electronically recorded the date and hour each time the container was opened. Longitudinal records showed that spot drug levels taken during clinic visits did not represent a steady state of medication; rather, compliance declined between doctor visits and increased again just before and after the visit. The fact that knowledge of a pending visit appeared to increase compliance was labeled "white coat compliance" in one editorial (Feinstein, 1990).

IMPLICATIONS OF COMPLIANCE IDEOLOGY FOR PATIENT CARE

Health care providers often use noncompliance like an epithet, obscuring the variability and denying the legitimacy of behaviors that differ from their clinical prescription. When physicians label their patients "noncompliant," they often distance themselves from their patients' actions, judging and labeling rather than analyzing and understanding. Compliance is successful as a descriptive term in clinical practice precisely because it assumes that physicians legitimately control patient behavior. Yet thinking about patient behavior in terms of "compliance" constrains communication by substituting a simple epithet for a complex act or series of acts over time. Professionals know that noncompliant patients have not followed clinical prescriptions, but they do not know what those patients have done instead. Most compliance research focuses only on the results of doctor-patient interactions, and it therefore misses this important larger context. As Zola (1966, 1981) pointed out, people often have many illnesses and attempts to alleviate symptoms before they see a doctor; these prior experiences are likely to influence compliance, but they usually are excluded from the examining room. Thinking about drug-taking behavior in terms of noncompliance thus impedes rather than facilitates communication: It marks a patient's "misbehavior" as being outside the boundaries of a physician's responsibility. The term rationalizes physician withdrawal and blames the patient rather than promoting a reexamination of clinical priorities. It further justifies the dominance of the physician in controlling the type and direction of information given during clinical interactions (Waitzkin, 1985).

If one takes an omniscient position outside the physician-patient relationship, one can see that noncompliance can be the behavioral result of many motivations. It can express someone's disagreement or dissatisfaction with clinical advice. It can be a rational response to a series of social realities competing with the clinical agenda (e.g., financial constraints, labeling as a patient, inability to function adequately under a medication's side effects, familial opposition to therapy). It can express a conscious preference of illness to health, be an immature response to adult responsibilities, and represent a manipulation of one's physical condition for other goals, or even a rejection of medical intervention altogether (Conrad, 1985; Taussig, 1980; Trostle, Hauser, & Susser, 1983; Udry & Morris, 1971). Thus, noncompliance is an unavoidable by-product of collisions between the clinical world and other competing worlds of work, play, friendship, and family life.

The compliance literature at its most coercive teaches physicians how to manipulate their patients' behavior without questioning their own beliefs or increasing their patients' understanding (for examples of this approach, see Benfari, Eaker, & Stoll, 1981; DiMatteo & DiNicola, 1982; Rodin & Janis, 1979). One extreme variant of this approach outlines how physicians can build up their own "motivating power," i.e., their ability to make patients internalize their recommendations, by using positive feedback and encouraging self-disclosure in their patients. Rodin and Janis (1979) conclude with what is essentially a recommendation to study how physicians can manipulate patients without being found out (p. 76):

> Clients are just as aware of the norms of social equity as practitioners, and they are likely to be suspicious when given overzealous unearned praise or compliments. Practitioners' attempts to use acceptance can have boomerang effects if they give so much praise that they are presumed to be ingratiating with a hidden manipulative intent. *The conditions under which acceptance by health-care practitioners will and will not be perceived as ingratiating by their patients need to be systematically investigated* [emphasis added].

This is a call to seek the limits of medical deception, for it never acknowledges that "motivating power" is being increased precisely *to facilitate* a "hidden manipulative intent." Physicians and other health care providers can teach patients techniques for self-assessment, behavioral change, and behavioral reinforcement; doing so provides patients with the tools to follow through with their professed desire to comply. Physicians can also give positive feedback with a coercive intent, a practice that has been labeled unethical by some compliance researchers (Jonsen, 1979; Sackett, 1976).

These excerpts highlight some of the basic assumptions of most compliance research. They show that a concern for compliance serves professional purposes and that the justifications for this concern change over time. These changes can even be seen in the ways the medical literature on patients' behavior is categorized. "Patient Compliance" first appeared as a medical subject heading in the *Index Medicus* in 1975, but was cross-referenced under the heading "Patient Dropouts" until 1981. In 1981, "Patient Dropouts" was replaced by the heading "Patient Non-Compliance." This substitution refined a relatively crude category, but both the old and the new categories still use professional norms from inside the clinic to define and pass judgment on health-related behavior outside the clinic.

COMPLIANCE AND PHYSICIAN BEHAVIOR

In 1981, Ley (1981) wrote an article entitled "Professional Non-compliance: A Neglected Problem." Since that time, studies of inappropriate prescribing by physicians and pharmacists have continued to grow in importance and number, though not at the same rate as studies of patient compliance. Methodological reviews of successful prescribing interventions have been undertaken (e.g., Soumerai, McLaughlin, & Avorn, 1989). An analysis of a prescribing intervention in Mexico (Bronfman, Castro, Guiscafré, Muñoz, & Gutiérrez, 1991) showed that patient compliance increased as an indirect effect of an intervention aimed at improving physician prescribing. These types of studies point out the necessity of increasing the quality of physician prescribing alongside attempts to increase compliance. They also suggest that researchers should pay more attention to possible unexpected effects on patients of interventions targeted solely at physicians.

IS THE IDEOLOGY OF COMPLIANCE APPLICABLE ACROSS CULTURES?

Can compliance research adequately conceptualize patient behavior in other cultures and other medical systems? Given the global spread of biomedicine, noncompliance with prescribed drug regimens is possible everywhere. But noncompliance with the advice of traditional healers is possible only when they recommend behaviors or materials to be prepared, consumed, or performed after a healing session. Bone-setting, massage, and spiritual healing all are performed primarily on afflicted persons or those around them. Because there is little room for patient initiative during these treatments, there is also little room for noncompliance. The analogue of noncompliance in this case would be the refusal to attend or to return to a specialist's care.

Compliance in urban North America usually refers to taking medications as ordered. In rural Africa, Asia, and Latin America, it may also mean preparing and drinking teas as ordered or performing specific ritual activities at "prescribed" times and places. A cross-cultural theory of health-related compliance would need to take these other activities and forms of authority into account. But such a cross-cultural theory of the differences between a healer's recommendations and a patient's actions must wait until the topic of compliance is separated from its association with professional biomedical care.

A review of compliance studies from developing countries found only 37 examples of such studies despite searching computer databases and following leads through personal networks (Homedes & Ugalde, 1993). The authors report these studies to be predominantly biomedical in orientation, but showing high levels of noncompliance across sites.

CONCLUSION

The topic of compliance is popular among physicians because it gives a focus to their interactions with "problem" patients, reflects their ideas about how patients should behave, and addresses their notions about the determinants of proper patient behavior. There was little research literature on patient compliance before the 1960s, but there is no reason to believe that patients before that time had obeyed doctors' orders in larger proportion or that practitioners before that time had no concerns about compliance. A number of factors must have combined to bring noncompliance to clinical attention: Increasing numbers of prescription drugs made noncompliance more possible and thus more visible; drug companies often mentioned compliance in their advertising; social scientists and clinicians convinced the growing biomedical research industry to examine the behavioral correlates of the problem; and health educators designed interventions. None of these factors should be singled out as the most important influence, but all have combined to create and sustain a long period of research on the topic.

Analyzing compliance as an ideology is useful because it helps explain why the more than 11,600 articles on the topic form a literature so contradictory and incomplete. Looking at patient behavior in terms of medical compliance perpetuates the notion that health care is (and ought to be) centered around proper use of physicians. The causes of problems in the physician-patient relationship are sought in patient behavior and beliefs. Researchers could hypothesize that all patients are potential noncompliers and that particular kinds of situations cause noncompliance. Instead, most of the research hypothesizes that there are noncompliant types of people and that with sufficient ingenuity their traits can be identified.

Descriptions of patient behavior and interventions designed to influence it have come full circle. Early in this century, companies manufacturing infant foods attempted to take product information and responsibility for care away from mothers. They gave doctors frank descriptions of how they might attempt to control their patients, and they loudly proclaimed their efforts to consolidate physician control over infant feeding practices. Patient education became accepted practice somewhat later, accompanied by attempts to increase patient responsibility and self-control, as well as attempts to bring patients subtly around to adopting physician desires as their own. Most recently, one can see the use of medical technology to reduce the need for patient initiative. For example, long-acting medications are recommended over short-acting, injections are recommended over pills, and office-centered interventions are valued over those in the home. These interventions may be effective, but they risk turning patients from responsible subjects into responsive objects, with information about advanced technologies again the primary domain of the physician.

If research on people's use of medications continues to be analyzed in terms of their compliance, then this research will continue to give a distorted picture of behavior. The word "compliant" has unfortunate connotations, but the underlying concept also needs reworking. It is valid to investigate what patients do with their medications and how they respond in daily life to the requests of medical professionals. However, these activities can be investigated far more comprehensively under rubrics such as "drug-taking behavior," "clinic attendance," or "medication consumption" than they can under the rubric of compliance. A behavioral definition can address the complexities introduced by self-care, care by nonmedical specialists, and care by nonspecialists. It must be flexible enough, however, to describe what strategies, if any, are adopted in place of those recommended by a healer.

FUTURE RESEARCH QUESTIONS

Most of these issues can be distilled into a series of empirical questions. For example, if medication use were better divided into component categories (e.g., taking medication as directed, taking it sporadically, regularly taking less, regularly taking more, discontinuing completely), would these component categories have stronger associations with predictor variables than the broader category of noncompliance? Are these subcategories associated with recourse to multiple sources of biomedical care, recourse to nonbiomedical care, or neither? What situations affect people's use of medications? Do people who modify or reject one medical regimen also modify or reject other medical regimens? Do they modify or reject other nonmedical regimens? Do rates or strategies of medication use vary across cultures? If variation exists, is it associated with different cultural rules about response to authority, different types of health systems, different expectations by medical professionals, or other factors?

These questions cannot be framed within the present definitions of compliance research. They still need to be asked and answered, however, to better portray the complexity and determinants of health-related behavior outside the examining room.

ACKNOWLEDGMENTS. This chapter is a revised version of J. Trostle, "Medical Compliance as an Ideology," *Social Science and Medicine*, *27*(12), 1299-1308, 1988, used here with permission from Pergamon Press. Support for the revision was provided by a grant from the Harvard Institute for International Development. The original paper was supported by the Epilepsy Foundation of America, the Wenner-Gren Foundation for Anthropological Research, the U.S. Berkeley Rennie Endowment, and the National Institute of Mental Health (MH09039-01 to -03). I am grateful to Andrew Noymer for his bibliographic and other research assistance. Lynn Morgan, Laura Nader, Fred Dunn, and two reviewers from *Social Science and Medicine* helped me to clarify prior drafts. An abridged version was presented in 1984 before the American Anthropological Association Annual Meeting.

REFERENCES

Apple, R. D. (1982).To be used only under the direction of a physician: Commercial infant feeding and medical practice, 1870-1940. *Bulletin of the History of Medicine*, *54*, 402-417.

Apple, R. D. (1987). *Mothers and medicine: A social history of infant feeding, 1890-1950*. Wisconsin Publications in the History of Science and Medicine, Number 7. Madison: University of Wisconsin Press.

Aronson, J. K., & Hardman, M. (1992). Patient compliance. *British Medical Journal*, *305*(6860), 1009-1011.

Barofsky, I. (1978). Compliance, adherence and the therapeutic alliance: Steps in the development of self-care. *Social Science and Medicine*, *12*, 369-376.

Becker, M. H., & Maiman, L. A.(1980). Strategies for enhancing patient compliance. *Journal of Community Health*, *6*, 113-131.

Benfari, R. C., Eaker, E., & Stoll, J. G. (1981). Behavioral interventions and compliance to treatment regimens. *Annual Review of Public Health*, *2*, 431-471.

Bissonette, R., & Seller, R. (1980). Medical noncompliance: A cultural perspective. *Man and Medicine*, *5*, 41-53.

Blackwell, B. (1992). Compliance. *Psychotherapy and Psychosomatics*, *58*, 161-169.

Bronfman, M., Castro, R., Guiscafré, H., Muñoz, O., & Gutiérrez, G. (1991). Prescripción médica y adherencia al tratamiento en diarrea infecciosa aguda: Impacto indirecto de una intervencón educativa. *Salud Pública de México*, *33*, 568-575.

Brown, E. R. (1979). *Rockefeller medicine men: Medicine and capitalism in America*. Berkeley: University of California Press.

Buchanan, N. (1982). Treatment of epilepsy: Whose right is it anyway? *British Medical Journal*, *284*, 173-174.

Conrad, P. (1979). Types of medical social control. *Sociology of Health and Illness*, *1*, 1-11.

Conrad, P. (1985). The meaning of medications: Another look at compliance. *Social Science and Medicine*, *20*, 29-37.

Cramer, J. A., Scheyer, R. D., & Mattson, R. H. (1990). Compliance declines between clinic visits. *Annals of Internal Medicine*, *150*, 1509-1510.

Crout, J. R. (1980). Self-medication: The government role, Part II. In *Self-medication: The new era—A symposium* (pp. 41-44). Washington, DC: The Proprietary Association.

David, M. S. (1968). Variations in patients' compliance with doctors' advice: An empirical analysis of patterns of communication. *American Journal of Public Health*, *58*, 274-288.

DiMatteo, M. R., & DiNicola, D. D. (1982). *Achieving patient compliance: The psychology of the medical practitioner's role*. New York: Pergamon Press.

Duffy, J. (1984). American perceptions of the medical, legal, and theological professions. *Bulletin of the History of Medicine*, *58*, 1-15.

Eraker, S. A., Kirscht, J. P., & Becker, M. H. (1984). Understanding and improving patient compliance. *Annals of Internal Medicine*, *100*, 258-268.

Evans, W. (1959). Faults in the diagnosis and management of cardiac pain. *British Medical Journal*, *1*(Jan. 31), 249-253.

Feinstein, A. R. (1990). On white-coat effects and the electronic monitoring of compliance. *Annals of Internal Medicine*, *150*, 1377-1378.

Freidson, E. (1970). *Profession of medicine: A study of the sociology of applied knowledge*. New York: Dodd, Mead.

Freidson, E. (1975). *Doctoring together: A study of professional social control*. New York: Elsevier-North Holland.

Garrity, T. F. (1981). Medical compliance and the clinician-patient relationship: A review. *Social Science and Medicine, 15*, 215-222.

Haug, M., & Lavin, B. (1983). *Consumerism in medicine: Challenging physician authority*. Beverly Hills, CA: Sage.

Hayes-Bautista, D. (1976). Modifying the treatment: Patient compliance, patient control and medical care. *Social Science and Medicine, 10*, 233-238.

Haynes, R. B. (1979). Introduction. In R. B. Haynes, D. L. Sackett, & D. W. Taylor (Eds.), *Compliance in health care* (pp. 1-10). Baltimore, MD: Johns Hopkins University Press.

Haynes, R. B., Sackett, D. L., & Taylor, D. W. (Eds.). (1979). *Compliance in health care*. Baltimore, MD: Johns Hopkins University Press.

Homedes, N., & Ugalde, A. (1993). Patients' compliance with medical treatments in the third world: What do we know? *Health Policy and Planning, 8*, 291-314.

Horwitz, R. I., & Horwitz, S. M. (1993). Adherence to treatment and health outcomes. *Annals of Internal Medicine, 153*, 1863-1868.

Jonsen, A. R. (1979). Ethical issues in compliance. In R. B. Haynes, D. L. Sackett, & D. W. Taylor (Eds.), *Compliance in health care* (pp. 113-120). Baltimore, MD: Johns Hopkins University Press.

Kasl, S. V. (1975). Issues in patient adherence to health care regimens. *Journal of Human Stress, 1*, 5-17.

Klein, R. (1973). *Complaints against doctors: A study in professional accountability*. London: Charles Knight.

Lasagna, L. (1973). Fault and default. *New England Journal of Medicine, 289*, 267-268.

Leventhal, H. (1985). The role of theory in the study of adherence to treatment and doctor-patient interactions. *Medical Care, 23*, 556-563.

Leventhal, H., Zimmerman, R., & Gutmann, M. (1984). Compliance: A self-regulation perspective. In W. D. Gentry (Ed.), *Handbook of behavioral medicine* (pp. 369-436). New York: Guilford Press.

Levin, L. (1980). Self-medication: The social perspective. In *Self-medication: The new era—A symposium* (pp. 44-57). Washington DC: The Proprietary Association.

Ley, P. (1981). Professional non-compliance: A neglected problem. *British Journal of Clinical Psychology, 20*, 151-154.

McKinlay, J. B., & Arches, J. (1985). Towards the proletarianization of physicians. *International Journal of Health Services, 15*, 161-195.

Morris, L. S., & Schulz, R. M. (1993). Medication compliance: The patient's perspective. *Clinical Therapeutics, 15*, 593-606.

Nichter, M., & Vuckovic, N. (1994). Agenda for an anthropology of pharmaceutical practice. *Social Science and Medicine, 39*, 1509-1525.

Richardson, M. A., Simons-Morton, B., & Annegers, J. F. (1993). Effect of perceived barriers on compliance with antihypertensive medication. *Health Education Quarterly, 20*, 489-503.

Robbins, J. A. (1980). Patient compliance. *Primary Care, 7*, 703-711.

Rodin, J., & Janis, I. L. (1979). The social power of health care practitioners as agents of change. *Journal of Social Issues, 35*, 60-81.

Roth, J. S. (1962). "Management bias" in social science study of medical treatment. *Human Organization, 21*, 47-50.

Sackett, D. L. (1976). Introduction. In D. L. Sackett, & R. B. Haynes, (Eds.), *Compliance with therapeutic regimens* (pp. 1-6). Baltimore, MD: Johns Hopkins University Press.

Sackett, D. L., & Snow, J. C. (1979). The magnitude of compliance and noncompliance. In R. B. Haynes, D. L. Sackett, & D. W. Taylor (Eds.), *Compliance in health care* (pp. 11-12). Baltimore, MD: Johns Hopkins University Press.

Schneider, J. W., & Conrad, P. (1983). *Having epilepsy: The experience and control of illness*. Philadelphia: Temple University Press.

Soumerai, S. B., McLaughlin, T. J., & Avorn, J. (1989). Improving drug prescribing in primary care: A critical analysis of the experimental literature. *Milbank Quarterly, 67*, 268-317.

Starr, P. (1982). *The social transformation of American medicine*. New York: Basic Books.

Stevens, R. (1971). *American medicine and the public interest*. New Haven, CT: Yale University Press.

Stimson, G. V. (1974). Obeying the doctor's orders: A view from the other side. *Social Science and Medicine, 8*, 97-104.

Stone, G. C. (1979). Patient compliance and the role of the expert. *Journal of Social Issues, 35*, 34-59.

Taussig, M. (1980). Reification and the consciousness of the patient. *Social Science and Medicine, 14B*, 3-13.

Temkin, O. (1964). Historical aspects of drug therapy. In P. Talalay (Ed.), *Drugs in our society* (pp. 3-16). Baltimore, MD: Johns Hopkins University Press.

Trostle, J. A., Hauser, W. A., & Susser, I. S. (1983). The logic of noncompliance: Management of epilepsy from the patient's point of view. *Culture, Medicine and Psychiatry, 7*, 35-56.

Udry, J. R., & Morris, N. M. (1971). A spoonful of sugar helps the medicine go down. *American Journal of Public Health, 61*, 30-33.

U.S. Department of Commerce. (1994). *Statistical abstract of the United States*. Washington, DC: U.S. Government Printing Office.

Vandereycken, W., & Meermann, R. (1988). Chronic illness behavior and noncompliance with treatment: Pathways to an interactional approach. *Psychotherapy and Psychosomatics, 50*, 182-191.

Van Kamerik, S. B. (1978). Why don't patients do what you tell them? *Legal Aspects of Medical Practice, 6*, 30-33.

Waitzkin, H. (1985). Information giving in medical care. *Journal of Health and Social Behavior, 26*, 81-101.

Weibert, R. T., & Dee, D. A. (1980). *Improving patient medication compliance*. Oradell, NJ: Medical Economics Company, Book Division.

Weintraub, M. (1976). Intelligent noncompliance and capricious compliance. In L. Lasagna (Ed.), *Patient compliance* (pp. 39-47). Mt. Kisco, NY: Futura Publishing.

Wright, E. C. (1993). Non-compliance—or how many aunts has Matilda. *Lancet*, *342*(Oct. 9), 909-913.

Zola, I. K. (1966). Culture and symptoms—an analysis of patients' presenting complaints. *American Sociological Review*, *31*, 615-630.

Zola, I. K. (1981). Structural constraints in the doctor-patient relationship: The case of noncompliance. In L. Eisenberg & A. Kleinman (Eds.), *The relevance of social science for medicine* (pp. 241-252). Dordrecht, The Netherlands: Reidel Press.

B. DISEASE-FOCUSED REGIMENS

ADHERENCE TO DISEASE-FOCUSED REGIMENS

The introductory material for Part III is equally suitable as a context for this section. The issues identified and the analysis of the concepts of compliance, adherence, and acceptance are just as applicable for discussions of adherence to specific disease-focused, largely medical regimens. Although the literature on "compliance" deals with a variety of health behaviors, including weight control and smoking reduction, it has historically been concerned primarily with proper acceptance of medication for diseases—particularly those that are seen as life-threatening, such as asthma, diabetes, hypertension, seizure disorders, and end-stage renal disease—and with patients' keeping of appointments. Stimson (1974) pointed out decades ago that much of the literature reflects attempts to discover the nature of the "flaws" in the patient that account for the failure to comply. Despite such admonition, the literature remains focused on the individual patient, as Dunbar-Jacob (1993) observed nearly 20 years later; the theoretical models used—e.g., the health belief model, common sense models, cost-benefit models, self-efficacy models, the theory of reasoned behavior—all focus on patient characteristics rather than on those of the provider or the system (e.g., Dunbar-Jacob, 1993). Much of the psychological literature on compliance or adherence is driven by intervention research based upon the models, rather than by an interest in finding out the wide range of factors—personal, family, social, and institutional—that affect adherence.

Research on compliance can be considered, for convenience, in terms of whether it focuses on the individual or on system factors or whether it addresses reconceptualization of compliance itself.

INDIVIDUAL AND FAMILY FACTORS

The Health Belief Model

Much research dealing with the individual is derived from the health belief model. In one early study, for example, a modified health belief model was shown to be a predictor of how well mothers will engage in recommended behaviors relating to their child's health, such as giving medications or keeping appointments (Becker, Drachman, & Kirscht, 1974). While this study introduced some health care system factors, such as whether the same physician treated the child previously, the major focus was nonetheless on the mothers' beliefs, such as whether she perceives that her child is resusceptible to the present illness, whether that illness is serious, and whether the prescribed medicine will be of benefit. Perceived benefits and perceived barriers were found to be the most important health belief model variables in the prediction of compliance with hemodialysis (Hartman & Becker, 1978). Later research continued to show some predictive value for perceived benefits and perceived barriers, particularly under conditions of low perceived threat (Aiken, West, Woodward, & Reno, 1994). Although some components of the model were significant predictors of acceptance of a recommendation for mammography screening in asymptomatic women, system factors, such as having a regular source of care, predicted more of the variance.

In other settings, however, the belief model was of limited value. It was a poor predictor of whether prescribed medications will be picked up from the pharmacist (Fincham & Wertheimer, 1985), and it was not a good predictor of children's acceptance of a mouth-rinse program, which was more solidly predicted by patterns of environmental reward contingency (Kegeles & Lund, 1984) and by perceptions of decisional control and student work characteristics (Burleson, Kegeles, & Lund, 1990).

Attribution Theory

Attribution theory provides another framework for adherence research. An extensive examination of the several components of adherence to dietary regimens among persons with hypertension revealed different types of attributes for "failures" to adhere to different dietary programs. While difficulty in dealing with environmental demands and social situations, and "lack of willpower," were common attributions among persons in the different treatment programs, those in the weight-loss and weight-loss plus sodium-reduction programs were more likely to use a characterological defect or an emotional status explanation, and more likely to consider their problems internal rather than external, than were persons in the sodium-reduction and sodium-reduction plus increased-potassium groups. Persons in these latter groups were more likely to use nonsocial situational attributions for their problems in adherence (Jeffrey, French, & Schmid, 1990). The terminology used in such report, however, conveys a sense of "self-serving" attributions, or an optimistic bias, as factors in understanding adherent behaviors. More important, the data showed no linkage between the nature of attributions and the actual degree of adherence to the programs. Research generated by attribution theory has also shown that levels of adherence to the different sets of demands within a diabetes regimen (e.g., weight control, carrying emergency glucose) were generally inconsistent, further arguing against consistent patient characteristics as barriers (Orme & Binik, 1989).

Other Approaches

In an effort to improve predictions about "self-management" of asthma in youngsters and adolescents, Matus, Kinsman, and Jones (1978) attempted to systematize the measurement of related attitudes. Their factor analyses showed seven clearly defined and stable clusters of attitudes to chronic asthma and hospitalization: minimization of severity, passive observance of illness, bravado, expectation of staff rejection, moralistic authoritarianism, stigma, and external control.

The Dishman (1982) study of compliance with an exercise regimen dealt with a large number of individual cognitive, motivational, and physiological characteristics, together with consideration of the exercise setting and the interaction between the person and the setting. Although self-motivation seemed to show some promise as a predictor of compliance, most of the variables had little or no predictive value.

An extensive examination of family risk factors revealed that having means of transportation was one of the most appreciable factors in appointment keeping at a pediatric otology clinic (Kavanagh, Smith, Golden, Tate, & Hinkle, 1991), pointing to the importance of larger social system determinants. Although ethnographic evidence is available to enlarge medical horizons about family barriers to adherence and to encourage physicians to take a "systems" perspective, the arguments generated by this evidence often are directed to systems beyond the physician's office (e.g., Stein & Pontious, 1985). Focusing primarily on individual and family characteristics seems to promise limited effectiveness in increasing compliance.

PROVIDER FACTORS

Moving beyond individual and family factors, the study by Lorber (1975) of how hospitalized surgical patients comply with—or disrupt—hospital routines demonstrated how such disruptions lead to differential responses by physicians and nurses, invoking labeling in terms of conformity or deviance. Lorber's analyses showed how the organization of tasks within the hospital setting, together with professionals' differential expectations for behavior and responses to pain for different categories of patients, enters into the labeling process.

Davis (1976) examined how the profession of dentistry functions as a social regulatory institution and reasoned that compliance with dental regimens must be understood in terms of the degree of congruity that exists between the components of the provider system and the culture of the patient. Evidence exists that providers fail to consider the ethnic backgrounds of geriatric patients and label as "noncompliant" behaviors that are ethnically appropriate but depart from those of the larger community and as "difficult" the patients who exhibit them (Fineman, 1991). Staff misperceptions of behavior in elderly patients often led to categorizing them as unwilling to comply and thus blameworthy (Fineman, 1991). Fineman demonstrates the subjective nature of such perceptions, arguing that compliance is a provider-constructed category of unacceptable behavior.

Borkman (1976) identified how professional-staff perceptions of patients' grasp of instructions and intelligence were related to adherence to hemodialysis regimens. Borkman noted that staff perceptions of patients' understanding led to self-fulfilling prophecies: Those who were perceived to have greater understanding could have been given more attention and more instruction.

Marlatt's relapse-prevention model (e.g., Curry, Marlatt, Gordon, & Baer, 1988) is a framework for understanding and reducing relapses in the process of changing lifestyle behaviors such as smoking. Relapse prevention is based on developing skills for recognizing and dealing with situations in which relapse is likely to occur.

The relative importance of structural aspects of the health care system in determining levels of appointment keeping is demonstrated by the Hertz and Stamps (1977) analysis of clients of a Model Cities Health Center. Hulka, Cassel, Kupper, and Burdette's (1976) systematic examination of how inadequate physician communications impede acceptance of medication by patients with diabetes mellitus and congestive heart failure further demonstrated the importance of the interaction between the system and the patient.

Interventions at the system level have also been examined by Reid (1979), who showed that instructional materials were moderately successful on a short-term basis in maintaining adherence to an exercise program by fire fighters; by Tagliacozzo, Luskin, Lashof, and Ima (1974), who showed that instructional interventions by nurses could improve compliance by increasing patients' understanding of their condition; by Bélisle, Roskies, and Lévesque (1987), who reported very modest success for a "relapse-prevention" program to improve adherence to an exercise regimen; and by Roberts, Wurtele, and Leeper (1983), who raised questions about the value of specific forms of reminders in increasing the return rate of patients for tuberculosis screening.

In comparison to the great number of studies reported on patient characteristics, studies exploring physician characteristics in relation to adherence are rare (e.g., DiMatteo et al., 1993). Patients of physicians who made definite future follow-up appointments, or who answered all of their patient's questions, tended to have higher levels of adherence to a range of regimens (DiMatteo et al., 1993). Ross (1991) demonstrated problems in adherence that stem from discrepancies in health professionals' knowledge and understanding of drugs. District nurses in Great Britain often did not know what drugs their patients were taking. Possibly this lack of knowledge was a result of limited information provided to them by hospitals or of communication barriers between nurses and physicians. Ross urges that responsibility for compliance be shared by professionals and not laid solely upon the patient.

Squier's (1990) integration of research literature from the social sciences led him to propose a critical characteristic for physicians and other practitioners: empathic understanding. The data underlying Squier's proposal suggests that such understanding would increase adherence to a range of treatment regimens, from psychotherapy to medical therapies.

Regardless of whether the behaviors are referred to as compliance, adherence, or acceptance; or of whether they are viewed in terms of physician, social, or patient control, the research and conceptualizations about how persons respond to medical or health regimens clearly indicate that a simple medical perspective is insufficient and that the problem will not be resolved by technology or simplistic interventions. The problem does not inhere in patient or client inadequacy; the problem is multifaceted and emerges from interactions with the system. On one hand, nonadherence or nonacceptance may not be a problem at all, but an appropriate means of adaptive behavior from the patient's perspective. On the other hand, when patients wish to adhere or accept, professionals must consider the importance of their own behavior, their communication, their role performance, other system dimensions, and other factors in order to increase the likelihood that such adherence or acceptance will occur.

However, the predominant cognitive theoretical models maintain a focus on the individual. Even movement toward conceptions such as self-regulation (e.g., Leventhal & Cameron, 1987) maintain a focus on the individual rather than on the health care system and the individual's interactions with it.

DISEASE-FOCUSED INTERVENTIONS

Although the focus of this *Handbook* was intended to emphasize determinants of adherence rather than the technology or packaging of programs or interventions, it was sometimes difficult to get contributors to deal explicitly with these determinants. Much of the research on adherence is done from a clinical perspective, emphasizing attempts at change and technologies of change. Much of the research is driven by psychological theory and thus does not reflect knowledge of a broader range of social factors that facilitate or impede adherence. While contributors were asked to discuss adherence as an outcome of institutional determinants, they understandably defined this request in terms of "programmatic" determinants. As appropriate, they were encouraged to add explicit discussion of personal, social, family, and cultural factors that influenced adherence, and the chapters *do* contain such material.

DETERMINANTS OF ADHERENCE TO DISEASE-FOCUSED REGIMENS

The distinction between disease-focused and lifestyle regimens is arbitrary and made for convenience. Many of the disease-focused regimens involve a considerable degree of lifestyle change, particularly in diet and exercise. At the same time, some theories—e.g., decisional balance, transtheoretical, stages of change—might be more suitable for understanding, predicting, and enhancing attempts at lifestyle change than for dealing with medical immediacy. Moreover, Leventhal and Cameron (1987) raise cogent questions about differences between factors that determine adherence in relation to prevention and those that determine adherence in relation to cure. Questions also arise about differences in factors that underlie adherence to a lifestyle change and those that underlie acceptance of a once-a-year screening or one-shot immunization.

In Chapter 7, Creer and Levstek present

insights into some personal determinants of adherence to an asthmatic regimen, as well as recommendations for provider actions from which one can infer provider and system factors that facilitate or impede adherence.

In Chapter 8, on self-regulation of heart disease and hypertension, Clark considers personal and social determinants, yet emphasizes the importance of the provider and the patient-provider interaction in increasing the patient's ability to engage in self-regulatory behavior.

Wysocki and Greco's Chapter 9, on adherence to a diabetes regimen in children, stresses the importance of the family context, the child's developmental level, and the interactions of the family and the provider. The family, rather than the provider, is considered the major agency for assuring adherence.

In contrast, in Chapter 10, on adherence to a diabetes regimen in adults, Fisher, Arfken, Heins, Houston, Jeffe, and Sykes stress not only the role of the provider, but also cultural, worksite, economic, and social factors that affect adherence.

In Chapter 11, on epilepsy, Dr. Iorio stresses a "framework of relationships" model that incorporates intervention strategies designed to change the antecedents of adherence, including personal beliefs, family practices, behaviors of providers, and institutional and community resources.

In addition to discussing patient beliefs, other personal characteristics, and social and demographic factors in Chapter 12, on adherence to renal dialysis regimens, Christensen, Benotsch, and Smith emphasize the interactions between the patient and the treatment context.

In Chapter 13, Champion and Miller discuss the factors that underlie acceptance of mammography and breast self-examination from the perspectives of both descriptive and intervention research, emphasizing the special importance of provider initiatives and recommendations in increasing acceptance of mammography.

The resurgence of tuberculosis as a major public health problem, after years in which it had not been one, adds special import to Chapter 14, in which Morisky and Cabrera stress provider responsibility and institutional access in increasing adherence to tuberculosis regimens and discuss the impact of stigmatization.

Barriers to acceptance of screenings for cervical, colorectal, skin, prostate, and testicular cancers are discussed in Chapter 15 by Rimer, Denmark-Wahnefried, and Egert, which stresses the importance of provider recommendation, convenience, and the embarrassment faced by persons undergoing certain of the screening procedures.

In Chapter 16, McCaul emphasizes the role of provider initiatives and monitoring in adherence to regimens for dental disease, particularly in relation to flossing.

REFERENCES

Aiken, L. S., West, S. G., Woodward, C. K., & Reno, R. R. (1994). Health beliefs and compliance with mammography-screening recommendations in asymptomatic women. *Health Psychology, 13*, 122-129.

Becker, M. H., Drachman, R. H., & Kirscht, J. P. (1974). A new approach to explaining sick-role behavior in low-income populations. *American Journal of Public Health, 64*, 205-216.

Bélisle, M., Roskies, E., & Lévesque, J.-M. (1987). Improving adherence to physical activity. *Health Psychology, 6*, 159-172.

Borkman, T. S. (1976). Hemodialysis compliance: The relationship of staff estimates of patients' intelligence and understanding to compliance. *Social Science and Medicine, 10*, 385-392.

Burleson, J. A., Kegeles, S. S., & Lund, A. K. (1990). Effects of decisional control and work orientation on persistence in preventive health behavior. *Health Psychology, 9*, 1-17.

Curry, S. J., Marlatt, G. A., Gordon, J., & Baer, J. S. (1988). A comparison of alternative theoretical approaches to smoking cessation and relapse. *Health Psychology, 7*, 545-556.

Davis, P. (1976). Compliance structures and the delivery of health care: The case of dentistry. *Social Science and Medicine, 10*, 329-337.

DiMatteo, M. R., Sherbourne, C. D., Hays, R. D., Ordway, L., Kravitz, R. L., McGlynn, E. A., Kaplan, S., & Rogers, W. H. (1993). Physicians' characteristics influence patients' adherence to medical treatment: Results from the medical outcomes study. *Health Psychology, 12*, 93-102.

Dishman, R. K. (1982). Compliance/adherence in health-related exercise. *Health Psychology, 1*, 237-267.

Dunbar-Jacob, J. (1993). Contributions to patient adherence: Is it time to share the blame? *Health Psychology, 12*, 91-92.

Fincham, J. E., & Wertheimer, A. I. (1985). Using the health belief model to predict initial drug therapy defaulting. *Social Science and Medicine*, *20*, 101-105.

Fineman, N. (1991). The social construction of noncompliance: Implications for cross-cultural geriatric practice. *Journal of Cross Cultural Gerontology*, *6*(2), 219-227.

Hartman, P. E., & Becker, M. H. (1978). Non-compliance with prescribed regimen among chronic hemodialysis patients: A method of prediction and educational diagnosis. *Dialysis and Transplantation*, 7, 978-985.

Hertz, P., & Stamps, P. L. (1977). Appointment-keeping behavior re-evaluated. *American Journal of Public Health*, *67*, 1033-1036.

Hulka, B. S., Cassel, J. C., Kupper, L. L., & Burdette, J. A. (1976). Communication, compliance, and concordance between physicians and patients with prescribed medications. *American Journal of Public Health*, *66*, 847-853.

Jeffrey, R. W., French, S. A., & Schmid, T. L. (1990). Attributions for dietary failures: Problems reported by participants in the hypertension prevention trial. *Health Psychology*, *9*, 315-329.

Kavanagh, K. T., Smith, T. R., Golden, G. S., Tate, N. P., & Hinkle, W. G. (1991). Multivariate analysis of family risk factors in predicting appointment attendance in a pediatric otology and communication clinic. *Journal of Health and Social Policy*, *2*(3), 85-102.

Kegeles, S. S., & Lund, A. K. (1984). Adolescents' acceptance of caries-preventive procedures. In J. Matarazzo, S. Weiss, J. Herd, N. Miller, & S. Weiss (Eds.), *Behavioral health: A handbook of health enhancement and disease prevention* (pp. 895-909). New York: Wiley.

Leventhal, H., & Cameron, L. (1987). Behavioral theories and the problem of compliance. *Patient Education and Counseling*, *10*, 117-138.

Lorber, J. (1975). Good patients and problem patients: Conformity and deviance in a general hospital. *Journal of Health and Social Behavior*, *16*, 213-225.

Matus, I., Kinsman, R. A., & Jones, N. F. (1978). Pediatric patient attitudes toward chronic asthma and hospitalization. *Journal of Chronic Disease*, *31*, 611-618.

Orme, C. M., & Binik, R. M. (1989). Consistency of adherence across regimen demands. *Health Psychology*, *8*, 27-43.

Reid, E. A. L. (1979). Exercise prescription: A clinical trial. *American Journal of Public Health*, *69*, 591-595.

Roberts, M. C., Wurtele, S. K., & Leeper, J. D. (1983). Experiments to increase return in a medical screening drive: Two futile attempts to apply theory to practice. *Social Science and Medicine*, *17*, 741-746.

Ross, F. M. (1991). Patient compliance—Whose responsibility? *Social Science and Medicine*, *32*, 89-94.

Squier, R. W. (1990). A model of empathic understanding and adherence to treatment regiments in practitioner-patient relationships. *Social Science and Medicine*, *30*, 325-339.

Stein, H. F., & Pontius, J. M. (1985). Family and beyond: The larger context of noncompliance. *Family Systems Medicine*, *3*(2), 179-189.

Stimson, G. V. (1974). Obeying doctor's orders: A view from the other side. *Social Science and Medicine*, *8*, 97-104.

Tagliacozzo, D. M., Luskin, D. B., Lashof, J. C., & Ima, K. (1974). Nurse intervention and patient behavior: An experimental study. *American Journal of Public Health*, *64*, 596-603.

7

Adherence to Asthma Regimens

Thomas L. Creer and Deirdre Levstek

INTRODUCTION

A number of effective medications have been introduced for the treatment of asthma in the past 25 years. Advances in the development of medications both to prevent and to treat ongoing attacks are the hallmark of the period. Despite considerable progress in treating asthma, however, the disorder is a health concern to more and more Americans. A number of factors contribute to the paradox of asthma, but none is more important than adherence to medication regimens. Medication adherence is best explained within a context that includes a description of epidemiological data, characteristics of asthma, and management of the disorder (Creer & Bender, 1993).

EPIDEMIOLOGY

Prevalence

Approximately 15 million individuals in the United States have asthma. On the basis of National Health Interview Survey data from 1980 through 1990, the age-adjusted prevalence rate of self-reported asthma increased by 38%; this figure included a 50% increase for females and a 27% increase for males (*MMWR*, 1992). According to the National Health Interview Survey, Taylor and Newacheck (1992) found a statistically significant increase from 3.2% in 1981 to 4.3% in 1988 in the prevalence of asthma in children younger than 18 years of age. It is known that racial or ethnic minorities who are poor and who live in urban environments are at risk for asthma (Weiss, Gergen, & Crain, 1992). Little is known about those who live in rural areas, in part because these populations are rarely studied.

Morbidity

Morbidity data reflect the quantitative and qualitative conditions or states influenced by asthma. A number of types of data were reported by the Centers for Disease Control (CDC) (*MMWR*, 1992). Physician visits for asthma as a first-listed diagnosis increased from 6.5 million in 1985 to 7.1 million in 1990. The age-adjusted rate of physician visits increased 35% for blacks, but decreased 8% for whites. For blacks, the rate of visits decreased 46% for males, but increased 98% for females. For whites, the rate decreased 23% for males, but increased 8% for females.

Thomas L. Creer and Deirdre Levstek • Department of Psychology, Ohio University, Athens, Ohio 45701-2979.

Handbook of Health Behavior Research II: Provider Determinants, edited by David S. Gochman. Plenum Press, New York, 1997.

Mortality

Mortality due to asthma pales beside that from other causes, particularly heart disease and cancer. There are, however, two reasons that deaths due to asthma are alarming (Creer & Bender, 1993). First, there has been a sharp increase in deaths from asthma in the past few years. As compiled by the CDC, the age-adjusted death rate for asthma as the underlying cause of death increased 46% from 1.3 per 100,000 to 1.9 per 100,000, from 1980 through 1989. The second reason is that with newer and more effective treatments for asthma, there should be a decrease, not an increase, in deaths from asthma. The puzzle of why increased deaths from asthma have occurred when better treatments for the disorder are available is exacerbated by the knowledge that, as pointed out by Ellis (1988), any mortality from a potentially reversible disorder such as asthma is unacceptable.

CHARACTERISTICS OF ASTHMA

Any description of asthma emphasizes the intermittent, variable, and reversible nature of the disorder.

Intermittency

The number of attacks varies from patient to patient and, for a given individual, from time to time. A patient may suffer several attacks over the span of a few days and then go several months or even years without suffering an attack. Another patient may experience asthma perennially and on most days throughout the year. The frequency of attacks experienced by patients is a function of several variables, including the number and types of stimuli that trigger their asthmatic episodes, the degree of hyperreactivity of their airways, the degree of control established over their asthma, health care variables including access to asthma specialists, and patient variables including medication compliance. Any of these variables may produce dramatic changes in an individual's asthma (Creer & Bender, 1993).

The intermittent nature of asthma has two implications for medication adherence (Renne & Creer, 1985). First, the intermittent nature of asthma means there may be long periods of time between attacks. When this pattern occurs, patients may forget how to manage asthmatic episodes and be unprepared to manage an attack when one occurs. Second, the intermittent nature of asthma generates different expectations in patients. Those with perennial asthma anticipate that they will experience asthma throughout the year; consequently, they are usually prepared to manage episodes when they occur. Those with intermittent asthma, however, may fail to anticipate what could be a severe asthmatic episode and therefore be unprepared to abort the attack.

Variability

The term *variability* can refer either to the severity of a patient's asthma or to the intensity of discrete attacks. Use of the term is therefore confusing in that it is not always clear whether severity refers to the patient's general condition or to specific attacks the patient experiences.

Two additional issues are raised by the ambiguity of the term variability. First, until recently, there was no consensual agreement on how to classify either a given attack or the asthma itself as mild, moderate, or severe. Although these comparative terms were used throughout the asthma literature, there were no established criteria for their use (Creer & Bender, 1993). This situation is changing, since both a national panel of experts (National Institutes of Health, 1991) and an international panel of experts (National Institutes of Health, 1992) offered a general classification of asthma severity and a guide for treatment of patients who experience mild, moderate, or severe asthma attacks.

Second, Renne and Creer (1985) pointed out that patients acquire different expectations as a function of the severity of their attacks. If their attacks are mild, they tend to anticipate that all future attacks will be mild and are unprepared to cope with more severe attacks if and when they occur. A single severe episode may lead to emotional reactions, such as panic, that accompany future attacks (Creer, 1979). Expectations that they will experience only mild asthma attacks may lead patients to delay seeking medical attention for severe episodes. Failure to seek prompt and aggressive medical action for attacks that increasingly intensify in severity is a frequently cited factor for deaths due to asthma (e.g., Sheffer & Buist, 1987).

Reversibility

Reversibility is a distinguishing characteristic of asthma; it differentiates the condition from other respiratory disorders, particularly emphysema, that are irreversible. Like other characteristics of asthma, however, reversibility too is ambiguous. First, reversibility may be relative. Although most patients show complete reversibility of airway obstruction with appropriate medical treatment, others do not achieve total reversibility of asthma even with intensive therapy (Loren et al., 1978). Second, the spontaneous remission of some attacks makes it impossible to prove a cause-effect relationship between changes in a patient's asthma and treatment for the disorder (Creer, 1982). Although outcome data may support the efficacy of a particular intervention, symptoms can remit spontaneously and coincidentally with treatment.

MEDICAL TREATMENT OF ASTHMA

Asthma was long considered a disorder of the nervous system and smooth muscle. In the past decade, however, it has been described primarily as an inflammatory process. Recognition that inflammation is significant in the pathogenesis of asthma changed the focus of asthma treatment toward prescribing some medications for maintenance or prevention therapy and other medications for treatment of acute exacerbations of asthma (National Institutes of Health, 1991, 1992).

Maintenance or Preventative Medications

Major types of medications used for maintenance or prophylactic purposes are cromolyn sodium and inhaled corticosteroids (Ellis, 1993; National Institutes of Health, 1991).

Cromolyn Sodium. When used prophylactically, cromolyn sodium inhibits both early- and late-phase allergen-induced asthma. It is effective in reducing acute airway narrowing after exercise and after exposure to cold, dry air and sulfur dioxide. The mechanism of action of cromolyn sodium is not fully understood, but it is thought that the medication stabilizes and prevents mediator release from mast cells. While cromolyn sodium is an ideal drug to use in preventing asthma attacks, particularly in children, it is not effective with all patients. Cromolyn sodium produces only minimal side effects.

Corticosteroids. Corticosteroids are the most effective anti-inflammatory medications for the treatment of asthma. Two main forms of corticosteroid therapy are available for asthma: oral and inhaled. Oral corticosteroid therapy is typically used only in the treatment of severe asthma. It helps prevent further exacerbations of attacks, and it decreases the morbidity associated with asthmatic episodes. A problem is that there are many adverse side effects associated with both short- and long-term use of oral corticosteroids. Inhaled corticosteroid therapy is safer and, in many cases, more effective for the treatment of asthma. Because of airway inflammation, inhaled corticosteroids are used as primary therapy for moderate and severe asthma (Ellis, 1993; National Institutes of Health, 1991).

Medications for Attack Management

Bronchodilators are used for managing acute attacks because they dilate the airways by relaxing bronchial smooth muscle. The types of bronchodilators used to manage acute attacks of asthma are β-adrenergic agonists and methylxanthines.

β-Adrenergic Agonists (β_2-Agonists). β_2-Agonists relax airway smooth muscle and may modulate mediator release from mast cells that contribute to inflammation. β-Adrenergic agonists are valuable in asthma therapy because of their action on β_2-adrenergic receptors (National Institutes of Health, 1991). Inhaled β_2-agonists are the medication of choice for acute exacerbations of asthma and for prevention of exercise-induced asthma.

Methylxanthines

Theophylline is the principal methylxanthine used in asthma therapy. While the precise manner in which the drug works is unclear, theophylline serves as a bronchodilator for mild to moderate asthma. When used as a sustained-release preparation, theophylline has a long duration of action; this property makes it particularly useful in the control of nocturnal asthma. The National Institutes of Health (1991) pointed out that when used in combination with usual doses of inhaled β_2-agonists, theophylline may produce additional bronchodilation. A number of side effects are produced by theophylline preparations. Furthermore, there are individual differences in eliminating these drugs from the body, as well as a large number of stimuli that interact with the agent to reduce or enhance theophylline clearance (Ellis, 1993; National Institutes of Health, 1991).

ADHERENCE AND ASTHMA

There is no single, clinically useful, and widely accepted definition of the concept of adherence. Generally speaking, adherence is the congruence between patient behaviors and advice or instructions provided by health care providers. Medication adherence or compliance is how closely a patient's medication-taking behaviors match instructions prescribed by the physician. There is no single criterion that defines adherence across situations or behaviors. Many researchers have committed what Dirks and Kinsman (1982) referred to as a "yes-no" fallacy by reducing multiple patterns of medication usage to a simplistic dichotomy of compliant or noncompliant patients. In reality, medication adherence of patients should be conceived of as a continuum ranging from total nonadherence to total adherence (Creer, 1993). At one end of the continuum are patients who fail to fill prescriptions and who rely upon hospital emergency rooms for treatment of their asthma. At the other end are patients, referred to by Kirschenbaum and Tomarken (1982) as "obsessive-compulsive self-regulators," who adhere to all instructions provided by health care providers all the time. There is uncertainty about the adherence of a given patient in that while a test may reveal the patient to be taking medications as prescribed, the individual's behavior is likely to be inconsistent over time (Spector et al., 1986).

Specific features of the health situation, such as the therapeutic levels required to achieve symptom relief, may be more useful in defining medication adherence than in setting arbitrary percentages for medication use (e.g., 80% of medication ingested equals adherence). Therefore, it is important to determine the minimum standard for a given setting and regimen that will result in the desired health outcome and to choose measurements appropriate for determining adherence in a given context (Rand & Wise, 1994; Turk & Meichenbaum, 1991). Results of studies that have specifically investigated adherence to asthma regimens range from 2% to 100% compliance; the overall rate of adherence across a sample of studies is less than 50% (Creer, 1993; Jerome, Wigal, & Creer, 1987).

Adherence Variables in Asthma

Adherence to prescribed medication can be influenced by a number of variables. Factors thought to affect compliance in patients with asthma, compiled from Creer (1979 1993), Creer & Kotses (1990), Spector (1985), Spector et al. (1986), and Sublett, Pollard, Kadlec, and Karibo (1979), are listed in Table 1. The factors are categorized into five groups: (1) patient variables, (2) parent variables (for childhood asthma), (3) communication patterns between physicians and patients and/or parents, (4) medication characteristics, and (5) the nature of asthma. Many of these variables merit comment.

Patient Variables. Patient variables found to be unrelated to adherence include intelligence, income, marital status, education, age (excluding extremes of age), sex, and economic status (Haynes, Taylor, & Sackett, 1979). Patient variables demonstrated to be associated with medication compliance in asthma are listed in Table 1. One set of variables that cries for investigation are the beliefs and expectations of patients. A promising approach is to determine the characteristics of patients who comply with medication instructions. Two investigations (Baum & Creer, 1986; LeBaron, Zeltzer, Ratner, & Kniker, 1985) reported the recruitment of subjects who were generally adherent to medical instructions. The high adherence of the subjects remained unchanged both when medications were introduced (LeBaron et al., 1985) and when the children received self-management training (Baum & Creer, 1986). This finding could reflect the expectations of subjects that their medication compliance would be assessed in the study (Renne & Creer, 1985), that adherence was socially desirable (Turk and Meichenbaum, 1991), or that they were compulsive self-regulators (Kirschenbaum & Tomarken, 1982).

Parent Variables. Characteristics of the parent of asthmatic children include such factors as failure to obtain medications, apathy, and the social stigma of having a child with asthma. A number of beliefs and expectations that interfere with the management of pediatric asthma were described by Creer and Bender (1995). In partic-

Table 1. Factors That Influence Medication Compliance in Asthma[a]

1. Patient variables
   a. Incorrect dosage of medicine
      i. Underuse of medicine
      ii. Overuse of medicine
      iii. Erratic use of medicine
   b. Refusing or vomiting medicine
   c. Indifference or unconcern
   d. Beliefs and expectations
   e. Social stigma
   f. Past experience
   g. Adolescence
   h. Failure to obtain medicine
   i. Social support
   j. Reinforcement contingencies
   k. Memory
   l. Misperception of severity of attack
2. Parent variables
   a. Misperception of severity of attack
   b. Spilled or broken bottles
   c. Failure to obtain medication
   d. Discontinuation due to side effects
   e. Apathy
   f. Social stigma
   g. Memory
   h. Beliefs and expectations
3. Communication between physicians and patients and/or parents
   a. Incomplete or inadequate instruction
   b. Poor communication patterns
   c. Failure to explain potential side effects
   d. Failure to analyze asthma-related behaviors in patients and/or parents
   e. Failure to monitor patients
   f. Incorrect medicine or dosage of medicine prescribed
   g. Misperception of severity of attack
4. Medication characteristics
   a. Taste
   b. Expense
   c. Schedule
   d. Side effects
   e. Duration of dose
   f. Route of delivery
   g. Multiple medications or multiple doses of a medication
   h. Incomplete labeling or dispensing of medicine
5. Nature of asthma
   a. Intermittent, variability, and reversible characteristics
   b. Preventative and as-needed medications

[a]Adapted from Creer and Kotses (1990).

ular, there are often sharp differences between parents in their perception of pediatric asthma (Creer, 1979). Mothers, perhaps because they provide much of the treatment for their child's asthma, generally view asthma as a physical disorder. Fathers, perhaps because of erroneous information they received from friends and coworkers, often view asthma as a psychosomatic condition. Conflicting beliefs about the nature of asthma can generate considerable intrafamily turmoil, which may influence medication adherence.

Communication between Physicians and Patients. Most communication factors enumerated in Table 1 concern how physicians communicate with their patients. In many instances, physicians provide inadequate instruction to their patients about how asthma should be treated. One variable not listed is the expertise of physicians in treating asthma. An increasing number of studies have indicated that patients who see asthma specialists obtain better care for their asthma than patients who seek care from nonspecialists (e.g., Zeiger et al., 1991). In addition, Kaliner, a leading expert on asthma at the National Institutes of Health, declared that increased mortality due to asthma was linked to the ignorance of many physicians who treat the disorder (Altman, 1993).

Medication Characteristics. In discussing why patients with asthma are nonadherent to medication instructions, it is fashionable to put all the blame on the patient. It is unfair to do so, in part because of characteristics of asthma medications and how they are dispensed. Two factors—expense and side effects—are variables that patients are unable to control. Unless they have health insurance that helps defray costs of medications, many cannot pay up to $200 a month for required asthma medications. At the same time, some asthma medications, particularly oral corticosteroids, have severe side effects. Consequently, it is common for patients to weigh the costs and benefits of controlling asthma by taking medications. Having done so, they may decide that the costs or side effects of medications are worse than the asthma (Creer, 1979).

Nature of Asthma. The intermittency of asthma affects medication adherence. Another factor is the confusion among patients with respect to taking maintenance or prophylactic medications, particularly during periods when they are not experiencing asthma. As noted, some medications were developed to prevent attacks. However, taking medications when not ill flies in the face of the repeated admonitions by medical personnel that one should take drugs only when one is sick. Reconciling the latter view with the need to take prophylactic medications generates considerable dissonance in many patients with asthma.

Education Variables and Asthma

All patients are entitled to know about their disorder and how it is treated. Only through education can patients become efficient consumers of health care services, as well as partners with medical personnel in establishing treatment goals and regimens. Despite the proliferation of asthma education programs in recent decades, there has been little formal evaluation of educational techniques in improving compliance (Creer, 1993). This lack has led reviewers to contend that educational efforts, in and of themselves, are unlikely to improve medication adherence in patients with asthma (Moran, 1987). Others (e.g., Spector et al., 1986) suggest that education be used in conjunction with other intervention procedures. Adding an educational component to other intervention strategies has generally been the approach to improving adherence in patients with asthma. Educational components that should be considered include those discussed below.

Instruction about Asthma and Its Treatment. The foundation of any approach to increase adherence in asthmatic patients is to convey knowledge of the disorder and how it is treated. This information should include a description of any drugs and their side effects, with an emphasis on pharmacokinetics (Moran, 1987). Physicians and other medical personnel must verbally communicate the behaviors they want the patient to perform. This task is difficult for many physicians and may result in incomplete patient instruction or poor physician-patient communication. The latter two situations were cited by Sublett et al. (1979) as two factors that contribute to noncompliance in children with asthma. Many experts, including Spector et al. (1986), advise that written materials be used to augment verbal instruction. Single-sheet handouts, provided by such organizations as the American Lung Association and pharmaceutical companies, are useful for this purpose.

Spector (1985) emphasized the importance of teaching patients to take medications as prescribed. Most investigator (e.g., Creer, 1979, 1993; Spector et al., 1986; Sublett et al., 1979) stress the importance of describing possible side effects of asthma medications. Patients should never be surprised by the side effects of medications prescribed to control their asthma. If they are surprised, they are likely to become noncompliant (Creer, 1979).

Use of Basic Vocabulary. It is imperative that clear instructions be provided to patients about what to do. In doing so, medical personnel must communicate with patients in a vocabulary the patients understand. It is necessary to provide ample opportunities for interaction if patients and medical personnel are going to arrive at a common goal and strategy for managing a patient's asthma. Patients cannot be considered as passive bystanders in developing a treatment program for any health problem. Rather, after educational preparation, treatment goals should be established collaboratively by patient and physician (Creer & Holroyd, in press). Three consequences of the joint establishment of goals are that it establishes positive outcomes; enhances the commitment of patients to perform self-regulatory skills, including medication adherence; and engenders expectancies on the part of patients that trigger their effort and performance (Ford, 1987; Karoly, 1993).

Categorizing Information. Categorizing information, an important element of patient and physician education, is often ignored. It was noted that two types of asthma medications are prescribed, either to prevent or to control attacks. Prophylactic or maintenance medications prevent asthma; bronchodilators abort attacks. The medications are not interchangeable; e.g., maintenance medications do not bring attacks under control. While the distinction between types of medications may seem simple, it is not, for one reason: Many physicians, particularly general practitioners who occasionally treat asthma, do not always prescribe the proper medication to patients.

Demonstrating Instrument Use. Creer (1993) pointed out several problems that arose in teaching children to take inhaled medications correctly. A number of studies demonstrated that most problems could be overcome by instruction and the use of behavioral techniques, including shaping and modeling. One barrier is the instruction provided to patients on how to use their inhalers correctly. Kesten, Zive, and Chapman (1993), for example, reviewed pharmacist knowledge and ability to use inhaled medications. They found that pharmacists' knowledge of inhalers was roughly proportional to the length of time the device had been available and that pharmacists required instruction regarding the devices. Hanania, Wittman, Kesten, and Chapman (1994) assessed the ability of respiratory therapists, physicians, and nurses to use three widely used inhaler devices. They found that many medical personnel responsible for instructing and monitoring patients in optimal use of inhalers lacked rudimentary skills with the devices. For example, the mean knowledge score regarding inhalers was 67% for respiratory therapists, 48% for physicians, and 39% for nurses.

Amirav, Goren, and Pawlowski (1994) examined the knowledge of 50 pediatric residents about metered-dose inhalers (MDIs) and space devices. Of the seven steps required to use the instruments, the residents demonstrated an average of 3.8 steps correctly. The most common errors included not shaking the MDI before use (18% correct) and insufficient breath holding (28% correct). In testing spacer use, the most common errors included not shaking the canister (16% correct) and incorrect number of activations and inhalations (12% correct). No wonder that in examining patients' use of an MDI, Goodman et al. (1994, p. 1259) concluded: "Our findings confirm those of others (i.e., proper use of the MDI is rare); 75% of the subjects did not perform an acceptable MDI maneuver as defined by standard criteria."

Asthmatic patients cannot be expected to adhere to a medication regimen involving inhalers if they are not taught to use the devices correctly.

Establishing Regular Tracking and Follow-up. Patients frequently misunderstand or forget the physician's instructions (Moran, 1987). Indeed, a major patient excuse for not adhering to medication instructions is that the patient forgot to take a dose as instructed (Creer, 1993). Spector (1985) employed several aids to increase adherence by an asthmatic patient, including: having the patient recite or paraphrase the physician's instructions; asking to see, during an office visit, all prescribed medications, drugs, and vitamins the patient is taking; and using medication charts.

A. M. Weinstein (1987) advocated the use of a written summary of asthma medications with patients. Advantages of such a summary are that it permits the patient's asthma to be treated promptly; reduces the uncertainty and panic often associated with asthma; specifies the dosage and timing of the patient's medications, including the order in which they are to be taken; emphasizes the possible side effects of each medication; reminds the patient what medications should be avoided, including over-the-counter drugs; and specifies the exact point during an attack at which the patient should notify the physician. These instructions are useful in helping patients remember their treatment regimens. Written instructions, when prominently displayed, also serve as discriminative stimuli to remind patients of the behaviors they should perform to achieve adherence (Creer et al., 1988).

Providing Constant Support and Reinforcement. All patients should be reinforced when they comply with medical instructions. Adherent behavior is often overlooked, in part because physicians tend to focus on patients who are nonadherent (Creer, 1993; Jerome et al., 1987). As with most behaviors, however, the continued performance of adherent behaviors rests upon periodic reinforcement by a patient's physician or a member of the medical team (Creer, 1993).

IMPROVING ADHERENCE

Two general approaches have been taken to improve medication adherence in patients with asthma (Creer, 1993): (1) altering treatment regimens and (2) applying behavioral techniques.

Altering Treatment Regimens

One approach to increasing medication compliance is to adjust treatment regimens so they are most convenient to patients. Specific actions that might be taken include those discussed below.

Dropping Ineffective Medications. Spector (1985) advocates dropping ineffective medications whenever possible. Many patients take over-the-counter medications that have little value in managing asthma and that may interfere with prescribed medical treatment. Examples include cough syrups and antihistamines. With a new prescription, patients may not require drugs they had been using to help control their asthma. Spector (1985) suggests that these medications be dropped from the patient's regimen with an explanation as to why they are no longer necessary.

Minimizing the Complexity of the Medication Regimen. A general rule in the treatment of asthma is that patients take only as much medication as necessary to produce and maintain improvement and that they reduce treatment when symptoms remit. The goal is to control the patient's asthma while permitting the patient to live as normal a life as possible (Chai & Newcomb, 1973). Tailoring treatment regimens for given patients is a dynamic process: There are times when medications may be reduced and times when medications may be increased. Whenever possible, physicians should avoid making treatment regimens too complex. This caveat acknowledges that the more complex a treatment regimen, the greater the probability that nonadherence may occur (Jerome et al., 1987).

Prescribing as few medications as possible is one method of reducing the complexity of treatment regimens. Minimizing the number of medications can be done by: (1) dropping one medication and increasing the dosage of a second medication, (2) keeping the number of other treatments to a minimum, (3) using longer-lasting preparations, (4) adding one medication at a time and evaluating its effects, and (5) introducing the simplest or most easily administered medication first. All of these methods have been shown to increase medication adherence (Creer, 1993).

Decreasing the Duration of Medication Use. Adherence is generally found to decrease when medications are prescribed over an extended period of time (Garfield, 1982). It is not always possible to decrease the duration of medication use and to control asthma, but whenever possible, it is a strategy taken by medical personnel.

Prescribing the Medications That Cause the Fewest Side Effects First. In prescribing medications, physicians initiate treatment with the safest agents and escalate treatment, if necessary, by increasing doses or adding more powerful, albeit more dangerous, medications. Matching treatment with asthma severity guides physicians in medication selection (Ellis, 1988). It is when asthma cannot be managed that more potent medications, particularly oral corticosteroids, are used.

Minimizing the Number of Lifestyle Changes. Patients are unlikely to adhere to regimens that require major lifestyle changes. To overcome this obstacle, physicians should consider how to introduce medications in a manner that does not necessitate lifestyle changes. For example, Spector et al. (1986) suggested that if a patient is to take a medication three times a day and the patient has three appropriately timed meals, it is better to prescribe that it be taken with meals than simply to prescribe that it be taken three times a day.

Reducing the Costs of Medications. A number of practical approaches can be taken by physicians to reduce the costs of asthma medications (Creer, 1979). These approaches include: (1) teaching patients to do comparative shopping for medications, (2) instructing families to obtain health insurance that assumes a major portion of medication expenses, (3) prescribing generic drugs when feasible, and (4) tailoring the drug regimen to fit the patient's pocketbook. Many physicians assist patients by providing office samples of medications or equipment for dispensing the medications. For indigent patients, governmental programs, including Social Security, may help defray the costs of asthma treatment.

Behavioral Techniques

Behavioral techniques are used to improve medication adherence in patients with asthma. These techniques include: (1) shaping, (2) negotiation and contracting, (3) modeling, (4) monitoring, and (5) self-management.

Shaping

Shaping involves the training of successive approximations to a target behavior. Two procedures described in altering treatment regimens—adding one medication at a time and introducing the medications that are simplest to take before medications that are more difficult to administer—are simple forms of shaping. Several studies have used shaping in a different manner, particularly with asthmatic children. Marion, Creer, and Burns (1983) targeted behaviors required to correctly use a hand-held nebulizer. Using shaping, modeling, and reinforcement, they taught children with asthma to correctly use the nebulizer during attacks. Renne and Creer (1976) observed that many children with asthma did not use a compressor-driven nebulizer correctly. A behavioral analysis of their children's behavior indicated that they had to coordinate three responses—diaphragmatic breathing, attending to the apparatus, and inhaling the dispensed medication correctly—in order for the apparatus to achieve this goal. The study resulted in a 100% improvement in the efficacy of medications administered via the nebulizer.

Negotiation and Contracting

Spector et al. (1986) repeatedly noted the role of negotiation with asthmatic patients in determining the types, doses, and schedule of medications. If medical personnel and patients are to agree jointly on treatment goals, negotiation must occur. Many physicians are concerned about negotiation because they realize they must direct and formulate any treatment regimen. At the same time, however, patients must perform whatever steps are needed if the regimen is to be successful. The purpose of negotiation is to arrive at a treatment strategy that patients will successfully pursue.

The outcome of negotiation between patients and medical personnel should be a written agreement or contract. With medication adherence, the contract should stipulate the reinforcement patients will receive contingent on their performing the stipulations of the contract. An example of such a contract between asthmatic children and their physicians was that employed at the National Asthma Center in Denver (Creer, 1979, 1993; Jerome et al., 1987). A contract was negotiated with all children several weeks before they were considered for discharge from the facility. Doctors and children agreed that the latter would demonstrate their ability to manage their medications in the proper dose according to the appropriate schedule. The reinforcement contingency was that the children would be discharged from the center to return to their homes. The procedure outlined in the contract became the foundation for successfully teaching medication-adherence skills to the youngsters before they returned home. A. G. Weinstein, Faust, McKee, and Padman (1992) and A. G. Weinstein (1995) developed similar programs for use with outpatients. It is anticipated that commitment, or the pledging or binding of an individual to behavioral acts, will be added to future contracts. Eliciting verbal or written commitment has been demonstrated to result in greater adherence to medical regimens (Putman, Finney, Barkley, & Bonner, 1994).

Modeling

Modeling has been used to teach asthmatic children to use nebulizers correctly (Croft, 1989; Marion et al., 1983). Croft (1989) had mothers of 20 2-year-old children model correct usage of a tube spacer. He reported that 15 of the 20 children learned to imitate their mothers' responses, with the result that 8 of the children used the spacer correctly to inhale their medications.

Monitoring

A number of techniques have been used to monitor medication adherence in patients with asthma.

Medication Checklists or Diaries. Many experts on asthma adherence advocate the use of medication checklists or charts by patients (Spector, 1985; A. G. Weinstein & Cuskey, 1985). The devices simplify data collection and provide uniformity in gathering information (Jerome et al., 1987). Asthma diaries also serve as discriminative stimuli to prompt adherence behaviors in patients (Kotses et al., 1995).

Telephone Contacts. A. G. Weinstein and Cuskey (1985) employed weekly telephone calls to track medication adherence in asthmatic children. This contact proved a useful means of monitoring the patients' behavior, and it prompted adherence.

Reviewing All Medications. Spector (1985) recommended that medical personnel periodically ask patients to bring in all medications they are taking, including vitamins, for review. This is a practical tactic for three reasons: (1) It permits determination of whether a prescription has actually been filled. (2) It provides physicians the opportunity to determine whether patients are taking a medication that interferes with asthma medications. (3) It allows physicians to determine if a medication should be changed or discontinued.

Providing Feedback. Spector et al. (1986) advocate providing patients with feedback on any test results to reward adherence when it is high and to stimulate adherence when it is low. Nides et al. (1993) found that patients who received feedback on their medication taking adhered more closely to medical instructions than did a group of control patients who did not receive feedback.

Observation. Some patients with asthma, particularly children, may deliberately discard their medications. An excellent example of this behavior was supplied by Spector (1985, p. 52): "One patient simply threw her pills down the toilet, others hid them in shirt pockets, bras, or other orifices other than the mouth. A few could be chewing gum when they received the pills so that both would land in the waste basket." These are behaviors commonly observed in children with asthma (Creer, 1979).

Self-Management

Almost two dozen programs for the self-management of childhood asthma have been developed and evaluated (Wigal, Creer, Kotses, & Lewis, 1990). The positive results obtained in these programs would not have been obtained had patients been nonadherent to medication instructions. Several other studies have demonstrated medication compliance resulting from self-management programs developed for adults. In implementing a self-management program, Kotses et al. (1995) found that medication adherence could be increased even in patients whose asthma was considered to be under good medical control. A specific self-management program is not what is important with respect to medication adherence and asthma. What is important is that self-management or self-regulation is necessary for medication adherence to occur. For this reason, the processes and skills of self-management should be considered. These skills include (Creer & Holroyd, in press): (1) goal selection, (2) information collection, (3) information processing and evaluation, (4) decision-making, (5) action, and (6) self-reaction.

RESEARCH AND METHODOLOGICAL ISSUES

This chapter describes the state-of-the-art knowledge of a number of topics regarding medication adherence and asthma. The discussion has not described several trends regarding these topics. These trends are relevant and must be considered as part of the context that affects determinants of adherence. Two major areas worthy of discussion are assessment and clinical issues.

Assessment of Adherence in Asthma

Assessment techniques used to measure adherence vary in precision, sensitivity, and specificity (Turk & Meichenbaum, 1991). There are two major categories of adherence measures: (1) measures that directly assess patient adherence in correctly using medications and (2) measures that indirectly assess adherence through patient reports, pill counts, liquid measurement, mechanical instruments, and treatment outcomes.

Direct Methods

Direct methods of measuring adherence in patients with asthma include biochemical analyses, biochemical tracers, and direct observations. There are advantages and disadvantages to these methods.

Biochemical Analyses. Analyses of blood, urine, or saliva directly confirm whether a patient has taken an asthma medication. Biochemical markers are invaluable with asthma medications, particularly theophylline, which must be administered in the correct dosage to control a patient's asthma without producing harmful side effects. Advantages of using biochemical analyses or assays are that they provide objective assessment of adherence; permit direct assessment of medication levels at or within specific time periods of time; and are adequately specific and sensitive in detecting individual differences in absorption, distribution, metabolism, and secretion of asthma medications, particularly theophylline.

There are several disadvantages of using biochemical assays (Creer, 1993): They require specialized equipment; pharmacokinetic interactions occur when asthma medications are taken concurrently with other drugs (Reed, 1991); the time when testing occurs, relative to taking an asthma medication, is significant; they are an intrusive process and, in the case of blood assays, painful; and finally, there are no standardized criteria for judging a patient's compliance.

Biochemical Tracers. Cluss, Epstein, Galvis, Fireman, and Friday (1984) and Cluss and Epstein (1985) described the use of a riboflavin tracer to asses medication compliance in asthmatic children. The method, whereby a patient's urine turns red-orange if medicine is taken, has a number of advantages including the fact that it is objective, direct, and produces quantifiable results. The disadvantages of the method are similar to those discussed for biochemical analyses.

Direct Observation. Observation of compliance in patients, particularly children, can be made by members of a patient's family or treatment team (Rapoff & Christophersen, 1982). Advantages of direct observation are that it is direct and objective, provides quantifiable data, and is more valid and reliable than estimates of adherence by clinicians or parents (Creer, 1993; Jerome et al., 1987). Observation can also take place in the patient's home or in medical settings. Disadvantages of direct observation include (Creer, 1993): (1) Observation may be obtrusive in that it disrupts the normal routine of children and their families, particularly when it occurs in a child's home (Renne & Creer, 1985); (2) reactivity can occur in that knowledge that someone is monitoring may change the patient's behavior; (3) it is difficult to teach the observer to observe and not interfere with the patient, particularly if the patient is a child (Rapoff & Christophersen, 1982); (4) observers require training and constant monitoring; and (5) observational methods are not feasible for extended use by physicians and other members of the medical team.

Indirect Measures

There are advantages and disadvantages to the use of indirect measures to assess medication adherence with asthma. Several of these advantages or disadvantages were described by Rapoff and Christophersen (1982) and Creer (1993).

Patient Self-Reports. Self-reports are the most common method used to assess medication adherence. There are four advantages to patient self-reports (Creer, 1993): (1) Invaluable information can be obtained from patients; (2) the collection of data can be tailored to the competencies of individual patients, including children; (3) the data can be easily obtained; and (4) self-report information can be the most accurate data gathered on compliance because only patients know the number of attacks they experienced and whether they adhered to treatment instructions. It should be noted, however, that self-reports are not suitable for all patients: If patients are accurate observers of their behavior, they gather valid and reliable data; if they are not, they generate data that not only are false, but also can lead to erroneous treatment decisions (Creer, 1979; Creer & Winder, 1986).

There are a number of disadvantages to using self-reports (Creer, 1993): (1) Patients may overestimate the self-administration of their medication; (2) patients may underreport nonadherence; (3) self-report data may be less accurate than more direct techniques for assessing compliance; (4) the collection of accurate self-report data requires the training of patients and the constant tracking of their performance by physicians; (5) external checks are needed to validate self-report information; (6) memory may distort self-report data; and (7) the skills of physicians and other medical personnel at eliciting information can influence the reliability and validity of self-report information. Other patient variables that influence compliance are social desirability and patient motivation. Rand and Wise (1994) argue that tailoring asthma diaries for asthma patients reduces the external validity and reliability of such instruments. This drawback holds when conducting research; it is not important, however, in collecting data from individual patients within a clinical context.

Medication Measurement. There are a number of advantages and disadvantages to assessing medications through pill counts, liquid measurement, canister weighing, tallying prescription refills, and other means. Advantages include (Creer, 1993; Jerome et al., 1987): (1) The data are objective; (2) they are easily obtained; (3) measurement is inexpensive; (4) it is superior to estimates of compliance; and (5) it complements other methods.

Disadvantages of the procedures include: (1) the unwillingness of patients to bring their medications to physicians for assessment; (2) pill counts and liquid assessment overestimate adherence; (3) differences caused by the use of teaspoons with different volumes to determine doses of liquid medications taken; (4) the boredom involved in counting pills or weighing canisters; (5) the inability to assess daily patterns of medication use with these measures; and, most important, (6) the fact that changes in any of these measures do not necessarily correlate with the behavior of patients. Patients may dump pills and liquid medication, often on the way to medical appointments; inhaled medications may be discharged into the air. The use of prescriptions can be accurate if patients obtain all their medications from a single source; inaccurate data may be obtained if they do not. Even if a prescription is filled, it is unknown whether patients actually take the medication as directed.

Mechanical Measures. Several mechanical measures can be used to assess compliance in patients with asthma. The most widely used piece of equipment is the nebulizer chronolog (Spector, 1985). This device surrounds the container of any commercial nebulizer; it is small, lightweight, and easily transportable. Each inhalation triggers a microswitch. The memory unit of the instrument measures each activation within plus or minus 4 minutes of the time of use.

A second instrument, the medication event monitoring system (MEMS), consists of a container with a computer chip embedded in its cap. When the cap is removed, the chip records the time and day.

A third device records the removal of individual pills from a blister sheet wired with loops carrying low-voltage current and including a chip with electronic memory that records the time of pill removal.

Advantages of using mechanical methods for assessing compliance are that they (1) are technically sophisticated, (2) provide objective data, (3) yield quantifiable information, (4) can be used over a long period of time; and (5) require minimal effort on the part of patients.

Disadvantages of mechanical devices are

that they are expensive and may produce reactivity. While Gong, Simmons, Clark, and Tashkin (1988) lauded the effectiveness, accuracy, and ability of the chronolog to monitor nebulizer use, 53% of the instruments they used malfunctioned during the course of their study. Sumartojo (1993) cited data from the Centers for Disease Control and Prevention indicating that in using the MEMS unit, patients lost or dismantled the caps, left bottles open if they found the caps difficult to operate, or opened the bottles frequently out of curiosity. Finally, the major disadvantage of mechanical devices is that they assess use of the dispenser, not medication adherence. On the basis of data obtained from the instruments alone, it is impossible to determine whether patients needed to take any medicine, whether they took medications as directed, or whether they took the medicine correctly.

Treatment Outcome. Two advantages of using treatment outcome in assessing adherence are (Creer, 1993; Jerome et al., 1987): (1) Because patients' asthma remains uncontrolled, physicians are often the first to suspect nonadherence; and (2) it is a method of assessment readily available to physicians.

Disadvantages of treatment outcome in measuring compliance include: (1) Treatment outcome often lacks validity; (2) it is not a robust measure of medication adherence; and (3) outcome measures of asthma can change independently of whether patients are compliant or noncompliant.

Assessment Issues

Two suggestions can be drawn from this discussion of the assessment of adherence in asthma. First, multiple methods of assessment should be used. Self-report methods must be one of the procedures selected, however. Second, patients should be asked to gather medication-adherence data over predetermined periods of time.

Assessment is a necessary component in any study of patient adherence, including compliance with a medication regimen. The level of compliance must be known if there are to be positive changes in the behavior of patients. The assessment of adherence in asthmatic patients is a direct outgrowth of the development of technology to measure the amount of theophylline in the blood of patients taking the medication to control their asthma. Eney and Goldstein (1976) reported that only 11% of their sample of asthmatic children had therapeutic levels of theophylline in their blood. This report was followed by a study by Sublett et al. (1979), who randomly selected 50 asthmatic children from 500 walk-in patients at a hospital emergency room and found that only 2% (1 child) of the youngsters had a blood theophylline level within an acceptable therapeutic range.

These classic studies objectively demonstrated that compliance with an asthma medication regimen was low, a fact that has never been disputed, although the proportion of those who are nonadherent may range anywhere from 2% to 100%. The trend since these two studies has been disturbing for four reasons. First, a cycle has been established in which, periodically, a review appears that decries the lack of adherence in patients with asthma. Systematic replication of findings is required in science, but the problem is that each review tends to describe what the authors apparently view as a new phenomenon. It is not, and the result is tantamount to yet another reinvention of the wheel.

Second, the assessment of medication compliance has often occurred without patients being aware that their adherence is being measured. Levine (1994) complained that assessing medication compliance without making patients aware of the assessment violates their right to informed consent.

Third, focusing almost entirely on assessment has distracted researchers from investigating techniques that could improve medication adherence. In addition, there have been no investigations on how to ensure that patients will continue to exercise whatever self-regulatory skills are required to control their asthma over time and across settings.

Finally, and most disconcerting, many recent studies have yielded redundant data with respect to the problem of medication compliance; these results, in turn, have mainly served to reinforce the view that noncompliance is mainly a patient problem. It is not. Adherence represents successful cooperation between medical personnel and patients; it is not the sole province of either patients or physicians, although, as will be noted, there has recently been a tilt toward suggesting that physician ignorance may represent a more serious impediment to medication adherence than previously recognized.

Clinical Issues

Physician Ignorance

Newer and more effective treatments are available for the treatment of asthma. Used correctly, these treatments can control asthma in most patients. However, Sublett et al. (1979) found that one patient with a theophylline level in the therapeutic range was prescribed a dose so high (20 μg/ml) that it could have resulted in seizures and possibly death. More recently, in his discussion of deaths from asthma, Kaliner (quoted in Altman, 1993) pointed out that primary care physicians underused specific treatments that allergists and other asthma specialists regard as the first line of treatment against asthma. In addition, Kaliner continued, primary care physicians tended to rely on drugs that provide only symptomatic relief for asthma and do not address additional measures, such as maintenance therapy, that might avoid unnecessary deaths from asthma (Altman, 1993). An additional problem is that many pharmacists, physicians, and others who treat asthma do not know how to correctly use the devices with which asthma medications are dispensed.

The problem of how to teach patients to take their medications properly has not been adequately addressed. Finkelstein (1994) described deaths in two elderly patients who incorrectly used a long-lasting preventative medication in an attempt to manage acute asthma. The mistake of using a preventative medication to manage acute episodes was blamed on the patients' age. In response, Palmer, Rickard, and Thompson (1994) indicated that there was a strong safety record for the medicine, salmeterol, and suggested that the problem was a lack of patient education in using the drug. This position was supported by Bone (1995), who reiterated the need for correct usage of salmeterol to prevent unnecessary deaths.

It is apparent to many, including behavioral and social scientists who have worked with asthma for a period, that many patients received inappropriate and inadequate treatment for their disorder. This raises a significant question for these scientists: *Do you want to teach asthmatic patients to be compliant to a regimen that may be harmful to them? Scientists should carefully consider their answer to this question before they agree to help improve patient compliance, particularly compliance with asthma treatments.*

Physician–Patient Cooperation

Fortunately, there is a bright spot regarding patient adherence to treatment regimens. A sizable number of asthma specialists report that they rarely experience problems with medication compliance in their patients. Several allergists and chest physicians who referred subjects to a study by Creer et al. (1988), for example, repeated this point. Corroborating evidence supported their reports in that their patients rarely used emergency rooms or were hospitalized for asthma.

In seeking the reasons these asthma specialists encounter few problems with compliance, there are indications that they employ similar strategies in treating asthmatic patients. Among their tactics are these: First, the physicians jointly establish treatment goals with their patients. After providing a solid foundation of knowledge about asthma and its management, the specialists use all forms of techniques, including negotiation and contracting, to help establish the goals of treatment with individual patients.

Second, the physicians teach patients to monitor their behavior and provide brief diaries or checklists to help patients gather data on themselves. The latter practice not only serves to prompt patients' behavior, but also helps them gather useful information on themselves and their asthma.

Third, the physicians teach patients to process and evaluate the information they have collected on themselves and their asthma. On the basis of these data, patients learn to make decisions about what actions to take in a number of diverse situations.

Fourth, the physicians teach patients the steps they should perform to manage their asthma. The steps are written as a guide that can be placed in a conspicuous place to remind patients how to manage attacks.

Finally, the specialists track their patients' behavior. These physicians realize that the management of asthma requires patients to be their partners, and they take every action to cement this interactive and collaborative relationship. This relationship requires, as Winder (1984) emphasized, that patients not only perform the ABCs of asthma control, but also that they add D—call the doc—any time they need additional information or assistance.

Using these common strategies has ensured that patients comply with medication instructions and that they do not needlessly suffer because of asthma. Similar tactics should be used by all physicians and medical personnel who treat asthma. If the strategies were applied consistently, patients would become true partners in the management of their asthma, and the problem of medication compliance and asthma could be relegated to a historical footnote.

REFERENCES

Altman, J. K. (1993). Rise in asthma deaths is tied to ignorance of many physicians. *The New York Times*, May 4, B8.

Amirav, I., Goren, A., & Pawlowski, N. A. (1994). What do pediatricians in training know about the correct use of inhalers and spacer devices? *Journal of Allergy and Clinical Immunology, 94*, 669-675.

Baum, D., & Creer, T. L. (1986). Medication compliance in children with asthma. *Journal of Asthma, 23*, 49-59.

Bone, R. G. (1995). Another word of caution regarding a new long-acting bronchodilator. *Journal of the American Medical Association, 273*, 967-968.

Chai, H., & Newcomb, R. W. (1973). Pharmacologic management of childhood asthma. *American Journal of Diseases of Children, 125*, 757-765.

Cluss, P. A., & Epstein, L. H. (1985). The measurement of medical compliance in the treatment of diseases. In P. Karoly (Ed.), *Measurement strategies in health psychology* (pp. 403-432). New York: Wiley.

Cluss, P. A., Epstein, L. H., Galvis, S. A., Fireman, P., & Friday, G. (1984). Effects of compliance for chronic asthmatic children. *Journal of Consulting and Clinical Psychology, 52*, 909-910.

Creer, T. L. (1979). *Asthma therapy: A behavioral health-care system for respiratory disorders*. New York: Springer.

Creer, T. L. (1982). Asthma. *Journal of Consulting and Clinical Psychology, 50*, 912-921.

Creer, T. L. (1993). Medication compliance and childhood asthma. In N. A. Krasnegor, L. Epstein, S. B. Johnson, & S. J. Yaffe (Eds.), *Developmental aspects of health compliance behavior* (pp. 303-333). Hillsdale, NJ: Erlbaum.

Creer, T. L., Backial, M., Burns, K. L., Leung, P., Marion, R. J., Miklich, D. R., Morrill, C., Taplin, P. S., & Ullman, S. (1988). Living with asthma. Part I. Genesis and development of a self-management program for childhood asthma. *Journal of Asthma, 25*, 335-362.

Creer, T. L., & Bender, B. A. (1993). Asthma. In R. J. Gatchel & E. B. Blanchard (Eds.), *Psychological disorders* (pp. 151-203). Washington, DC: American Psychological Association.

Creer, T. L., & Bender, B. A. (1995). Pediatric asthma. In M. C. Roberts (Ed.), *Handbook of pediatric psychology* (2nd ed.) (pp. 219-240). New York: Guilford Publications.

Creer, T. L., & Holroyd, K. A. (in press). Self-management. In A. Baum, C. McManus, S. Newman, J. Weinman, & R. West (Eds.), *Cambridge handbook of psychology, health and medicine*. Cambridge, England: Cambridge University Press.

Creer, T. L., & Kotses, H. (1990). An extension of the Reed and Townley conception of the pathogenesis of asthma: The role of behavioral and psychological stimuli and responses. *Pediatric Asthma, Allergy, and Immunology, 2*, 169-184.

Creer, T. L., & Winder, J. A. (1986). Asthma. In K. A. Holroyd & T. L. Creer (Eds.), *Self-management of chronic disease: Handbook of clinical interventions and research* (pp. 269-303). Orlando, FL: Academic Press.

Croft, R. D. (1989). 2-Year old asthmatics can learn to operate a tube spacer by copying their mothers. *Archives of Disease in Childhood, 64*, 742-743.

Dirks, J. F., & Kinsman, R. A. (1982). Bayesian prediction of noncompliance: As-needed (PRN) medication usage patterns and the battery of asthma illness behavior. *Journal of Asthma, 19*, 25-31.

Ellis, E. F. (1988). Asthma in infancy and childhood. In E. Middleton, Jr., C. E. Reed, E. F. Ellis, N. F. Adkinson, Jr., & J. W. Yunginger (Eds.), *Allergy: Principles and practice* (pp. 969-998). St. Louis, MD: C. V. Mosby.

Ellis, E. F. (1993). Asthma in infancy and childhood. In E. Middleton, Jr., C. E. Reed, E. F. Ellis, N. F. Adkinson, Jr., J. W. Yunginger, & W. W. Busse (Eds.), *Allergy: Principles and practice* (pp. 1225-1262). St. Louis, MD: C. V. Mosby.

Eney, R. D., & Goldstein, E. O. (1976). Compliance of chronic asthmatics with oral administration of theophylline as measured by serum and salivary level. *Pediatrics, 57*, 513-517.

Finkelstein, F. N. (1994). Risks of salmeterol? *New England Journal of Medicine, 331*, 1314.

Ford, D. H. (1987). *Humans as self-constructing living systems: A developmental perspective on behavior and personality*. Hillsdale, NJ: Erlbaum.

Garfield, E. (1982). Patient compliance: A multifaceted problem with no easy solution. *Current Comments, 37*, 5-14.

Gong, H., Jr., Simmons, M. S., Clark, V. A ., & Tashkin, D. P. (1986). Metered-dose inhaler usage in subjects with asthma: Comparison of nebulizer chronolog and daily diary recordings. *Journal of Allergy and Clinical Immunology, 82*, 5-10.

Goodman, D. E., Israel, E., Rosenberg, M., Johnston, R., Weiss, S. T., & Drazen, J. M. (1994). The influence of age, diagnosis, and gender on proper use of metered-dose inhalers. *American Journal of Respiratory and Critical Care Medicine, 150*, 1256-1261.

Hanania, N. A., Wittman, R., Kesten, S., & Chapman, K. R. (1994). Medical personnel's knowledge of and ability to use inhaling devices: Metered-dose inhalers, spacing chambers, and breath-actuated dry powder inhalers. *Chest, 105*, 111-116.

Haynes, R. B., Taylor, D. W., & Sackett, D. L. (1979). *Compliance with therapeutic regimens*. Baltimore, MD: Johns Hopkins University Press.

Jerome, A., Wigal, J. K., & Creer, T. L. (1987). A review of medication compliance in children with asthma. *Pediatric Asthma, Allergy, and Immunology, 1*, 193-211.

Koroly, P. (1993). Mechanisms of self-regulation: A systems view. *Annual Review of Psychology, 44*, 23-52.

Kesten, S., Zive, K., & Chapman, K. R. (1993). Pharmacist knowledge and ability to use inhaled medication delivery systems. *Chest, 104*, 1737-1742.

Kirschenbaum, D. S ., & Tomarken, A. J. (1982). On facing the generalization problem: The study of self-regulatory failure. In P. C. Kendall (Ed.), *Advances in cognitive-behavioral research and therapy: Vol. 1* (pp. 119-200). New York: Academic Press.

Kotses, H., Bernstein, I. L., Bernstein, D. I., Reynolds, R. V. C., Korbee, L., Wigal, J. K., Ganson, E., Stout, C., & Creer, T. L. (1995). A self-management program for adult asthma. Part I. Development and evaluation. *Journal of Allergy and Clinical Immunology, 95*, 529-540.

LeBaron, S., Zeltzer, L. K., Ratner, P., & Kniker, W. T. (1985). A controlled study of education for improving compliance with cromolyn sodium (Intal): The importance of physician-patient communications. *Annals of Allergy, 55*, 811-818.

Levine, R. J. (1994). Monitoring for adherence: Ethical considerations. *American Journal of Respiratory and Critical Care Medicine, 149*, 287-288.

Loren, M. L., Leung, P. K., Cooley, R. L., Chai, H., Bell, T. D., & Buck, V. M. (1978). Irreversibility of obstructive changes in severe asthma in children. *Chest, 74*, 126-129.

Marion, R. J., Creer, T. L., & Burns, K. L. (1983). Training asthmatic children to use a nebulizer correctly. *Journal of Asthma, 20*, 183-188.

MMWR (Morbidity and Mortality Weekly Report). (1992). *Asthma—United States, 1980-1990*. Atlanta, GA: Centers for Disease Control and Prevention.

Moran, M. G. (1987). Treatment noncompliance in asthmatic patients: An examination of the concept and reviews of the literature. *Seminars in Respiratory Medicine, 8*, 271-277.

National Institutes of Health. (1991). Expert Panel Report. *Guidelines for the diagnosis and management of asthma*. DHHS Publication No. 91-3042. Washington, DC: U.S. Government Printing Office.

National Institutes of Health. (1992). *International consensus report on diagnosis and treatment of asthma*. Washington, DC: U.S. Department of Health and Human Services.

Nides, M. A., Tashkin, D. P., Simmons, M. S., Wise, R. A., Li, V. C., & Rand, C. S. (1993). Improving inhaler adherence in a clinical trial through the use of the nebulizer chronolog. *Chest, 104*, 501-507.

Palmer, J. B. D., Rickard, K. A., & Thompson, J. R. (1994). Risks of salmeterol? *New England Journal of Medicine, 331*, 1314.

Putnam, D. E., Finney, J. W., Barkley, P. L., & Bonner, M. J. (1994). Enhancing commitment improves adherence to a medical regimen. *Journal of Consulting and Clinical Psychology, 62*, 191-194.

Rand, C. S., & Wise, R. A. (1994). Measuring adherence to asthma medication regimens. *American Journal of Respiratory and Critical Care Medicine, 149*, S69-S76.

Rapoff, M. A., & Christophersen, E. R. (1982). Improving compliance in pediatric practice. *Pediatric Clinics of North America, 29*, 339-357.

Reed, C. E. (1991). Pharmacologic basis of the treatment of the allergic patient. *Immunology and Allergy Clinics of North America, 11*, 1-15.

Renne, C. M., & Creer, T. L. (1976). Training children with asthma to use inhalation therapy equipment. *Journal of Applied Behavioral Analysis, 9*, 1-11.

Renne, C. M., & Creer T. L. (1985). Asthmatic children and their families. In M. L. Walraich & D. K. Routh (Eds.), *Advances in developmental and behavioral pediatrics* (pp. 41-81). Greenwich, CT: JAI Press.

Sheffer, A. L., & Buist, A. S. (1987). Proceedings of the asthma mortality task force. *Journal of Allergy and Clinical Immunology*, *80*, 361-514.

Spector, S. L. (1985). Is your asthmatic patient really complying? *Annals of Allergy*, *55*, 552-556.

Spector, S. L., Lewis, C. E., Feldman, C. H., Haynes, R. B., Hindi-Alexander, M., Kinsman, R. A., Menendez, R. A., & Sbarbaro, J. A. (1986). Workshop 6: Compliance factors. *Journal of Allergy and Clinical Immunology*, *78*, 529-533.

Sublett, J. L., Pollard, S. J., Kadlec, G. J., & Karibo, J. M. (1979). Non-compliance in asthmatic children: A study of theophylline levels in pediatric emergency room populations. *Annals of Allergy*, *43*, 95-97.

Sumartojo, E. (1993). When tuberculosis treatment fails: A social behavioral account of patient adherence. *American Review of Respiratory Diseases*, *147*, 1311-1320.

Taylor, W. R., & Newacheck, P. W. (1992). Impact of childhood asthma on health. *Pediatrics*, *90*, 657-662.

Turk, D. C., & Meichenbaum, D. (1991). Adherence to self-care regimens. In J. J. Sweet, R. H. Rozensky, & S. M. Tovian (Eds.), *Handbook of clinical psychology in medical settings* (pp. 249-266). New York: Plenum Press.

Weinstein, A. G. (1995). Clinical management strategies to maintain drug compliance in asthmatic children. *Annals of Allergy, Asthma, and Immunology*, *74*, 304-310.

Weinstein, A. G., & Cuskey, W. (1985). Theophylline compliance in asthmatic children. *Annals of Allergy*, *54*, 19-24.

Weinstein, A. G., Faust, D. S., McKee, L., & Padman, R. (1992). Outcome of short-term hospitalization for children with severe asthma. *Journal of Allergy and Clinical Immunology*, *90*, 66-75.

Weinstein, A. M. (1987). *Asthma: The complete guide to self-management of asthma and allergies for patients and their families*. New York: McGraw-Hill.

Weiss, K. B., Gergen, P. J., & Crain, E. R. (1992). Inner-city asthma: The epidemiology of an emerging U.S. public health concern. *Chest*, *101*, 362S-367S.

Wigal, J. K., Creer, T. L., Kotses, H., & Lewis, P. D. (1990). A critique of 19 self-management programs for childhood asthma. Part I. The development and evaluation of the programs. *Pediatric Asthma, Allergy, and Immunology*, *4*, 17-39.

Winder, J. A. (1984). Keep asthma patients in your practice and out of the ER. *Practice/84*, *1*, 19-25.

Zeiger, R. S., Heller, S., Mellon, M. H., Wald, J., Falkoff, R., & Schatz, M. (1991). Facilitated referral to asthma specialist reduces relapses in asthma emergency room visits. *Journal of Allergy and Clinical Immunology*, *87*, 1160-1168.

8

Self-Regulation and Heart Disease

Noreen M. Clark

INTRODUCTION

Heart disease continues to be one of the three leading causes of mortality among Americans and tops the list of causes of death in people over 65 years of age (Institute of Medicine, 1990). Personal health care expenditures for cardiovascular disease in 1980 totaled $33 billion (HCFA, 1989), and costs have continued upward since that time (Wittels, Hay, & Gotto, 1990). Prevention and control of almost all forms of heat disease (including coronary artery disease, angina, arrhythmia, valve disease, and congestive heart failure) as well as hypertension, a prominent risk factor for heart disease and stroke, largely require that individuals manage their ways of life. This management generally entails, among other things, modifying diets, changing exercise habits, taking medicine, giving up smoking, and avoiding stress. Obviously, the extent to which people can do these things is influenced by external factors (e.g., one's job, the material resources that are available). It has been persuasively argued (Israel & Schurman, 1990) that more effective approaches to prevention and control of heart disease might involve changing working conditions (e.g., reducing stressful situations), laws (e.g., curtailing cigarette production), and policies (e.g., providing reduced insurance premiums for healthful behavior).

Nonetheless, in the past decade, most effort in the health care community has been directed toward helping individuals change their lifestyles to reduce their risk of heart disease, or to manage it effectively if disease is already apparent. This chapter will focus primarily on these health behavior change strategies. The chapter has three goals. First is to review and summarize the recent research related to the social and behavioral aspects of heart disease and interventions to prevent or control it. The review, although comprehensive, is not exhaustive and is offered to provide examples of progress that has been made and questions that remain. The second goal is to discuss an interesting theoretical approach for understanding heart disease prevention and control, i.e., how individuals can be helped to be more self-regulating concerning diet, exercise, medicine taking, and other aspects of lifestyle management. This view of self-regulation in heart disease is offered to illustrate how theoretical understanding of patient behavior is evolving and suggests that interventions will improve as theories do. The third goal is to comment on the

Noreen M. Clark • School of Public Health, University of Michigan, Ann Arbor, Michigan 48109-2029.

Handbook of Health Behavior Research II: Provider Determinants, edited by David S. Gochman. Plenum Press, New York, 1997.

type of research that is needed to move the field along in coming years and contribute to reducing the effects of heart disease on individuals and families.

In order to address these goals, the discussion in this chapter is organized around six questions for which there are some empirically derived answers: What predicts adherence to a heart-related medical regimen, including risk-reducing behavior? How does communication between the individual and the health care provider influence adherence? How does social support influence adherence to clinical advice and other heart disease prevention and management behaviors? Can predictions be made about which people are likely to engage in behavior that puts them at greater risk than others of heart problems? How can behavioral and educational interventions improve the outlook for those at risk of heart disease? How can interventions improve the health status and functioning of people who have heart disease?

REVIEW OF EXISTING STUDIES

The Problem and Predictors of Adherence

The extent of the problem of patients not following their health care providers' recommendations has been well documented (M. H. Becker, 1990), especially regarding long-term therapies. Heart disease prevention and management, including hypertension control, are no exceptions. The incidence of noncompliance or nonadherence in hypertensive patients, for example, has been shown to range between 5% and 60% (Breckenridge, 1983). Further, rates of adherence, even when good, have been shown to erode over time among patients with hypertension (NHLBI, 1982) and among those with active heart disease. One study showed for the latter group that by the third year of treatment, noncompliance (failure to use or incorrect use of digoxin) was almost 40% (Maenpaa, Manninen, & Heinonen, 1987). Further, 10-15% of patients with hypertension are entirely lost to follow-up in the first year of therapy (Luscher, Vetter, Siegenthaler, & Vetter, 1985).

Few demographic factors have been associated with noncompliance related to heart disease; that is, it is impossible to predict by virtue of these factors which patients will comply and which will not. Some limited generalizations about age can be made. Contrary to what some may believe, advancing age does not appear to have a negative influence on adherence to clinicians' advice and heart medicine prescriptions. In general, older individuals are in fact likely to be more compliant with hypertension regimens. This appears to be the case even though studies have shown that knowledge levels of older adults (e.g., 70 years and older) about hypertension are lower than those of younger patients (Carney, Gillies, Smith, & Taylor, 1993). Indeed, better compliance for older individuals is evident, even in the group over 80 years of age, whether measured by self-report, pill counts, or urine assays (Black, Brand, Greenlick, Hughes, & Smith, 1987). In addition, older individuals are significantly more likely than younger ones to change their adherence behavior following education related to heart disease (Morisky, Levine, Green, & Smith, 1982). But one can also find the occasional study in which even age does not predict compliance. In an investigation by Balazovjech & Hnilica (1983), compliance with medical regimens among hypertensive patients over 60 years of age was poorer than average.

Beyond these limited observations about age, adherence to the heart regimen cannot be anticipated by individual characteristics or other demographic characteristics. Neither has it been possible to predict on the basis of personality or psychological profiles which patients will comply with medical advice. For example, in a study of 40 heart patients classified according to Myers-Briggs Type Indicator Exam (which categorizes individuals by their systemic preferences for responding to tasks and problems), results of the exam did not accurately predict either patient compliance or noncompliance (Wilson, Robinson, & Orlando, 1982). This is not to say that psychosocial factors are not associated with compliance in heart disease. Researchers in a study of 50 hypertensive patients followed them over a 10-week period and assessed their compliance through self-reports, pill counts, and monitoring medical appointments. Data analyses revealed that adherence could be predicted by higher levels of knowledge about the treatment regimen, stronger social support, and greater expectancy for one's internal control over health matters in general and hypertension in particular. Compliance in turn was associated, as one would hope, with lower blood pressure (Stanton, 1987).

Individuals' beliefs about their susceptibility to heart-related problems, the seriousness of the problems, and the cost and benefits of recommended actions (Janz & Becker, 1984) can influence compliance. In a study of 120 cardiac patients, these health belief model variables predicted compliance and noncompliance 65% of the time, although the model explained only 5% of the variance. When demographic factors, health behaviors, and health beliefs were considered together, compliance and noncompliance were predicted 74% of the time, and 21% of the variance was explained (Oldridge & Streiner, 1990).

It is safe to say that accepting clinical recommendations in order to prevent or manage heart disease is a highly individualistic phenomenon. The observation by McKenney (1981) after extensive review of compliance enhancing strategies in hypertension, seems relevant: It is unlikely that any one intervention method will work with all patients, since compliance behavior is very complex and multifaceted. Nonetheless, a factor that is salient in many, if not most, studies of adherence with heart disease regimens is the behavior of the health care provider treating the patient. The way health professionals communicate with and educate heart patients appears to influence the patients' compliance behavior.

Patient–Provider Relationships and Compliance

The relationships between people who need to reduce their risk for heart problems or actively manage disease and the health professionals assisting them have been studied fairly extensively. These relationships and the interactions resulting from them appear to be significant in enhancing compliance. M. H. Becker (1987) identified relationship factors in general that increase adherence to the medical regimen. One of these, reducing the complexity of the medical regimen, is an important element of the physician-patient relationship. Physicians have more options in prescribing regimens for heart patients than they are sometimes willing to accept. One approach is to recommend the ultimate and optimum therapeutic plan. Often, however, these regimens are complicated and costly, requiring patient dedication and frequent taking of medicine. Many patients simply will not follow demanding recommendations to the letter. Another approach is to pare down the regimen, maintaining as much effectiveness as possible while making it significantly less demanding of patients. Such a therapy seems to stand a better chance of being followed (Moore, 1988).

The point is that factors other than education and counseling by professionals significantly affect what patients do. Nonetheless, education also exerts an influence. Studies have demonstrated empirically that physicians' advice and counseling can have a positive effect on their heart patients' health status. For example, Zismer, Gillum, Johnson, Becerra, and Johnson (1982) assessed a patient education program offered by physicians in private practice to their hypertensive patients. After 6 months, blood pressure levels in the treatment group receiving the education fell. In the control group, blood pressure levels rose over the same time period.

At a minimum, education from the physician might be expected to increase a patient's understanding of a condition, an important accomplishment. In a study of 100 individuals with hypertension, initially thought to be in control because of compliance with the medicine regimen, lack of information about the correct use of the drugs was shown to be a factor in the erosion of compliance in the group over time and the subsequent increase in blood pressure (Ogunyemi, 1983).

Studies have demonstrated that in fact some patients get more and better information or education from their health care providers than do other patients. In a study of over 2000 patients with hypertension, whether or not patients recalled receiving advice from their physicians could be predicted by their demographic characteristics. Patients demographically similar to physicians, i.e., male, younger, more educated, and white, reported receiving more information from the physician. Patients receiving less information were likely not to resemble the physician. These patients included less educated younger patients with high sodium intake, younger less educated women, overweight black patients, and older women who exercised less than average (Tschann, Adamson, Coates, & Gullion, 1988). An analysis of the speech content of 11 physicians seeing hypertensive patients in 267 encounters showed that physicians generally asked few questions and gave few instructions to patients continuing the same regimen as usual. However, instructions increased significantly for new patients and those with changed regimens (Scherwitz, Hennrikus, Yusim, Lester, and Vallbona, 1985).

That hypertensive patients continuing their usual regimens received little education may well be associated with the eroding rates of compliance by these patients over time, a fact noted previously. It may be the case that their physicians believe these patients do not need or want advice. Kottke, Foels, Hill, Choi, and Fenderson (1984), in a study of family practice physicians, found that only 10% gave nutrition counseling to 80% or more of their patients. While physicians perceived that giving such advice was appropriate to their clinical goals, they perceived that patients did not want and would not follow their advice, and this perception inhibited the physicians' behavior. Yet *most* patients want information, and generally they prefer that it come from a physician rather than another type of provider, as discussed in more detail below.

Patients with heart-related problems may see the situation somewhat differently from other types of patients and from their care providers. In a study of 216 patients with hypertension, diabetes, or a nonchronic illness, Dawson (1985) found that hypertensive patients perceived their physicians to be the least empathetic and at the same time attributed the greatest importance to physician discussions of their therapy. The mismatch between patients' and providers' perceptions about their relationships also extends to the degree they value shared decision making (Strull, Lo, & Charles, 1984).

The communication style of the health care provider has also proven to be important to patients. Orth, Stiles, Scherwitz, Hennrikus, and Vallbona (1987) showed that the blood pressure of hypertensive patients was more likely to decrease when, during the encounter with their health care providers, the patients were able to express themselves in their own words (versus, for example, using medical terms) and providers were able to give relevant information based on these expressed concerns.

The communication task becomes even more complex when family members are involved in counseling. Montgomery and Amos (1991) studied 35 heart patients (mostly male) and 29 spouses to discern priority questions and concerns. Patients were most interested in health care providers' counseling related to compliance with and the benefits of the recommended diet. Spouses were most interested in learning about food selection.

Despite the problems associated with interactions with their physicians, heart patients, if given the choice, seem to want information from them rather than from other types of health professionals. In a study of coronary artery disease patients, physicians were clearly the educators of choice (Karlik, Yarcheski, Braun, & Wu, 1990). This preference seems to obtain even though research has shown that among physicians, physician assistants, dieticians, nurses, and counselors, no professional group consistently possessed the most or the fewest patient counseling skills (Russell, Insull, & Probstfield, 1985). The investigators in this study also noted that the ability of each of these groups to counsel was less strong than their ability to conduct patient interviews (Russell et al., 1985). Further, patients appear to prefer to receive information about their antihypertensive regimens from their clinicians rather than from their pharmacists (DeTullio et al., 1986).

Some of the characteristics of clinicians who are more successful in educating their patients have been identified. For example, physicians' attributes (e.g., medical specialty, job satisfaction) and practice style predicted patients' adherence to treatment in a 2-year study of 186 physicians and their diabetes, hypertension, and heart disease patients (DiMatteo et al., 1993).

Considering that many attributes of physicians that enhance patient compliance and health status should be modifiable through education, it is surprising that education for physicians is rarely assessed on the basis of what happens to their patients. The fact that physicians' prescribing and medical treatment behavior can be changed through education has been established to a degree (Clark et al., 1995), and at least one example exists of continuing education related to medical dimensions of disease as a route to improving *physician* management of hypertension (Jennett, Wilson, Hayton, Mainprize, & Laxdal, 1989). However, only one study is available in which physician education was assessed to determine whether it led to improved health status of *patients* with hypertension or heart disease. In this case, the education did not emphasize the medical issues but the social-behavioral ones. Inui, Yourtee, and Williamson (1976) provided education for physicians based on the health belief model. The intention was to provide clinicians with a way to understand their patients' concerns and tailor counseling to address them. A sample of the physicians' patients with hypertension were followed and compared with hypertensive patients of the control group physicians. Subsequent to the education, patients of program physicians used their antihypertension drugs more correctly and continuously and exhibited lower levels of blood pressure than did patients of control group doctors.

To summarize, quite a bit is known about heart physician-patient relationships. Modes of physician communication influence patient compliance, and effective communication and education by the physician in the office can lead both to better compliance and to lowering of blood pressure levels of hypertensive individuals. Some health care providers are better educators than others, and some of their positive attributes can be described. Some professionals are better accepted as educators by patients than others. Few patients get from physicians the level of education they need or want. Finally, education for physicians related to their role as counselor and communicator appears to result in better health status for patients with hypertension, although this premise has been tested in only one study.

Social Support

The extent and quality of social support available to people trying to reduce the risk of heart problems or manage a heart condition appears to influence their success.

The *degree* of social support one receives from a spouse has been shown to influence compliance with the heart-related medical regimen. In one study (Doherty, Schrott, Metcalf, & Iasiello-Vailas, 1983), adherence to a preventive regimen among those men having low levels of social support averaged 70%, compared to 96% in the group perceiving high levels of social support from their spouses.

The *type* of social support appears to be important in achieving heart health. O'Reilly and Thomas (1989) studied 290 participants who had taken part in a large trial of cardiovascular disease risk reduction. Three years after completion of the trial, they were screened once again to determine whether they were maintaining their risk-reducing behavior. There were small but significant differences between maintainers and nonmaintainers regarding their social support and social networks. Maintainers had significantly higher levels of four types of social support: information/advice, appraisal, emotional support, and availability. In addition, compared to nonmaintainers', maintainers' social networks were more family-centered and denser (i.e., more proximate members).

At least one study (Morisky, Demuth, Field-Fass, Green, & Levine, 1985) has demonstrated improvements in compliance and health status as a result of educating people in the social support network to be more helpful to hypertensive patients in managing their regimens. The study randomly assigned families to a control or intervention group in which family members were interviewed and counseled and provided with written educational materials. Patients were followed for 3 years to assess long-term outcomes. Patients whose family members took part in the social support training were significantly more likely to keep medical appointments and have their weight and blood pressure levels under control.

To summarize, it seems that social support is an important element in adherence to heart regimens and improved patient health status. Interventions to enhance the ability of those in the social network to aid patients may contribute to positive outcomes for the patients.

Predicting Risk

Those interested in the psychosocial aspects of heart disease and development of behavioral/educational interventions certainly want to know whether those at risk of problems related to heart disease can be identified before the fact. Can risk be assessed? Does one know to whom programs might best be targeted? The topic of risk assessment has received a fair amount of attention by researchers and one can say, cautiously, that the answer to each of these questions is "Maybe." To answer another way: "Yes, to some extent."

Various categories of predictors of risk have been examined, primarily the following: demographic characteristics such as age and gender, personality type, psychosocial factors, and behavior. For example, older age is clearly a factor in developing heart problems. The relative risk of cardiovascular disease is greater among the elderly at every level of blood pressure (NHBPEP), 1994). It is also argued that equivalent blood pressure reduction is likely to produce greater benefit in the elderly than in younger patients at every level of blood pressure.

It is the behavioral risk factors that are of greatest interest in the context of this chapter. Among these factors, of course, smoking is the behavior most frequently associated with risk of succumbing to heart disease and complications subsequent to treatment if one has active disease (Fava et al., 1992). An interesting possibility related to smoking and heart disease is that the more individuals smoke, the less healthful in general their lifestyles become. This degradation in lifestyle may increase their risk even more.

A large number of surveys and paper-and-pencil tests to assess cardiovascular risk behavior have been developed since the 1970s (King, Martin, Morrell, Arena, & Boland, 1986). Whether these assessments correlate prospectively with actual documented cases of disease remains in question. The most frequent way patients discover they are at risk, however, is not through standardized structural risk appraisal questionnaires, but on conversation with their physicians. Two factors have been evident in recent studies: (1) Some patients are unaware that they are at risk of heart disease and (2) when they assess their health condition, they come up with priority problems that differ from the priorities their physicians deem important for them. For example, Shankar, Russell, Southard, and Schurman (1982) studied a sample of 19,210 adult inpatients discharged from Maryland community hospitals. One in four had either a diagnosis of hypertension or an elevated diastolic blood pressure ($\leq$100 mm Hg). Among patients with elevated blood pressure, 44% were subsequently diagnosed with hypertension. Race and sex differences were significant. In general, white males were least likely to be diagnosed or treated or to receive information about their hypertension. Levenkron and Greenland (1988) assessed 241 patients with a structured cardiovascular risk appraisal form (RISKO) and told them which factors constituted their greatest personal risk for heart disease. In 63% of the cases, patients selected as a priority risk-reducing behavior one that was different from the one specified as most important by the physician in the appraisal process. The researchers suggested that these findings underscore the need for physicians to negotiate with their patients the target behaviors for change.

Since the 1970s, health professionals appear to have succeeded in alerting most Americans to the need for cardiovascular risk reduction. Two national programs, both sponsored by the National Institutes of Health, have focused on public education for high blood pressure and cholesterol prevention. While rigorous evaluative trials of these mass media campaigns have been impossible to conduct, an impressive body of evidence exists to suggest that they have been in large part responsible for the increase in public awareness of heart disease (Eppler, Eisenberg, Schaeffer, Meischke, & Larson, 1994). But, of course, awareness is not enough—an observation that brings us to the crucial question: Can behavioral and educational programs have an effect on behavior? This question can be split in two as it regards heart disease: First, can interventions reduce risk among those with no disease? Second, can they improve perceptions of well-being, the daily functioning, and the health status of those who already have a heart condition?

Risk-Reduction Programs

This discussion is concerned with whether or not programs elicit new behavior on the part of individuals. It does not consider the larger epidemiological question of whether engaging in specific behaviors generates sufficient clinical benefit to prevent the onset of disease or to change its course in populations at risk. The latter is an important issue that has, of course, received extensive attention (e.g., see Sleight, 1991), but it is a subject beyond the scope of this chapter. Of interest here is the extent to which programs improve adherence to specific recommendations people receive, i.e., to control blood pressure, use medicines preventively, be sufficiently physically active, quit smoking, drink alcohol in moderation, and follow a prudent diet.

Can specific risk-reducing behavior be developed or strengthened through targeted interventions? In the main, a reasonable body of evidence supports the contention that behavioral and educational programs make a difference. For example, Gonzalez-Fernandez, Rivera, Torres, Quiles, and Jackson (1990) identified 47 hypertensive patients among those hospitalized for other non-hypertension-related illness and randomly assigned half to receive education. Eight weeks later, compliance and both systolic and diastolic blood pressure improved in the treatment group. Similar results were evident in a study by Muhlhauser et al. (1993), who examined education for 200 hypertensive patients in ten general practice settings, five of which were randomly selected as the experimental sites. Blood pressure (systolic and diastolic) and the number of antihypertensive drugs per patient in the treatment group decreased significantly, although a large number (approximately 40%) of study patients were lost to follow-up. Body weight did not differ between groups.

Various *types* of risk-reducing interventions have been tested, with generally favorable results. Group programs have been frequent and shown to be successful (Nugent, Carnahan, Sheehan, & Meyers, 1984). For example, Gleichman et al. (1989) involved a group of 29 hypertensive patients in a weekly meeting group format for almost 2 years. Each session entailed education (regarding nutrition and lifestyle) and exercise training. Subsequently, there was a significant decrease in systolic and diastolic blood pressure at rest and during exercise. There were no dramatic changes in fat as a percentage of total calorie intake. Cholesterol levels were reduced. Since no control group was employed, these participants were essentially a self-selected group, and as Martinez-Amenos, Fernandez Terre, Mota Vidal, and Alsina Rocasalbas (1990) have demonstrated, education tends to work for those who want to participate in it.

A group approach did not succeed, however, in a study reported by German et al. (1994). They compared two intervention models, both of which involved individual education with family support. One used, in addition, group education. Only in the individual-education group did blood pressure drop over the 6-month study period.

Several investigators have tried *combinations of approaches* in risk-reduction education and have realized some success. Rehder, McCoy, Blackwell, Whitehead, and Robinson (1980) combined counseling with provision of a special medication container for 100 hypertensive patients. Patients were randomly assigned to receive counseling, container, or both, or to serve as control. At the end of 3 months, findings showed that both the combined intervention and the container alone improved compliance. It was in the container-alone group, however, that there was a decrease in diastolic blood pressure. Binstock and Franklin (1988) assigned 112 individuals to receive education alone, home blood pressure monitoring, patient-provider contracts, pill packs, or a combination of these. One year later, there was no significant change in blood pressure for the group that received education only. Across techniques among those who complied with their regimen, blood pressure did decrease. There were too few subjects to detect differences among the types of groups, but investigators concluded that the education provided alone was insufficient to influence compliance.

Morisky et al. (1983) conducted a 5-year study of 400 hypertensive patients introduced sequentially into a program consisting of the following elements: (1) an exit interview/counseling after a clinic visit, (2) a home visit to encourage compliance, and (3) invitations to small group sessions to increase the patients' confidence and ability to manage hypertension. They also employed a control group. At 3 years and again at the 5-year follow-up point, program participants exhibited a positive change in their weight and blood pressure control. The hypertension-related mortality rate was 53.2% less for experimental group members compared to control.

In another study of 453 patients (Sclar et al., 1991), a combination of strategies, including a patient kit (i.e., a supply of medication, hypertension newsletter, information on nutrition and lifestyle changes, and a description of the change program objectives), reminder phone calls, and monthly newsletters, led patients randomly assigned to the program to secure more hypertensive medication whether they were new or continuing clinic patients.

In summary, there is good evidence that risk-reducing educational interventions, particularly related to blood pressure, can be successful, although data are inconclusive about whether or not individual or group approaches are superior. In some cases, but not all, combinations of strategies have proven effective. Some evidence suggests that lay educators can be as effective as or even more effective than health professionals in assisting hypertensives to lower their blood pressure. How long-lasting the effect of education is largely remains an unanswered question. Morisky et al. (1983), who provided an intensive intervention of long duration, noted change persisting as long as 5 years. At least one team (Ferran Mercade, Casabella Abril, Parcet Solsona, 1990) has suggested that after 6 months, there are no differences in blood pressure of intervention or control groups. When a cholesterol-lowering diet is the route to risk reduction, the same decay of initial success has been noted (Witschi, Singer, Wu Lee, & Stare, 1978).

While many questions remain about the type of educational interventions for risk reduction that are successful and the durability of their effects, it is clear that some programs work and work very well. After a look at interventions designed specifically for people with active heart disease, the chapter will offer some speculations on improving the "hit" rate, i.e., generating more robust interventions that are more likely to achieve success.

Interventions to Improve the Functioning of People with Heart Disease

Frequently, people with some form of organic heart disease must follow regimens very similar to those followed by people who are trying to reduce their risk of disease. But the situation is in a sense more compelling, for these are individuals who have experienced a heart-related trauma or have been given a confirming diagnosis by their physicians. Managing heart disease can be accompanied by fear, anxiety, frustration, and, not uncommonly, depression. For many individuals, there is no "cure"; rather, there is the need to modify one's lifestyle over the long term and try to avoid a debilitating or even terminal event. For many individuals who are managing heart disease at home, it is a daily endeavor undertaken more or less (according to severity of disease) in partnership with a physician.

Because heart disease and the people who have it vary greatly, the outcomes of an intervention for people with heart disease are likely to be very person-specific. They are likely to include a range of physical benchmarks, e.g., from simply being able to ambulate to engaging in significant levels of exercise; or psychological ones, e.g., from a lower degree of depression to robust mental and emotional health; or social ones, e.g., from being somewhat less socially isolated to full integration in a social network. Increasingly, even for physicians, the success of a heart disease education program is being measured by the extent to which it brings participants to an optimum level of functioning and enhances the quality of life.

Studies have examined socioeconomic and psychological factors as barriers to management of heart disease, factors that might be considered in designing interventions. Findings must be treated very cautiously, however, since there are few investigations on these topics. One group of investigators (Conroy et al., 1986) who studied 299 middle-aged male survivors of unstable angina or myocardial infarction found a significant correlation between failure to follow their regimens and socioeconomic status (SES). Men of lower SES were more likely to smoke, have higher weekly alcohol intake, and take significantly longer than men of higher SES to return to work. However, there was no significant association between SES and 3-year mortality from cardiac conditions. Godin, Valois, Jobin, and Ross (1991) studied 161 cardiac patients to understand their intentions to engage in adequate exercise. They found three categories of psychosocial barrier: difficulties in time management, difficulties in psychological adaptation to illness and management requirements, and a behavior they termed "laziness."

Rehabilitation and Exercise Programs. Much of the available heart disease literature focuses on cardiac rehabilitation programs (Pashkow, 1993) as the route to disease management. These interventions have traditionally aimed at building a patient's tolerance for exercise through training and have involved a significant degree of education related to other aspects of disease management.

As with the cardiovascular risk-reduction programs described previously, at least two questions can be posed: Do patients stick with these programs and if they do, what benefits do they reap? A program example is provided by Niebauer et al. (1994), who provided education regarding low-fat diets and conducted fairly aggressive physical training, using fitness equipment (e.g., treadmills) for 36 middle-aged men with coronary heart disease randomly assigned to a weekly program or control group. They were observed for 6 years. Cholesterol levels decreased and physical performance significantly increased over time for the program group compared to control. The researchers believed the progression of disease to be slowed in the intervention group. Meta-analyses of rehabilitation programs like this one suggest that they reduce overall cardiovascular death by about 20% and sudden death by about 37% during the year after an acute myocardial infarction (Pashkow, 1993).

Cardiac rehabilitation programs have generated other outcomes as well. Roviaro, Holmes, and Holmsten (1984) found in a controlled study of 28 male cardiac patients that the physical performance and blood pressure of men in the program group improved over 4 months, and in addition, the men were more compliant with treatment regimens and had more positive self-perceptions (self-concept, progress toward personal goals) and psychosocial functioning (decreased employment-related stress, more enjoyment of leisure time, more sexual activity).

Programs involving relatively less strenuous physical activity also appear to produce desired outcomes. Moderate exercise, combined with education for other lifestyle changes, has been shown to improve health status. Ornish et al. (1990) conducted a controlled clinical trial, involving 28 male cardiac patients in a program group and 20 in a control group. They showed, after only 1 year, that a program providing education and training focused on a low-fat vegetarian diet, smoking cessation, stress management, and moderate exercise reduced stenosis in the experimental group compared to control and, in the researcher's view, caused regression of severe atherosclerosis without use of lipid-lowering drugs.

Post-myocardial infarction (MI) stress-monitoring and -management programs may have long-term effects. Frasure-Smith and Prince (1989) found in a controlled trial with 461 male patients that a stress-management program reduced cardiac deaths by 50% 1 year following the program and during the 6 subsequent years, there were fewer MI reoccurrences among treated patients.

However, the selection of patients for traditional cardiac rehabilitation programs of the type described thus far is an exceedingly important part of the process. Some individuals, because of age, severity of disease, comorbidities, or other factors, simply will not be good candidates for conventional programs.

Evaluations demonstrating such promising results from cardiac rehabilitation have been conducted, in the main, with middle-aged and, generally, white men. The interventions have demanded almost zealous adherence and, with few exceptions, have required fitness conditioning through aerobic exercise such as running or using treadmills or other forms of training equipment. An important consideration is how heart disease management programs, including the traditional cardiac rehabilitation model, help other populations, e.g., women, the elderly, different ethnic or cultural groups, and the less motivated.

Women

Caution must be used in considering the case of women and heart disease management, since few data are available. Most observers agree that we know little about the differences between men and women in the psychosocial and clinical aspects of heart disease (R. C. Becker, 1990). Many in the scientific community have recognized that the etiology of heart disease, its natural history, its epidemiology, and the social and behavioral aspects of its management are all likely to differ significantly between men and women. However, what these differences are and how they affect individual patients are not at all well understood.

Those interested in the way social and behavioral aspects of heart disease management are influenced by gender have only three or four studies to rely on. Cannistra, Balady, O'Mally, Weiner, and Ryan (1992) studied 51 middle-aged women and 174 men. Most were white and had had an MI or revascularization and were participating in a cardiac rehabilitation program. To begin, women's cardiovascular risk profile was significantly less favorable than men's; e.g., they exhibited higher levels of cholesterol, diabetes, and hypertension. Initial exercise capacity was less for women. Following the program, however, women were found to be equally compliant with the recommended regimen and to experience a training effect similar to that of men, achieving the same improvements in functional capacity. O'Callahan et al. (1984) studied a somewhat similar population, 227 middle-aged males and 37 females in a supervised program. They found that women dropped out of the program more and attended less. Following the program, exercise duration for both men and women increased, but the absolute values were consistently higher in men. Blood pressure levels did not change for either group.

Older Adults

When it comes to older adults, who often are not good candidates for conventional cardiac rehabilitation programs (because of comorbidities, or a frail condition, or inability to engage in strenuous activity), the data are also scarce. A number of differences in disease management between men and women have been noted in at least one study. Sharpe, Clark, and Janz (1991) studied 323 older individuals with various forms of heart disease, all over 65 years of age and none participating in a conventional cardiac rehabilitation program. Men reported different symptom pattens than women, and were more likely to comply with clinical recommendations for physical activity and be more physically active in general. There were no differences in the emotional well-being and psychological functioning of women and men (as measured by the Sickness Impact Profile), but women reported significantly more stress associated with carrying out their household management tasks. Clark et al. (1992) conducted a clinical trial of heart disease self-management education tailored for 636 older adults. Program activities centered on the elements of the regimen the physician recommended to the patient. They found that the program affected male and female participants differently. Both groups improved significantly in psychosocial functioning postprogram. However, while males experienced modest but significant gains in physical activity as a result of participation, no gains at all in this area were noted for women.

In a series of focus groups conducted with older women with heart disease, Clark, Janz, Dodge, and Garrity (1994a) identified the following ten themes that captured the barriers reported by these older adults in trying to follow the regimens prescribed by their physicians and manage the problems heart disease causes in daily life: differentiating changes due to aging from changes due to the heart condition, determining the seriousness of heart-related symptoms, setting priorities and making choices, handling fears and anxieties, maintaining independence, reaching self-acceptance, feeling undervalued, dealing with a retired spouse, managing the burden and responsibility of caring for others, and evaluating and responding to advice and help from family and friends.

The paucity of information about heart disease management for important subgroups of the population such as women and the elderly is vexing. The dearth of data related to management in various cultural/racial/ethnic groups is particularly serious. There is little information on which to form the most tentative opinion. The need for research on these important subpopulations is discussed in more detail in a later section.

SELF-REGULATION: AN EXAMPLE OF A THEORETICAL APPROACH TO IMPROVING INTERVENTIONS

One can conclude from the data on the effect of behavioral and educational interventions for cardiovascular risk reduction and heart disease management that they contribute to enhanced functioning and well-being. But as one reviews the available work, with the exception of fitness training components, there is a troubling lack of information in most articles regarding the actual content and processes comprising heart-related interventions. One can therefore only make guesses about the level of sophistication of these programs. It may be that the interventions offered to improve heart health described in the literature are more grounded in theory than descriptions make them seem. On the other hand, the full potential of social-behavioral interventions may not yet have been realized because programs have not been designed to take optimum advantage of what is known about changing behavior.

The advantage of, indeed the necessity for theory-based programs related to heart disease is supported in two very nice discussions in the literature in which authors have looked across programs to identify the elements that have engendered success. Mullen, Mains, and Velez (1992) conducted a meta-analysis of 28 controlled heart-related studies that demonstrated some measurable change in blood pressure levels, exercise, diet, and mortality. They attempted to describe the characteristics of the programs that had influenced patient behavior and health status. Certain specific educational principles drawn from learning theory were evident. These principles included providing reinforcement to the patients' efforts to change, giving feedback on progress, offering the opportunity for individualization of learning, facilitating behavior change by providing skills and access to resources, and making continual efforts to address patients' needs and abilities.

In a similar vein, Garrity and Garrity (1985) reviewed seven successful research projects that employed a variety of intervention strategies intended to improve compliance with heart-related therapeutic regimens as well as blood pressure control. They identified four themes associated with success: the "active patient theme," which emphasized the need for self-care; the "social support theme," which emphasized support from significant people in the patients' social environment in helping to meet the illness management challenge; the "fear arousal theme," which attempted to heighten the patients' concern about the potential consequences of the disease; and the "patient instruction theme," which was the effort to transmit needed information about the illness or regimen. The most effective behavior change strategies were those used in the active patient theme, especially contingency contracting, and those associated with the social support theme.

The assumptions represented in these themes derive from theoretical perspectives that are reasonably well developed and have been tested empirically. Social support, for example, has been associated not only with better management of heart disease but also with a range of problems (health-related and non-health-related) that individuals must handle in the course of daily life (Israel & Schurman, 1990). Fear arousal is a theoretical concept that has given rise to important studies in health behavior and the formulation of principles to guide intervention development (Job, 1988; Sutton, 1982). Instruction of patients is a theme built on communication theory, such as work exploring the dynamics of sending and receiving verbal and written messages (McGuire, 1989). Patient instruction is also informed by work examining the interaction of beliefs held by the patients and their behavior exemplified, for example, in the health belief model (Janz & Becker, 1984).

While one or two authors have explored aspects of patienthood through the notion of the "activated patient" (DeFriese, Woomert, Guild, Steckler, & Konrad, 1989), the idea of the individual patient as the primary actor (as opposed to the health professional) managing his or her health or disease is more fully addressed in the constructs of social cognitive theory (Bandura, 1986). Since the "active patient" theme appears to be highly important in successful heart health interventions and since social cognitive theory is a useful theoretical framework for both predicting behavior and explaining how to change it, both of these viewpoints are used as a starting point for suggesting a direction for future work. *Self-regulation* is seen as the vehicle through which heart-related behavior change is achieved, i.e., how patients are "activated."

There are at least two important assumptions pertinent to understanding heart disease prevention and management based on this perspective. First, individuals mobilize their resources and behave in certain ways in order to reach end points. Second, the process by which they learn to reach these outcomes entails self-regulation (Clark & Starr, 1994). One observes oneself and others, makes judgments from these observations, tries out behavior, and reacts to the behavioral experience (Clark & Zimmerman, 1990). The two most important reactions (Bandura, 1986) are the belief that one is capable of carrying out the behavior (often called "self-efficacy") and the belief that the behavior is linked to the desired result (often called the "outcome expectation"). Figure 1 attempts to illustrate these assumptions.

Both intrapersonal and external factors interact to produce behavior. Individual behavior is influenced by intrapersonal factors—knowledge, attitudes, beliefs, and feelings—that are influenced by external factors in the social environment. The external factors include, for example, role models from whom potential prevention and management strategies can be learned (usually vicariously through observation), technical advice and service from health professionals, social support from significant others, money and material resources to obtain care and maintain an adequate physical environment, and so on. It also must be noted that while intrapersonal factors

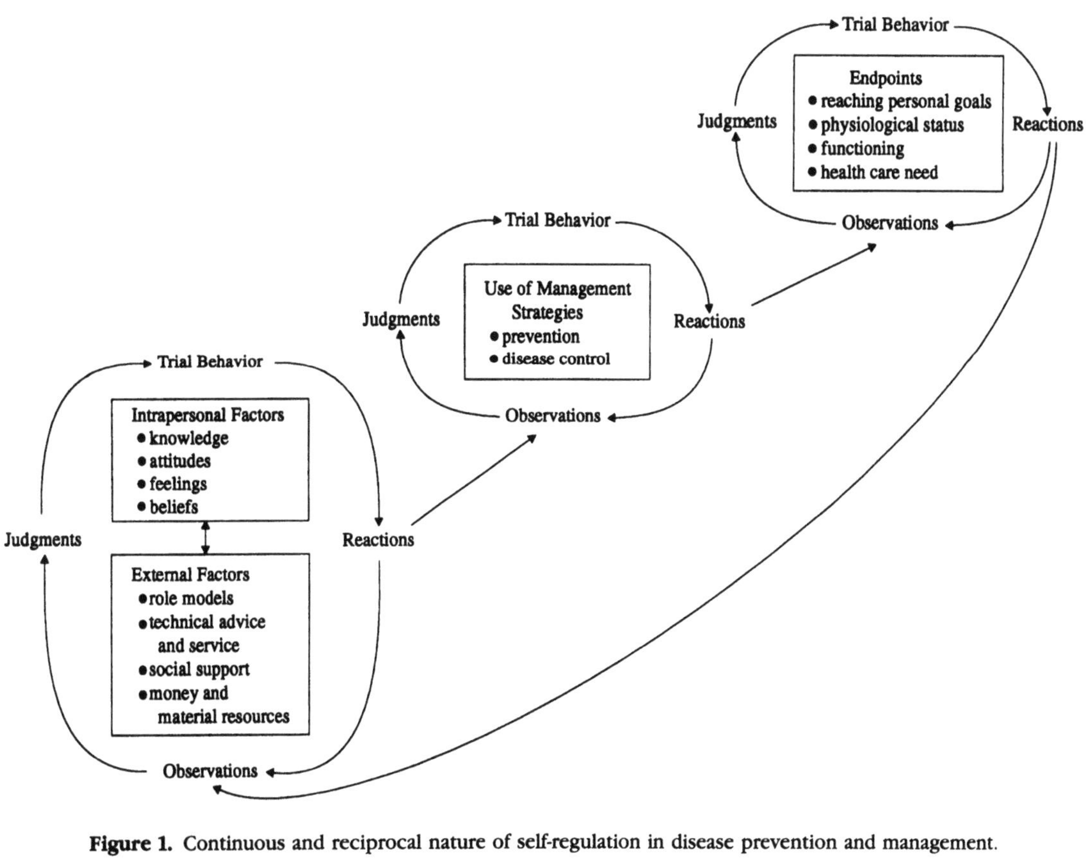

Figure 1. Continuous and reciprocal nature of self-regulation in disease prevention and management.

are the basis for action, they also can change as a *result* of behavior; thus, the determinants are reciprocal (Bandura, 1986). Use of management strategies represents conscious manipulation of situations, i.e., efforts to enhance daily life or reduce the impact of disease on it. That is, the use of strategies to prevent or control disease grows out of the experience of being self-regulating regarding intrapersonal and external factors (Clark & Starr, 1994).

Having tried and reacted favorably to disease prevention or management strategies, one will continue the process of self-regulation to determine whether over time the strategies continue to produce results. Management strategies are not ends in themselves, but means to ends. These end points include outcomes of importance to the individual, e.g., personal goals, physiological status, physical and psychosocial functioning, and appropriate use of health care services. An example would be a middle-aged man who enjoys being physically active, believes he is susceptible to heart problems, thinks lowering his cholesterol will help, and so seeks advice from his physician and support from his family, develops a strategy for managing his diet, and as a result feels enabled to continue his golf or tennis or skiing, i.e., to reach his personal goal. Through self-regulation, i.e., his observations, judgments, trials of new behavior, and reactions, intrapersonal and external factors are mobilized, strategies tested, and end points confirmed. Self-regulation, therefore, is pervasive, operating through the initial stages of mobilizing resources to using management strategies and, finally, to realizing desired outcomes.

While these elements of self-regulation have been empirically examined primarily in school-based learning, they provide a model for understanding health behavior (Clark & Starr, 1994). One preliminary health-related study, though not conducted in heart disease, is promising and suggests that predicted links between elements of self-regulation and more effective use of management strategies do indeed exist (Clark et al., 1994b).

If this model accurately describes the constituent parts of self-regulation and explains how new health behavior comes about, there is a related and crucial question: Can individuals concerned with heart health and managing disease be taught to be more self-regulating, i.e., to increase their ability to observe, judge, try new behavior, and react? While data are as yet scant, at least one study with older cardiac patients suggests that the answer may be yes (Clark, Janz, Dodge, & Sharpe, 1992). Another controlled study (McAuley, Courneya, Rudolph, & Lox, 1994) of behavior specific to heart health showed that bolstering individuals' feelings of self-efficacy while they participated in a walking program significantly increased frequency and duration of exercise in the early and middle stages of the intervention (but not in the final month). Research seems warranted to verify the hypothesized elements of self-regulation as they operate in prevention and management of heart disease and to test interventions that enhance these elements.

Other theoretical approaches to behavior change also appear to be promising for heart disease education and deserve attention. These include, for example, the stages of change model (Prochaska, DiClemente, Velicer, Ginpel, & Norcross, 1985) and models for examining the interaction of stress and social support in health behavior developed by Israel, House, Schurman Heaney, and Mero (1989). A point to emphasize is that there are at least two challenges for those interested in designing interventions to prevent or control heart disease. The first is to use existing theory more effectively as a basis for programs. The second is to conduct research that will yield more robust theoretical explanations of how to change health behavior. Of course, other research efforts are also needed.

FUTURE DIRECTIONS: RESEARCH AND METHODOLOGICAL ISSUES

While the decade since the mid-1980s has provided a fair amount of knowledge about the social and behavioral aspects of heart disease, it has also revealed how much is not yet known. This section will describe several categories of needed research, work that should lead to a fuller understanding of psychosocial factors in heart disease as they relate to interventions to prevent or manage it. Moreover, the strides made in prevention and control of this health problem may well apply to other chronic conditions and enrich health programs more generally. The four categories of needed research are: the theoretical bases for interventions, differences among populations, aspects and elements of effective programs, and outcomes—what will be accepted as indicators of success.

Theoretical Bases of Interventions

Programs for behavior change in heart disease, obviously, must be based on the best epidemiological data and the most current clinical information, i.e., the therapeutic regimens most likely to benefit patients and those trying to avoid disease. But it is equally important that programs be based on extant understanding of behavior change. This understanding comes from the theories that both predict behavior and explain how it can be transformed. Much more empirical research is needed related to heart disease that explicitly examines existing theoretical models, as well as work to create new theoretical perspectives and approaches. No less important is to ensure that all the interventions are solidly built on extant theory and are not simply a hodgepodge of techniques and activities. A good theory is one that works. A good intervention is one that can be explained in theoretical terms so it can be strengthened, replicated, and, when worthy, disseminated.

Reaching Different Populations

Current knowledge about how to tailor heart disease prevention and control programs to differing populations is not at all extensive. Nor are the effects of different programs on these populations known. There is a particular lack of understanding about disease management. Very few examples concerning women are available. Some work with African-Americans, primarily through their churches, has been reported (Stillman, Bone, Rand, Levine, & Becker, 1993), programs for children in school have been undertaken (Perry et al., 1990), and examples for workers in various occupational settings have been described (Heirich, Foote, Erfurt, & Konopka, 1993). One safe assumption is that interventions are most powerful when they closely reflect the perspectives, experience, and psychosocial dimensions of the participants (Bandura, 1986). As many have noted, this makes the fact that most heart-related work has focused on white men even more problematic, given the increasing diversity of American society.

There are at least two ways to think about approaching the need for more gender- and culture-specific heart health programs. One is to identify settings in which studies can be introduced to focus on certain population groups. Evaluations of programs conducted in African-American churches is a good example of this approach (Stillman et al., 1993). Another is to conduct large enough studies in settings with sufficient numbers of people in different populations to enable subgroup comparisons. Studies in clinical settings used equally by men and women are one example of this approach (Sharpe et al., 1991). Regardless, more data are needed on many salient populations: women, the elderly, African-Americans, Latinos, Asians, Native Americans, children, and low-income people, to name a few. An important point, of course, is that none of these groups is homogeneous. Within given categories (e.g., African-American or Latino), one finds great variety and a large number of subcultures (Jackson, Tucker, & Bowman, 1983). Addressing variations in the heart health experience is very complex, but researchers must begin to tease out critical population differences to move toward better interventions.

A group different from those mentioned above, but one that cannot be overlooked, is the population of health care providers. Of the few things that can be said with certainty from the review of data in this chapter, one is that physicians have influence on their patients' behavior. There is a great need for studies that examine how interventions can influence clinical practice, especially by enhancing the counseling and educational skills of health professionals. There must also be studies to determine whether programs to change the behavior of physicians have an effect on the behavior and health status of patients. Achieving change in clinical practice has no import without benefit for the patient.

Elements of Effective Programs

As concluded from the literature review presented in this chapter, little is known about the aspects of interventions that make them successful. The most basic questions remain: What core content is needed in various types of prevention or heart disease management interventions? What processes and methods best engender self-management? Which produce effective social support? Are these processes best provided to individuals or to groups or in some combination? What combinations of external factors are crucial to success (e.g., organizational arrangements in the health care facility, behavior of service providers, resources available in the community)?

Further, while observers for many years have been calling for multifactorial designs in our social-behavioral intervention research (Green & Figa-Talamanca, 1974), such research in heart disease has not come very far. Most programs continue to be the "box" into which a variety of activities are poured, and when success is seen, it often cannot be accounted for very precisely. Of course, there are excellent exceptions (Janz, Becker, & Hartman, 1984), but these have generated limited information (e.g., patient-provider contracts generally work in combination with some other approach), and much more needs to be known.

Outcomes

Finally, there is the question of what will be accepted as indicators of success of heart health interventions. And the related issue: How durable is success? For many years, clinicians were satisfied when their patients improved on physiological or clinical markers (e.g., reduced cholesterol values, lowered blood pressure, maintenance of a given drug regimen). Sometimes these things meant success to patients. Sometimes they didn't. More and more clinicians, behavioral scientists, and patients alike deem other benchmarks to be of equal or greater importance. How fully functioning physically, psychologically, and socially are cardiac patients and those trying to prevent disease? What is the quality of their lives? How can quality be assessed in terms important to patients versus professionals (i.e., can we generate patient-defined quality-of-life measures)? There are available an increasing number of indices and scales, relevant but not necessarily specific to heart disease, that measure functioning (Bergner et al., 1981) and quality of life (Beckman & Frankel, 1985). Some have been developed for particular populations, primarily the elderly (George & Fillenbaum, 1985). There are at least two ways to derive heart-specific measures. One is to test these existing scales on populations who are at risk or are managing disease. Another is to develop new scales for populations of people explicitly trying to prevent heart disease or groups of cardiac patients. Both efforts are to be encouraged. There is a great need to understand what is unique in functioning and quality of life for heart health so programs can be designed to reach these ends and success can be recognized when programs achieve it.

Also needed are longitudinal program evaluations. These will tell what happens not just in 1 year after interventions, but 5 and 10 and perhaps even more years later. Researchers need to know the most effective time lines for activities of people at different stages in the life span. What is the best pattern for education and fitness training of children over time? What is the ideal time frame for interventions to help middle-aged people as they move through the years to old-old age? What are examples of the immediate, intermediate, and ultimate outcomes to be expected along the way? What are the most important outcomes for subpopulations at different ages or developmental phases?

Finding answers to these questions—indeed to all the questions raised in this chapter—will be a complex undertaking, requiring multidisciplinary teams of investigators approaching problems from various theoretical perspectives. But such questions as these pose exciting challenges for social and behavioral researchers in heart disease. Much more important, answering them is crucial to reducing the catastrophic effect, on an alarming number of Americans, of one of the leading causes of their premature death and disability.

REFERENCES

Balazovjech, I., & Hnilica, P., Jr. (1993). Compliance with antihypertensive treatment in consultation rooms for hypertensive patients. *Journal of Human Hypertension*, 7(6), 581-583.

Bandura, A. (1986). *Social foundations of thought and action*. Englewood Cliffs, NJ: Prentice-Hall.

Becker, M. H. (1987). Improving patient compliance to prescribed therapy. *Cardiovascular Review and Reports*, *8*, 57-59.

Becker, M. H. (1990) Theoretical models of adherence and strategies for improving adherence. In S. A. Schumaker et al. (Eds.), *The handbook of health behavior change* (pp. 5-43). New York: Springer.

Becker, R. C. (1990). Cardiovascular disease in women: Clinical highlights and future directions. *Cardiology*, 77(Suppl. 2), 1-5.

Beckman, H., Frankel, R. (1985). Collecting quality of life data from patients with cardiovascular disease. *Quality of Life and Cardiovascular Care*, *1*(7), 336-341.

Bergner, M., Bobbitt, R. A., et al. (1981). The Sickness Impact Profile: Development and final revision of a health status measure. *Medical Care*, *19*, 787-805.

Binstock, M. C., & Franklin, K. L. (1988). A comparison of compliance techniques on the control of high blood pressure. *American Journal of Hypertension*, *1*(3/Pt. 3), 1925-1945.

Black, D. B., Brand, R. J., Greenlick, M., Hughes, G., & Smith, J. (1987). Compliance to treatment for hypertension in elderly patients: The SHEP pilot study. *Journal of Gerontology*, *42*(5), 552-557.

Breckenridge, A. (1983). Compliance of hypertensive patients with pharmacological treatment. *Hypertension*, *5*(5/Pt. 2), III85-89.

Cannistra, L. B., Balady, G. J., O'Mally, C. J., Weiner, D. A., & Ryan, T. J. (1992). Comparison of the clinical profile and outcome of women and men in cardiac rehabilitation. *American Journal of Cardiology*, *69*(16), 1274-1279.

Carney, S., Gillies, A., Smith, A., & Taylor, M. (1983). Hypertension education: Patient knowledge and satisfaction. *Journal of Human Hypertension*, 7(5), 505-508.

Clark, N. M., Evans, D., Zimmerman, B. J., Levison, M. J., & Mellins, R. B. (1994b). Patient and family management of asthma: Theory based techniques for the clinician. *Journal of Asthma*, *3*(16).

Clark, N. M., Janz, N. K., Becker, M. H., Schork, M. A., Wheeler, J., Liang, J., Dodge, J. A., Keteyian, S., Rhoads, K. L., & Santinga, J. T. (1992). Impact of self-management education on the functional health status of older adults with heart disease. *Gerontologist*, *32*(4), 438-443.

Clark, N. M., Janz, N. K., Dodge, J. A., & Garrity, C. R. (1994a). Managing heart disease: A study of the experience of older women. *Journal of the American Medical Women's Association*, *49*(6), 202-206.

Clark, N. M., Janz, N. K., Dodge, J. A., & Sharpe, P. A. (1992). Self-regulation in health behavior: The "take PRIDE" program. *Health Education Quarterly*, *19*(3), 341-354.

Clark, N. M., Nothwehr, F., Gong, M., Evans, D., Maiman, L. A., Hurwitz, M. E., Roloff, D., & Mellins, R. B. Physician-patient partnership in managing chronic illness. *Academic Medicine*, *70*(11), 957-959.

Clark, N. M., & Starr, N. S. (1994). Management of asthma by patients and families. *American Journal of Respiratory and Critical Care Medicine*, *149*, S54-66.

Clark, N. M., & Zimmerman, B. J. (1990). Social cognitive view of self-regulated learning about health. *Health Education Research*, *5*(3), 371-379.

Conroy, R. M., Cahill, S., Mulcahy, R., Johnson, H., Graham, I. M., & Hicky, N. (1986). The relation of social class to risk factors, rehabilitation, compliance and mortality in survivors of acute coronary heart disease. *Scandinavian Journal of Social Medicine*, *14*(2), 51-56.

Dawson, C. (1985). Hypertension: Perceived clinician empathy and patient self-disclosure. *Research in Nursing and Health*, *8*(2), 191-198.

DeFriese, G. H., Woomert, A., Guild, P. A., Steckler, A. B ., & Konrad, T. R. (1989). From activated patient to pacified activist: A study of the self-care movement in the United States. *Social Science and Medicine*, *29*(2), 195-204.

DeTullio, P. L., Eraker, S. A., Jepson, C., Becker, M. H., Fujimoto E., Diaz, C. L., Loveland, R. B., & Strecher, V. J. (1986). Patient medication instruction and provider interactions: Effects on knowledge and attitudes. *Health Education Quarterly*, *13*(1), 51-60.

DiMatteo, M. R., Sherbourne, C. D., Hays, R. D., Ordway, L., Kravitz, R. L., McGlynn, E. A., Kaplan, S., & Rogers, W. H. (1993). Physicians' characteristics influence patients' adherence to medical treatment. *Health Psychology*, *12*(2), 93-102.

Doherty, W., Schrott, H. G., Metcalf, L., & Iasiello-Vailas, L. (1983). Effect of spouse support and health beliefs on medication adherence. *Journal of Family Practice*, *17*(5), 837-841.

Eppler, E., Eisenberg, M. S., Schaeffer, S., Meischke, H., & Larson, M. P. (1994). 911 and emergency department use for chest pain: Results of a media campaign. *Annals of Emergency Medicine*, *24*(2), 202-208.

Fava, M., Littman, A., Lamon-Fave, S., Milani, R., Shera, D., MacLaughlin, R., Cassem, E., Leaf, A., Marchio, B., Bolognesi, E., et al. (1992). Psychological, behavioral, and biochemical risk factors for coronary artery disease among American and Italian male corporate managers. *American Journal of Cardiology*, *70*(18), 1412-1416.

Ferran Mercade, M., Casabella Abril, B., Parcet Solsona, J., Fernandez Ferre, L. I., & de la Torre Casteneda, M. (1990). Health education in arterial hypertension: The evaluation of a course aimed at poorly controlled hypertensives. *Atención Primaria*, 7(3), 194, 196-198.

Frasure-Smith, N., & Prince, R. (1989). Long-term follow-up of ischemic heart disease: Life Stress Monitoring Program. *Psychosomatic Medicine*, *51*(5), 485-513.

Garrity, T. F., & Garrity, A. R. (1985). The nature and efficacy of intervention studies in the National High Blood Pressure Education Research Program. *Journal of Hypertension*, *3*(1), 591-595.

George, L. K., & Fillenbaum, C. G. (1985). The OARS methodology: A decade of experience in geriatric assessment. *Journal of the American Geriatrics Society*, *33*, 607, 615.

German, C., Heierle, C., Zunzunegui, M. V., Contreras, E., Blanco, P., Ruiz, E., & Salas, A. (1994). The control of arterial hypertension in primary care: The evaluation of a program of self-care. *Atención Primaria*, *13*(1), 3-7.

Gleichman, U. M., Philippi, H. H., Gleichman, S. I., Laun, R., Mellwig, K. P., Frohnapfel, F., & Liebermann, A. (1989). Group exercise improves patient compliance in mild to moderate hypertension. *Journal of Hypertension*, 7(3), 577-580.

Godin, G., Valois, P., Jobin, J., & Ross, A. (1991). Prediction of intention to exercise of individuals who have suffered from coronary heart disease. *Journal of Clinical Psychology*, *47*(6), 762-772.

Gonzalez-Fernandez, R. A., Rivera, M., Torres, D., Quiles, J., & Jackson, A. (1990). Usefulness of a systematic hypertension in -hospital educational program. *American Journal of Cardiology*, *65*(20), 1384-1386.

Green, L. W., & Figa-Talamanca, I. (1974). Suggested designs for evaluation of health education programs. *Health Education Monographs*, *2*, 34-60.

HCFA (Health Care Finance Administration). (1989). *Health care utilization and costs of adult cardiovascular conditions, United States, 1980*. Series C, Analytical Report No. 7 PHS, CDC. Hyattsville, MD: National Center for Health Statistics.

Heirich, M. A., Foote, A., Erfurt, J. C., & Konopka, B. (1993). Work-site physical fitness programs: Comparing the impact of different program designs on cardiovascular risks. *Journal of Occupational Medicine*, *35*(5), 510-517.

Institute of Medicine. (1990). *Health people 2000: Citizens chart the course*. Washington, DC: National Academy Press.

Inui, T. S., Yourtee, E. L., & Williamson, J. W. (1976). Improved outcomes in hypertension after physician tutorials. *Annals of Internal Medicine*, *84*, 646-651.

Israel, B. A., House, J. S., Schurman, S. J., Heaney C. A., & Mero, R. P. (1989). The relation of personal resources, participation, influence, interpersonal relationships, and coping strategies to occupational stress, job strains, and health: A multivariate analysis. *Work and Stress*, *3*(2), 163-194.

Israel, B. A., & Schurman, S. J. (1990). Social support, control and the stress process. In K. Glanz, F. Lewis, & B. Remer (Eds.), *Health behavior and health education: Theory, research, and practice* (pp. 187-215). San Francisco: Jossey-Bass.

Jackson, J. S., Tucker, M. B., & Bowman, P. J. (1992). Conceptual and methodological problems in survey research on black Americans. In W. T. Liu (Ed.), *Methodological problems in minority research*. Chicago: Pacific/Asian American Mental Health Research Center.

Janz, N. K., & Becker, M. H. (1984). The health belief model: A decade later. *Health Education Quarterly*, *11*, 1-47.

Janz, N. K., Becker, M. H., & Hartman, P. E. (1984). Contingency contracting to enhance patient compliance: A review. *Patient Education and Counseling*, *5*, 165-178.

Jennett, P. A., Wilson, T. W., Hayton, R. C., Mainprize, G. W., & Laxdal, O. E. (1989). Desirable behaviors in the office management of hypertension addressed through continuing medical education. *Canadian Journal of Public Health*, *80*(5), 359-362.

Job, S. F. S. (1988). Effective and ineffective use of fear in health promotion campaigns. *American Journal of Public Health*, *78*(2), 163-167.

Karlik, B. A., Yarcheski, A., Braun, J., & Wu, M. (1990). Learning needs of patients with angina: An extension study. *Journal of Cardiovascular Nursing*, *4*(2), 70-82.

King, A. C., Martin, J. E., Morrell, E. M., Arena, J. G., & Boland, M. J. (1986). Highlighting specific patient education needs in aging cardiac population. *Health Education Quarterly*, *13*(1), 29-38.

Kottke, T. E., Foels, J. K., Hill, C., Choi, T., & Fenderson, D. A. (1984). Nutrition counseling private practice: Attitudes and activities of family physicians. *Preventive Medicine*, *13*(2), 219-225.

Levenkron, J. C., & Greenland, P. (1988). Patient priorities for behavioral change: Selecting from multiple coronary dis-

ease risk factors. *Journal of General Internal Medicine*, *3*(3), 224-229.
Luscher, T. F., Vetter, H., Siegenthaler, W., & Vetter, W. (1985). Compliance in hypertension: Facts and concepts. *Journal of Hypertension*, *3*(1), S3-9.
Maenpaa, H., Manninen, V., & Heinonen, O. P. (1987). Comparison of the digoxin marker with capsule counting and compliance questionnaire methods for measuring compliance to medication in a clinical trial. *European Heart Journal*, *8*(Suppl. I), 39-43.
Martinez-Amenos, A., Fernandez Terre, M. L., Mota Vidal, C., & Alsina Rocasalbas, J. (1990). Evaluation of two educative models in a primary care hypertension programme. *Journal of Human Hypertension*, *4*(4), 362-364.
McAuley, E., Courneya, K. S., Rudolph, D. L., & Lox, C. L. (July 1994). Enhancing exercise adherence in middle-aged males and females. *Preventive Medicine*, *23*, 498-506.
McGuire, W. J. (1989). Theoretical foundations of campaigns. In R. Rice & C. Atkin (Eds.), *Public communication campaigns* (pp. 43-65). Beverly Hills, CA: Sage.
McKenney, J. M. (1981). Methods of modifying compliance behavior in hypertensive patients. *Drug Intelligence and Clinical Pharmacy*, *15*(1), 8-14.
Montgomery, D. A ., & Amos, R. J. (1991). Nutrition information needs during cardiac rehabilitation. *Journal of the American Dietetic Association*, *91*(9), 1078-1083.
Moore, M. A. (1988). Improving compliance with antihypertensive therapy. *American Family Physician*, *37*(1), 142-148.
Morisky, D. E., DeMuth, N. M., Field-Fass, M., Green, L. W., & Levine, D. M. (1985). Evaluation of family health education to build social support for long-term control of high blood pressures. *Health Education Quarterly*, *12*(1), 35-50.
Morisky, D. E., Levine, D. M., Green, L. W., Shapiro, S., Russell, R. P. & Smith, C. R. (1983). Five year blood pressure control and mortality following healthy education for hypertensive patients. *Journal of American Public Health*, *73*(2), 153-162.
Morisky, D. E., Levine, D. M., Green, L. W., & Smith, C. R. (1982). Health education program effects on the management of hypertension in the elderly. *Archives of Internal Medicine*, *142*(10), 1835-1838.
Muhlhauser, I., Sawicki, P. T., Dedjurgeit, U., Jorgens, V., Trampisch, H. J., & Berger, M. (1993). Evaluation of a structured treatment and teaching programme on hypertension in general practice. *Clinical and Experimental Hypertension*, *15*(1), 125-142.
Mullen, P. D., Mains, D. A., & Velez, R. (1992). A meta analysis of controlled trials of cardiac patient education. *Patient Education and Counseling*, *19*(2), 143-162.
NHBPEP (National High Blood Pressure Educational Program Working Group Report on Hypertension in the Elderly). (1994). *Hypertension*, *23*(3), 275-285.
NHLBI (National Heart, Lung and Blood Institute). (1982). Report of the Working Group: Management of patient compliance in the treatment of hypertension. *Hypertension*, *4*(3), 415-423.
Niebauer, J., Hambrecht, R., Marburger, C., Schlierf, G., Kubler, W., & Schuler, G. (1994). Low fat diet and physical training in coronary heart disease: Long-term results of secondary prevention. *Deutsche Medizinische Wochenschrift*, *119*(1-2), 7-12.
Nugent, C. A., Carnahan, J. E., Sheehan, E. T., & Meyers, C. (1984). Salt restriction in hypertensive patients: Comparison of advice, education, and group management. *Archives of Internal Medicine*, *144*(7), 1415-1417.
O'Callahan, W. G., Teo, K. K., O'Riordan, J., Webb, H., Dolphin, T., & Horgan, J. H. (1984). Comparative response of male and female patients with coronary artery diseases to exercise rehabilitation. *European Heart Journal*, *5*(8), 649-651.
Ogunyemi, O. (1983). Reasons for failure of antihypertensive treatment. *British Medical Journal* (Clinical Research Edition), *286*(6382), 1956-1957.
Oldridge, N. B., & Streiner, D. L. (1990). The health belief model: Predicting compliance and dropout in cardiac rehabilitation. *Medicine and Science in Sports and Exercise*, *22*(5), 678-683.
O'Reilly, P., & Thomas, H. E. (1989). Role of support networks in maintenance of improved cardiovascular health status. *Social Science and Medicine*, *28*(3), 249-260.
Ornish, D., Brown, S. E., Scherwitz, L. W., Billing, J. H., Armstrong, W. T., Ports, T. A., McLanahan, S. M., Kirkeeide, R. L., Brand, R. J., & Gould, K. L. (1990). Can lifestyle changes reverse coronary heart disease? The Lifestyle Heart Trial. *Lancet*, *336*(8208), 129-133.
Orth, J. E., Stiles, W. B., Scherwitz, L., Hennrikus, D., & Vallbona, C. (1987). Patient exposition and provider explanation in routine interviews and hypertensive patients' blood pressure control. *Health Psychology*, *6*(1), 29-42.
Pashkow, F. J. (1993). Issues in contemporary cardiac rehabilitation: A historical perspective. *Journal of the American College of Cardiology*, *21*, 822-834.
Perry, C. L., Stone, E. J., Parcel, G. S ., Ellison, R. C., Nader, P. R., Webber, L. S., & Luepker, R. V. (1990). School-based cardiovascular health promotion: The Child and Adolescent Trial for Cardiovascular Health (CATCH). *Journal of School Health*, *60*(8), 406-413.
Prochaska, J. O., DiClemente, C. C., Velicer, W. F., Ginpel, S., & Norcross, J. C. (1985). Predicting change in smoking status for self changers. *Addictive Behaviors*, *10*, 395-406.
Rehder, T. L., McCoy, L. K., Blackwell, B., Whitehead, W., & Robinson, A. (1980). Improving medication compliance by counseling and special prescription container. *American Journal of Hospital Pharmacy*, *37*(3), 379-385.
Roviaro, S., Holmes, D. S., & Holmsten, R. D. (1984). Influence of a cardiac rehabilitation program on the cardiovascular, psychological and social functioning of cardiac patients. *Journal of Behavioral Medicine*, *7*(1), 61-81.

Russell M. L., Insull, W., & Probstfield, J. (1985). Examination of medical professions for counseling on medication adherence. *American Journal of Medicine*, *78*(2), 277-282.

Scherwitz, L., Hennrikus, D., Yusim, S., Lester, J., & Vallbona, C. (1985). Physician communication to patients regarding medications. *Patient Education and Counseling*, 7(2), 121-136.

Sclar, D. A., Chin, A., Skaer, T. L., Okamoto, M. P., Nakahiro, R. K., & Gill, M. A. (1991). Effect of health education in promoting prescription refill compliance among patients with hypertension. *Clinical Therapeutics*, *13*(4), 489-495.

Shankar, B. S., Russell, R. P., Southard, J. W., & Schurman, E. W. (1982). Patterns of care for hypertension among hospitalized patients. *Public Health Reports*, *97*(6), 521-527.

Sharpe, P. A., Clark, N. M., & Janz, N. K. (1991). Differences in the impact and management of heart disease between older men and women. *Women and Health*, *17*(2), 25-43.

Sleight, P. (1991). Cardiovascular risk factors and the effect of interventions. *American Heart Journal*, *121*(3/Pt. 2), 990-994.

Stanton, A. L. (1987). Determinants of adherence to medical regimens by hypertensive patients. *Journal of Behavioral Medicine*, *10*(4), 377-394.

Stillman, F. A., Bone, L. R., Rand, C., Levine, D. M., & Becker, D. M. (1993). Heart, body and soul: A church-based smoking cessation program for urban African-Americans. *Preventive Medicine*, *22*(3), 335-349.

Strull, W. M., Lo, B., & Charles, G. (1984). Do patients want to participate in medical decision making? *Journal of the American Medical Association*, *252*(21), 2990-2994.

Sutton, S. R. (1982). Fear arousing communications: A critical examination of theory and research. In J. R. Eiser (Ed.), *Social psychology and behavioral medicine*. New York: Wiley.

Tschann, J. M., Adamson, T. E., Coates, T. J., & Gullion, D. S. (1988). Behaviors of treated hypertensive patients and patient demographics. *Journal of Community Health*, *13*(1), 19-32.

Wilson, T. A., Robinson, J. D., & Orlando, J. B. (1982). A pharmacy student searches for psychological predictors of patient compliance. *American Journal of Pharmaceutical Education*, *46*(1), 46-48.

Witschi, J. C., Singer, M., Wu Lee, M., & Stare, F. J. (April 1978). Family cooperation and effectiveness in a cholesterol lowering diet. *Journal of the American Dietetic Association*, *72*(4), 384-389.

Wittels, E. H., Hay, J. W., & Gotto, A. M., Jr. (1990). Medical costs of coronary artery disease in the United States. *American Journal of Cardiology*, *65*(7), 432-440.

Zismer, D. K., Gillum, R. F., Johnson, C. A., Becerra, J., & Johnson, T. H. (1982). Improving hypertension control in a private medical practice. *Archives of Internal Medicine*, *142*(2), 297-299.

9

Self-Management of Childhood Diabetes in Family Context

Tim Wysocki and Peggy Greco

INTRODUCTION

This chapter surveys self-management of insulin-dependent diabetes mellitus among children and adolescents and emphasizes the critical role of family context in the acquisition and maintenance of these behaviors. Self-management refers to the responsibility assumed by patients and families in monitoring, evaluating, and adjusting diabetes treatment. This chapter reviews an extensive literature that illustrates that a wide range of cognitive, affective, behavioral, and social variables influence the effectiveness of self-management of diabetes by youngsters and their families. The chapter begins with a review of the pathophysiology of the disease and a summary of its medical management. From there, the chapter turns to a task analysis of the demands placed upon the family by virtue of parenting a child with IDDM and a review of the research pertinent to these responsibilities. Next, a model of family contributions to the cultivation of sophisticated diabetes self-management is proposed. The chapter concludes with a research agenda that addresses important knowledge gaps revealed in the foregoing discussion.

INSULIN-DEPENDENT DIABETES MELLITUS (IDDM)

Pathophysiology

Insulin-dependent, or Type I, diabetes mellitus (IDDM) is a common pediatric endocrine disorder, with a prevalence of 1 per 600 youths (American Diabetes Association, 1988; Travis, Brouhard, & Schreiner, 1987). The disease results from the autoimmune destruction of pancreatic islet cells that secrete the hormone insulin. The trigger for the autoimmune process that culminates in IDDM has yet to be specified, but it is known that the disease may have an insidious onset of as long as 5 years, during which islet cell antibodies appear and insulin secretion declines. There is a genetic susceptibility to IDDM, but the mechanisms of genetic transmission have yet to be specified.

Tim Wysocki and Peggy Greco • Nemours Children's Clinic, 807 Nira Street, Jacksonville, Florida 32207.

Handbook of Health Behavior Research II: Provider Determinants, edited by David S. Gochman. Plenum Press, New York, 1997.

The primary function of insulin is to promote cellular intake of glucose from the blood. Thus, insulin deficiency results in chronically high blood glucose levels (hyperglycemia). Eventually, there is insufficient insulin to sustain bodily needs and the overt symptoms of polydipsia (excessive drinking), polyuria (excessive urination), polyphagia (excessive eating), dehydration, weight loss, and fatigue lead to the diagnosis of IDDM. The onset of IDDM may occur at any age through early adulthood, but it happens most commonly in middle childhood (7-11 years old). It is now possible to identify individuals at elevated genetic risk for developing IDDM, and this capability may lead eventually to preventive interventions. IDDM differs from the more common adult-onset form of diabetes, non-insulin-dependent diabetes mellitus (NIDDM, or Type II), in that NIDDM is characterized by insulin resistance, rather than insulin deficiency, and NIDDM can often be controlled through diet or exercise and oral medications. The psychological concomitants of NIDDM are reviewed by Fisher and colleagues in Chapter 10.

Medical Management

Despite rapidly advancing knowledge of the etiology, IDDM is still not preventable or reversible. Pancreas transplantation is feasible, but it is reserved for patients with advanced diabetic complications. Research is ongoing to perfect transplantation of insulin-producing islet cells, but clinical application of this technique is still years away.

Current therapy for IDDM approximates normal glucose metabolism through insulin replacement in accord with the patient's caloric intake and activity. Patients take two or more daily subcutaneous injections of insulin, typically about 30 minutes before meals. Available insulin preparations differ in speed of onset and duration of action. Patients typically mix short-acting and longer-acting types of insulin in each injection to ensure continuous availability of insulin. There are also "insulin pumps" that provide a constant basal infusion of short-acting insulin and bolus infusions administered by the patient just before meals, but insulin pumps are infrequently prescribed for children and adolescents. Regardless of mode of administration, insulin dosages are adjusted to each patient's diet and exercise habits.

There are varied dietary management methods, but all attempt to balance insulin availability with food intake and exercise to achieve near-normal blood glucose levels. The American Diabetes Association (1994a) recommends a meal plan that is guided by an individualized assessment of nutritional needs and an emphasis on accommodating the diet to the patient's previous food preferences. Less emphasis is placed on restricting intake of refined sugar and on achieving generic food composition goals compared to past practices. Day-to-day consistency in diet composition is a more important goal of modern nutritional management of IDDM.

Regular aerobic exercise is also an important component of IDDM management because it reduces insulin needs and promotes cardiovascular health. The exercise regimen is important because IDDM is a risk factor for atherosclerosis.

Since the metabolic effects of the diabetes regimen vary, patients practice self-monitoring of blood glucose (SMBG) several times daily to evaluate regimen adequacy and the need for treatment adjustments. SMBG tests consist of pricking a finger to obtain a small blood sample, placing blood on a reagent strip, and inserting the strip into a blood glucose meter. Some meters store test results in memory, while with others the results must be recorded in a logbook. A typical SMBG routine consists of testing before meals and bedtime, a schedule that yields only a crude approximation of normal physiological function.

SMBG may also help in determining proper insulin doses. Many patients use a "sliding scale" insulin algorithm in which the dosage for each injection is specified by the preceding test result. Others may self-adjust insulin dosages, diet, or exercise to compensate for blood glucose fluctuations. Patients and families must also be able to correct elevated blood glucose levels that may occur when the patient is suffering from an infection or has encountered significant psychological stress. There is research in progress on the development of noninvasive, continuous methods of monitoring blood glucose levels. Although significant technical obstacles remain, such methods may soon be available. Glycemic control is also monitored with glycohemoglobin (GHb) assays, which estimate average blood glucose level over the prior 2-3 months.

Patient and family education about the disease and its treatment is critical to effective diabetes management. Inpatient diabetes education programs delivered just after diagnosis may include several days of intensive education on the pathophysiology of the disease and the "survival skills" needed for safe and healthy daily living with IDDM. The initial program may be bolstered by follow-up sessions with a diabetes educator and a dietitian.

Complications

IDDM has many short-term and long-term complications that create a psychological burden. Short-term complications are due to variability in insulin action, dietary intake, activity level, and psychological stress; all of which can cause either insulin excess or insufficiency.

Insulin excess may result in abnormally low blood glucose (hypoglycemia), which is often manifested as disorientation, dizziness, sweating, tremors, and other idiosyncratic symptoms. If not remedied by the ingestion of carbohydrates, a hypoglycemic episode can deteriorate to seizures and loss of consciousness. Hypoglycemic episodes may also precipitate accidents and may lead to social embarrassment. Patients and parents must learn to manage hypoglycemia, preferably by anticipating and preventing its occurrence. There is evidence that severe hypoglycemia can be predicted from SMBG data and that psychological factors may also influence the frequency of these episodes (Cox et al., 1994).

Insulin insufficiency results in abnormally high blood glucose levels (hyperglycemia), and the symptoms seen at diagnosis may recur. It may also result in diabetic ketoacidosis, an altered metabolic state that can culminate in diabetic coma and death. Diabetic ketoacidosis is a common reason for hospitalization of youth with IDDM, and many patients present in this condition at diagnosis. Hyperglycemia is more difficult to detect and prevent than hypoglycemia; mild hyperglycemia, even if chronic, may not produce salient, aversive symptoms.

Long-term complications of IDDM include cardiovascular disease, blindness (retinopathy), kidney failure (nephropathy), and nerve damage (neuropathy). IDDM may also complicate pregnancy in women and cause impotence in men. There have been many advances in the early detection of these complications and improved methods of early treatment. However, 40-50% of patients are likely to develop one or more of these complications, typically more than 15 years after diagnosis. The life expectancy of individuals with IDDM is reduced significantly. Hence, IDDM and its complications have major public health significance given the fiscal and human costs that they entail.

Diabetes Control and Complications Trial

It was suspected that chronic hyperglycemia causes the long-term complications of IDDM, but this was not proven until the mid-1990s. The National Institutes of Health funded the 10-year Diabetes Control and Complications Trial (DCCT) to determine whether the maintenance of near-normoglycemia could prevent the development and/or slow the progression of long-term diabetic complications (DCCT Research Group, 1993, 1994). Over 1400 highly selected patients, including 195 adolescents, were randomized to conventional medical care or to intensive therapy. The intensive regimen included three or more daily insulin injections or the use of an insulin pump, six to eight daily SMBG tests, monthly as opposed to quarterly clinic visits, weekly telephone contact with a nurse, active use of SMBG data for daily treatment adjustments, and services from dietitians and psychologists. The multidisciplinary DCCT teams were instructed to do whatever was necessary to promote and maintain adherence to the intensive regimen.

The DCCT intensive regimen reduced GHb by 1.5-2.0% compared with conventional treatment. Normoglycemia was maintained by only a minority of patients in the intensively treated group, but these patients enjoyed 50-70% reductions in the onset or progression of diabetic retinopathy, nephropathy, and neuropathy. Comparable results were obtained with adolescents.

The clinical implications of the DCCT will be felt for years. The DCCT was, in essence, a behavioral intervention, since its striking findings were achieved solely with current medical technology supplemented by extensive reliance on compliance-enhancement and stress-management interventions, patient education, and social support. However, the cost and feasibility of intensive therapy will present formidable obstacles to its clinical translation. The findings that intensive therapy resulted in a threefold increase in the frequency of severe hypoglycemia and greater weight gain compared with conventional treatment will also present barriers to its dissemination. Hence, clinical translation of the DCCT requires more efficient delivery of intensive therapy and effective response to its attendant increased risks of severe hypoglycemia and weight gain. The DCCT enrolled a highly select sample of patients, and more obstacles may be encountered as intensive therapy is disseminated broadly. Also, since the DCCT enrolled only patients over 13 years of age, the feasibility and efficacy of intensive therapy with younger children are unknown. Given the striking findings of the DCCT, psychologists, psychiatrists, and social workers who work with this population can expect increased involvement in efforts to promote adherence, self-management, and problem solving among patients with IDDM and their families.

FAMILY RESPONSIBILITIES IN RESPONDING TO THE CHALLENGE OF IDDM

This summary of the medical aspects of IDDM illustrates that the family is critical to effective diabetes care (Blechman & Delamater, 1993; Lorenz & Wysocki, 1991). This section surveys ten responsibilities that are imposed on families by IDDM that may affect treatment adherence, health status, and coping with diabetes and summarizes pertinent research in each area.

Responsibility 1: Families must acquire and refine knowledge of IDDM sufficient to allow implementing the insulin, diet, exercise, and SMBG aspects of treatment carefully, safely, and effectively.

Youths and their parents should have adequate knowledge about IDDM as a disease process and understand the role of each treatment component. The importance of adequate knowledge is highlighted by the finding that family knowledge can affect both adherence (Hanson, Henggeler, & Burghen, 1987a) and metabolic control (Gray, Marrero, Godfrey, Orr, & Golden, 1988).

Knowledge is certainly a prerequisite to adequate diabetes management, but it does not guarantee that treatment recommendations will be implemented properly. A classic study of in-home observation of diabetes skills (Watkins, Williams, Martin, Hogan, & Anderson, 1967) showed that 80% of adult patients make errors in insulin administration, 50% erred in regard to insulin dosage, 75% tested urine incorrectly, and 75% made errors in meal spacing. Poor knowledge of diabetes care was associated with worse diabetes management.

These findings have been mirrored in studies of children and adolescents (e.g., Johnson et al., 1982; Weissberg-Benchell, Glasgow, Tynan, Wirtz, & Turek, 1995). Weissberg-Benchell et al. (1995) found that 25% of adolescents with IDDM admitted to missing an insulin injection, 81% ate inappropriate food, and 29% made up BG test results because they had not actually conducted a BG test.

The importance of knowledge in preventing diabetes mismanagement as described above has been demonstrated by studies postulating a relationship between diabetes knowledge and regimen adherence. Christensen (1983) noted a strong relationship between diabetes knowledge and extent of participation in diabetes care for school-age children with diabetes. Adequate knowledge may also be reflected in better metabolic control (e.g., Harkavy, 1981). This relationship between knowledge and health outcome has been somewhat elusive, however, possibly due to methodological weaknesses. An increasing number of studies have made efforts to use standardized tests of diabetes knowledge, have attempted to identify specific components of knowledge in addition to global scores, and have considered possible factors that may moderate the relationship between knowledge and metabolic control. These methodological advances may result in increased accuracy in measuring diabetes knowledge and its effects on health outcome.

Few diabetes educational programs have been specifically designed (and/or empirically evaluated) for children and adolescents with IDDM. Most commonly, youths with diabetes and their families receive instruction at the time of diagnosis and at diabetes summer camps. Although patient knowledge may increase at summer camps (e.g., Harkavy et al., 1983), learning may be related to the child's age. Harkavy and colleagues noted that 12- to 14-year-olds benefited from instruction during diabetes summer camp, while 10- to 11-year-olds did not.

Responsibility 2: Families must maintain an appropriate balance of parent and child responsibilities for diabetes management tasks.

Modern therapy for IDDM promotes the gradual transfer of diabetes responsibilities from parent to child in accord with the child's psychological maturity (American Diabetes Association, 1983). An appropriate balance of self-care independence and psychological maturity is felt to result in IDDM-specific self-sufficiency and to maximize treatment safety and efficacy (Cerreto & Travis, 1984; Follansbee, 1989; Johnson, 1984, 1988; La Greca, Follansbee, & Skyler, 1990). Deviation from this balance may have adverse effects. Allen, Tennen, McGrade, Affleck, and Ratzan (1983) and La Greca et al. (1990) found that children with higher degrees of responsibility, particularly for insulin administration, were in poorer diabetic control. Ingersoll, Orr, Herrold, and Golden (1986) concurred, noting that adolescents with IDDM are often entrusted with insulin self-regulation without regard to their cognitive maturity. Swift, Seidman, and Stein (1967) cautioned, however, that constraining the *capable* child from assuming legitimate self-care autonomy could discourage the child from accepting that responsibility later.

A survey of 229 diabetes professionals about the typical ages at which children master 38 IDDM skills (Wysocki, Meinhold, Cox, & Clarke, 1990) revealed substantial variability among professionals about the ages at which they expect skill mastery by children with IDDM. In a later survey of 490 parents of youths with IDDM (Wysocki, Meinhold, et al., 1992), parents and professionals agreed about the sequence in which the various skills were mastered, but disagreed significantly about the ages at which specific IDDM skills are mastered. Compared to professionals' estimates, parents reported earlier mastery of skills that either were rote or resulted in immediate aversive consequences if not completed correctly. Parents reported later mastery of skills that required more planning and self-regulation by the adolescent, of skills for which the aversive consequences of errors were delayed, and of tasks that were not required often.

A cross-sectional study of 100 youths with IDDM further explored the relationship between self-care autonomy and diabetes outcomes (Wysocki et al., 1995). For each child, an "Autonomy/Maturity Ratio" was calculated as a measure of the extent to which the child's IDDM independence was balanced with the child's measured psychological maturity. Using a tertile split, participants were divided into groups based on their Autonomy/Maturity Ratio scores as follows: Constrained Self-Care Autonomy (degree of self-care autonomy less than expected for child's maturity), Appropriate Self-Care Autonomy (self-care autonomy appropriate for child's maturity), and Excessive Self-Care Autonomy (degree of self-care autonomy greater than expected for child's maturity). These groups differed on treatment adherence and hospitalizations: Excessive Self-Care Autonomy was associated consistently with adverse diabetes outcomes, while Constrained Self-Care Autonomy had no evident adverse effects. Results also indicated that the probability of excessive self-care autonomy increased with the child's age. These findings sound a note of caution regarding the encouragement of maximal self-care autonomy among adolescents with IDDM and imply that families who maintain more parental involvement in diabetes care during adolescence may enjoy better outcomes.

Responsibility 3: Families must assure that the IDDM treatment and monitoring regimen is carried out as planned so that the adequacy of the regimen can be evaluated and refined as needed.

Many behavioral, psychological, and medical factors can contribute to the metabolic status of children with IDDM, but one of the most critical of these factors is compliance with this complex and demanding regimen. As the DCCT demonstrated, compliance with an intensive regimen may prevent or forestall some of the short- and long-term complications of diabetes (DCCT Research Group, 1993, 1994). Consequences of noncompliance may include exacerbation of disability and progression of disease (Epstein & Cluss, 1982). Further, noncompliance impedes accurate monitoring of the effectiveness of the prescribed diabetes regimen.

In clinical and research settings, most health care professionals rely on patients' and/or parents' reports of compliance. Patients may be asked to rate their adherence to specific components of the diabetes regimen (e.g., Hanson et al., 1987a; Israel, Berndt, & Barglow, 1986; La Greca & Skyler, 1991), may record diabetes adherence behaviors (i.e., keeping a home diary), or may be interviewed about diabetes-related activities (Johnson, Silverstein, Rosenbloom, Carter, & Cunningham, 1986; Reynolds, Johnson, & Silverstein, 1990). Despite variation in self-report assessment methods, most of these tools recognize the importance of conceptualizing adherence as an interdependent network of regimen behaviors rather than a single behavior (R. E. Glasgow, McCaul, & Schafer, 1987; R. E. Glasgow, Wilson, & McCaul, 1985; Johnson et al., 1986). Children and adolescents may be adhering to one aspect of the regimen, such as insulin administration, but not others, such as blood glucose testing and exercise.

Adherence to particular aspects of the diabetes regimen relates inversely to the degree of lifestyle change required by the task (R. E. Glasgow et al., 1987) and to the number and severity of barriers that interfere with task compliance (R. E. Glasgow, McCaul, & Schafer, 1986). Dietary and exercise tasks require the greatest amount of lifestyle change and have been associated with a high frequency of barriers by adolescents with IDDM (R. E. Glasgow et al., 1986); it is in these two areas that noncompliance is most often noted.

Compliance has also been associated with many family variables such as knowledge of IDDM (Hanson et al., 1987a), family relations (Hanson et al., 1987a), environmental support (McCaul, Glasgow, & Schafer, 1987), family communication (Bobrow, AvRuskin, & Siller, 1985), and family conflict (Hauser et al., 1990). Given these associations, it is apparent that family-focused interventions are important for addressing problems with diabetes management. Gray et al. (1988) proposed a stepwise intervention that addresses the family's understanding of diabetes care principles, dysfunctional family patterns, conflict resolution skills, and children and adolescents' ability to manage their diabetes.

Gross and colleagues have also published a series of intervention studies that demonstrate the effectiveness of behavioral approaches to problems with compliance (Gross, Magalnick, & Richardson, 1985; Gross, 1987). After participating in social skills training in a group setting, children and adolescents with diabetes demonstrated an improvement in their abilities to cope with stressful disease-related social situations (Gross, Heimann, Shapiro, & Schultz, 1983; Gross et al., 1985). However, these changes were not reflected in improved metabolic control.

Despite the presumed influence of compliance on metabolic functioning, research has not revealed a consistently robust relationship between these two variables (e.g, Johnson, Freund, Silverstein, Hansen, & Malone, 1990; Johnson et al., 1992; K. E. Glasgow et al., 1987). Possible reasons for these findings include: (1) Discrepant time frames over which adherence and metabolic control are measured. Adherence tends to be measured over a shorter period of time (e.g., 3 days within a 2-week period [Johnson et al., 1986]) than most typical measures of metabolic control, which represent functioning over a 2- to 3-month period. (2) Regimen instructions and measures used to assess adherence may not correspond (e.g., child is told to "cut down on meat intake" and adherence is measured as the percentage of calories from fat [R. E. Glasgow et al., 1985]). (3) Children or adolescents may be adhering to regimen prescriptions that are inappropriate or that are inaccurately recalled. (4) Measures of adherence may be biased by a social desirability response set. These methodological problems may dilute the statistical relationship between compliance and metabolic control, but do not reduce the importance of assessing and working to improve compliance in youths with IDDM.

Responsibility 4: Families must cultivate and use appropriate diabetes problem-solving skills through some combination of self-regulation of the regimen or timely consultation with health care providers.

SMBG data are collected to permit health care providers to evaluate and adjust the treatment regimen, to enable the family to anticipate and prevent hypoglycemia and hyperglycemia, and to increase awareness of the glycemic effects of daily activities (American Diabetes Association, 1987, 1994b). SMBG may therefore be used to help prevent short-term diabetic complications, to optimize diabetic control, and to maximize flexibility in daily living. Despite their central role in IDDM management, the nature and correlates of family use of SMBG data have been researched infrequently.

Delamater, Davis, et al. (1988) found that families of adolescents with IDDM rarely used SMBG data for adjusting insulin doses or injection–meal intervals. The benefit of doing so is clear; Peyrot and Rubin (1988) found that adults who reported more frequent use of SMBG data for insulin self-regulation were in better diabetic control.

Wysocki, Hough, Ward, Allen, and Murgai (1992) reported a prospective study of use of SMBG data by 47 families of youths with IDDM. Patients used reflectance meters with memory, and parents completed a daily dairy of their use of SMBG data. Parents recorded occurrences of specific categories of uses of SMBG data, such as: adjustments in insulin, diet, or exercise; confirmation and/or management of hypoglycemia; and decisions to complete urine ketone tests. Families reported an average of 4.85 actions taken in response to SMBG results. At least one treatment action was reported by 74% of the families. Half of the reported actions consisted of responses to hypoglycemia; among the remainder, only 18% were proactive efforts to prevent hypoglycemia or hyperglycemia. Families who reported more frequent use of SMBG data had less parent–child conflict about IDDM, better diabetes knowledge, and better treatment adherence. This study suggests that training in proactive use of SMBG data may enhance IDDM self-management, that reflectance meters with memory provide a rich source of behavioral and medical data, and that family conflict may obstruct diabetic control by impeding family use of SMBG data.

Several studies have evaluated interventions designed to promote IDDM problem-solving based on SMBG data. Delamater et al. (1990) reported 2-year follow-up data for a sample of 36 youths with IDDM who were randomized at diagnosis to either conventional therapy (CT), supportive counseling (SC), or self-management training (SMT). SMT yielded significantly lower GHb levels than the other two groups at Year 1, but the effect at Year 2 remained significant only for the difference between the SMT and CT groups. Similarly, Anderson, Wolf, Burkhart, Cornell, and Bacon (1989) described a peer group intervention targeting family use of SMBG data and showed that this treatment improved diabetic control compared to standard care.

Interactions between health care providers and patients surrounding the analysis and interpretation of SMBG data are also important. Only one study has investigated this topic even though a key component of the DCCT intensive therapy regimen was frequent consultation with health care professionals about regulation of the treatment regimen based on SMBG results. Marrero et al. (1989) reported that patient and physician collaboration in the computerized review of recent SMBG results was an effective and valued educational experience. This would seem to be a fruitful area of inquiry that would complement additional studies of families' utilization of SMBG data.

Responsibility 5: Families must recognize and respond adequately to general and diabetes-related psychological stressors that may impede diabetic control directly and interfere with treatment adherence and diabetes problem solving.

It is important for youths with IDDM and their families to accept that it is difficult to adhere to the diabetes regimen. R. E. Glasgow et al. (1986) assessed the frequency of barriers—environmental and cognitive events that are obstacles to regimen adherence—in adolescents and adults with IDDM. They noted that there are many barriers to adherence and that the greatest number of barriers are reported for those treatment aspects that require greater lifestyle changes, such as dietary and exercise adherence. Further, the number of barriers reported was directly related to actual regimen adherence; the greater the number of obstacles reported for a particular aspect of the diabetes regimen, the more likely the youth with IDDM would have difficulty adhering to that particular aspect.

Stress may also affect glycemic control and adherence; neuroendocrine responses to stress can directly alter metabolic functioning. Support for this process was provided by Chase and Jackson (1981), who noted that the frequency of stressful events reported by children with IDDM was associated with the physiological measures of metabolic control, triglyceride concentration, cholesterol, and serum glucose. Hanson et al. (1987a) also showed a direct effect of stress on metabolic control in adolescents with IDDM.

Although it has been postulated that stress can have either direct effects, through physiological mechanisms, or mediated effects, through processes such as regimen adherence (e.g., Aikens, Wallander, Bell, & Cole, 1992), there has been inconsistent support for adherence as a mediating variable. Hanson et al. (1987a) noted that chronic stress and adherence were both *directly* linked to metabolic control, rather than the relationship between stress and metabolic control being mediated by adherence. Likewise, in a test of their model, Aikens et al. (1992) found no empirical support for adherence as a mediator of the relationship between stress and metabolic control.

Adolescents and families under stress may have a harder time managing the adolescents' diabetes. In a retrospective study of psychosocial stress factors in children and adolescents with IDDM, White, Kolman, Wexler, Polin, and Winter (1984) noted that stress in families with limited problem-solving skills is a major factor in poorly controlled diabetes. As the authors point out, the presence of stress itself does not always result in poor diabetic control; how families respond to stressors also determines the concomitants of stress. This idea has received empirical support; patients who are in poor metabolic control have been found to use maladaptive ways of coping with stress to a greater extent than youths in good metabolic control (Delamater, Kurtz, Bubb, White, & Santiago, 1987; Hanson, Henggeler, &

Burghen, 1987b; Hanson et al. 1989). Thus, adolescents and their families not only need to recognize the presence and effects of stress, but also may benefit both psychologically and physiologically by learning to cope with it in adaptive ways.

Responsibility 6: Families must maintain effective communication about diabetes management and encourage open expression about emotional adjustment to the disease.

The treatment, monitoring, and lifestyle demands imposed by IDDM pervade daily life. Many studies have shown that certain dimensions of family function are important predictors of the efficacy of family adaptation to these demands (Blechman & Delamater, 1993; Lorenz & Wysocki, 1991).

For example, Bobrow et al. (1985) found that mother-daughter conflict was associated with poorly controlled IDDM. Hanson et al. (1987a) reported that parental support and adolescent social competence buffered the adverse effects of stress on glycemic control. Wysocki (1993) found that family communication, problem-solving, and conflict resolution skills were important correlates of treatment adherence, diabetic control, and adolescents' affective adjustment to IDDM. Anderson, Miller, Auslander, and Santiago (1981) reported that youths in poor diabetic control had families who reported more conflict and less cohesion than those in fair or good diabetic control. Anderson, Auslander, Jung, Miller, and Santiago (1990) found that disagreement about parent-child responsibility for diabetes tasks was predictive of diabetic control. Greater disagreement was associated with poorer diabetic control.

These cross-sectional studies yielded consistent results, but their findings have been bolstered further by the work of Hauser and Jacobson and their group on a longitudinal study of children enrolled at diagnosis of IDDM. Reports from this series indicate that premorbid family function was a significant predictor of initial coping with the diagnosis (Wertlieb, Hauser, & Jacobson, 1986), adherence over intervals as long as 4 years (Hauser, Jacobson, Wertlieb, Brink, & Wentworth, 1985; Hauser et al., 1986, 1990; Jacobson et al., 1986, 1987, 1990), and diabetic control over the same intervals (Hauser, DiPlacido, Jacobson, Willett, & Cole, in press; Jacobson et al., 1994). The prospective nature of these studies bolsters the conclusion that family function is associated causally with diabetes outcomes, rather than simply being a correlate of those outcomes.

Responsibility 7: Families must encourage children with IDDM to develop disease-specific social skills and to obtain positive social support from family members and friends.

Family dysfunction can be associated with poor compliance and health status, while positive family communication may be beneficial (e.g., Bobrow et al., 1985; Hanson et al., 1987a; Hauser et al., 1990; Minuchin, Rosman, & Baker, 1978). In addition to the specific skills of communication and problem solving previously discussed, social support can be important for the child's general and disease-specific functioning. Social support has been defined as "an individual's access to emotional, intellectual, and material assistance from other persons when beleaguered" (Blaney, 1985, p. 272). Thus, as pertains to the youth with IDDM, social support refers to the ways in which the child or adolescent is aided in coping with diabetes. Social support may be offered by family members or by friends; children and adolescents value both of these sources of support (Greco et al., 1991; La Greca et al., 1995).

Diabetes-specific social support provided by family members may vary by regimen task; family members appear to offer the most support for maintaining a meal plan and for insulin administration (Greco et al., 1991; La Greca et al., 1995). The *type* of support offered from family members also differs from that provided by friends; family members are more likely to offer tangible support such as reminding about tasks, assisting with tasks, or doing diabetes-related tasks for the child, while peer support is primarily oriented toward companionship and emotional support (La Greca et al., 1995). The value of tangible support offered by family members is evidenced by better treatment adherence for those adolescents reporting higher levels of family support (La Greca et al., 1995). The support offered by friends also varies by diabetes task; friends are more likely to offer support for exercising than for other aspects of the regimen (La Greca et al., 1991, 1995). Friends are most likely to support an adolescent with diabetes by "joining in" or providing companionship; they may exercise or eat a snack with the adolescent.

Despite the importance of peer interactions, and the amount of time that older youths spend with their peers, adolescents appear to be reluctant to talk about diabetes with their friends (Jacobson et al., 1986). Thus, although adolescents with diabetes report that they consider support from friends helpful, this source of support is unavailable for adolescents who have not informed their peer group about their diabetes. Improving their social skills in this context can be beneficial and may even impact glycemic control, as demonstrated in an intervention study by Kaplan, Chadwick, and Schimmel (1985). The value of effective communication about diabetes between children and their friends is thus underscored by the findings that adolescents with diabetes considered peer support beneficial (e.g., La Greca et al., 1995) and that improved social skills may be reflected in adherence (Citrin, La Greca, & Skyler, 1985; Gross, 1987) as well as better glycemic control (Kaplan et al., 1985).

Responsibility 8: Families must recognize that IDDM may threaten the psychological adjustment of all family members and respond effectively to this threat.

In addition to recognition that IDDM may represent a threat to the psychological adjustment of patients themselves, there is a growing recognition that the diabetes treatment burden may also have adverse psychological effects on other family members, particularly mothers. Given the importance of family cooperation and support for effective diabetes management, families must also recognize and contend with these risks.

There is ample evidence that mothers assume the brunt of the behavioral and emotional burden of diabetes management. Studies by Hodges and Parker (1987), Banion, Miles, and Carter (1983), Wysocki, Huxtable, Linscheid, and Wayne (1989), and Hauenstein, Marvin, Snyder, and Clarke (1989) confirmed that mothers of children with IDDM report more parenting stress than do mothers of healthy children, that the uncertainties associated with IDDM are important contributors to that stress, and that parenting these children is more complex and challenging. Thus, it is not surprising that mothers show an elevated incidence of depression during the first year of IDDM (Kovacs et al., 1985) and that maternal depressive symptoms may re-emerge several years after diagnosis as a manifestation of a diabetes-specific "burnout" syndrome (Kovacs et al., 1990). The extent to which maternal stress, anxiety, and depression adversely affect IDDM management is unknown, but it is likely that these symptoms could impede adherence and self-regulation in some families.

The role of fathers in IDDM management, as in most arenas of pediatric psychology, has been researched infrequently. Kovacs et al. (1985) found that fathers did not demonstrate increased depressive symptomatology during the first year after diagnosis of childhood IDDM. Wysocki (1993) reported that father-adolescent communication and problem-solving skills were as robust predictors of adolescents' diabetic control and treatment adherence as were mother-adolescent interactions, but fathers' reports about other aspects of parent-adolescent relationships were weaker correlates of diabetes outcomes compared with mothers' reports. Hanson, Henggeler, Rodrigue, Burghen, and Murphy (1988) found that youths from father-absent families were at risk of poorer glycemic control. No studies have explored the impact of fathers' involvement in IDDM management on diabetes outcomes or determined whether it serves as a protective factor for the emergence of maternal depression. Given the important role of social support as a determinant of health outcomes in a wide variety of medical conditions, it is likely that families with more paternal involvement in daily disease management would enjoy better diabetic control and easier adaptation to the family demands imposed by IDDM.

There has also been increased recent interest in interactions between youths with IDDM and their siblings, since brothers and sisters may be in a unique position to influence diabetes management, either positively or negatively. Resentment about inequitable parental attention given to the child with IDDM, the imposition of dietary constraints on the entire family, and the impact of IDDM on family finances could aggravate conflicts among healthy siblings and children with diabetes. Alternatively, disease-specific social support from siblings may have positive effects on children with IDDM in terms of treatment adherence, managing hypoglycemia, and facilitating adaptation to diabetes within the peer group. A few studies have explored relationships among youths with IDDM and their siblings (e.g., Hanson et al., 1992), but none has been concerned with whether brothers and sisters exhibit clinically significant psychological sequelae attributable to diabetes.

Responsibility 9: Families must encourage appropriate interactions with health care professionals and internalization of protective health values.

Every child with IDDM must be prepared to face a lifetime of interactions with health professionals, and ideally to cultivate a productive therapeutic partnership that is founded on mutual trust and effective communication. Similarly, each child with IDDM should develop beneficial health-related values and beliefs that will guide a lifetime of choices and decisions. Whether intentionally or not, each family teaches its children how to interact with health care providers and encourages its children to adopt positive or negative health-related values, all of which are likely to exert lasting influences on adjustment to IDDM, adaptation to its treatment demands into adult life, and, ultimately, health outcomes.

Despite the potential importance of these processes, little research has been done on the factors that influence children's socialization as health care consumers, their internalization of attitudes toward health care delivery and health professionals, and their achievement of autonomous relationships with health care providers. As with other aspects of children's internalization of social attitudes, norms, and values, it is very likely that parental modeling plays a primary role, but this question has not been investigated.

Wysocki, Hough, Ward, and Green (1992) studied psychological adjustment, diabetes self-management, health care use, and diabetic control in 81 young adults with IDDM (18–23 years old). Mildly elevated scores on the Health Care Orientation subscale of the Psychological Adjustment to Illness Scale (DeRogatis, 1983) suggested that in comparison with adult medical patients, young adults with IDDM demonstrated more denial of the disease process and resistance to lifestyle changes imposed by the disease. Little evidence of clinically significant psychopathology was found, but a prior history of poor adjustment to IDDM in earlier adolescence was predictive of persistent poor diabetic control, discontinuous health care utilization, and early diabetic nephropathy. This work suggests that the IDDM adjustment difficulties that are common among adolescents may not be benign or transient and that prevention and intervention efforts should be directed at high-risk youths and their families.

The few studies that have been done on health care utilization during the transition to adulthood suggest that young adults visit health care providers infrequently for routine or proactive services and are far more prone to utilize health care services episodically or in response to specific crises (Bartsch, Barnes, Jarrett, & Lindsay, 1987; Frank, Perlman, & Ehrlich, 1991; Wysocki, Hough, Ward, & Green, 1992).

Recently, there has been extensive research attention devoted to interactions between patients and health care providers and the impact of these factors on treatment adherence and other health-related behaviors (e.g., Kaplan, Greenfield, & Ware, 1989; Suchman, Roter, Green, & Lipkin, 1993; Tabak, 1987). Little of this research has focused on pediatric health care interactions and their influence on IDDM self-management skills. Delamater, Kurtz, White, & Santiago (1988) found that social demand characteristics of typical clinical encounters between youths with IDDM and their physicians may influence many children to report erroneous blood glucose test results, presumably to avoid disapproval or criticism. Wilson and Endres (1986) earlier reported a high frequency of distorted SMBG results recorded in children's logbooks compared with automated recording of true test results by reflectance meters with memory. Thus, clinical encounters with children with IDDM carry the potential for generating considerable counterproductive and deceptive interaction between youths and health professionals (Weissberg-Benchell et al., 1995). Research is clearly needed to analyze encounters among health care providers and youths with IDDM and their families, particularly since these variables affect the therapeutic utilization of SMBG data during health care interactions.

Responsibility 10: Parents must advocate for the needs of children with IDDM in schools and other broader social systems.

In addition to interacting comfortably with health professionals in a way that facilitates good diabetes care, youths and their families must also learn to advocate for the child's special needs in other social systems. The social systems in which the child with diabetes functions may benefit from (1) general information about IDDM, (2) a description of the child's regimen and the impact that it will have in that setting, (3) discussion of barriers within that particular setting that may interfere with adequate performance of the regimen, and (4) a means for addressing problems that may arise periodically within the system.

The degree to which the parent or youth takes responsibility for this process depends on factors discussed above related to maturity as well as age. Anderson et al. (1990) devised a measure of family sharing of diabetes responsibilities, part of which examines the sharing of information about diabetes in social systems other than the family. Adolescents and their mothers were asked to rate who takes responsibility for informing friends, relatives, and teachers about diabetes, as well as who explains school absences. Older children assumed greater responsibility for informing others about their diabetes in multiple contexts, as did girls as compared to boys. The authors postulated that this pattern reflected a general shift of responsibility for IDDM-related tasks as children mature. Gender differences in maturation rate and parental expectations for responsibility are consistent with girls assuming greater responsibility for sharing information about their diabetes in various social contexts than did boys.

The assumption is that the child will benefit from the sharing of information and advocating for the diabetes regimen in various social contexts, but this assumption has not been evaluated empirically. Until contradictory data are presented, families should assume a positive benefit of advocating for their child's diabetes-related needs while remaining sensitive to individual differences (e.g., age, maturation, shyness or embarrassment over disclosure) that might influence this process.

A DEVELOPMENTAL MODEL OF DIABETES SELF-MANAGEMENT

The preceding section summarized an array of tasks that are imposed on families who have a child with IDDM. It should not be surprising that a minority of families achieve this idealized adaptation to IDDM and that some others fall far short of these ideals. This section of the chapter will integrate the major themes established by existing psychological research on IDDM into a model of the development of competent diabetes self-management and of its effects on health status and affective adjustment to the disease.

There is abundant evidence that demographic factors, psychological stress, and aspects of family function are associated with adjustment to IDDM and diabetic control. Many of these asso-

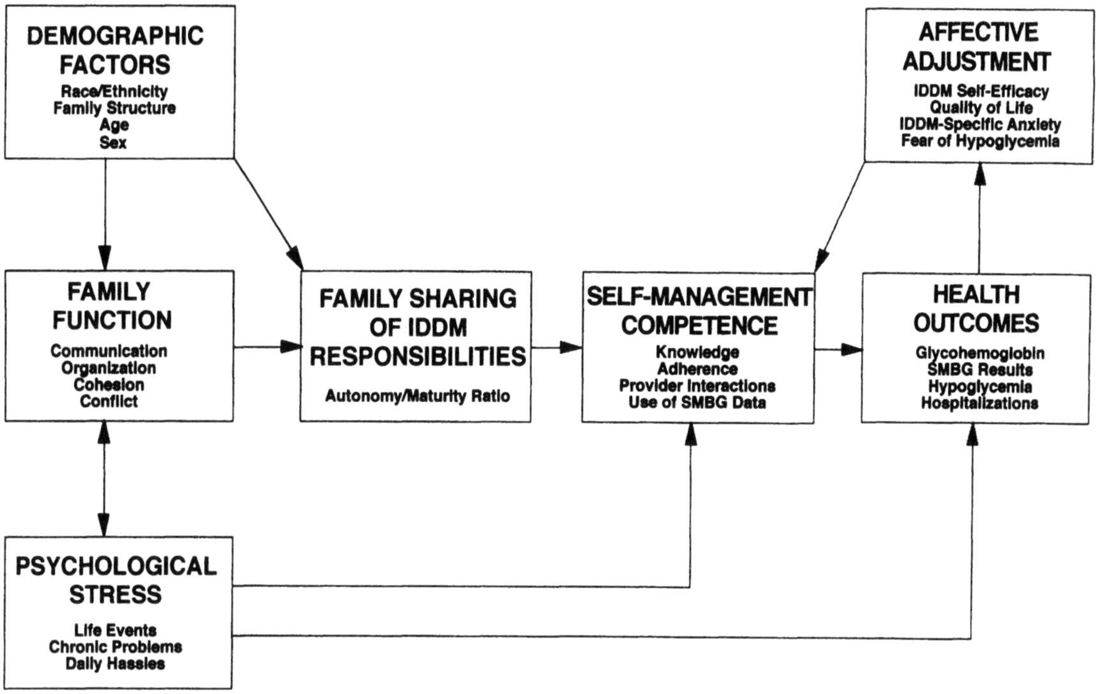

Figure 1. Model depicting the associations among demographic factors, family function, psychological stress, parent-child division of IDDM responsibilities, and self-management competence with health outcomes and affective adjustment to the disease.

ciations are probably indirect, mediated by other variables. This section offers a conceptual model of the behavioral and psychological mechanisms that influence these associations. Figure 1 depicts a framework that relates several contextual variables (demographic factors, family function, and psychological stress) that may influence the extent to which the child deviates from developmentally appropriate IDDM self-care autonomy. The magnitude of this deviation is then presumed to affect the family's self-management competence through effects on treatment adherence, family-provider interactions, and use of SMBG data for treatment adjustments. Self-management success or failure then accrues affective and attitudinal consequences that influence subsequent self-management behaviors. Examples of IDDM-specific affective and attitudinal reactions include quality of life, health beliefs, anxiety about complications, fear of hypoglycemia, and IDDM self-efficacy. Psychological stress enters the model at several points by affecting family function and self-management competence and influencing diabetic control directly. The model expands upon previous conceptualizations in that deviation from developmentally appropriate self-care autonomy has a central role and family self-management competence is conceptualized as a cluster of four skills. The model incorporates current research on the development of IDDM self-care autonomy and begins to explain why previous studies have failed to reveal highly consistent associations between treatment adherence and health status in IDDM.

There is a vast literature on the cross-sectional and longitudinal associations of the model's contextual factors with treatment adherence, diabetic control, and psychological adjustment of youths with IDDM. Many studies have reported associations of various demographic factors with IDDM treatment adherence and metabolic control. Age (e.g., Amiel, Sherwin, Simonson, Lauritano, & Tamborlane, 1986; Johnson, 1984, 1988), racial/ethnic background (Delamater, Albrecht, Postellon, & Gutai, 1991; Hanson et al., 1987b), family structure (Hanson et al., 1988), and socioeconomic status (A. M. Glasgow et al., 1991) have all been implicated as correlates of diabetes outcomes.

Many studies have documented the importance of family function as a predictor of IDDM outcomes (Blechman & Delamater, 1993; Lorenz & Wysocki, 1991). The dimensions of family function that have emerged most consistently in the research literature as affecting IDDM outcomes are family communication skills and the degree of family conflict and cohesion. These variables may affect diabetic control by influencing family adaptation to stress (e.g., Hanson et al., 1987a) or by affecting the family's IDDM self-management and problem-solving skills (Hanson, et al., 1987a; Wysocki, 1993; Wysocki, Green, & Huxtable, 1989; Wysocki, Hough, Ward, Allen, & Murgai, 1992).

Stress may have direct, psychophysiological effects on metabolic control as well as indirect, behavioral effects on diabetes outcomes through influences on family self-management competence. Family relations play a key role in cultivating coping skills that may buffer the effects of stress on diabetic control (Delamater et al., 1991; Hanson et al., 1987a; Hauser et al., 1993; Mengel et al., 1992; Wertlieb et al., 1986).

The model attributes crucial status to children's deviation from developmentally appropriate self-care autonomy. Several studies have implicated excessive IDDM self-care autonomy as a risk factor for poor diabetic control and treatment adherence (Allen et al., 1983; Ingersoll et al., 1986; La Greca et al., 1990; Wysocki et al., 1995). Other research shows that mothers bear the brunt of the psychological burden of IDDM management (Banion et al., 1983; Hodges & Parker, 1987; Hauenstein et al., 1989; Kovacs et al., 1985, 1990; Wysocki, Huxtable, et al., 1989) and suggests that paternal involvement in IDDM management may facilitate diabetes outcomes and reduce depression and "burnout" among mothers (Hanson et al., 1988).

This chapter portrays self-management competence as a multifactorial construct composed of the adequacy of the family's IDDM knowledge, treatment adherence, family-provider interactions, and use of SMBG data for treatment adjustments. Each component is presumed to contribute hierarchically to IDDM outcomes. Thus, diabetes knowledge is prerequisite to adequate treatment adherence; adequacy of treatment adherence affects the productivity of the family-provider interactions; efficacy of the family-provider alliance influences the therapeutic use of SMBG data, which, in turn, mediates the ultimate effects of self-management on health outcomes. This sequential process implies that competent self-management of IDDM is achieved only if all of these elements are in place concurrently over a sufficient period of time.

The chapter has reviewed research on the nature and determinants of diabetes knowledge and skills, leading to the conclusion that accurate diabetes knowledge is a necessary, but insufficient, precursor of acceptable treatment adherence and diabetic control. The review further indicates that adherence to the IDDM regimen is a labile, multifactorial construct, rather than a unitary or stable personality trait, and that there is not a simple one-to-one correspondence between IDDM treatment adherence and diabetic control. Finally, the review of the few available studies of family use of SMBG data for daily diabetes problem solving reveals that proactive utilization of SMBG data is uncommon and that interventions focusing on these sophisticated skills have shown considerable promise in promoting diabetic control.

IDDM SELF-MANAGEMENT: A RESEARCH AGENDA

The survey of research included in this chapter and the formulation of a model that attempts to integrate that research show that much has been learned about the psychological factors that influence health and psychological outcomes in IDDM, but that much remains to be clarified. The three broad areas discussed in this section represent particularly exciting avenues for future exploration.

Maintenance of Parental Involvement in Diabetes Management

Several studies support the conclusion that many typical adolescents are not fully competent to manage IDDM completely independently and that excessive self-care autonomy relative to psychological maturity is associated negatively with treatment adherence, GHb, and hospitalization rates. Thus, maintenance of parental involvement in diabetes management during adolescence may protect against the deterioration in treatment adherence and diabetic control that typify that period. But the precise nature of that parental involvement, and of the factors that affect it, remain to be specified.

Factors That Affect Higher-Level IDDM Self-Regulation Skills

As was discussed earlier in this chapter, research on the relationship between treatment adherence and diabetic control has largely neglected the importance of families' day-to-day self-regulation of the IDDM treatment regimen. Instead, adherence has been conceptualized as simply following the instructions given by health professionals. While this may be an important requisite, adequate treatment adherence when so defined, like diabetes knowledge, may be insufficient to ensure the achievement and maintenance of health status objectives. This chapter argues for a broader conceptualization of IDDM self-management that incorporates diabetes knowledge, treatment adherence, interactions with health care providers, and active use of SMBG data.

There has been only very limited research conducted on IDDM self-management conceptualized in this way, but the research that has been done suggests significant underutilization of SMBG data for treatment adjustments, particularly in a proactive sense (Delamater, Davis, et al., 1988; Wysocki, Hough, Ward, Allen, & Murgai, 1992). Research on factors that affect the frequency and proficiency of family self-regulation of the diabetes regimen is desperately needed. Little is known about the contribution of interactions between families and their health care providers to the therapeutic use of SMBG data. This process would seem to play a particularly important role in the management of those children whose families lack the prerequisite cognitive or motivational attributes needed to support effective higher-level diabetes self-management.

Enhancement of Efficiency and Cost-Effectiveness of Intensive Therapy

The high cost of DCCT-style intensive therapy relative to standard medical care for IDDM, the observation that this investment is not recovered for years, and the short-term focus on health care cost containment efforts make it very unlikely that funding sources will support the widespread implementation of intensified IDDM therapy. But these same observations imply that research oriented toward enhancing the efficiency of intensive therapy would be valued.

There are at least three distinct avenues that such research could pursue. First, intensive therapy in the DCCT combined several intervention components including intensified insulin regimens, more frequent SMBG, more frequent and personal interaction with health professionals, emphasis on active use of SMBG data, and access to psychological services. Component analyses of intensive therapy could identify its critical elements, possibly permitting the design of a less expensive, but equally effective, treatment.

Second, many patients in the DCCT intensive therapy group failed to approach normoglycemia, while another substantial group of patients in the conventional therapy group did achieve near-normoglycemia. Empirically validated identification of patients who are likely to benefit from intensive therapy and to fare poorly without it could permit targeted allocation of those resources that are available for clinical translation of the DCCT findings.

A third research strategy would be to identify behaviors that predict successful intensive therapy rather than try to identify stable traits of patients. For example, research could focus on such behaviors as parent-child division of IDDM responsibilities, frequency and proficiency of families' active use of SMBG data for self-regulation, diabetes problem-solving and communication skills, and patient-family-provider interactions as predictors of benefit from intensive therapy. This information could be helpful in optimizing treatment outcomes among those who initiate intensified therapy.

SUMMARY

This chapter began with a treatment of the physiological and medical aspects of IDDM and offered a concise illustration of the complex demands that are imposed upon the families of children with this disease. It surveyed the pertinent research, identified salient gaps in that literature, and provided an integrative model. It is hoped that this discussion will serve as a useful introduction to this field for beginning students and researchers and as a plausible guide to future research for more advanced investigators.

REFERENCES

Aikens, J. E., Wallander, J. L., Bell, D. S. H., & Cole, J. A. (1992). Daily stress variability, learned resourcefulness, regimen adherence, and metabolic control in Type I diabetes mellitus: Evaluation of a path model. *Journal of Consulting and Clinical Psychology*, *60*, 113-118.

Allen, D. A., Tennen, H., McGrade, B. J., Affleck, G., & Ratzan, S. (1983). Parent and child perceptions of the management of juvenile diabetes. *Journal of Pediatric Psychology*, *8*, 129-141.

American Diabetes Association. (1983). *Curriculum for youth education*. Alexandria, VA: American Diabetes Association.

American Diabetes Association. (1987). Consensus statement on self-monitoring of blood glucose. *Diabetes Care*, *10*, 95-99.

American Diabetes Association. (1988). *Physician's guide to insulin-dependent diabetes (Type I): Diagnosis and treatment*. Alexandria, VA: American Diabetes Association.

American Diabetes Association. (1994a). Nutrition recommendations and principles for people with diabetes mellitus. *Diabetes Care*, *17*, 519-522.

American Diabetes Association. (1994b). Consensus statement: Self-monitoring of blood glucose. *Diabetes Care*, *17*, 81-86.

Amiel, S.A., Sherwin, R. S., Simonson, D. C., Lauritano, A. A., & Tamborlane, W. V. (1986). Impaired insulin action in puberty: A contributing factor to poor glycemic control in adolescents with diabetes. *New England Journal of Medicine*, *315*, 215-219.

Anderson, B. J., Auslander, W. F., Jung, K. C., Miller, J. P., & Santiago, J. V. (1990). Assessing family sharing of diabetes responsibilities. *Journal of Pediatric Psychology*, *15*, 477-492.

Anderson, B. J., Miller, B., Auslander, W. F., & Santiago, J. V. (1981). Family characteristics of diabetic adolescents: Relationships to metabolic control. *Diabetes Care*, *4*, 586-594.

Anderson, B. J., Wolf, F. M., Burkhart, M. T., Cornell, R. G., & Bacon, G E. (1989). Effects of peer group intervention on metabolic control of adolescents with IDDM: Randomized outpatient study. *Diabetes Care*, *12*, 179-184.

Banion, C., Miles, M., & Carter, M. (1983). Problems of mothers in the management of children with diabetes. *Diabetes Care*, *6*, 548-551.

Bartsch, C., Barnes, B., Jarrett, L., & Lindsay, R. (1989). Where did they go? Life after teen diabetes clinic. *Diabetes*, *38*(Suppl. 2), 40A (abstract).

Blaney, P. H. (1985). Stress and depression in adults: A critical review. In T. M. Field, P. M. McCabe, & N Schneiderman (Eds.), *Stress and coping* (p. 272). Hillsdale, NJ: Erlbaum.

Blechman, E. A., & Delamater, A. M. (1993). Family communication and Type I diabetes: A window on the social environment of chronically ill children. In R. E. Cole & D. Reiss (Eds.), *How do families cope with chronic illness?* (pp. 1-24). Hillsdale, NJ: Erlbaum.

Bobrow, E. S., AvRuskin, T. W., & Siller, J. (1985). Mother-daughter interaction and adherence to diabetes regimens. *Diabetes Care*, *8*, 146-151.

Cerreto, M. C., & Travis, L. B. (1984). Implications of psychosocial and family factors in the treatment of diabetes. *Pediatric Clinics of North America*, *31*, 689-710.

Chase, H. P., & Jackson, G. G. (1981). Stress and sugar control in children with insulin-dependent diabetes mellitus. *Journal of Pediatrics*, *98*, 1011-1013.

Christensen, K. (1983). Self-management in diabetic children. *Diabetes Care*, *6*, 552-555.

Citrin, W., La Greca, A. M., & Skyler, J. S. (1985). Group intervention in Type I diabetes mellitus. In P. I. Ahmed & N. Ahmed (Eds.), *Coping with juvenile diabetes* (pp. 181-204). Springfield, IL: Charles C. Thomas.

Cox, D. J., Kovatchev, B. P., Julian, D. M., Gonder-Frederick, L. A., Polonsky, W. H., Schlundt, D. G., & Clarke, W. L. (1994). Frequency of severe hypoglycemia in insulin-dependent diabetes mellitus can be predicted from self-monitoring blood glucose data. *Journal of Clinical Endocrinology and Metabolism, 79*, 1659-1662.

Delamater, A. M., Albrecht, D. R., Postellon, D. C., & Gutai, J. P. (1991). Racial differences in metabolic control of children and adolescents with Type I diabetes mellitus. *Diabetes Care, 14*, 20-25.

Delamater, A. M., Bubb, J., Davis, S., Smith, J. A., Schmidt, L., White, N. H., & Santiago, J. V. (1990). Randomized prospective study of self management training with newly diagnosed diabetic children. *Diabetes Care, 13*, 492-498.

Delamater, A. M., Davis, S., Bubb, J., Smith, J., White, N. H., & Santiago, J. V. (1988). Self monitoring of blood glucose by adolescents with diabetes: Technical skills and utilization of data. *Diabetes Educator, 15*, 56-61.

Delamater, A. M., Kurtz, S., Bubb, J., White, N. H., & Santiago, J. V. (1987). Stress and coping in relation to metabolic control of adolescents with Type I diabetes mellitus. *Journal of Developmental and Behavioral Pediatrics, 8*, 136-140.

Delamater, A. M., Kurtz, S. M., White, N. H., & Santiago, J. V. (1988). Effects of social demand on reports of self-monitored blood glucose in adolescents with Type I diabetes mellitus. *Journal of Applied Social Psychology, 18*, 491-502.

DeRogatis, L. (1983). *Psychosocial Adjustment to Illness Scale*. Baltimore, MD: Clinical Psychometrics Research.

Diabetes Control and Complications Trial Research Group. (1993). Diabetes Control and Complications Trial: The effect of intensive treatment of diabetes on the development and progression of long term complications in insulin-dependent diabetes mellitus. *New England Journal of Medicine, 329*, 977-986.

Diabetes Control and Complications Trial Research Group. (1994). Effect of intensive treatment on the development and progression of long term complications in adolescents with insulin-dependent diabetes mellitus. *Journal of Pediatrics, 125*, 177-188.

Epstein, L. H., & Cluss, P. A. (1982). A behavioral medicine perspective on adherence to long-term medical regimens. *Journal of Consulting and Clinical Psychology, 50*, 950-971.

Follansbee, D. M. (1989). Assuming responsibility for diabetes management: What age, what price? *Diabetes Educator, 15*, 347-352.

Frank, M., Perlman, K., & Ehrlich, R. (1990). Factors contributing to noncompliance with medical follow-up after discharge from a pediatric diabetes clinic. *Diabetes, 39* (Suppl. 1), 55A (abstract).

Glasgow, A. M., Weissberg-Benchell, D. R., Tynan, W. D., Epstein, S. F., Driscoll, C., Terek, J., & Beliveau, E. (1991). Re-admissions of children with diabetes mellitus to a children's hospital. *Pediatrics, 88*, 98-104.

Glasgow, R. E., McCaul, K. D., & Schafer, L. C. (1986). Barriers to regimen adherence among persons with insulin-dependent diabetes. *Journal of Behavioral Medicine, 9*, 65-77.

Glasgow, R. E., McCaul, K. D., & Schafer, L. C. (1987). Self-care behaviors and glycemic control in type I diabetes. *Journal of Chronic Disease, 40*, 399-417.

Glasgow, R. E., Wilson, W., & McCaul, K. D. (1985). Regimen adherence: A problematic construct in diabetes research [Editorial]. *Diabetes Care, 8*, 300-301.

Gray, D. L., Marrero, D. G., Godfrey, C., Orr, D. P., & Golden, M. P. (1988). Chronic poor metabolic control in the pediatric population: A stepwise intervention program. *Diabetes Educator, 14*, 516-520.

Greco, P., La Greca, A. M., Auslander, W. F., Spetter, D., Skyler, J. S., Fisher, E., & Santiago, J. V. (1991). Family and peer support of diabetes care among adolescents. *Diabetes, 40*(Suppl 1), 537A (abstract).

Gross, A. M. (1987). A behavioral approach to the compliance problems of young diabetics. *Journal of Compliance in Health Care, 2*, 7-21.

Gross, A. M., Heimann, L., Shapiro, R., & Schultz, R. M. (1983). Children with diabetes: Social skills training and hemoglobin A1c levels. *Behavior Modification, 7*, 151-163.

Gross, A. M., Magalnick, L. J., & Richardson, P. (1985). Self management training with families of insulin-dependent diabetic children: A controlled long-term investigation. *Child and Family Behavior Therapy, 7*, 35-50.

Hanson, C. L., Cigrang, J. A., Harris, M. A., Carle, D. L., Relyea, G., & Burghen, G. (1989). Coping styles in youths with insulin-dependent diabetes mellitus. *Journal of Consulting and Clinical Psychology, 57*, 644-651.

Hanson, C. L., Henggeler, S. W., & Burghen, G. (1987a). Social competence and parental support as mediators of the link between stress and metabolic control in adolescents with insulin-dependent diabetes mellitus. *Journal of Consulting and Clinical Psychology, 55*, 529-533.

Hanson, C. L., Henggeler, S. W., & Burghen, G. (1987b). Race and sex differences in metabolic control of adolescents with IDDM: A function of psychosocial variables? *Diabetes Care, 10*, 313-318.

Hanson, C. L., Henggeler, S. W., Harris, M. A., Cigrang, J. A., Schinkel, A. M., Rodrigue, J. R., & Klesges, R. C. (1992). Contributions of sibling relations to the adaptation of youths with insulin-dependent diabetes mellitus. *Journal of Consulting and Clinical Psychology, 60*, 104-112.

Hanson, C. L., Henggeler, S. W., Rodrigue, J. R., Burghen, G. A., & Murphy, W. D. (1988). Father-absent adolescents with insulin-dependent diabetes mellitus: A population at special risk? *Journal of Applied Developmental Psychology, 9*, 243-252.

Harkavy, J. M. (1981). *A study of the relationship of knowledge, behavior and control in juvenile diabetes*. Unpublished master's thesis. Gainesville: University of Florida.

Harkavy, J., Johnson, S. B., Silverstein, J. H., Spillar, R., McCallum, M., & Rosenbloom, A. (1983). Who learns what at diabetes summer camp? *Journal of Pediatric Psychology, 8*, 143-153.

Hauenstein, E., Marvin, R., Snyder, A., & Clarke, W. L. (1989). Stress in parents of children with diabetes mellitus. *Diabetes Care, 12*, 18-23.

Hauser, S. T., DiPlacido, J., Jacobson, A. M., Willett, J., & Cole, C. (1993). Family coping with an adolescent's chronic illness: An approach and three studies. *Journal of Adolescence, 16*, 305-329.

Hauser, S. T., Jacobson, A. M., Lavori, P., Wolfsdorf, J. I., Herskowitz, R. D., Milley, J. E., Bliss, R., Wertlieb, D., & Stein, J. (1990). Adherence among children and adolescents with insulin-dependent diabetes mellitus over a four year longitudinal follow-up: Immediate and long-term linkages with the family milieu. *Journal of Pediatric Psychology, 15*, 527-542.

Hauser, S. T., Jacobson, A. M., Wertlieb, D., Brink, S., & Wentworth, S. (1985). The contributions of family environment to perceived competence and illness adjustment in diabetic and acutely ill children. *Family Relations, 34*, 99-108.

Hauser, S. T., Jacobson, A. M., Wertlieb, D., Weiss-Perry, B., Follansbee, D., Wolfsdorf, J. I., Herskowitz, R. D., Houlihan, J., & Rajapark, D. C. (1986). Children with recently diagnosed diabetes: Interactions with their families. *Health Psychology, 5*, 273-296.

Hodges, L., & Parker, J. (1987). Concerns of parents with diabetic children. *Pediatric Nursing, 13*, 22-24.

Ingersoll, G., Orr, D. P., Herrold, A., & Golden, M. P. (1986). Cognitive maturity and self management among adolescents with insulin-dependent diabetes mellitus. *Journal of Pediatrics, 108*, 620-623.

Israel, C., Berndt, D. J., & Barglow, P. (1986). Development of a self-report measure of adherence for children and adolescents with insulin-dependent diabetes. *Journal of Youth and Adolescence, 15*, 419-428.

Jacobson, A. M., Hauser, S. T., Lavori, P., Willett, J., Cole, C., Wolfsdorf, J. I., Dumont, R. D., & Wertlieb, D. (1994). Family environment and glycemic control: A four-year prospective study of children and adolescents with IDDM. *Psychosomatic Medicine, 17*, 267-274.

Jacobson, A. M., Hauser, S. T., Lavori, P., Wolfsdorf, J. I., Herskowitz, R. D., Milley, J., Bliss, R., Gelfand, E., & Wertlieb, D. (1990). Adherence among children and adolescents with IDDM over a four-year longitudinal follow-up: The influence of patient coping and adjustment. *Journal of Pediatric Psychology, 15*, 511-526.

Jacobson, A. M., Hauser, S. T., Wertlieb, D., Wolfsdorf, J., Orleans, J., & Vieyra, M. (1986). Psychological adjustment of children with recently diagnosed diabetes mellitus. *Diabetes Care, 9*, 323-329.

Jacobson, A. M., Hauser, S. T., Wolfsdorf, J., Houlihan, J., Milley, J. E., Herskowitz, R. D., Wertlieb, D., & Watt, E. (1987). Psychologic predictors of compliance in children with recent onset of diabetes. *Journal of Pediatrics, 110*, 805-811.

Johnson, S. B. (1984). Knowledge, attitudes and behavior: Correlates of health in childhood diabetes. *Clinical Psychology Review, 4*, 503-524.

Johnson, S. B. (1988). Diabetes mellitus in childhood. In D. Routh (Ed.), *Handbook of pediatric psychology* (pp. 9-31). New York: Guilford Press.

Johnson, S. B., Freund, A., Silverstein, J. H., Hansen, C. A., & Malone, J. I. (1990). Adherence-health status relationships in childhood diabetes. *Health Psychology, 9*, 606-631.

Johnson, S. B., Kelly, M., Henretta, J. C., Cunningham, W., Tomer, A., & Silverstein, J. H. (1992). A longitudinal analysis of adherence and health status in childhood diabetes. *Journal of Pediatric Psychology, 17*, 537-553.

Johnson, S. B., Pollak, T., Silverstein, J. H., Rosenbloom, A., Spillar, R., McCallum, M., & Harkavy, J. (1982). Cognitive and behavioral knowledge about insulin-dependent diabetes mellitus among children and their parents. *Pediatrics, 69*, 708-724.

Johnson, S. B., Silverstein, J. H., Rosenbloom, A., Carter, R., & Cunningham, W. (1986). Assessing daily management in childhood diabetes. *Health Psychology, 5*, 545-564.

Kaplan, R. M., Chadwick, M. W., & Schimmel, L. E. (1985). Social learning intervention to improve metabolic control in Type 1 diabetes mellitus. *Diabetes Care, 8*, 152-155.

Kaplan, S., Greenfield, S., & Ware, J. (1989). Assessing the effects of physician-patient interactions on the outcomes of chronic disease. *Medical Care, 27*(Suppl. 3), S110-127.

Kovacs, M., Finkelstein, R., Feinberg, T. L., Crouse-Novak, M., Paulauskas, S., & Pollock, M. (1985). Initial psychologic responses of parents to the diagnosis of insulin-dependent diabetes mellitus in their children. *Diabetes Care, 8*, 568-575.

Kovacs, M., Iyengar, S., Goldston, D., Obrosky, D. S., Stewart, J., & Marsh, J. (1990). Psychological functioning among mothers of children with insulin-dependent diabetes mellitus: A longitudinal study. *Journal of Consulting and Clinical Psychology, 58*, 159-165.

La Greca, A. M., Auslander, W. F., Greco, P., Spetter, D., Fisher, E. B., & Santiago, J. V. (1995). I get by with a little help from my family and friends: Adolescents' support for diabetes care. *Journal of Pediatric Psychology, 20*, 449-476.

La Greca, A. M., Auslander, W. F., Spetter, D., Greco, P., Skyler, J. S., Fisher, E. B., & Santiago, J. V. (1991). Adolescents with IDDM: Family and peer support of diabetes care. *12th Annual Proceedings of the Society of Behavioral Medicine*, 110 (abstract).

La Greca, A. M., Follansbee, D. M., & Skyler, J. S. (1990). Developmental and behavioral aspects of diabetes management in youngsters. *Children's Health Care, 19*, 132-139.

La Greca, A. M., & Skyler, J. S. (1991). Psychosocial issues in IDDM: A multivariate framework. In P. McCabe, N. Schneiderman, T. Field, & J. Skyler (Eds.), *Stress, coping, and disease* (pp. 169-190). Hillsdale, NJ: Erlbaum.

Lorenz, R. A., & Wysocki, T. (1991). From research to practice: The family and childhood diabetes. *Diabetes Spectrum, 4*, 261-292.

Marrero, D. G., Kronz, K. K., Golden, M. P., Wright, J. C., Wright, J. C., Orr, D. P., & Fineberg, N. S. (1989). Clinical evaluation of computer-assisted self-monitoring of blood glucose system. *Diabetes Care*, *12*, 351-356.

McCaul, K. D., Glasgow, R. E., & Schafer, L. C. (1987). Diabetes regimen behaviors predicting adherence. *Medical Care*, *25*, 868-881.

Mengel, M. B., Blackett, P. R., Lawler, M. K., Volk, R. J., Viviani, N. J., Stamps, G., Dees, M. S., Davis, A. B., & Lovallo, W. R. (1992). Cardiovascular and neuroendocrine responsiveness in diabetic adolescents within a family context: Association with poor diabetic control and dysfunctional family dynamics. *Family Systems Medicine*, *10*, 5-33.

Minuchin, S., Rosman, B., & Baker, L. (1978). *Psychosomatic families*. Cambridge, MA: Harvard University Press.

Peyrot, M., & Rubin, R. R. (1988). Insulin self-regulation predicts better glycemic control. *Diabetes*, *37*(Suppl 1), 53A (abstract).

Reynolds, L. A., Johnson, S. B., & Silverstein, J. H. (1990). Assessing daily diabetes management by 24 hour recall interview: The validity of children's reports. *Journal of Pediatric Psychology*, *15*, 493-509.

Suchman, A., Roter, D., Green, M., & Lipkin, M. (1993). Physician satisfaction with primary care office visits. *Medical Care*, *31*, 1083-1092.

Swift, C. F., Seidman, F., & Stein, N. (1967). Adjustment problems in juvenile diabetes. *Psychosomatic Medicine*, *29*, 555-571.

Tabak, E. R. (1987). The relationship of information exchange during medical visits to patient satisfaction: A review. *Diabetes Educator*, *13*, 36-40.

Travis, L. B., Brouhard, B. H., & Schreiner, B. J. (1987). *Diabetes mellitus in children and adolescents*. Philadelphia: W. B. Saunders.

Watkins, J. D., Williams, T. F., Martin, D. A., Hogan, M. D., & Anderson, E. (1967). A study of diabetic patients at home. *American Journal of Public Health*, *57*, 452-459.

Weissberg-Benchell, J., Glasgow, A.M., Tynan, W. D., Wirtz, P., Turek, J., & Ward, J. (1995). Adolescent diabetes management and mismanagement. *Diabetes Care*, *18*, 77-82.

Wertlieb, D., Hauser, S. T., & Jacobson, A. M. (1986). Adaptation to diabetes: Behavior symptoms and family context. *Journal of Pediatric Psychology*, *11*, 463-479.

White, K., Kolman, M. L., Wexler, P., Polin, G., & Winter, R. J. (1984). Unstable diabetes and unstable families: A psychosocial evaluation of children with recurrent diabetic ketoacidosis. *Pediatrics*, *73*, 749-755.

Wilson, D. P., & Endres, R. K. (1986). Compliance with blood glucose monitoring in children with Type I diabetes mellitus. *Journal of Pediatrics*, *108*, 1022-1024.

Wysocki, T. (1993). Associations among parent-adolescent relationships, metabolic control and adjustment to diabetes in adolescents. *Journal of Pediatric Psychology*, *18*, 443-454.

Wysocki, T., Green, L. B., & Huxtable, K. (1989). Blood glucose monitoring by diabetic adolescents: Compliance and metabolic control. *Health Psychology*, *8*, 267-284.

Wysocki, T., Hough, B. S ., Ward, K. M., Allen, A. A., & Murgai, N. (1992). Use of blood glucose data by families of children and adolescents with IDDM. *Diabetes Care*, *15*, 1041-1044.

Wysocki, T., Hough, B. S ., Ward, K. M., & Green, L. B. (1992). Diabetes mellitus in the transition to adulthood: Adjustment, self-care and health status. *Journal of Developmental and Behavioral Pediatrics*, *13*, 194-201.

Wysocki, T., Huxtable, K., Linscheid, T. R., & Wayne, W. (1989). Adjustment to diabetes mellitus in preschoolers and their mothers. *Diabetes Care*, *12*, 524-529.

Wysocki, T., Meinhold, P. A., Cox, D. J., & Clarke, W. L. (1990). Survey of diabetes professionals regarding developmental changes in diabetes self care. *Diabetes Care*, *13*, 65-68.

Wysocki, T., Meinhold, P. A., Abrams, K., Barnard, M. U., Clarke, W. L., Bellando, B. J., & Bourgeois, M. J. (1992). Parental and professional estimates of self-care independence of children and adolescents with IDDM. *Diabetes Care*, *15*, 43-52.

Wysocki, T., Taylor, A., Hough, B. S., Linscheid, T. R., Yeates, K. O., & Naglieri, J. A. (1995). Deviation from developmentally appropriate self-care autonomy: Associations with diabetes outcomes. *Diabetes*, *44*(Suppl. 1), 97A (abstract).

10

Acceptance of Diabetes Regimens in Adults

Edwin B. Fisher, Jr., Cynthia L. Arfken, Joan M. Heins, Cheryl A. Houston, Donna B. Jeffe, and Roslyn K. Sykes

OVERVIEW

Diabetes affected an estimated 14 million people in the United States as of 1993 (American Diabetes Association [ADA], 1993a). There are several types of diabetes. As a group, they raise virtually all the issues of prevention, management, and adjustment dealt with in health psychology (Fisher, Delamater, Bertelson, & Kirkley, 1982), and they raise these issues across the life span, from a family's reaction to a young child's diagnosis with a lifelong, life-threatening disease to blindness and amputations among adults. Parallel with the complexity of the disease and the diversity of its effects, acceptance in diabetes is complex, entailing a number of skills and tasks. Acceptance is also influenced by a wide range of factors, from the economic and cultural to the personal. This complexity of acceptance and the multiple influences on it are a theme of this chapter.

Emphasizing the complexity of diabetes helps place acceptance in its psychological and social contexts (B. J. Anderson et al., 1982). For example, when it is recognized that frequent changes in professionals' recommendations for diabetes management reinforce patients' *rational* skepticism regarding the utility of a current prescription, then variability in adherence is seen as reflecting important aspects *of diabetes*, not only the conscious or unconscious choices of the individual. Even individual characteristics, such as a tendency to "act out" against restrictions or rigid prescriptions, may be exacerbated by the many demands imposed by diabetes management; again, the acting out may reflect the diabetes as much as the individual.

A powerful context for this chapter is the Diabetes Control and Complications Trial (DCCT) (DCCT Research Group, 1993). The DCCT showed that maintaining blood sugars close to the normal range of 70–140 milligrams per deciliter (mg/dl) led to 76% lower risk for developing diabetic eye disease, 54% lower risk for existing eye disease progressing, 39% lower risk of developing kidney

Edwin B. Fisher, Jr., Cynthia L. Arfken, Joan M. Heins, Cheryl A. Houston, Donna B. Jeffe, and Roslyn K. Sykes • Center for Health Behavior Research and Diabetes Research and Training Center, Washington University, St. Louis, Missouri 63108.

Handbook of Health Behavior Research II: Provider Determinants, edited by David S. Gochman. Plenum Press, New York, 1997.

disease, 54% lower risk of kidney disease progressing, and 60% lower risk for developing clinical neuropathy. Critically, the DCCT identified diabetes management to maintain blood sugars as close as possible to normal (*euglycemia*) as the cause of these long-term benefits. Thus, a number of sections in this chapter refer to the DCCT, and an extended description sets forth the positive example of diabetes acceptance it provides.

The following two sections describe the nature of diabetes and its care and management. The chapter then includes a section reviewing various perspectives from which to consider acceptance of diabetes, including those of the individual, the clinician, and the population at large, and a section on "naturally occurring" influences on diabetes acceptance, ranging from broad economic and cultural influences to personality variables. Interventions to encourage acceptance of diabetes in clinical, educational, and community settings receive extended review before concluding sections on special populations (underserved/disadvantaged groups, older adults, and adults with insulin-dependent diabetes mellitus) and on research issues.

NATURE OF DIABETES

Most cases of diabetes can be assigned to one of two categories, Type I or insulin-dependent diabetes mellitus (IDDM), which usually develops in childhood or adolescence, and Type II or non-insulin-dependent diabetes (NIDDM), which usually develops in adulthood. IDDM accounts for the vast majority of diabetes among children and adolescents and is therefore a focus of Chapter 9. In contrast, NIDDM accounts for the majority of diabetes among adults and is the focus of much of this chapter. In IDDM, the insulin-producing cells are destroyed by an autoimmune process leading to a sudden, intense onset. IDDM is characterized by absolute deficiency of insulin production with lifelong daily administration of insulin required along with a regulated diet and exercise program (ADA, 1994a). Approximately 2-10% of people with diabetes have IDDM (ADA, 1993a).

The more common type of diabetes, affecting 90-98% of people with diabetes, is NIDDM. This disease is characterized by two defects, impaired insulin secretion and decreased tissue sensitivity to insulin, termed ***insulin resistance*** (ADA, 1994b). People with NIDDM secrete insulin, but metabolic regulation of the timing and amount secreted is impaired. This regulatory defect creates a cyclic effect, with a delay in insulin secretion fostering a high postmeal blood glucose level that stimulates excessive insulin secretion, triggering a compensatory release of glucose from the liver, which often exacerbates hyperglycemia. The incidence of NIDDM increases with age, so it is more prevalent among older adults. It also is associated with obesity and a sedentary lifestyle, and so disproportionately affects disadvantaged minorities. Approximately half of those with NIDDM are not diagnosed and are unaware of having the disease. Too often, they have developed diabetic complications by the time they are diagnosed.

Many adults with NIDDM end up using insulin to manage their diabetes and therefore pursue a regimen quite similar to that for IDDM. Also, with improvements in diabetes care, more and more individuals with IDDM are surviving into full adulthood. Thus, much of the material on diabetes in adults is based on those with both IDDM and NIDDM. Specific ways in which the issues developed in this chapter influence those with IDDM are discussed in the later section on special populations.

Because they share an absolute or relative inability to metabolize glucose, the several types of diabetes all may lead to hyperglycemia—high blood glucose. Hyperglycemia is accompanied by a marked propensity to develop short- or long-term complications, which can include kidney failure, blindness, amputations, and cardiovascular disease (ADA, 1994a,b). At the opposite end of the glycemia spectrum, when the energy requirement balance is upset due to overabundance of insulin or exercise and too little food, hypoglycemia results. If the symptoms are not addressed, hypoglycemia can lead to impaired judgment or unawareness of surroundings, convulsions, and collapse. In a negative-feedback pattern, cognitive effects of hypoglycemia lessen the ability to perceive and address it (ADA, 1994a). Because it can be a frequent complication of efforts to keep blood sugar levels near normal, hypoglycemia has been described as the limiting factor in treating diabetes (Cryer, Fisher, & Shamoon, 1994).

In addition to hyperglycemia, hypoglycemia, and their associated symptoms, people with diabetes are also vulnerable to chronic complications. These complications involve the circulatory (both small and large vessels), renal, nervous, and optic systems. In concrete terms, people with diabetes are at increased risk for heart disease, stroke, renal disease including end-stage renal disease, amputations, impotence, skin ulcers and infections, gastroparesis, and vision disorders including blindness. Important for acceptance, blood sugar can be managed and hyperglycemia minimized, thereby reducing these complications (DCCT Research Group, 1993).

Metabolic Control and Its Measurement

Metabolic or "diabetic" control is usually thought of as the level of blood sugar relative to a normal 24-hour range of 70-140 mg/dl. Nevertheless, the reader should be aware of the importance of other dimensions of diabetes management, such as regular eye examinations, foot care, and quality of life.

Research in diabetes has benefited from the availability of measures that reflect average blood sugar over several months. These are known as glycosylated hemoglobin (GHb) measures. They are based on the binding of glucose to hemoglobin in the blood. Because this process is directly proportional to the level of glucose circulating in the blood and is slow and stable, GHb reflects blood sugar levels over an appreciable period of time. This measure contrasts with direct measures of blood sugar, which change throughout the day and reflect only recent diabetes management. Since the erythrocytes that carry hemoglobin have an average life span of 120 days, GHb represents general levels of control over a period of several months (Goldstein et al., 1995). The DCCT results also showed that GHb predicts risk of long-term diabetes complications. With caution, changes in GHb may also be interpreted as an indirect or rough measure of adherence. However, psychological variables associated with adherence may not be associated with GHb (Wilson et al., 1986) since GHb is determined not only by adherence but also by other aspects of disease state and metabolism.

There are several assays of GHb and several components of it. GHb values must therefore be evaluated using the validated ranges for a specific test and, preferably, the laboratory performing the test.

TREATMENT AND REGIMENS FOR DIABETES MANAGEMENT

To control the interrelated metabolic derangements of NIDDM, therapy is designed to maximize the effect of endogenous insulin by decreasing insulin resistance. Although the pathology of NIDDM is complex, many individuals can achieve good metabolic control using nutrition and exercise. Modification in food intake can be used to compensate for the alteration in insulin secretion, and a consistent exercise program improves tissue sensitivity to insulin. A majority of individuals with NIDDM are overweight, a condition that increases insulin requirements, insulin resistance, and glucose production. Caloric restriction and exercise to promote a weight loss of 5-10% of body weight generally improves metabolic control. When diet and exercise do not result in desired blood glucose levels, oral hypoglycemic agents that stimulate glucose metabolism are added to the regimen.

People with NIDDM may achieve good diabetes control with oral diabetes medication initially, but experience a loss of effect later. This failure may be due to poor adherence to diet and exercise, problems associated with oral medications for diabetes or for other conditions, progressive loss of insulin secretory capacity, or increased insulin resistance. When oral agents do not control hyperglycemia, exogenous insulin is added to the diet-exercise regimen in place of or in addition to the oral diabetes medication. Thus, many NIDDM patients are treated with exogenous insulin, resulting in treatment regimens similar to therapy for IDDM.

The DCCT was carried out with adolescents and adults with IDDM. However, the relationship between improvement in glycemic control and reduced complications approached linearity, suggesting that even modest improvements in metabolic control confer some benefit. Thus, the benefits should also apply to NIDDM, since there is no reason that the complications of hyperglycemia or benefits of metabolic control should be dependent on the reason for high blood sugar, i.e., IDDM versus NIDDM. However, consideration of the major risks of NIDDM tempers encouragement of achieving metabolic control with the same intensive insulin therapy as used in DCCT. NIDDM influences mortality primarily through cardiovascular disease. Hyperinsulinemia is also a cardiovascular risk. Thus, achieving metabolic control by utilizing greater quantities of insulin may accomplish the desired metabolic control, but still pose risks for the cardiovascular diseases for which NIDDM is already a risk (Crofford, 1995). Thus, accomplishment of metabolic control in NIDDM is probably better pursued through diet and exercise than through intensive insulin regimens.

Diabetes therapy makes a large number of demands on the patient. These demands range from altering daily patterns of eating and activities to mastering complicated techniques needed for insulin administration. Few other diseases rely on patient decision making and performance to the extent required in diabetes management. Individuals with diabetes are asked to evaluate their food intake and activity levels, self-administer their oral medication or insulin medication at specified times, and evaluate therapeutic effectiveness by self-monitoring of blood glucose, with the possible added responsibility of making changes in any or all of their diet, exercise, and medications on the basis of blood glucose values.

Though the multiple elements of diabetes therapy create a threat to regimen adherence, it is diet that patients mention as the most difficult when discussing adherence (Lockwood, Frey, Gladish, & Hiss, 1986). Studies of adherence rates across different management tasks confirm this view (Ary, Toobert, Wilson, & Glasgow, 1986; Hanestad & Albreksten, 1991). Difficulty with dietary adherence appears to be a problem not simply of comprehension or of skills in estimating food intake, but of changing a behavior that occurs frequently, must be modified rather than extinguished, and is tied to numerous social, cultural, and emotional determinants. The challenges posed by the modification of eating behavior alone ensure that difficulties with regimen adherence will occur for almost all persons with NIDDM independent of the number of components in their treatment plan.

PERSPECTIVE ON ACCEPTANCE

Adults accept, manage, cope with, react to, and participate in the management of diabetes in a social context that includes the clinicians who treat them and the broader public whose attitudes toward disease and concerns about cost of its treatment influence those with diabetes. Diabetes is reviewed here from each of these perspectives.

Clinician's Perspective

It is first necessary to define the term *clinician* as used in this context. Patients with NIDDM are most often managed in primary care settings, but should have access as needed to a team that includes a diabetologist or endocrinologist as well as a nurse, a dietitian, and a psychologist or social worker, all with experience in diabetes management. Ideally, those with IDDM are routinely managed by such a team, but economic and geographic limitations often result in their receiving care, also, through primary care settings. Because of emphasis on team care, and the frequent overlapping roles of dietitians, nurses, and physicians in working with patients to plan diet, exercise, and insulin administration, the term *clinicians* is used to denote these and other professionals, including social workers and psychologists, who provide direct patient care, including patient education and counseling, in a clinical setting. We only refer to "physicians" when intending to limit a comment to that group. The term *health professionals* is used more broadly to refer to those in public health as well as clinical settings.

In treating diabetes, the clinician must attend not only to complex metabolic interactions among diet, exercise, insulin secretion, insulin resistance, and injected insulin, but also to the patient's needs for education and support in managing all of these aspects in daily life, the extent to which the patient's circumstances may or may not support the clinician's recommended treatment, monitoring and treatment of likely complications of diabetes, and the patient's short- and long-term psychological reactions to all of these, including bouts of hypoglycemia, resistance and denial, and, not uncommonly, clinical depression. Clearly, diabetes poses a burden for the clinician as well as the patient. How the clinician responds to this burden is important, since research shows that the clinician's behavior (particularly communication style) is an important element in the patient's willingness and ability to follow treatment advice (Cassell, 1985), while lack of communication, impersonality, and lack of warmth have been shown to have adverse affects on patient adherence (Rosenstock, 1985).

It is important for patients and clinician to agree on goals for adherence and current status (Pendleton, House, & Parker, 1987). Just in terms of adherence, patients' judgments often differ significantly from those of objective measures (House, Pendleton, & Parker, 1986). In a weight loss program for NIDDM, 68% of participants felt they were adherent, although objective measures put adherence at 52%. The objective measures dropped to 31% adherence by the end of the study as the self-reports remained around the initial level (Wing Epstein, Nowalk, Koeske, & Hagg, 1986).

How nonadherence is evaluated is also a source of difference between clinician and patient. Clinicians tend to view nonadherence as "the patient's problem," with the clinician's role being to treat and cure disease as well as to present information and teach relevant skills, after which it is the patient's responsibility to comply (Meichenbaum & Turk, 1987). Other aspects of the clinician's perspective include the belief that adherence procedures will not work and that the patient is too old, too young, too uneducated, or too unsophisticated to follow adherence procedures. Although such views may sound primitive, consider that they share the assumptions guiding much research in the area. Studies of adherence tend to focus on relationships between poor diabetes control and patients' personality characteristics, rather than on clinicians' beliefs or behaviors (Bradley & Marteau, 1986).

The effect of the clinician's general approach to adherence and the patient may be considerable. More truthful reporting of blood glucose monitoring followed low-demand instructions that emphasized modest expectations ("Sticking to the diabetes regimen 100% of the time is impossible") and an objective of finding out "how things really are...." This approach was compared to high-demand instructions that emphasized the clinician as evaluator: "... important ... so that we can see exactly how well you are doing" (Delamater, Kurtz, White, & Santiago, 1988, pp. 494-495).

Patient's Perspective

Diabetes management places complex burdens on the patient, and complexity is associated with low adherence rates across a variety of diseases and health problems (Haynes, Taylor, & Sackett, 1979). Thus, adherence to the diabetes regimen is demanding and difficult (Goodall & Halford, 1991). Yet the number of components of an individual's regimen is not, itself, associated with lower quality of life. However, perceived *difficulties* in regimen adherence have been associated with lower levels of self-assessed life satisfaction and emotional well-being (Hanestad & Albreksten, 1991).

The patient's view of diabetes management is confused by several areas of uncertainty. As noted earlier, good management is not a guarantee that complications will not develop. Further, over the course of a number of years with the disease, recommended management practices will change. Some of this change will reflect the natural evolution of the disease. For instance, after a number of years, individuals often must begin taking exogenous insulin to supplement deficient insulin production. But changes also occur with changes in knowledge, such as in types of insulin (animal, synthetic) and insulin management (single versus multiple daily injections, use of a "pump" for continuous insulin infusion mimicking the natural delivery from the pancreas). There have also been changes in approaches to dietary management. Many individuals with diabetes recall days when they were encouraged to eat high levels of protein and minimize carbohydrate intake. More recently, recognition of heart disease as a major risk in NIDDM and recognition of the role of dietary fat in heart disease has led to encouragement of reduction of fat and increased consumption of complex carbohydrates. The potential for confusion and loss of faith in the "best advice available" when that advice changes repeatedly compromises important incentives for acceptance.

Population's Perspective

If large numbers of people with diabetes were to control obesity, reduce cholesterol levels, exercise, stop smoking, and improve control of blood glucose levels, complications of diabetes would decrease. One study suggested that half of NIDDM cases and major complications could be prevented by following such advice (Carter Center of Emory University, 1985). Such an improvement would result in enormous savings in disease and health care costs across the population (ADA, 1993b).

For the individual, adherence problems and factors other than lifestyle may also influence whether or not complications are averted. However, enough people have diabetes and the benefits of management are sufficiently reliable that even modest improvements in adherence by large numbers of people would have an appreciable effect on the number and severity of complications. Not everyone has to achieve ideal or very good control for there to be a major public health impact. This realization mirrors public health approaches to other health risks, such as high cholesterol (Jeffery, 1989). It leads to thinking about public health efforts to promote improvements in diabetes acceptance in large numbers, as opposed to ideal management in the individual.

Patient's versus Population's Perspective

The advantages and disadvantages of diabetes management may be very different for the individual than for society. From the societal perspective, efforts at diabetes management, aggregated across millions of individuals, pay off in substantial reductions in health costs. But for the individual, even good metabolic control leaves reduction in complications still uncertain, calling into question the rationality of extensive management efforts at the cost of other sources of enjoyment. Consider the individual contemplating results of the DCCT. At a cost of extensive effort and a two- to threefold increase in the frequency of hypoglycemia, the individual can reduce long-term chances of complications. Although the reduced complications in the DCCT were remarkably striking and significant when viewed as incidence figures across groups of participants, they take on a different perspective when weighed for the individual (Fisher, 1988).

"NATURALLY OCCURRING" INFLUENCES

Whether or not a person accepts a regimen prescribed by a health professional for diabetes management is influenced by a variety of personal characteristics as well as by environmental factors, which may facilitate or constrain behavior in a number of ways and over which individual persons may have little or no control. Thus, McLeroy, Bibeau, Steckler, and Glanz (1988) described an ecological perspective of multiple factors influencing health behaviors: intrapersonal (characteristics of individual persons), interpersonal (primary social networks, such as families and friends), institutional (policies and rules that circumscribe behavior within formal structures, such as schools or the workplace), community (organizational/group networks and standards, formal and informal), and public policy (local, state, and federal). From a similar perspective, the following sections discuss the influence of culture, worksites, economic, and other aspects of access to care, social and family influences, and personal influences.

Culture

Various components of acceptance of diabetes management may be influenced by a culture's general beliefs and attitudes about susceptibility to illness, control of future outcomes, seriousness of an illness, acceptance of responsibility for one's own health, active management versus fatalism in the face of chronic disease, the value of folk or traditional medicine, and efficacy of Western medical care. Additionally, acceptance of diabetes will be influenced by a culture's more specific characteristics such as practices surrounding food, cultural norms for body image, self-medication with insulin, and use of technological innovations, such as blood glucose monitoring, and the importance of chronic complications such as blindness, sexual dysfunction, and amputation.

That cultural influences may have complex effects is illustrated by fatalism versus belief in one's own ability to control one's health. From a number of Eurocentric, Western, or middle-class perspectives, disease should be actively managed and controlled. Belief in such control has been related to risk reduction and adherence to various regimens (e.g., Christensen, Smith, Turner, Holman, & Gregory, 1990). At times in life when disease cannot be controlled, however, as often happens in the course of diabetes, a more fatalistic acceptance may provide some advantage in terms of emotional adjustment or quality of life (Haire-Joshu, Strube, & Yost, 1987). Thus, viewing a culture's fatalistic approach to disease as simply a barrier to acceptance may distract the clinician from recognizing strengths with which to work.

Worksite

A worksite's organizational culture modifies the attitudes and beliefs of individual members, directs rules and regulations, and shapes interpersonal relationships. For individuals with diabetes, organizational culture can influence their willingness to disclose diabetes, ability to follow their treatment regimen, and the way other members relate to them. Because of the number of hours on the job, the influence of the organization is of particular importance. An understanding of organizational characteristics that may affect worker health behaviors can help clinicians counsel their patients on ways to integrate demands of the job and of diabetes management.

Culture, structure, and size are among organizational characteristics that influence employer–employee relationships including actions related to health. Size appears to be an important variable. Large companies have the capacity to invest more in employee health through benefits and resources (e.g., cafeteria, worksite wellness program). However, accommodations for individual health needs may be more limited in larger than in smaller companies due to the expedience of general rules versus individual decisions, the organizational distance between employee and policy maker, and the tendency for larger organizations to adopt more formal, less flexible structures.

In one study, over two thirds of human resource managers from large companies (>500 employees) reported not knowing whether anyone in their company needed special consideration because of diabetes, in contrast to only 14% of those from medium and 16% of those from small companies (25–99 employees) (Padgett, Heins, & Nord, 1995).

What types of accommodations facilitate diabetes management at work? A survey of endocrinologists identified a work schedule with inflexible timing of meals and breaks as a condition that makes diabetes management difficult (Heins, Arfken, Nord, Houston, & McGill, 1994). When asked about changes that would make diabetes management easier, the physicians had a wide range of suggestions, with the majority (64%) related to work environment, e.g., social environment, physical facilities, and policies/regulations.

What can employees with diabetes and their clinicians do to improve the work environment to enhance diabetes management? One approach is to educate employers about the types of accommodations that would facilitate diabetes management at work. In one study (Heins et al., 1994), human resource managers felt that their supervisors were sensitive to the needs of employees with chronic diseases, including diabetes. A majority indicated, however, that the type of allowances important to diabetes management (e.g., ability to set break and lunch schedule or to take them as needed) currently were not being made in their company. Identifying job modifications that would enhance diabetes management now has legal support. The Americans with Disabilities Act prohibits employment discrimination against qualified individuals with disabilities and requires employers to make reasonable accommodations to enable disabled workers to perform essential job functions (Equal Employment Opportunity Commission, 1992). While the Disabilities Act provides legal recourse, it also can create an atmosphere that will promote collaboration of clinicians, worker, and employer to improve the climate of the workplace to support health behaviors important for diabetes management.

Economic Influences

In 1992, direct and indirect costs amounted to $6229 for each person with NIDDM (ADA, 1993b). Individual costs related to diabetes vary widely. For the individual with NIDDM controlled with diet and exercise, health costs may not differ widely from those of individuals without diabetes. Even with NIDDM, however, these costs may include additional doctor visits, laboratory work, periodic home glucose testing, periodic eye screening, modest additional cost for diet, and perhaps increased costs of health and life insurance. The progression of diabetes may necessitate the use of additional, costly medications and doctor visits. Should complications of diabetes develop, major increases in costs are incurred for laser therapy, renal dialysis, transplantation, vascular surgery, and many other measures (Quickel, 1994).

Financial resources have major impacts on adherence. An individual who does not have money to buy special foods, medications, or a glucose-monitoring device may not be able to adhere to a recommended self-management regimen. Services not reimbursed by some insurance plans include recommended annual eye exams, insulin, meters and strips for blood glucose self-monitoring, and patient education (Bransome, 1992). Medicaid has funding constraints, so that some services may not be covered. In view of the higher prevalence of diabetes in minority groups, these inadequacies will have special effects on diabetes care.

With the movement toward capitated payment systems in the United States, the incentive for health care plans may be to maintain the health of patients through preventive educational practices. But since capitated payment systems are most profitable when the patients are healthy, plans may seek not to educate patients, but rather to exclude diabetic and other patients with costly diseases. They reportedly discourage enrollment by offering benefit packages that are especially unattractive to those with diabetes.

Social and Family Influences

The role of social factors in diabetes was underscored in a 54-month, prospective study of diabetic adults (W. Davis, Hess, & Hiss, 1988). A measure of the social impact of diabetes completed at baseline included items such as "My diabetes and its treatment keep me from ... having enough money," "... going out or traveling as much as I want," or "... having good relationships with people." In a Cox regression model, the social impact variable was the second most predictive of subsequent mortality; the most predictive was age. Social impact was more predictive of subsequent mortality than clinical measures such as renal function or glycated hemoglobin, gathered at baseline.

A number of studies have found associations between social support and diabetes management (e.g., Lloyd, Wing, Orchard, & Becker, 1993; Ruggiero, Spirito, Coustan, McGarvey, & Low, 1993). Hopper and Schechtman (1985) simply asked individuals if they had someone available to offer support, "someone you could count on to help ... if you had a crisis with diabetes." A "yes" was significantly associated with lower fasting blood sugars, i.e, better metabolic control. In addition to facilitating management, social support is associated with better emotional status among diabetic adults, including buffering the effects of stress (Griffith, Field, & Lustman, 1990) and diabetes-related restrictions in daily activities (Littlefield, Rodin, Murray, & Craven, 1990).

Nevertheless, social support should not be viewed as a panacea. Among adults with NIDDM who were asked about different strategies for coping with temptations to overeat, the only strategy that was *not* related to successful avoidance of overeating was social support, such as talking with a friend (Grilo, Shiffman, & Wing, 1993).

Research has also explored more specific aspects of support, including effects on emotional adjustment as well as adherence, and specific types and paths of support's influence. Connell, Davis, Gallant, and Sharpe (1994) found two paths linking social support to depression among diabetic adults. The first was a direct path, in which greater perceived support was associated with lower levels of depression. The second was an indirect path. Perceived support was associated with lower perceived threat from diabetes, such things as threats to continuation of daily activities and social functioning. Lower levels of perceived threat were then also associated with lower levels of depression.

In another approach to understanding specific paths by which support influences management, directive support (i.e., taking over responsibility for tasks or for choosing goals, as opposed to more reciprocal or nondirective support) was found to be related to *poorer metabolic control* (as measured by GHb), and nondirective support (cooperating, sharing activities, expressing understanding of emotions without trying to alter them) tended to be associated with *better metabolic control* and was associated with lower levels of depression (Fisher et al., 1991).

Whether social support is associated with adherence and management or emotional adjustment was found to vary by sex among older adults. Among men, social support was correlated with adherence, which in turn was correlated with metabolic control, which in turn was correlated with morale. Among women, support was not correlated with adherence, adherence was not correlated with metabolic control, and metabolic control was not correlated with morale. However, general perceived social support was associated with general morale (Connell, Fisher, & Houston, 1992). Counter to popular views that social support is important for women and *un*important for men, these data indicate that social support may be important for both men and women but via different paths.

An important locus of support for many adults is the family. Although based primarily on children and adolescents, a fairly reliable relationship appears to exist among disease management and several family factors. Encouragement of independence and open expression of emotion, family cohesion, low levels of family conflict, and communication and cooperation, as well as financial resources, have all been associated with better metabolic control as measured by GHb, while marital stress has been associated with poorer control (e.g., B. J. Anderson, Miller, Auslander, & Santiago, 1981).

Family influences can also be detrimental, such as the criticality, hostility, and emotional overinvolvement of expressed emotionality (Leff & Vaughn, 1985). In a study of participants in the DCCT, family members' criticality was associated with poorer metabolic control (Koenigsberg, Klausner, Pelino, Rosnick, & Campbell, 1993). Several authors have noted that ambiguities and risks of disease can lead family members to make attempts at support that end up being detrimental (e.g., Coyne, Ellard, & Smith, 1990).

The two patterns of findings—(1) that open expression of feelings, low levels of conflict, and encouragement of independence are related to better management and adjustment and (2) that criticality, hostility, and emotional overinvolvement are related to poorer management and adjustment—suggest an important set of common family factors. These factors might either facilitate or complicate not only diabetes management and adjustment but also management of and adjustment to a wide range of chronic diseases and psychological disorders.

Family, social, and cultural influences may also interact. With older adults, dietary inadequacies are associated with living alone (M. A. Davis, Murphy, & Neuhaus, 1988). But other evidence suggests that patients who live alone have better than average adherence (Kouris, Wahlwvist, & Worsley, 1988) and, by inference, that living with others makes adherence difficult. Living alone may avoid the problems of large households in which food available must meet the needs of growing children and adolescents and older adults (Kumanyika & Ewart, 1990). For women who serve as the gatekeepers of food for their families, reluctance of other family members to change dietary habits can interfere with adherence (Axelson, 1986).

Personal Influences

S. M. Dunn and Turtle (1981) concluded that there is no personality type that distinguishes patients with diabetes from other chronically ill patients or from the population at large. They further argued that poor metabolic control is not attributable to a particular type of "deviant personality." However, they did find beneficial effects "of a stable personality and a stable home environment on the control of diabetes and on its prognosis" (S. M. Dunn & Turtle, 1981, p. 644; see also Peyrot & McMurry, 1992).

Although the search for a "diabetic personality" is unlikely to be renewed, research has identified psychological problems that are more common among those with diabetes. Depression is especially prevalent among persons with diabetes (Gavard, Lustman, & Clouse, 1993) and has been linked to both poorer adherence to diabetes management (e.g., McGill et al., 1992) and poorer glycemic control (e.g., Lustman, Griffith, Clouse, & Cryer, 1986).

The health belief model (Rosenstock, 1990) continues to find support in diabetes research. In one study, variables based on this model accounted for about 50% of the variance in patients' reports of their own diabetes management (e.g., Wilson et al., 1986). In another, better adherence was associated with perceived severity of illness and perceived benefits of treatment (Brownlee-Duffeck et al., 1987).

Specific rather than global effects characterize prediction of adherence. Adherence to one aspect of the regimen is not highly associated with adherence to others (e.g., Ary et al., 1986). Regimen-specific, as opposed to broad, dispositional measures of health beliefs and social support are most highly related to self-care behaviors, such as glucose testing or exercise (Wilson et al., 1986). Predictors of one aspect of adherence may be different from predictors of other aspects; adherence to diet was associated with seriousness of illness and the number of tests ordered, but adherence to exercise was associated with the level of health distress (DiMatteo et al., 1993).

Ruggiero (1994) and her colleagues have worked to adapt models of stages of change (Prochaska, DiClemente, & Norcross, 1993) to diabetes. This approach also emphasizes specific behaviors or regimen elements, not a global state of readiness. Thus, one may be in the maintenance stage of, say, drinking sugar-free soft drinks, but a precontemplator when it comes to exercise or glucose monitoring. This focus on specific regimen tasks makes the model appropriate to the diverse and varied tasks of diabetes management. At the same time, the diversity of tasks poses substantial challenge to applying the model to all of them.

Other individual characteristics that have been associated with metabolic control are concurrent illness, age (e.g., Wilson et al., 1986), stress (e.g., Aikens, Wallander, Bell, & Cole, 1992), hormonal fluctuations (e.g., in pregnancy [see Coustan, 1985]), anger (P. F. Dunn & Alexander, 1994), and poor impulse control, mood instability, and tendencies toward dependent, manipulative interpersonal relationships (e.g., Lustman, Frank, & McGill 1991).

PLANNED INFLUENCES

There is evidence that glycemic control has improved over the past decade, at least among those with IDDM (Arfken, Schmidt, McGill, White, & Santiago, 1996). The DCCT established that improving glycemic control reduces complications. Numerous studies have examined and found different interventions to reduce hyperglycemia. These interventions include self-monitoring of blood glucose, regimens for more physiological insulin replacement, new dietary recommendations, extensive patient and professional education, and better GHb measures of blood glucose that can prompt more aggressive treatment efforts among patients with high values.

The Diabetes Control and Complications Trial as an Example of a Successful Program

As noted in the Overview, the DCCT was an extended, multicenter clinical trial that demonstrated the benefits of improved metabolic control in terms of reduced complications of diabetes. In the experimental condition, participants followed a regimen that included (1) multiple insulin injections or use of an insulin infusion pump attached subcutaneously, (2) blood glucose monitoring four times daily and appropriate adjustment of insulin, (3) dietary management, (4) exercise, and (5) adjustment of insulin in light of stress, intercurrent disease, and other incidental factors. Those in the standard care condition received what was judged to be the standard of care at the time of the trial's planning and inception from 1982 to 1985: injections of insulin a maximum of two times per day with blood glucose monitoring once per day. Mean blood sugar accomplished in the experimental group over the duration of the trial was 155 mg/dl in comparison to 231 mg/dl in the standard care (DCCT Research Group, 1993).

It is important to note that the DCCT employed no medical tactics or technologies that were not widely available in the early 1980s and that had not been individually validated in previous research. Thus, the DCCT was not so much a test of an innovative treatment as a test of a comprehensive effort to utilize available treatments to achieve sustained metabolic control and evaluate its worth. As such, it stands as a substantial model of how to utilize available treatment to promote sustained adherence.

The DCCT achieved remarkable levels of adherence. In monitoring of adherence during the trial's first year, adherence levels were 97% for visits completed according to protocol, 84–90% for self-monitoring of blood glucose, 99% for completion of capillary blood collections, and 96% for completion of end-of-year assessments of main study variables (DCCT Research Group, 1989). Over the 6.5 years of the trial, 97% of participants were retained (DCCT Research Group, 1993). This remarkable level of adherence and retention relied upon a comprehensive array of patient education procedures that had at their center the eager interest, responsiveness, and continuous, 24-hour-a-day availability of professional staff. Key elements in this array included careful patient education in an initial inpatient hospital stay, then weekly until the patient was "comfortable and confident with ... [the] regimen." Another key element was the individualization of treatment. Although the general parameters of the regimen in the experimental condition were followed, there was substantial flexibility for adjustment according to individual needs. Self-monitoring, insulin management, and diet counseling were all pursued from an individualized, problem-solving approach.

Perhaps the most critical of the interventions in the DCCT was the ongoing support it provided. It included extensive individualized as well as group contact as well as the availability of project staff by phone 24 hours per day. The staff member on call was well trained in the regimen, including insulin adjustments for which participants might be seeking guidance. Importantly, though, much of this contact with participants was of a more general, supportive nature, addressing frustrations with the trial and problems in maintaining adherence, as well as general life issues participants may have faced. As a participant quoted in the *New York Times* article reporting on the DCCT results put it: "The team was the strongest part of the program. They are really there to help us through the tough times" (*The New York Times*, June 14, 1993).

The importance of support is reflected in a study to identify participants' views of critical aspects of the DCCT (K. Davis, Heins, & Fisher, 1996). Preliminary findings included two key features. First was the general quality of care provided. Aspects of this care included feedback and monitoring of management, basic problem-solving and self-management counseling, and the expertise and professionalism of staff. The second key feature was the accessibility and availability of staff as well as their encouragement and supportiveness.

A critical challenge to dissemination of DCCT findings is providing support for diabetes acceptance. Interpersonal support was a key element of the comprehensive patient education and disease-management instruction it provided. But such support is in danger of being overlooked because of the difficulty in articulating what it entails and because it is a "soft" approach in a health care culture that values technological innovations and in a national culture that values the independent heroics of the individual.

Clinical Care and Prescription

Diabetes requires flexible and responsive medical care, since not only the patient's disease but also circumstances and needs change. Paradoxically, the demands on the patient tend to increase with improved technology. For instance, the regimen tested in the DCCT entailed measurement of blood glucose levels several times daily and then adjustment of insulin dosages in light of blood sugar, exercise and activity, and recent and planned food intake. While advantageous for the patient in terms of risks of complications, this procedure poses considerably greater burden than a plan of one dose of insulin per day and avoidance of sweets. With increased burden on the patient comes increased need for patient education and regular monitoring and support by clinicians. Noting that the needs of professional and patient are not met by the acute care model of care delivery, Etzwiler (1994) emphasized that it is imperative to introduce a comprehensive chronic disease model that recognizes the patient as "primary provider" of 90–99% of required care. The patient should have access to appropriate supplies and services and a therapeutic treatment plan that is negotiated individually according to his or her own needs and resources. Greater patient involvement in asking questions and taking an active role in medical visits, along with physician responsiveness to the patient's questions, are associated with better metabolic control among clinic patients (Greenfield, Kaplan, & Ware, 1985).

The basic therapeutic approach should be grounded in education, but education alone is not sufficient to ensure successful incorporation of recommended therapeutic modalities. Medical aspects of the regimen need to be planned with likelihood of adherence in mind. Attention to barriers to adherence needs to consider the range of psychological, social, and other factors noted above. In light of the importance of ongoing support, care needs to be delivered by easily available individuals who can address or gain ready answers to questions regarding the regimen, as well as provide understanding of and interest in the many ways in which diabetes influences patients' lives.

Patient Education

Conventional patient education programs focused on knowledge of disease and regimen (Resler, 1983). More recent approaches have recognized the importance of changing patients' behavior and so have integrated assessment of individual learning needs, planning teaching/learning strategies, identifying appropriate behavioral goals and objectives, implementing educational strategies to promote behavior change, and evaluating outcomes (Houston & Haire-Joshu, 1996), with the expectation that once this education occurs, regimen adherence will soon follow. Research indicates, however, that the combination of information and training of skills still does not guarantee behavior change (Padgett, Mumford, Hynes, & Carter, 1988).

Because an individual's behavior and the environment influence each other, current models of education also stress the need to change the systems and environments in which the individual with diabetes lives. For example, failure to check blood glucose levels routinely may be labeled as nonadherence. However, a variety of factors may contribute to this "failure." The individual may not understand the relationship between diet, exercise, medication, and blood glucose level or may find blood glucose monitoring painful. The clinician may not have stressed the importance of blood glucose monitoring or may have given vague management recommendations. The individual may lack physical access to skilled medical personnel to provide feedback about self-management skills or may be unable to pay for blood glucose monitoring supplies due to lack of adequate insurance coverage. Glasgow (1995) has discussed how (1) the patient, (2) the community, (3) the health care system, (4) the interaction between patient and provider, and (5) the interaction between short-term effects of treatment and regimen adjustment all contribute to the ongoing course and quality of diabetes management.

Results of the DCCT indicate that diabetes education programs can be effective when they address multiple levels of influence, including teaching specific skills necessary to apply management strategies, encouraging self-efficacy, and providing incentives, praise, and encouragement by professionals. In addition to the DCCT, other programs have also demonstrated benefits of patient education regarding diet, exercise, and insulin management; behavioral self-management approaches to diet and exercise; and behavioral and cognitive approaches to stress and other barriers to adherence. Such programs have shown benefits in terms not only of improved metabolic control but also of quality of life (Rubin & Peyrot, 1992). A state-of-the-art, 5-day, 24-hour outpatient group program offered instruction and guidance in intensive insulin therapy, blood glucose monitoring three or four times per day, five injections of insulin per day, and adjustment of dosage by patients. Although the study was not controlled, mean GHb among participants fell from 8.7 mg/dl to 7.5 mg/dl ($p = 0.001$) (Pieber et al., 1995).

Peyrot and Rubin (1994) evaluated the importance of behavior change in patient education. They identified three levels of behavioral change in response to a patient education program: no change, improved *either* in self-monitoring of blood glucose *or* in exercise, and improvement in *both* self-monitoring and exercise or in insulin administration. Beneficial changes in GHb were greatest in the group that made the most substantial management changes and least among those making no change.

A model for diabetes care suggested by Fisher (1995) is based on the fact that most diabetic adults are treated by primary care physicians rather than specialists and on studies of brief counseling and appropriate referral to promote smoking cessation in primary care (Fisher, Lichtenstein, Haire-Joshu, Morgan, & Rehberg, 1993). By analogy, primary care of diabetic patients could include (1) brief review of metabolic control; (2) inquiry as to problems in diet, exercise, or insulin management; (3) brief instruction in ways to improve management; and (4) referral for patient education or nutritional or psychological counseling when indicated by a patient's knowledge deficit or behavioral or emotional problems.

Psychological Factors in Patient Education, Counseling, and Support

Lustman et al. (1995) evaluated a tricyclic antidepressant, nortriptyline, in terms of its benefits in both reducing depression and improving metabolic control among both depressed and nondepressed adults with diabetes. Interestingly, the nortriptyline was well tolerated by both groups, including the nondepressed. Among the depressed, those receiving nortriptyline showed significantly greater reductions in depression than those receiving placebo. Further, reductions in depression were associated with improved metabolic control as measured by GHb. Such findings should serve as an important opening wedge for health psychology research. An immediate and important question is whether other approaches to treating depression, such as cognitive behavior therapy, could be effective in improving mood and metabolic control.

Depression may cut across a number of chronic diseases. Other psychological interventions have addressed problems peculiar to acceptance of diabetes. Perhaps most specific to the disease is the problem of hypoglycemia. In addition to the intrinsically unpleasant nature of hypoglycemia, adherence and tight metabolic control are discouraged by the consequences of hypoglycemia, including social embarrassment as well as more concrete concerns, such as risks of automobile accidents. These concerns are heightened by encouragement to manage diabetes so as to keep blood sugars low, i.e., closer to hypoglycemia, the risks of which are documented in the two- to threefold increased frequency of hypoglycemia observed in the intensive treatment group of the DCCT.

In an admirably systematic series of studies, Cox, Gonder-Frederick, and their colleagues (Cox, Gonder-Frederick, Julian, & Clarke, 1994) have developed a treatment to prevent hypoglycemia and hyperglycemia. Blood Glucose Awareness Training (BGAT) includes education, skills training, and practice in (1) increased sensitivity to symptoms of hypo- and hyperglycemia so that they may serve as stimuli for appropriate action; (2) identification of external events such as insulin administration, exercise, or changes in diet that may increase the likelihood of hypo- or hyperglycemia; and (3) appropriate responses to internal and external cues in order to prevent hypo- and hyperglycemia. Studies have replicated findings that patients can improve their ability to identify symptoms of hypo- and hyperglycemia and that BGAT reduces not only hypo- and hyperglycemic events but also important sequelae such as automobile accidents (Cox et al., 1994) and motor vehicle violations (Cox et al., 1995). BGAT thus stands as a model for intervention development in health psychology. Understanding of the specific psychological and behavioral problems associated with the disease led to careful application of psychological procedures (training and rehearsal in self-management procedures to establish appropriate, preventive responses to internal and external cues of untoward events), resulting in improvements not only in terms of meaningful disease events but also in terms of real-world consequences such as motor vehicle accidents.

The potential benefits of such psychological intervention in terms of costs as well as the welfare of patients and others whom they may affect are substantial.

Both as an antecedent to diabetes and a problem in its management, obesity is a major challenge for applications of psychology. Wing and her colleagues have conducted a series of studies developing and evaluating behavioral weight loss programs for individuals with NIDDM. The most effective of these programs have evolved into a year-long program that includes self-monitoring; behavioral self-control strategies for coping with temptations; behavioral strategies for limiting cues associated with eating; nutrition education, including concrete skills in shopping, food preparation, and food storage; exercise; and group support. This research has also explored the inclusion of very-low-calorie diets in the year-long program. Such programs are able to promote average weight losses in the range of 20–30 pounds (Wing, 1993). These results are especially impressive given the findings that even modest weight losses or calorie restriction or both can have appreciable benefits on metabolic control (Wing et al., 1994).

Motivation and the Patient's Role

The patient's role in decisions has been emphasized in programs to enhance adherence and disease management (e.g., Etzwiler, 1994). The American Diabetes Association's Standards of Medical Care for Patients with Diabetes Mellitus (ADA, 1994c, p. 618) note:

> Patient self-management should be emphasized. To this end, the management plan should be formulated in collaboration with the patient, and the plan should emphasize the involvement of the patient in problem solving as much as possible. A variety of strategies and techniques should be employed to provide adequate education and development of problem-solving skills in the various aspects of diabetes management.

By participating fully in the process of setting self-management goals, planning appropriate interventions, and evaluating the effectiveness of these interventions, patients become active participants in their own care rather than passive recipients of professional prescriptions. In motivational terms, patient participation in this process enables the patient to feel more like an Origin than a Pawn (deCharms, 1968). Emphasis on the patient's own goals and choices can be especially effective in encouraging patients to take an active, responsible role in the management of chronic disease (Haire-Joshu, 1988; Tinker, Heins, & Holler, 1994). Stressing the active role of the patient in care, R. M. Anderson, Funnell, and their colleagues (1995, p. 943) showed that an educational program to "enhance the ability of patients to identify and set realistic goals; ... apply a systematic problem-solving process to eliminate barriers to achieving those goals; ... manage the stress caused by living with diabetes ...; ... identify and obtain appropriate social support; and ... improve their ability to be self motivated" improved attitudes and self-efficacy as well as GHb.

Problems emerge if there is a mismatch between the clinician's recommendation and the patient's motivation to follow it. One way this mismatch may develop is in the *assumption* of shared objectives and goals. The clinician may assume that the patient is ready to focus substantial energy on achieving metabolic control, while the patient may seek amelioration of complications amid a life already filled with other priorities. Without an emphasis on the patient's role in choosing objectives and goals, such disjunctions between patient and clinician are likely to remain unrecognized.

A caveat on self-management is in order at this point. An individual's motivation or ability to do something often becomes enmeshed in an ideology of personal responsibility. In this ideology, success and failure may both be attributed to personal effort, skill, and knowledge without taking environmental and social influences into consideration. Failure in particular is often explained by "blaming the victim," i.e., the person who failed. For instance, recall the findings noted above that physicians tend to view adherence as the patient's responsibility. Professionals need to be clear about what is meant by autonomy or self-management. Emphasis on the patient's choice and responsibility and active engagement of the patient in planning management goals and strategies may enhance acceptance. However, *explaining* the choices the individual ends up making as the *effects* of the patient's responsibility (1) is circular (e.g., "She chose it because she had the opportunity to make her own choice"); (2) ignores important social, organizational, economic, or clinical and educational influences; (3) may lead to blaming the victim and viewing professionals as having nothing further to contribute; and (4) distracts from the many important things that those around the individual can do to assist diabetes management.

Community Approaches

Community-based programs may focus directly on the interpersonal, social, and logistic factors that influence acceptance of diabetes care. An important component of many community programs is the use of peers as change agents. Adapting this approach to prevention of diabetes, the "Eat Well, Live Well Program" trains women from low-income, African-American neighborhoods to implement a basic nutrition lifestyle intervention that includes dietary skills (such as reading food labels), education about meal planning and preparation, and general support (Auslander, Haire-Joshu, Houston, & Fisher, 1992). In comparison to dietary education offered at a neighborhood health center, this intervention led to greater improvements in skills to read food labels, knowledge about fat content of food, and total knowledge of nutrition (Auslander, Haire-Joshu, Houston, & Daily, 1994). A full test of the intervention's ability to encourage improved nutrition habits and reduced diabetes risk was under way in the mid-1990s. Other examples of possible community approaches to diabetes include screening programs such as for diabetic retinopathy (Stepien, Bowbeer, & Hiss, 1992), outpatient diabetes education programs at community hospitals and clinics (Rubin, Peyrot, & Saudek, 1993), diabetes education newsletters (R. M. Anderson et al., 1994), and support groups.

To assist individuals interested in diabetes programming at the community level, a course called Diabetes Today! has been developed by the Centers for Disease Control and Prevention. Based on the Planned Approach To Community Health (PATCH) approach (Buckner, Miner, Kreuter, & Wilson, 1992), this program covers strategies and methods for identifying and involving community members, conducting a community needs assessment, selecting target groups, prioritizing diabetes-related community needs, planning intervention strategies, and evaluating the resulting program. The program emphasizes integrating community values into the program's goals, objectives, educational messages, and materials. Diabetes Today! is currently the basis for a test of community approaches to care of NIDDM among adults in North Carolina, sponsored by the Centers for Disease Control and Prevention.

Challenges to community programs include competing community problems. Particularly in low-income minority neighborhoods, poverty, drug use, and crime may be greater priorities. In rural areas, lack of local health care resources may pose challenges. Other problems include lack of program funds and logistic barriers such as lack of transportation, all of which may be accentuated by diabetes being a disease of low to moderate prevalence and therefore one difficult to raise on local agendas. Coalitions with groups interested in other diseases, especially those that share objectives with diabetes (e.g., improved nutrition to prevent heart disease), may be an effective strategy.

Standards of Care

There is considerable inconsistency in the way physicians treat diabetes. Some differences are associated with type of training (e.g., general practitioner, internist) and some with physician attitudes toward tight blood glucose control (Tuttleman, Lipsett, & Harris, 1993). The DCCT added weight to the position that therapy to achieve as near normal blood glucose as possible reduces complications of diabetes (DCCT Research Group, 1993). But feasibility of efforts to promote tight blood glucose control has been questioned from perspectives of the increased risk of hypoglycemia, patients' willingness to adhere to an intensive regimen, and costs (Farkas-Hirsch & Hirsch, 1993).

Concern over what constitutes good care has led to development of guidelines or standards for treatment of complications, patient education, and medical treatment of NIDDM, IDDM, and pregnancy complicated by diabetes. Studies show, however, that practice guidelines have not made major changes in physician behaviors (Lomas et al., 1989). In a study of the effects of guidelines on treatment of NIDDM, most pronounced deficiencies persisted in education, adherence, risk prevention, and follow-up (Stolar & Endocrine Fellows, 1995).

The apparent benefits of patient education and behavioral contributions to them have been recognized in recently developed National Standards for Diabetes Self-Management Education Programs, developed by representatives of several organizations at the request of the National Diabetes Advisory Board (Funnell & Haas, 1995). Among the 15 content areas that the standards identify are attention to "stress and psychosocial adjustment," "family involvement and social support," and "behavior change strategies, goal-setting, risk factor reduction, and problem solving" (Funnell & Haas, 1995, p. 104). The diabetes community's recognition of the importance of educational and behavioral aspects of care for a clearly biological disease is worth noting.

Unfortunately, actual diabetes care does not reflect recognition of patient education. For instance, Hiss, Anderson, Hess, Stepien, and Davis (1994) reviewed changes in care patterns in Michigan communities across the decade from 1981 to 1991 for patients with NIDDM not on insulin, NIDDM and on insulin, and IDDM. Among patients with NIDDM but not on insulin, the percentage who had received patient education *declined* from 53% to 41% ($p = 0.02$); for those on insulin, the decline was 83% to 74% ($p = 0.03$). Regular medical visits are important opportunities for patient education and adjustment of management plans, but office visits per year decreased across the decade for all three groups of patients. Given the complex nature of the treatment of IDDM, it is disturbing that in another study (Coonrod, Betschart, & Harris, 1994), only 59% of those with IDDM reported ever attending a "diabetes education class," ever attending a "course or class in how to manage diabetes," or ever receiving "any education program or class about diabetes." For patients with NIDDM and not on insulin therapy, the proportion reporting patient education was only 24%.

The emergence of managed care as the dominant form of health delivery may strengthen the effect of policies and guidelines at the system level. If practice guidelines are used to define allowable services, they should prompt delivery of the care the guidelines define. Moreover, concern for cost containment through long-term savings from patient education may encourage care systems to emphasize these services. For instance, the demonstrated benefit of early detection and treatment of diabetic eye disease has led many managed care plans to include annual eye exams among their defined services for diabetes.

SPECIAL POPULATIONS

Underserved or Disadvantaged Groups

The prevalence of NIDDM varies by ethnic group from nearly zero in a small community of Melanesians studied in the highlands of Papua New Guinea (King et al., 1984) to highs of 39% and 45%, respectively, in male and female Pima Indians aged 25 years and over (Knowler, Bennett, Hamman, & Miller, 1978). Differences also have been noted in the prevalence between ethnic groups residing in the same country, such as among American Indians (Knowler et al., 1978), Hispanics (Gardner et al., 1984), and the European and African populations of the United States (Harris, Hadden, Knowler, & Bennett, 1985).

In the United States, NIDDM is more prevalent among the Pima Indians of Arizona and among Hispanic and African-American populations (ADA, 1993a). Bennett, Burch, and Miller (1971) identified obesity, large families, inbreeding, and important changes in lifestyle as contributing factors to the exploding incidence and prevalence of NIDDM among the Pimas. Stern and Haffner (1990) studied NIDDM in Mexican-Americans from San Antonio and Mexico City. They concluded that disproportionate incidence is related to environmental factors commonly associated with the phenomenon of "modernization" and "Westernization," namely, dietary change and adoption of sedentary lifestyles. Dietary change and sedentary lifestyle appear also to raise risks for NIDDM among those moving to industrialized societies, such as immigrants to the United States.

Of course, economics and the cost of treatment play a major role in diabetes care among many disadvantaged groups. NIDDM among African-Americans is associated with lower socioeconomic status and with obesity (Auslander et al., 1992). A recent study among insulin-using, urban African-Americans found that stopping insulin administration was the cause of 67% of cases of diabetic ketoacidosis and that the reason for stopping insulin in 50% of cases was lack of money to buy insulin or to get transportation to the hospital to obtain it (Musey et al., 1995).

Because of the effects of culture on diet, consumption of appropriate traditional, ethnic, and cultural foods should be encouraged (ADA, 1992). Culturally specific nutrition counseling to prevent problems with dietary adherence would also apply for African-Americans with limited incomes, low educational attainment, ambivalence about weight control, multiple health problems, and high-fat, high-sodium, low-fiber diets or food preferences.

Kumanyika and Ewart (1990) found that weight-control regimens require African-Americans to evaluate and restructure established eating and physical activity patterns. They stated that publicly funded health clinics, which may be the predominant setting of care in urban communities where most African-Americans live, are associated with poorer adherence to treatment regimens than private practice settings. Reasons for this difference may include discontinuity of care, waiting times, or aspects of staff behavior. The Diabetes Assessment, Nursing, Nutrition, and Dental Evaluation (DANNDE) project utilized techniques such as small groups, education materials designed specifically for the target population, frequent weighing, and familiar care providers to improve dietary adherence among Mexican-Americans (Elshaw, Young, Saunders, McGurn, & Lopez, 1994).

Older Adults

The prevalence of NIDDM increases dramatically with age, from 3-5% among those between the ages of 30 and 40 to 10% by the age of 60 and 16-20% by the age of 80 (Bennett, 1984). Data from the 1982 Health and Nutrition Examination Survey (HANES II) indicated that 17% of Caucasians and 25% of African-Americans between the ages of 65 and 74 years had diabetes.

Concerns about the problems of NIDDM in the older adult are heightened by the fact that the proportion of the population age 65 and older is increasing and is expected to be about 20% by the year 2020 (Lipson, 1986). Therefore, a substantial proportion of persons seeking treatment for NIDDM in the future will be older. As a result, health professionals are likely to be counseling more adults with diabetes who are over age 60. These professionals' attitudes, beliefs, and knowledge about aging will influence the care they provide.

The primary treatment for the older individual with NIDDM is diet, including weight maintenance or loss and decreased intake of saturated fat and cholesterol, as well as exercise, medication, blood glucose monitoring, and foot and eye care. Adherence may be especially challenging due to many of the physical, psychosocial, and economic changes associated with aging. Physical changes such as altered metabolic function, altered mobility, and multiple disease states are common in the older adult (Connell, 1991). Changes in vision and diminished hearing can complicate adherence to medication and blood glucose monitoring.

Psychosocial factors, such as depression, marital status, and social support, may take on special influence in the older adult. For example, dietary restrictions may discourage individuals from eating in restaurants or at friends' homes. Especially for those who live alone, this consequence may exacerbate social isolation and loneliness, which in turn may further reduce incentives for adherence (Fisher, 1996). Further, the demands of the entire regimen may fall on spouses, especially wives, exacerbating their burdens as caregivers.

Economic issues must also be considered for this population. Health care costs have continued to increase in this country while insurance benefits, particularly among older persons, have decreased. Diabetes is an expensive disease to manage. Medication, monitoring supplies, physician visits, and hospitalizations contribute to the cost and are often inadequately covered by older adults' insurance.

Adults with Insulin-Dependent Diabetes Mellitus

Little research has been conducted comparing acceptance by adults with IDDM versus NIDDM. However, several factors distinguish adults with IDDM. They usually have had diabetes longer. Because duration is a risk factor for complications, they are more likely to have developed complications. Relative to adolescents, the possibility of complications and awareness of others with complications may be more salient and threatening. This knowledge may foster a sense of wondering "When is it my turn?" even if complications have not already developed. If complications do develop, they may add more physical and emotional challenges to self-management.

By definition, people with IDDM are dependent on insulin and must therefore constantly be vigilant about their regimen. They can never take a "vacation" from the disease, which someone on diet or oral agents might do. Living with IDDM means arranging eating and exercise every day, with less flexibility than someone without IDDM. Scheduling eating, exercise, and insulin creates difficulties for children and adolescents; adults may also have to juggle work and family responsibilities. Some adults become especially cautious to avoid hypoglycemic events at work or in public; e.g., they avoid interviews or public speaking or job assignments in which their performance is easily observed at times when their blood sugar may be low or when they might need to administer insulin.

Increased awareness of the results of the DCCT may add an additional burden of increased pressure to manage diabetes more carefully. But even though the DCCT showed that good management reduces the probability of complications, complications may still occur regardless of management efforts and success. Resulting frustration may be especially intense. Awareness of the extent to which complications remain unpredictable may also undermine acceptance.

RESEARCH ISSUES

Consistent with the emphasis in this chapter on the breadth and complexity of acceptance of diabetes, research recommendations address needs in understanding relationships among different influences on acceptance and measures of outcomes related to it. This chapter has discussed diverse influences on acceptance and interventions to promote it. Understanding the relationships and interactions among them will be a challenge for the future. Identifying how patient education and community health promotion may reinforce or obviate each other, or how different components of patient education and support may be important or unnecessary, will help bring about more of the potential benefits of acceptance and effective diabetes management amid tremendous pressures to eliminate costly and unnecessary services. The chronic nature of diabetes introduces another dimension of complexity. Researchers have hardly begun to identify the interactions and aggregate effects of patient care, education, and support over the many years that people have to manage and accept diabetes.

Better articulation of the utility of a range of interventions for diabetes management, then, raises a complementary issue: that of identifying ways to tailor therapy, education, and counseling according to individual characteristics. The range of pertinent characteristics is great, from differences in metabolic defects to differences in learning styles.

Regarding outcomes, the availability of GHb as a measure of glucose control has provided an objective, common yardstick for educational, behavioral, and clinical research in diabetes and has stimulated many research endeavors. However, multiple factors other than patient acceptance influence GHb. Also, broader aspects of acceptance, emotional status, and quality of life are important end points in addition to metabolic control. Thus, GHb needs to be viewed as but one important outcome in research on acceptance in diabetes, and models for integrating GHb and other outcome measures need to be developed.

A research area of great importance is establishing the usefulness of educational, psychological, and related interventions for diabetes acceptance. Because the interventions themselves may be hard to define (e.g., provision of emotional support), and because some of their benefits may be hard to define (e.g., enhanced quality of life) or much delayed (e.g., reduced likelihood of blindness or other long-term complications), establishing their worth is challenging. Even if their worth is established, a further challenge lies in defining them in a way that facilitates widespread application without diluting their important components or the quality of their implementation.

SUMMARY AND CONCLUSIONS

This chapter has emphasized two broad dimensions: the range of factors that affect diabetes care, including the economic, cultural, and social circumstances of the individual along with the individual's own psychological characteristics; and the range of effects of diabetes on people's lives, including the quality of their psychological and social experiences as well as their physical health. Given the DCCT's demonstration that diabetes acceptance and blood glucose control can improve the course and reduce the complications of diabetes, and in the face of uncertainty as to how evolving systems of health care will meet the needs of those with diabetes, the social and behavioral sciences provide a growing base for assisting patients in managing their disease and taking advantage of state-of-the-art care, and for shedding light on how professionals, family, and friends can provide support and understanding to enhance the lives of those with diabetes.

REFERENCES

Aikens, J. E., Wallander, J. L., Bell, D. S., & Cole, J. A. (1992). Daily stress variability, learned resourcefulness, regimen adherence, and metabolic control in type I diabetes mellitus: Evaluation of a path model. *Journal of Consulting and Clinical Psychology*, *60*(1), 113-118.

American Diabetes Association. (1992). Clinical practice recommendations: Nutritional recommendations and principles for individuals with diabetes mellitus. *Diabetes Care*, *15*(4, Suppl. 2), 21-28.

American Diabetes Association. (1993a). *Diabetes: 1993 vital statistics*. Alexandria, VA: American Diabetes Association.

American Diabetes Association. (1993b). *Direct and indirect cost of diabetes in the United States in 1992*. Alexandria, VA: American Diabetes Association.

American Diabetes Association. (1994a). *Medical management of insulin-dependent (Type I) diabetes* (2nd ed.). Alexandria, VA: American Diabetes Association.

American Diabetes Association. (1994b). *Medical management of non-insulin-dependent (Type II) diabetes* (3rd ed.). Alexandria, VA: American Diabetes Association.

American Diabetes Association. (1994c). Standards of medical care for patients with diabetes mellitus. *Diabetes Care*, *17*, 616-623.

Anderson, B. J., Auslander, W., Epstein, M., Fisher, E., Flavin,

K., Hershey, P., Hopper, S., & Warren-Boulton, E. (1982). The importance of social contexts in diabetes management. In R. Mazze (Ed.), *Proceedings of fourth annual conference on diabetes education*. U.S. Department of Health and Human Services, Public Health Service, National Diabetes Information Clearinghouse.

Anderson, B. J., Miller, J. P., Auslander, W. F., & Santiago, J. (1981). Family characteristics of diabetic adolescents: Relationship to metabolic control. *Diabetes Care, 4*, 586-591.

Anderson, R. M., Funnell, M. M., Butler, P. M., Arnold, M. S., Fitzgerald, J. T., & Feste, C. C. (1995). Patient empowerment: Results of a randomized controlled trial. *Diabetes Care, 18*, 943-949.

Arfken, C. L., Schmidt, L. E., McGill, J. B., White, N. H., & Santiago, J. V. (1996). Major decrements in glycated hemoglobin levels between 1978 and 1989 in patients with insulin-dependent diabetes mellitus. *Journal of Diabetes and Its Complications, 10*, 2-17.

Ary, D., Toobert, D., Wilson, W., & Glasgow, R. E. (1986). Patient perspective on factors contributing to nonadherence to diabetes regimen. *Diabetes Care, 9*, 168-172.

Auslander, W., Haire-Joshu, D., Houston, C., & Daily, M. (1994). *Increasing diet-related skills and knowledge among low-income African American women at risk for NIDDM*. Paper presented at the annual meeting of the Society for Behavioral Medicine, Boston, MA.

Auslander, W. F., Haire-Joshu, D., Houston, C. A., & Fisher, E. B. (1992). Community organization to reduce risk of non-insulin dependent diabetes among low-income African American women. *Ethnicity and Disease, 2*(2), 176-184.

Axelson, M. L. (1986). The impact of culture on food-related behaviors. *Annual Review of Nutrition, 6*, 345-363.

Bennett, P. H. (1984). Diabetes in the elderly: Diagnosis and epidemiology. *Geriatrics, 39*(5), 37-41.

Bennett, P. H., Burch, T. A., & Miller, M. (1971). Diabetes mellitus in American (Pima) Indians, *Lancet, 2*, 125-128.

Bradley, C., & Marteau, T. M. (1986). Towards an integration of psychological and medical perspectives of diabetes management. In K. G. M. M. Alberti & L. P. Krall (Eds.), *The diabetes annual* (2nd ed.). New York: Elsevier.

Bransome, E. D. (1992). Financing the care of diabetes mellitus in the U.S.: Background, problems, and challenges. *Diabetes Care, 15*(Suppl. 1), 1-5.

Brownlee-Duffeck, M., Peterson, L., Simonds, J., Goldstein, D., Kilo, C., & Holette, S. (1987). The role of health beliefs and regimen adherence and metabolic control of adolescents and adults with diabetes mellitus. *Journal of Consulting and Clinical Psychology, 55*, 139-144.

Buckner, W. P., Miner, K. R., Kreuter, M. W., & Wilson, M. G. (1992). Planned approach to community health. *Journal of Health Education* (Special Issue), *23*(3), 131-192.

Carter Center of Emory University. (1985). Closing the gap: The problem of diabetes mellitus in the United States. *Diabetes Care, 8*, 391-406.

Cassell, E. J. (1985). *Talking with patients: Vol. 1. The theory of doctor-patient communication*. Cambridge, MA: MIT Press.

Christensen, A. J., Smith, T. W., Turner, C. W., Holman, J. M., Jr., & Gregory, M. C. (1990). Type of hemodialysis and preference for behavioral involvement: Interactive effects on adherence in end-stage renal disease. *Health Psychology, 9*, 224-236.

Connell, C. M. (1991). Psychosocial contexts of diabetes and older adulthood: Reciprocal effects. *Diabetes Educator, 17*, 364-371.

Connell, C. M., Davis, W. K., Gallant, M. P., & Sharpe, P. A. (1994). Impact of social support, social cognitive variables, and perceived threat on depression among adults with diabetes. *Health Psychology, 13*(3), 263-273.

Connell, C. M., Fisher, E. B., & Houston, C. A. (1992). Relationship between social support, diabetes outcomes, and morale among older men and women. *Journal of Aging and Health, 4*, 77-100.

Coonrod, B. A., Betschart, J., & Harris, M. I. (1994). Frequency and determinants of diabetes patient education among adults in the U.S. population. *Diabetes Care, 17*(8), 852-858.

Coustan, D. R. (1985). Management of the pregnant diabetic. In J. M. Olefsky & R. Sherwin (Eds.), *Contemporary issues in endocrinology and metabolism* (pp. 311-330). New York: Churchill Livingstone.

Cox, D. J., Gonder-Frederick, L., Julian, D. M., & Clarke, W. (1994). Long-term follow-up evaluation of blood glucose awareness training. *Diabetes Care, 17*(1), 1-5.

Cox, D., Gonder-Frederick, L., Kovatchev, B., Polonsky, W., Schlundt, D., Julian, D., & Clarke, W. (1995). *Reduction of severe hypoglycemia (SH) with blood glucose awareness training (BGAT-2)*. Paper presented at the annual meeting of the American Diabetes Association, Atlanta, GA.

Coyne, J. C., Ellard, J. H., & Smith, D. A. F. (1990). Social support, interdependence, and the dilemmas of helping. In B. R. Sarason, I. G. Sarason, & G. R. Pierce (Eds.), *Social support: An interactional view* (pp. 129-149). New York: Wiley.

Crofford, O. B. (1995). Diabetes control and complications. *Annual Review of Medicine, 46*, 267-279.

Cryer, P. E., Fisher, J. N., & Shamoon, H. (1994). Hypoglycemia. *Diabetes Care, 17*(7), 734-755.

Davis, K., Heins, J., & Fisher, E., Jr. (1996). Provider characteristics helping participants adhere to Intensive Therapy in the DCCT. *Diabetes, 45*(Suppl. 2), 43A.

Davis, M. A., Murphy, S. P., & Neuhaus, J. M. (1988). Living arrangements and eating behaviors of older adults in the United States. *Journal of Gerontology, 43*, 96-98.

Davis, W., Hess, G., & Hiss, R. (1988). Psychosocial correlates of survival in diabetes. *Diabetes Care, 11*, 538-545.

deCharms, R. (1968). *Personal causation*. New York: Academic Press.

Delamater, A. M., Kurtz, S., White, N., & Santiago, J. V. (1988).

Effects of social demand on reports on self-improved blood glucose in adolescents with Type I diabetes mellitus. *Journal of Applied Social Psychology, 18*, 491-502.

Diabetes Control and Complications Trial Research Group. (1989). Implementation of a multicomponent process to obtain informed consent in the diabetes control and complications trial. *Controlled Clinical Trials, 10*, 83-96.

Diabetes Control and Complications Trial Research Group. (1993). The effect of intensive treatment of diabetes on the development and progression of long-term complications in insulin-dependent diabetes mellitus. *New England Journal of Medicine, 329*(14), 977-986.

DiMatteo, M. R., Sherbourne, C. D., Hays, R. D., Ordway, L., Kravitz, R. L., McGlynn, E. A., Kaplan, S., & Rogers, W. H. (1993). Physicians' characteristics influence patients' adherence to medical treatment: Results from the medical outcomes study. *Health Psychology, 12*(2), 93-102.

Dunn, P. F., & Alexander, D. (1994). Could anger be a glycemic control issue? The effect of health-care teamwork in assessment and intervention: A biopsychosocial approach. *Diabetes Spectrum*, 7(1), 64-66.

Dunn, S. M., & Turtle, J. R. (1981). The myth of the diabetic personality. *Diabetes Care, 4*(6), 640-646.

Elshaw, E. B., Young, E. A., Saunders, M. J., McGurn, W. C., & Lopez, L. C. (1994). Utilizing a 24-hour dietary recall and culturally specific diabetes education in Mexican Americans with diabetes. *Diabetes Educator, 20*(3), 228-235.

Equal Employment Opportunity Commission. (1992). *A technical assistance manual of the employment provisions (Title I) of the Americans with Disabilities Act*. Pittsburgh: Superintendent of Documents.

Etzwiler, D. D. (1994). Diabetes translation: A blueprint for the future. *Diabetes Care, 17*, 1-4.

Farkas-Hirsch, R., & Hirsch, I. B. (1993). The question answered: Now what? *Diabetes Care, 17*, 237-238.

Fisher, E. B., Jr. (1988). Community and ethics in lifestyle changes. In *Proceedings of XXIst Conference of the Council for International Organizations of Medical Sciences*, Nordwijk aan Zee, The Netherlands. Geneva: World Health Organization.

Fisher, E. B., Jr. (1995). *Interventions for adults*. Paper presented at an invited symposium, "Behavioral Medicine Interventions: Implementation and Reimbursement," A. Delamater, Chair, at the annual meeting of the American Diabetes Association, Atlanta, GA.

Fisher, E. B., Jr. (1996). A behavioral-economic perspective on the influence of social support on cigarette smoking. In L. Green & J. H. Kagel (Eds.), *Advances in behavioral economics: Vol. 3. Substance use and abuse* (pp. 207-236). Norwood, NJ: Ablex Publishing.

Fisher, E. B., Jr., Delamater, A. M., Bertelson, A. D., & Kirkley, B. G. (1982). Psychological factors in diabetes and its treatment. *Journal of Consulting and Clinical Psychology, 50*, 993-1003.

Fisher, E., Greco, P., Spetter, D., Quillian, R., Skyler, J., & La Greca, A. (1991). *Specific and general characteristics of social support in diabetes care: Relationship with adherence and metabolic control*. Paper presented at the joint meeting of the American Diabetes Association and the International Diabetes Federation, June, Washington, DC.

Fisher, E. B., Jr., Lichtenstein, E., Haire-Joshu, D., Morgan, G. D., & Rehberg, H. R. (1993). Methods, successes, and failures of smoking cessation programs. In *Annual Review of Medicine* (pp. 481-513). Palo Alto, CA: Annual Reviews.

Funnell, M. M., & Haas, L. B. (1995). National standards for diabetes self-management education programs. *Diabetes Care, 18*(1), 100-116.

Garner, L. I., Jr., Stern, M. P., Haffner, S. M., Gaskill, S. P., Hazuda, H. P., Relethford, J. H., & Eifler, C. W. (1984). Prevalence of diabetes in Mexican-Americans: Relationship to percent of gene pool derived from Native American sources. *Diabetes, 33*, 86-92.

Gavard, J. A., Lustman, P. J., & Clouse, R. E. (1993). Prevalence of depression in adults with diabetes: An epidemiological evaluation. *Diabetes Care, 16*(8), 1167-1178.

Glasgow, R. E. (1995). A practical model of diabetes management and education. *Diabetes Care, 18*(1), 117-126.

Goldstein, D. E., Little, R. R., Lorenz, R. A., Malone, J. I., Nathan, D., & Peterson, C. M. (1995). Tests of glycemia in diabetes. *Diabetes Care, 18*, 896-909.

Goodall, T. A., & Halford, W. K. (1991). Self-management of diabetes mellitus: A critical review. *Health Psychology, 10*(1), 1-8.

Greenfield, S., Kaplan, S. H., & Ware, J. E. (1985). Expanding patient involvement in care. *Annals of Internal Medicine, 102*(4), 520-528.

Griffith, L. S., Field, B. J., & Lustman, P. J. (1990). Life stress and social support in diabetes: Association with glycemic control. *International Journal of Psychiatry in Medicine, 20*(4), 365-374.

Grilo, C. M., Shiffman, S., & Wing, R. R. (1993). Coping with dietary relapse crises and their aftermath. *Addictive Behaviors, 18*(1), 89-102.

Haire-Joshu, D. (1988). Motivation and diabetes self-care: An educational challenge. *Diabetes Spectrum, 1*(5), 279-282.

Haire-Joshu, D., Strube, M., & Yost, J. (1987). *Illness knowledge and reactions to illness among Type I diabetic patients*. Paper presented at the annual meeting of the American Diabetes Association, Indianapolis, IN.

Hanestad, B. R., & Albreksten, G. (1991). Quality of life, perceived difficulties in adherence to a diabetes regimen, and blood glucose control. *Diabetes Medicine, 8*, 759-764.

Harris, M. I., Hadden, W. C., Knowler, W. C., & Bennett, P. H. (1985). International criteria for the diagnosis of diabetes and impaired glucose tolerance. *Diabetes Care, 8*, 562-567.

Haynes, R. B., Taylor, D. W., & Sackett, D. L. (1979). *Compliance in health care* (pp. 49-62). Baltimore, MD: Johns Hopkins University Press.

Heins, J. H., Arfken, C. L., Nord, W. R., Houston, C. A., &

McGill, J. B. (1994). The Americans with Disabilities Act. *Diabetes Care, 17*, 453.

Hiss, R. G., Anderson, R. M., Hess, G. E., Stepien, C. J., & Davis, W. K. (1994). Community diabetes care: A 10-year perspective. *Diabetes Care, 17*(10), 1124-1134.

Hopper, S., & Schechtman, K. (1985). Factors associated with diabetic control: Utilization patterns in a low-income, older adult population. *Patient Education and Counseling, 7*, 275-288.

House, W. C., Pendleton, L., & Parker, L. (1986). Patients' versus physicians' attributions for diabetic patients' noncompliance with diet [letter and comments]. *Diabetes Care, 9*(4), 434.

Houston, C. A., & Haire-Joshu, D. (1996). Application of health behavior models to promote behavior change. In D. Haire-Joshu (Ed.), *Management of diabetes mellitus: Perspectives of care across the lifespan*. St. Louis, MO: C. V. Mosby.

Jeffery, R. W. (1989). Risk behaviors and health: Contrasting individual and population perspectives. *American Psychologist, 44*, 1194-1202.

King, H., Heywood, P., Zimmet, P., Alpers, M., Collins, V., Collins, A., King, L. F., & Raper L. R. (1984). Glucose tolerance in a highland population in Papua New Guinea. *Diabetes Research, 1*(1), 45-51.

Knowler, W. C., Bennett, P. H., Hamman, R. F., & Miller, M. (1978). Diabetes incidence and prevalence in Pima Indians: A 19-fold greater incidence than in Rochester, Minn. *American Journal of Epidemiology* 108, 497-504.

Koenigsberg, H. W., Klausner, E., Pelino, D., Rosnick, P., & Campbell, R. (1993). Expressed emotion and glucose control in insulin-dependent diabetes mellitus. *American Journal of Psychiatry, 150*(7), 1114-1115.

Kouris, A., Wahlwvist, M. L., & Worsley, A. (1988). Characteristics that enhance adherence to high-carbohydrate/high-fiber diets by persons with diabetes. *Journal of the American Dietetic Association, 88*(11), 1422-1425.

Kumanyika, S. K., & Ewart, C. K. (1990). Theoretical and baseline considerations for diet and weight control of diabetes among blacks. *Diabetes Care, 13*(11), 1154-1162.

Leff, J. P., & Vaughn, C. (1985). *Expressed emotion in families: Its significance for mental illness*. New York: Guilford Press.

Lipson, L. G. (1986). Diabetes in the elderly: Diagnosis, pathogenesis, and therapy. *American Journal of Medicine, 80*(5A), 10-21.

Littlefield, C. H., Rodin, G. M., Murray, M. A., & Craven, J. L. (1990). Influence of functional impairment and social support on depressive symptoms in persons with diabetes. *Health Psychology, 9*(6), 737-749.

Lloyd, C. E., Wing, R. R., Orchard, T. J., & Becker, D. J. (1993). Psychosocial correlates of glycemic control: The Pittsburgh Epidemiology of Diabetes Complications (EDC) study. *Diabetes Research and Clinical Practice, 21*, 187-195.

Lockwood, D., Frey, M. L., Gladish, N. A., & Hiss, R. G. (1986). The biggest problem in diabetes. *Diabetes Educator, 12*, 30-33.

Lomas, J., Anderson, G. M., Domnick-Pierre, K., Vayda, E., Enkin, M. W., & Hannah, W. J. (1989). Do practice guidelines guide practice? The effect of a consensus statement on the practice of physicians. *New England Journal of Medicine, 321*, 1306-1311.

Lustman, P. J., Frank, B. L., & McGill, J. B. (1991). Relationship of personality characteristics to glucose regulation in adults with diabetes. *Psychosomatic Medicine, 53*(3), 305-312.

Lustman, P. J., Griffith, L. S., Clouse, R. E., & Cryer, P. E. (1986). Psychiatric illness in diabetes: Relationship to symptoms and glucose control. *Journal of Nervous and Mental Disorders 174*, 736-742.

Lustman, P. J., Griffith, L. S., Clouse, R. E., Freedland, K. E., McGill, J. B., & Carney, R. M. (1995). *Improvement in depression is associated with improvement in glycemic control.* Paper presented at the annual meeting of the American Diabetes Association, Atlanta, GA.

McGill, J. B., Lustman, P. J., Griffith, L. S., Freedland, K. E., Gavard J. A., & Clouse, R. E. (1992). Relationship of depression to compliance with self-monitoring of glucose. *Diabetes 41*, 84A.

McLeroy, K. R., Bibeau, D., Steckler, A., & Glanz, K. (1988). An ecological perspective on health promotion programs. *Health Education Quarterly, 15*, 351-377.

Meichenbaum, D., & Turk, D. C. (1987). *Facilitating treatment adherence: A practitioner's guidebook*. New York: Plenum Press.

Musey, V. C., Lee, J. K., Crawford, R., Klatka, M. A., McAdams, D., & Phillips, L. S. (1995). Diabetes in urban African-Americans. I. Cessation of insulin therapy is the major precipitating cause of diabetic ketoacidosis. *Diabetes Care, 18*(4), 483-489.

Padgett, D. L., Heins, J. M., & Nord, W. R. (1995). Employers' perceptions of diabetes in the workplace. *Diabetes Spectrum, 8*, 10-15.

Padgett, D., Mumford, E., Hynes, M., & Carter, R. (1988). Meta-analysis of the effects of educational and psychosocial interventions in the management of diabetes mellitus. *Journal of Clinical Epidemiology, 41*, 1007-1030.

Pendleton, L. P., House, W. C., & Parker, L. E. (1987). Physicians' and patients' views of problems of compliance with diabetes regimens. *Public Health Reports, 102*(1), 21-26.

Peyrot, M. F., & McMurry, J. F. (1992). Stress buffering and glycemic control: The role of coping styles. *Diabetes Care, 15*(7), 842-846.

Peyrot, M., & Rubin, R. R. (1994). Modeling the effect of diabetes education on glycemic control. *Diabetes Educator, 20*(2), 143-148.

Pieber, T. R., Brunner, G. A., Schnedl, W. J., Schattenberg, S., Kaufmann, P., & Krejs, G. J. (1995). Evaluation of a structured outpatient group education program for intensive insulin therapy. *Diabetes Care, 18*(5), 625-630.

Prochaska, J. A., DiClemente, C. C., & Norcross, J. C. (1993). In search of how people change: Applications to addictive behaviors. *Diabetes Spectrum*, *6*(1), 25-33.

Quickel, K. E., Jr. (1994). Economic and social costs of diabetes. In C. R. Kahn & G. C. Weir (Eds.), *Joslin's diabetes mellitus* (pp. 586-604). Philadelphia: Lea and Febiger.

Resler, M. M. (1983). Teaching strategies that promote adherence. *Nursing Clinics of North America*, *18*, 799-811.

Rosenstock, I. M. (1985). Understanding and enhancing patient compliance with diabetic regimens. *Diabetes Care*, *8*(6), 610-616.

Rosenstock, I. M. (1990). The health belief model: Explaining health behavior through expectancies. In K. Glanz, F. M. Lewis, & B. K. Rimer (Eds.), *Health behavior and health education: Theory, research and practice* (p. 39-62). San Francisco: Jossey-Bass.

Rubin, R. R ., & Peyrot, M. (1992). Psychosocial problems and interventions in diabetes. *Diabetes Care*, *15*(11), 1640-1657.

Rubin, R. R., Peyrot, M., & Saudek, C. D. (1993). The effect of a diabetes education program incorporating coping skills training on emotional well-being and diabetes self-efficacy. *The Diabetes Educator*, *19*, 210-214.

Ruggiero, L. (1994). *Readiness for change: Application to diabetes management*. Paper presented at the American Diabetes Association Annual Convention, New Orleans, June.

Ruggiero, L., Spirito, A., Coustan, D., McGarvey, S. T., & Low, K. G. (1993). Self-reported compliance with diabetes self-management during pregnancy. *International Journal of Psychiatry in Medicine*, *23*(2), 195-207.

Stepien, C. J., Bowbeer, M. A., & Hiss, R. G. (1992). Screening for diabetic retinopathy in communities. *The Diabetes Educator*, *18*, 115-120.

Stern, M. P., & Haffner, S. M. (1990). Type II diabetes and its complications in Mexican Americans. *Diabetes—Metabolism Reviews*, *6*(1), 29-45.

Stolar, M. W., & Endocrine Fellows Foundation Study Group. (1995). Clinical management of the NIDDM patient: Impact of the American Diabetes Association practice guidelines, 1985-1993. *Diabetes Care*, *18*, 701-707.

Tinker, L. F., Heins, J. M., & Holler, H. J. (1994). Commentary and translation: 1994 Nutrition recommendations for diabetes. *Journal of the American Dietetic Association*, *94*(5), 507-511.

Tuttleman, M., Lipsett, L., & Harris, M. I. (1993). Attitudes and behaviors of primary care physicians regarding tight control of blood glucose in IDDM patients. *Diabetes Care*, *16*, 765-772.

Wilson, W., Ary, D. V., Biglan, A., Glasgow, R. E., Toobert, D. J., & Campbell, D. R. (1986). Psychosocial predictors of self-care behaviors (compliance) and glycemic control in non-insulin dependent diabetes mellitus. *Diabetes Care*, *9*, 614-622.

Wing, R. R. (1993). Behavioral treatment of obesity: Its application to type II diabetes. *Diabetes Care*, *16*(1), 193-199.

Wing, R. R., Blair, E. H., Bononi, P., Marcus, M. D., Watanabe, R., & Bergman, R. N. (1994). Caloric restriction per se is a significant factor in improvements in glycemic control and insulin sensitivity during weight loss in obese NIDDM patients. *Diabetes Care*, *17*(1), 30-36.

Wing, R., Epstein L. H., Nowalk, M. P., Koeske, R., & Hagg, S. (1986). Behavior change, weight loss and psychosocial improvements in type II diabetes patients. *Journal of Consulting and Clinical Psychology*, *53*, 111-122.

11

Epilepsy Self-Management

Colleen Di Iorio

INTRODUCTION

Tony, a 32-year-old male, is pleasant, articulate and handsome. Dressed in his dark suit, white shirt, and conservative tie, he looks like any other business executive. Tony related that he has had seizures since he was 6 years old. Over time, the seizure types and medications have changed. A few years ago, Tony elected to stop taking all his antiepileptic medication because of intolerable side effects. Currently, he has several partial seizures and one or two complex partial seizures per year. When he feels a seizure coming on, he begins to count backward in Italian. He explains that he does not know the Italian language very well, and counting backward forces him to concentrate on the task. He believes that focusing on counting serves as a distraction and prevents him from having a seizure.

Tony works for a soft drink firm, where he spends a large portion of his time working alone with computers. Several times per week, however, he meets with the rest of his project team. These meetings are a source of anxiety for Tony, since he fears he may have a seizure in front of his colleagues. Neither the members of his team, his immediate boss, nor the company executives know that he has epilepsy. He wants to move to another division within the company, and he fears that disclosure at this time would ruin his chances for a transfer and might even lead to dismissal. Although Tony has occasionally thought of pursuing a managerial position with the company and believes that he has the ability, he fears the added stress might bring on more seizures. Thus, he has elected to continue in his less challenging position.

Tony dates infrequently. Because he does not have a driver's license, he must use public transportation or cab service on a date. He notes that most women view this with suspicion. Currently, he does not date because of the hassle. When not working, he takes long walks, reads, and watches television.

The actions Tony takes to control his seizures and live with his disorder are referred to as *self-management behaviors*. Given the variety of strictures that Tony and others with epilepsy must follow to control seizures effectively and lead productive, worthwhile lives, self-management often presents a unique and complex challenge.

This chapter focuses on epilepsy self-management with a special emphasis on antiepileptic medication compliance—an area in which extensive research has been conducted. The objectives of this chapter are to: (1) present an overview of epilepsy; (2) define self-management and a central component, medication compliance; (3) critically evaluate current measures of epilepsy compliance and self-management; (4) identify health behavior models used to explain epilepsy self-management behaviors; (5) identify

Colleen Di Iorio • Rollins School of Public Health, Emory University, Atlanta, Georgia 30322.

Handbook of Health Behavior Research II: Provider Determinants, edited by David S. Gochman. Plenum Press, New York, 1997.

interventions to enhance epilepsy self-management practices; and (6) present directions for further study.

OVERVIEW OF EPILEPSY

Epilepsy is a disorder in which the normal pattern of nerve cell activity within the brain is disrupted. The regular conduction of nerve impulses is replaced by rapid and abnormal discharges that are manifested as seizures. Epilepsy is a general term for a variety of seizure disorders that are classified by factors such as type, severity, and chronicity of seizures. Approximately 1.7 million Americans, or 1 in 150, has epilepsy (Annegers, 1993). Epilepsy is usually diagnosed in childhood before the age of 20. As the American population ages, however, new diagnoses of epilepsy in persons over the age of 65 are becoming more common (Scheuer & Cohen, 1993). Idiopathic epilepsies and those with a genetic predisposition are most commonly diagnosed in childhood, whereas adult-onset epilepsy is most likely attributed to a specific cause such as head trauma, brain tumors, arteriovenous malformations, and cerebral infections. Cerebral vascular disease and degenerative brain disorders are the most common causes of epilepsy in people over 55 years of age.

Although it was once thought that people with epilepsy would never achieve total seizure control, today the outlook is brighter. Over 60% of individuals with epilepsy can achieve seizure control on medications, and many will be able to discontinue medications altogether (Hauser, 1993). Medical management of epilepsy is contingent upon the diagnosis of the correct epilepsy syndrome, seizure type, cause of seizures, and triggering factors as well as the use of the appropriate type and amount of medication (Wannamaker, Dreifuss, Booker, & Willmore, 1984). Because the effects of having epilepsy are so pervasive, medical management must take into consideration the educational, occupational, psychosocial, and emotional needs of individuals. Moreover, because the daily management of epilepsy, like that of many chronic disorders, is not under the control of the health care team but rests with the patient, health providers must collaborate with patients on treatment decisions. Patients, in turn, must learn about epilepsy and assume responsibility for its daily management. Therapy is successful when seizures are eliminated or significantly reduced and the patient reports leading a satisfactory and worthwhile life.

SELF-MANAGEMENT DEFINED

Broadly speaking, epilepsy self-management is the sum total of steps a person takes to control seizures and to control the effects of having a seizure disorder. The types of self-management practices employed to control epilepsy are quite diverse. Commonly listed self-management practices include taking medications as prescribed; avoiding factors that trigger seizures, such as flickering lights; and following safety precautions such as not driving when seizures are not under control or not taking a bath when home alone (Di Iorio, Faherty, & Manteuffel, 1992). Other practices include managing one's supply of drugs to avoid running out, consulting with health professionals about the treatment plan or unexpected problems, and monitoring seizure frequency.

Behavioral techniques used to control seizures constitute another type of self-management behavior. Lifestyle adjustments such as eating regular meals and getting adequate sleep, for example, are relatively simple behavioral techniques. More elaborate behavioral strategies include relaxation and stress management therapy (Legion, 1991). Trial-and-error approaches to controlling seizures may lead to such actions as exemplified by Tony's counting backward in Italian.

Still other practices less frequently addressed in the epilepsy self-management literature are those that are self-initiated and arise from personal representations about epilepsy and illness. For example, a person who believes that seizures are the result of an imbalance in body temperature would avoid extremes of heat or cold to control seizures. Another person who believes that illness is a manifestation of personal wrongdoing might seek to make amends as a means to control seizures.

Compliance in Epilepsy

The one aspect of epilepsy self-management that has received the most attention in the epilepsy literature is compliance with the prescribed medical regimen, and the aspect of compliance that has been examined in greatest detail is medication taking. The emphasis on the study of medication compliance is not without merit, since statistics show that taking medication as ordered is greatly effective in controlling seizures. Approximately 50% of persons with epilepsy who take medication on a regular basis can realize complete seizure control without side effects, and another 30% can achieve seizure control with an occasional seizure or minimal drug side effects or both (Cereghino, McNamara, Goldensohn, Porter, & Wannamaker, 1981). Only 20% of persons with epilepsy cannot achieve effective seizure control within the constraints of the currently available drug protocols.

Despite the good news for 80% of persons with epilepsy, statistics show that approximately 30-60% of all individuals prescribed antiepileptic drugs (AEDs) do not take them as ordered (Leppik & Schmidt, 1988). Thus, a large percentage of persons with epilepsy are not receiving protective benefits of medication because they fail to follow their prescriptions (Green & Simons-Morton, 1988).

Multidimensional Compliance in Epilepsy

Sackett and Haynes (1976) defined compliance as the degree of correspondence between the physician's prescription and the patient's behavior. This definition has been used to frame most of the epilepsy compliance studies. While this definition of compliance seems to allow for the study of degrees of compliance and multiple behaviors, by convention, participants in epilepsy compliance studies have been classified as either compliant (those who follow the prescribed medication regimen) or noncompliant (those who do not). In recent years, this classification has become problematic, as clinicians and researchers alike become more aware of the multiplicity of behaviors used to control seizures and the variety of drug use patterns observed among persons with epilepsy.

The inadequacy of the conceptualization of compliance as applied to epilepsy research was addressed at the First International Conference on Compliance in Epilepsy (Schmidt & Leppik, 1988).Conference participants agreed that the study of epilepsy compliance required a multidimensional approach (Leppik & Schmidt, 1988). Their efforts led to a refined definition of compliance in epilepsy. The multidimensional definition includes three major components: the type of behavior, the extent of compliance, and the degree of intention. Realizing that previous epilepsy compliance studies focused almost exclusively on medication compliance, the participants recommended that researchers examine other medically prescribed self-management practices such as getting adequate sleep and rest and avoiding contact with seizure-triggering factors. Recognizing the limitations of previous studies in which subjects were classified as either compliant or noncompliant, the conference participants recommended a five-category classification: consistent overcomplier, consistent undercomplier, irregular irregular user, sporadically irregular user, and cyclically irregular user.

In an attempt to include the patient's perspective in the equation of compliance, the conference participants added the dimension of intention, which can be patient-controlled or structural. Patient-controlled intentions that arise from personal belief systems can be categorized as either rational, such as a pregnant woman's fear of taratogenicity with use of AEDs, or irrational, such as fear of medication. Structural problems such as memory deficits and financial problems can also interfere with attempts to maintain compliance.

Although this new definition of compliance is reflective of the medical model of compliance, in which the physician prescribes and the patient follows, epilepsy researchers and clinicians alike are beginning to recognize the importance of the patient's perspective for understanding illness-related behaviors.

MEASURES OF SELF-MANAGEMENT

Since most studies of epilepsy self-management have been limited to medication compliance, this section focuses almost entirely on different approaches to measuring medication compliance. However, attempts to measure the more expansive area of epilepsy self-management practices are included as well.

Although the conceptual definition of compliance proposed by Sackett and Haynes (1976) has been used to frame most epilepsy compliance studies, the operational definitions of compliance have varied across studies. For example, investigators have employed different assessment methods, including pill counts, serum drug concentrations, and self-reports, to assess compliance (Cramer, 1991). Investigators have also employed a variety of approaches to classifying patients as compliant and noncompliant. Classification schemata include the percentage definition, the category definition, and the index definition (Dunbar, 1979). Using the percentage definition, patients are classified according to the degree to which they followed the prescribed regimen. Using the category definition, patients are classified as compliant or noncompliant on the basis of some predetermined criterion such as serum drug levels. The third approach, the index definition, requires a rating of several different types of compliant behaviors. The classification schemata used for epilepsy studies are discussed below within the context of assessment methods.

Pill Counts

A relatively easy way to assess compliance is to count the number of antiepileptic pills taken during a given segment of time and compare the count to the number prescribed. Although pill counts can indicate the percentage of prescribed medication used, other aspects of medication-taking behavior such as time of dosing and number of pills taken each time cannot be measured. To improve the accuracy of the standard pill-counting technique as a measure of compliance, Cramer, Mattson, Prevey, Scheyer, and Ouellette (1989) introduced an automated monitoring system. The medication event monitor system (MEMS) consists of an electronic device attached to the medication bottle and is used to record the date and time of every opening of the pill container. The data cannot reveal how many pills are extracted at each opening, nor can they reveal whether the pills are actually ingested.

Monitoring prescription refills is another method in which a variation of pill counts is used to measure compliance. However, because of the different ways in which patients obtain and use drugs, prescription refills are not always a reliable measure of actual medication ingestion.

Antiepileptic Drug Blood Levels

The most direct and preferred method of assessing medication compliance is to measure the amount of antiepileptic drug in the blood. Patients are generally classified as compliant if their AED levels are within the therapeutic range and noncompliant if their AED levels are lower than the therapeutic range. The manner in which AED levels were used to assess compliance has varied among epilepsy studies.

More often than not, a single AED level taken at the time of a clinic visit is used as a measure of medication compliance. While a single AED level provides information about current drug use, it provides little information about previous drug use and cannot be used to make judgments about long-term medication-taking behavior. Cramer, Scheyer, and Mattson (1990) found that participants were more likely to take their medication as ordered on the 10 days closest to a clinic visit and that compliance rates dropped significantly 1 month later. As expected, AED levels taken at a clinic visit correlated strongly with compliance rates measured closest to the time of the clinic visit. The findings demonstrate that it is possible for patients to have therapeutic levels at the time of a clinic visit, but not be totally complaint with the medication regimen at other times between visits. The concern that patients may be inappropriately classified as compliant or noncompliant on the basis of a single AED level taken during a clinic visit led Leppik, Cloyd, Sawchuk, and Pepin, 1979) to propose the use of more than one blood sample in compliance classification.

Self-Report

Asking people if they follow all aspects of their prescribed medical regimen is the easiest way to assess compliance. Despite the ease of administration, self-reports of adherence to medical regimens are generally suspect because of the belief that patients are likely to overestimate their actual degree of adherence (Cramer & Mattson, 1991). Moreover, it is well known that other forms of response bias may add to measurement error in self-report assessments (Nunnally & Bernstein, 1994). Despite limitations of interviews or questionnaires as measures of compliance, self-reports are one of the few means of collecting information on self-management practices other than medication taking and the only means of collecting information on patients' perceptions of their situation.

Several investigators have employed interview strategies and questionnaires to learn about self-management practices other than medication taking. Trostle, Hauser, and Susser (1983) conducted extensive interviews with seven persons with epilepsy to examine the beliefs, practices, and experiences of persons with epilepsy. Peterson, McLean, and Millingen (1982) and Stanaway, Lambie, and Johnson (1985) each constructed questionnaires to assess self-management practices including medication taking. Neither research team, however, provided information about the psychometric properties of their questionnaires—making replication of the studies difficult.

Di Iorio et al. (1992) have designed an instrument to measure epilepsy self-management practices. The Epilepsy Self-Management Scale (ESMS) is composed of 26 items related to medication taking, safety precautions, and general self-management issues. Items assessing medication compliance include "I take my seizure medication the way my doctor orders it." Other items measure compliance with safety recommendations ("I use power tools such as electric saws, hedge trimmers, and knives") and compliance with lifestyle adjustments ("I eat regular meals"). Each item is rated on a 5-point scale from *never* (1) to *always* (5). Total scores for the scale are found by first reverse scoring the negatively worded items and then adding item responses. Total possible scores range from 26 to 130, with higher scores representing more positive self-management practices. The scale has been used in three studies of epilepsy self-management (Di Iorio et al., 1992; Di Iorio, Faherty, & Manteuffel, 1994; Di Iorio, Hennessy, & Manteuffel, 1996). Across these studies, the reliability coefficients for the total scale have ranged from 0.81 to 0.84, suggesting consistency across samples and moderate to high levels of internal consistency.

Factor analysis techniques were employed to assess the underlying dimensions of the scale (Di Iorio, Hennessy, & Manteuffel, 1996). Four strong factors emerged, which were given the following tentative names: Consulting with the Physician, Maintaining Regular Practices, Managing Drug Scarcity, and Skipping Medication. The first factor, Consulting with the Physician, includes items assessing a person's tendency to check with the doctor before making changes in the regimen or when noticing changes in one's condition such as having more seizures than usual. The second factor, Maintaining Regular Practices, includes items assessing consistency of practices such as eating regular meals or taking medications at the same time every day. Managing Drug Scarcity, the third factor, measures the extent to which one spreads out doses to conserve medication. The fourth factor, Skipping Medication, assesses the degree to which a person skips doses of medicine. Although different aspects of medication taking emerged as separate factors, items related to safety recommendations did not combine to form cohesive factors. Thus, it is necessary to refine the safety items and continue to systematically test the items until a useful measure of this aspect of self-management is developed as well.

Treatment Outcome

Although treatment outcome seems to be an appropriate measure of medication adherence, treatment outcome cannot be used as a marker of compliance in epilepsy (Gordis, 1976). Although those who take their medications as ordered are more likely to achieve seizure control than those who deviate from the treatment plan, the relationship between medication use and seizure occurrence is not a simple linear one. A multiplicity of factors such as seizure types, epilepsy syndromes, and seizure triggers interact in complex ways to cause seizure activity (Cloyd, 1988).

Persons who must take high levels of an AED to achieve seizure control generally are sensitive to low levels of the drug and are likely to have a seizure if the levels fall below the minimum effective dose. These individuals may be compliant, but when they drift below the minimum effective dose level because of timing of drug administration, changes in metabolic needs, or interaction with a newly prescribed drug, a breakthrough seizure may occur (Cloyd, 1988). Moreover, the degree of compliance required to achieve seizure control varies with the type of medication (Cloyd, 1988). Because of the long half-life of phenobarbital, for instance, a person can miss several doses during a month and still maintain therapeutic blood levels. In contrast, missing a dose of valproic acid, a drug with a short half-life, is more likely to result in subtherapeutic blood levels and a greater likelihood of seizure activity.

A study by Barry and Hauser (1994) demonstrated the lack of a linear association between therapeutic levels and seizure occurrence. It is generally believed that persons who experience status epilepticus (continuous seizure activity) have not taken their medications as prescribed and therefore have non-therapeutic antiepileptic drug levels. Barry and Hauser (1994) found that 48% of their sample of 65 patients admitted to the hospital in status epilepticus had therapeutic levels for all AEDs on admission, and 65% had therapeutic levels of at least one AED. Only 15% of patients had subtherapeutic AED levels before and at the time of status, and 25% who previously had therapeutic levels had low levels of at least one drug at the time of status. The study demonstrated that there are other factors besides low AED levels that can precipitate status and that seizure activity is a poor marker of medication noncompliance.

MODELS OF SELF-MANAGEMENT

During the 1950s, the first model to explain preventive health behavior was introduced. Since that time, a plethora of models to explain different types of health behaviors have been proposed by members of health disciplines, including public health, nursing, psychology, sociology, and medicine. Although a few models have been used by epilepsy researchers as frameworks for exploring determinants of medication compliance and general self-management behaviors, most epilepsy research in this area has not been conceptualized within any one model. This section begins with a discussion of epilepsy compliance research that was not conceptualized within a specific health behavior model, follows with a discussion of epilepsy compliance research that was framed within health behavior models, and ends with a discussion of general self-management behaviors framed within social cognitive theory.

Medical Model

Studies in which an atheoretical approach is applied to the study determinants of health behaviors are often said to be following the medical model. This approach is relatively unstructured and characterized by the exploration of easily quantifiable factors such as patient- and illness-centered variables. The results of studies using the medical model are presented within five general categories of interest: (1) demographic characteristics, (2) illness- and regimen-related variables, (3) patient-provider interaction, (4) cognitive-perceptual factors, and (5) reasons for noncompliance.

Demographic Characteristics

Most epilepsy compliance investigators who have examined demographic characteristics such as age, gender, race, marital status, income, and education have found no significant correlations between them and measures of compliance (Di Iorio, Faherty, & Manteuffel, 1991; Dowse & Futter, 1991; Friedman et al., 1986; Hazzard, Hutchinson, & Krawiecki, 1990). Dodrill, Batzel, Wilensky, and Yerby (1987) found no differences on age and gender, but did find that persons classified as compliant had slightly higher educational levels than those who were classified as noncompliant.

Mattson, Cramer, Collins, and the Veterans Administration Epilepsy Cooperative Study Group (1988) found that participants missing no doses were significantly older than those missing two or more doses and also had higher mean Wechsler Adult Intelligence Scale IQ scores. Moreover, younger subjects and those with prior psychological or alcohol problems, currently unemployed, and without other medical problems were more likely to miss their clinic appointments. The difference between the results of this latter study and those of other studies may be ascribed to differences in sample composition. Subjects were chosen on the basis of highly selective criteria to participate in an experimental drug trial, and several strategies were used to enhance compliance. Persons participating in the other studies were primarily clinic patients approached to participate during their regularly scheduled appointments.

Illness-Related and Regimen-Related Variables

The search for determinants of medication compliance among illness- and regimen-related variables has not fared any better than that among demographic characteristics. The results of studies examining the relationship between epilepsy-related factors and compliant behaviors have been inconsistent and even contradictory. Eisler and Mattson (1975) found that a longer length of seizure disorder was associated with compliance, whereas Takaki, Kurokawa, and Aoyama (1985) and Loiseau and Marchal (1988) showed that a longer time on medication and a longer duration of illness were associated with noncompliance. In contrast, Di Iorio et al. (1991) and Dowse and Futter (1991) found no difference in length of seizure disorder between compliers and noncompliers.

The inconsistencies found in examining epilepsy-related variables are in contrast to the consistency concerning the complexity of the medication regimen. Persons with epilepsy who take fewer drugs and fewer doses of drugs have been shown to use drugs more regularly than those prescribed multiple drugs and complex dosage schedules (Eisler & Mattson, 1975; Takaki et al., 1985). Cramer et al. (1989) conducted a well-controlled study using an automated monitoring device to record pill-bottle openings. The overall compliance rate for participants taking one dose per day was 87%. Compliance rates dropped with increasing doses per day to 39% for participants taking pills four times per day. A few studies revealed no differences in complexity of drug regimen between compliers and noncompliers (Di Iorio et al., 1991; Dodrill et al., 1987; Kurokawa et al., 1988). An examination of these particular samples reveals, however, that most respondents were on monotherapy, making comparisons based on complexity of regimen inconclusive. The results of studies examining complexity of regimen have been so compelling that epilepsy practitioners strive to prescribe the simplest medication schedule possible for patients.

Patient–Provider Interaction

Patient-provider interaction has been a topic of considerable interest in compliance research. It is generally asserted that more positive patient-provider relationships are associated with compliant behavior (Becker & Maiman, 1975). Two general areas of patient-provider interaction have been examined in epilepsy compliance studies: degree of supervision of medication taking and patient satisfaction with care. Gibberd, Dunne, Handley, and Hazleman (1970) found that inpatients with epilepsy had higher serum phenytoin levels than a comparable group of outpatients. The researchers attributed this difference to the degree of supervision of medication taking. They subsequently increased the supervision of the outpatients by increasing the frequency of visits and the blood samples. With more frequent visits, serum concentrations of phenytoin increased, suggesting that more supervision facilitated adherence to the medication regimen. Chandra, Dalvi, Karnad, Kshirsagar, and Shah (1993) admitted 20 patients suspected of noncompliance to a hospital ward for 5 days. AED serum levels of all patients were in the nontherapeutic range before admission, but by the 5th day after admission, 14 patients had serum AED levels in the therapeutic range, suggesting previous undermedication. Kurokawa et al. (1988) also found that compliance was related to degree of supervision in children with epilepsy. Adherence rates as measured by serum drug levels increased when parents supervised their children's medication taking. AED levels were highest when children were hospitalized and nurses were responsible for drug administration.

The degree of patient satisfaction with health care providers and its association with compliant behavior were assessed in two studies. Hazzard et al. (1990), in a study of 35 children, found that children who were compliant reported greater satisfaction with their medical care than noncompliers. Their parents also reported higher degree of satisfaction with medical care than parents of children who were noncompliant. In contrast, Peterson et al. (1982) found that adult compliers were no more satisfied with the doctor's explanation of their illness than were their noncompliant counterparts.

Cognitive–Perceptual Factors

Only a few investigators using the medical approach to studies have addressed the association between cognitive-perceptual factors and epilepsy self-management. Variables assessed under this rubric include worry about health, emotional adjustment, perception of financial distress, presence of regular responsibilities, perceived benefits of treatment, uncertainty, social support, health conception, and health locus of control. Dodrill et al. (1987) found that compliance was not related to emotional adjustment as hypothesized or to the actual cost of medication among adults with epilepsy. Compliance, instead, was linked to the perception of financial distress; those who perceived less distress were more likely to be compliant. The explanation of compliance was further enhanced by knowledge of life responsibilities. Participants who were less distressed and had more regular responsibilities in life were more likely to be compliant.

Perception was also a key component of a study by Stanaway et al. (1985), who found that adults with epilepsy who perceived a greater benefit to treatment were more likely to have therapeutic serum levels. Hazzard et al. (1990) expected to find that the children of parents who worried about their children's health would be more compliant. Instead, they found that less adherent children had parents who reported worrying more about their children's health. Moreover, parents who reported greater anxiety placed more restrictions on their children's behavior. This latter finding corresponds to that of Friedman et al. (1986), who found that children with fewer restrictions placed upon them were more compliant than those with more behavioral restrictions. Hazzard et al. (1990) also examined the association between compliance and health locus of control, but found no substantial differences in control beliefs between those who were regular compliers and those who were not.

Uncertainty about illness has also been associated with compliant behavior in epilepsy management. Di Iorio et al. (1991) found that respondents who reported great uncertainty about their illness were likely to have subtherapeutic AED levels. The investigators noted that the greater uncertainty expressed by the noncompliers may be due to an unclear appraisal of the illness, which may in turn lead to testing one's own beliefs about one's condition. In the same study, respondents reporting more assistance from their social networks were more likely to have nontherapeutic AED levels, suggesting noncompliance. This finding is opposite that which was predicted, and the researchers proffered the view that other variables not yet identified may serve to mediate or modify the effect of social support on compliance behavior. In contrast to significant differences in dimensions of social support and uncertainty, there were no differences between compliers and noncompliers in their personal beliefs about the clinical dimension of health.

Reasons for Noncompliance

A few investigators sought to explore reasons for noncompliance. In these studies, participants were asked why they did not take their medications as ordered. While the most common reasons given were forgetfulness and not understanding the need for medication, other responses indicated some conscious deliberation about the course of action. For example, some persons stopped taking medication to test to see whether they still needed it (Stanaway et al., 1985). Some did not like taking the medication or felt that it was too much trouble or no longer effective. Others were bothered by side effects or feared addiction (Eisler & Mattson, 1975; Kurokawa et al., 1988). In contrast to those who altered their patterns of drug use, persons who took medications as ordered seemed to be motivated by the threat of seizures. These individuals reported the experience of having a seizure when off their medications and expressed fear of having another seizure. They also noted more positive support from family and health care providers (Eisler & Mattson, 1975).

In an interesting study of medication self-regulation, Trostle (1988) interviewed 127 adults with epilepsy about their recent past and present use of antiepileptic drugs. Trostle (1988) found that almost 60% of those interviewed had intentionally altered their medication regimens without prior approval by their physicians. Some participants had stopped taking medication altogether, others had changed the dosage for more than 2 weeks, and still others were taking more or less than prescribed. The participants offered specific reasons for medication self-regulation ranging from fear of harm to the fetus during pregnancy to the perceived need for more medication when they felt that a seizure was imminent. Other reasons for regulating their medication included intolerable side effects, dislike of dependence on medication, desire to see how they responded off the medication, and the perceived feeling of doing well. Trostle (1988) also found that while participants may not have been taking medications as the doctor ordered, some had constructed elaborate sets of health practices designed to prevent seizures and were compliant with their self-prescribed regimens. So while physicians often labeled them as noncompliant because they were not taking their medications as ordered, these individuals believed that they were compliant because they consistently followed their own regimens.

Health Belief Model

The health belief model (e.g., Rosenstock, 1966) is based on value expectancy and motivation theories. This model differs from the medical model in two important ways. First, the health belief model identifies important theoretical constructs in the enactment of health behaviors and states the relationship among the constructs. This theoretical approach to the study of determinants of health behaviors allows for a systematic test of proposed relationships. Results of studies based on the model can be used to modify the model and ultimately lead to a refined understanding of why people choose to participate in health-related activities. The health belief model also differs from the medical model by acknowledging that a person's perceptions and other defining characteristics such as age and gender can serve as a basis for behavior.

In 1975, Becker and Maiman (1975) suggested that the model could be used, with modifications, to understand patient compliance with prescribed therapies. The modified model is composed of three major components: readiness to undertake recommended compliance behaviors, modifying and enabling factors, and the compliant behavior of interest. Each component is represented by more specific concepts. Readiness to undertake recommended compliance behaviors is an expansion of the perceived susceptibility and seriousness components in the original model through the addition of more specific measures of the value of the medical regimen, motivations to comply, value of illness-threat reduction, perceived susceptibility, and probability that compliant behavior will reduce the threat. The second major component of the revised model, modifying and enabling factors, is represented by five general categories: demographic, structural, attitudinal, interactional, and enabling factors. This component deals primarily with barriers and benefits to the recommended action. Examples of specific variables measured are age, treatment complexity, cost, duration, and side effects; type and quality of the doctor-patient relationship; patient satisfaction; social pressure; and prior experience with the recommended action and illness.

The combined findings of two studies of parents of children with epilepsy revealed that motivation was an important component of compliance (Shope, 1988) as measured by a clinician's evaluation of the correlation between the prescribed dose of medication and the blood levels of the drug and by AED levels. Compliers were likely to seek information and do more special things to keep their children healthy. They were also less likely than noncompliant parents to run out of medication for several days, miss a dose, or be out of medicine at clinic visits, and more likely to try to make up a missed dose. Compliers also seemed to feel that their children were more susceptible to seizures, since they reported more recent and greater frequency of seizures. In contrast to the model's prediction, none of the measures of probability that compliant behavior would reduce the threat of seizures was associated with compliance. The results related to measures of barriers were somewhat inconsistent with the model's prediction. Parent compliers noted greater difficulty in affording medications and were less likely to be on government assistance. However, compliance was associated with more satisfaction with the clinic visit. With regard to the doctor-patient relationship, compliers noted that they saw the same doctor whom they described as friendly and respectful. They also reported fewer weeks since their last visit than those who were noncompliant. Compliers were more likely to have someone to remind them to take their medication and to have had a seizure while off their medicine. Noncompliers noted higher goals for their children and a history of not giving medication for a day or more.

The seriousness and susceptibility aspects of the health belief model seemed to be more predictive of compliance among adults than among parents. Shope (1988) found that adult compliers were more likely than noncompliers to seek information, to feel more susceptible to seizures, and to feel that the treatment was effective. As with the parent sample, the results related to barriers were inconsistent. Adults with more complex treatments, greater concerns about side effects, and friends who questioned the treatment were more likely to comply. These findings were inconsistent with the model's prediction. Compliers, however, were more likely to report having had a seizure while off their medication.

Ferguson (1982) contacted 87 of the 177 adults who participated in Shope's adult study 2 years after the first data collection and found that most of the health belief variables assessed at time 1 were significantly correlated to the time 2 measures. Variables that were related to compliance at the second assessment were total number of seizures, perceived inefficacy of the regimen, and past experience without medication. That is, respondents who had a greater number of seizures and perceived the regimen to be more effective were more likely to be compliant. Path models were tested to determine the direct and indirect effects of the variables on compliance. The tendency to disclose seizures, a commitment to the regimen, and health beliefs functioned as intermediate variables for age, income, and recency of seizures in explaining compliance.

Bryant and Ereshefsky (1981) conducted a final study conceptualized within the health belief framework in which participants were classified as compliant if they had therapeutic levels of phenytoin at two testings taken at least 3 months apart and a clinic attendance rate of 80% over the previous 18 months. These investigators developed a loosely constructed questionnaire, the items of which did not have one-to-one correspondence with the variables in the health belief model. The investigators found that noncompliant participants expressed more negative attitudes about medication taking than did compliant participants. Noncompliant participants were more likely to be undecided about the value of their medications and to alter their medication regimen when they felt sick. Compliers, in contrast, expressed more positive attitudes about their relationships with their health care providers and were more likely to have a supportive social network, as evidenced by having someone to talk with about their seizures and acknowledging their epileptic condition to their employer.

The small number of studies framed within the health belief model provide at best preliminary support for some of the propositions of the model. Taken together, the findings suggest that readiness-to-act variables are important in explaining epilepsy compliant behaviors. More specifically, participants who felt susceptible to seizures and exhibited greater awareness of consequences of taking medication, greater awareness of concern for health in general, and better monitoring skills were more likely to comply. Evidence for the influence of suggested modifying factors is inconsistent. Satisfaction with the physician and support from family and friends seem to be important determinants of compliance; however, evidence regarding barriers to compliance is less convincing. Compliers tended to express the existence of more barriers than did noncompliers. This finding is opposite that in a general review of studies conducted by Janz and Becker (1984). They found that perceived barriers was the most powerful of the health belief model constructs across the 29 studies evaluated.

Framework of Relationships Model

In 1978, Green and Roter published a model for compliance behavior entitled "The Framework of Relationships between Compliance and Behavioral Antecedents" (later changed to "The Framework of Relationships between Health Education, Compliance, and Outcomes in Epilepsy") (Green & Simons-Morton (1988)). Based on a combination of a family utilization of health services model, the health belief model, and a health education model, the framework offers another approach to understanding complaint behavior. The major propositions of the model are that compliant behaviors depend on certain antecedent behaviors and that these antecedent behaviors can be modified by educational interventions. The model also suggests that adequate resources are necessary for effective education and that the ultimate outcome of compliant behavior is seizure reduction.

The antecedents to compliant behavior in this model are similar to the proposed determinants of behavior outlined in the modified version of the health belief model. These factors include, for example, perceived resuceptibility to seizures, benefits of treatment, barriers to compliant behaviors, and satisfaction with medical care. However, Green and Roter (1978) placed a greater emphasis on access to health care than did Becker and Maiman (1975). Adequate referral, health insurance, and general availability of medical care were proposed by Green and Roter (1978) to be essential to understanding compliant behavior.

In contrast to the medical model and the health belief model, both of which focus on determinants of health behavior, the framework of relationships model goes one step further and incorporates educational strategies designed to influence antecedents of compliant behavior. Three essential strategies proposed are direct communication with patients, indirect communication with patients, and structural reorganization.

The first strategy, communicating directly with patients, can influence personal beliefs about epilepsy, its treatment, and the consequences of noncompliance. Direct communication involves tailoring instruction to the needs of the individual, teaching problem-solving skills, and enhancing one's confidence in one's ability to manage epilepsy and its consequences.

A second educational strategy designed to influence determinants of compliant behavior is communicating indirectly with patients through the family and health care providers. The additional emotional and instrumental support received from knowledgeable family members is expected to enhance a person's adherence to the medical regimen. Likewise, education for nurses, physicians, and other health care workers can enhance their awareness of the patients' predicaments regarding living with epilepsy. The resulting sensitivity to the patient's situation is expected to enhance relationships between patients and health providers.

Finally, a third strategy, structural reorganization through the mobilization of institutional and community resources, can indirectly foster compliance by removing barriers that limit access to treatment. At the community level, education of the public can dispel the myths and ignorance surrounding epilepsy, remove the stigma, and foster acceptance of people with epilepsy within the community.

The framework of relationships between compliance and its behavioral antecedents was acknowledged in a report by the Commission for the Control of Epilepsy and Its Consequences (1978), which became the basis for the development of a two-day training program for people with epilepsy and their families (Helgeson, Mittan, Tan, & Chayasirisobhon, 1990). This program has been used extensively throughout the United States, and the effects of the program on patient outcomes were assessed by Helgeson et al. (1990). Using an experimental design, subjects were randomly assigned to either the treatment group or the control group. Subjects in the treatment group participated in the two-day training program, which was designed to meet medical education and psychosocial treatment needs. Four months later, subjects in the treatment group knew significantly more about epilepsy and its treatment, expressed less fear of seizures, reported less use of hazardous medical self-management practices, and showed an improvement in medication compliance as measured by AED blood levels compared to the control group. There was no difference in the frequency of seizures between the groups at the 4-month posttreatment visit.

Although the authors stated that the treatment program was initiated as a response to the report in which the framework of relationships between compliance and its behavioral antecedents in relation to epilepsy first appeared, it is unclear how closely the training program was modeled after the framework (Helgeson et al., 1990). The published results of the study lacked sufficient detail to determine whether the framework was adequate to understand medication compliance among people with epilepsy and whether the educational strategies were sufficient to promote compliant behavior. Thus, as with the health belief model, additional research is required to determine whether the components of the model are adequate for understanding epilepsy compliant behavior or whether modifications are in order.

Social Cognitive Theory

In contrast to the health belief model and the framework for relationships among health education, compliance, and outcomes in epilepsy, social cognitive theory was not developed to explain health behavior per se. Rather, social cognitive theory originated in psychology as an outgrowth of social learning theory and as an attempt to explain performance of a wide range of behaviors. Early success of the theory as a basis for changing phobic behaviors brought the theory to the attention of health behavior researchers. Ewart, Taylor, Reese, and DeBusk (1983) found that the model provided accurate prediction of persistence in physical activity among heart attack victims, and Godding and Glasgow (1985) found a similar level of prediction for smoking cessation. Social cognitive theory has now been used to explain a wide range of health behaviors including AIDS risk-reduction practices (O'Leary, Goodhart, Jemmott, & Boccher-Lattimore, 1992), diabetes self-management (Glasgow et al., 1989), and chronic pain management (Jensen, Turner, & Romano, 1991).

Social cognitive theory proposes that behavior is determined by three sets of interacting factors: internal personal factors, environmental factors, and the behavior itself (Bandura, 1986). The internal personal factors that have been examined most closely are self-efficacy and outcome expectancies. Self-efficacy refers to one's confidence in one's ability to enact a specific behavior. According to the theory, individuals with high levels of self-efficacy are likely to overcome barriers to behavioral performance and to persevere until their behavioral goals are achieved. Outcome expectancy refers to the perceived value of a given behavioral outcome. Individuals who associate more positive outcomes with a specific behavior are more likely to engage in that behavior than are those who envision more negative behavioral outcomes. Other factors within the self-system that have been studied in relation to behavioral performance include self-esteem, anxiety, personal goals, and peer norms.

According to the theory, the environmental system includes everything that is not a part of the self-system. The most important components of the environmental system are family, friends, and associates who observe and evaluate one's behavior. At another level, community and societal expectations also play important roles in behavioral enactment. The environmental players often serve as powerful determinants of the type of behaviors that one engages in and the quality of the resultant behavior.

Social cognitive theory served as the framework for a study on epilepsy self-management conducted by Di Iorio et al. (1992). Self-management was defined as a set of skills and techniques used to control the frequency of seizures and was measured by the Epilepsy Self-Management Scale (ESMS). The ESMS, a researcher-developed epilepsy self-efficacy scale, and the Personal Resource Questionnaire—a measure of social support—were sent to members of a local epilepsy foundation. A total of 98 individuals returned completed questionnaires, representing a 24% response rate. As predicted by the theory, self-efficacy was positively related to self-management practices; i.e., respondents who were more confident in their ability reported more frequent practice of self-management strategies. General social support was also correlated with self-management, suggesting that the presence of a strong support system fosters the use of self-management practices. Using regression analysis, self-efficacy explained a significant amount of variance in self-management practices, but in the regression analysis, the contribution of social support was weak and nonsignificant. Further testing suggested that self-efficacy may serve as a mediator of social support; i.e., individuals with strong support systems may already have higher levels of self-efficacy, which in turn would influence self-management practices. The researchers also suggested developing more sensitive measures of support specific to the needs of persons with epilepsy.

In 1994, Di Iorio, Faherty, and Manteuffel (1994) reported the results of a second study designed as a partial replication and extension of the first study. The major findings of the first study were replicated; i.e., self-efficacy was significantly correlated with self-management and explained a significant amount of variance in self-management practices. Contrary to the first study, however, social support was not significantly related to self-management practices, but a more specific measure of epilepsy support was significantly correlated with self-management, suggesting that support received to implement the regimen was more important in helping participants manage their epilepsy than were more global supportive relationships.

In a third study, Di Iorio, Hennessy, and Manteuffel (1996) expanded the study of self-management practices by including additional variables derived from social cognitive theory. In addition to general social support, regimen-specific support and self-efficacy, anxiety, and outcome expectancies were measured. With the assistance of a local chapter of the Epilepsy Foundation of America, questionnaires were sent to members who participated in job training sessions. Questionnaires were received from 195 individuals, representing an approximate 50% response rate.

Using propositions derived from social cognitive theory, a proposed structural model was developed to test a model of self-management related to medication management. The major findings demonstrate that people with strong support networks do not always rely on others to assist them with epilepsy-related tasks. Indeed, for some, having someone to remind them to take their medications increased negative views about medications. Rather, their confidence in taking prescription medications was associated with more positive views of medications. Medication management was also associated with anxiety. Respondents who reported higher levels of anxiety were less able to manage their medications.

SELF-MANAGEMENT INTERVENTIONS

The previous section addressed the search for indicators of self-management practices. Understanding factors associated with the use of effective self-management practices is key to the development of studies to test the effectiveness of strategies to promote self-management. In this section, two general classifications of interventions related to epilepsy self-management practices are presented. The first type includes interventions designed to improve medication compliance; the second is composed of testing the effectiveness of selected self-management strategies in reducing seizure frequency.

Not surprisingly, investigators assessing epilepsy self-management programs have concentrated on interventions to enhance medication compliance. Early studies on interventions to foster compliance with medication taking focused on supervision and reminder systems. The results of these generally showed that oral and written instructions, more frequent visits with the physician (Lund, Jorgensen, & Kuhl, 1964; Wannamaker, Morton, Gross, & Saunders, 1980), greater physician supervision (Dawson & Jamieson, 1971; Gibberd et al., 1970), and reminder systems such as medication containers (Lund, 1973) generally enhanced medication compliance rates. Other investigators focused on the effect of educational counseling on medication compliance, including Peterson, McLean, & Millingen (1984), who found that educational counseling and reminder systems improved compliance rates.

Behavioral strategies designed to reduce seizure frequency constitute the second group of interventions examined in the epilepsy self-management literature (Parker & Baer, 1986). Behavioral self-management strategies that have been tested include biofeedback (Kuhlman, 1978) and relaxation therapy (Temkin & Davis, 1984). The participants in these types of studies generally reported an improvement in symptoms. However, the small sample sizes and in some studies the lack of control groups preclude definitive conclusions about the efficacy of the treatments. Additional study is necessary to determine whether the effects of biofeedback and relaxation can be attributed to the treatments or to other factors such as the placebo effect, bias in recording seizures, or improved medication compliance.

DIRECTIONS FOR FUTURE RESEARCH

The study of epilepsy self-management, including compliance, is relatively recent, and much of what is known about self-management has been generated from research conducted since the 1960s. This chapter has detailed a number of studies that have explored determinants of and interventions to promote self-management. The success of this work is reflected in the practices of epilepsy clinicians: Health care providers attempt to control patients' seizures using the simplest medication regimen possible. They also recommend that their patients use medication reminder systems and seizure calendars to help manage their epilepsy. Centers for the study and treatment of epilepsy have been created throughout the United States. These centers provide comprehensive care, including the education of the patient, family, and community. Likewise, the Epilepsy Foundation of America includes information about self-management practices in its mailings to interested individuals.

Participants at the International Conference on Compliance in Epilepsy (Schmidt & Leppik, 1988) recognized the contributions of previous compliance research, but also identified the need to explore self-management practices beyond medication compliance. To meet this goal, there is a need for high-quality descriptive studies to discover the broad range of self-management practices employed by people to control their seizures. Moreover, because illness- and sick-role behavior is often bound within one's culture (Kleinman, 1987), single-culture and single-ethnic descriptive studies are necessary to provide greater understanding of a person's choice of self-management strategies. Likewise, cross-cultural and cross-ethnic studies will yield a better appreciation of the similarities and differences in approaches to epilepsy self-management among various groups. Trostle et al. (1983) pointed out that self-management practices must also be examined within the context of the family and social networks. Family dynamics play an important role in how individuals choose to manage or not to manage their seizures, and this area deserves more study as well.

Research and Methodological Issues

To date, epilepsy self-management studies have been framed within three conceptual frameworks. Although the investigators have used the models to select variables for study, for the most part they have failed to suggest how these models can be modified on the basis of their findings. Such feedback is necessary to refine models and ultimately lead to a useful model of epilepsy self-management.

Conceptual issues related to self-management deserve attention as well. The term *self-management* is often used interchangeably with other terms such as *self-care* and *self-regulation*. The multidimensional definition of epilepsy compliance proposed in 1988 (Schmidt & Leppik, 1988) overlaps to some extent the definition of self-management. Future endeavors could be directed toward reconciling these differences and making a clear statement about the meaning of epilepsy self-management.

For the most part, studies exploring epilepsy self-management have been limited to samples derived from clinic populations. Patients who arrive for regularly scheduled appointments may differ in several respects from the entire population of people with epilepsy, including those who do not seek care on a regular basis

(Haynes, 1976). For example, participants recruited from a clinic are more likely to be compliant at least in keeping clinic appointments than are participants recruited from throughout a community; these two populations may differ in other ways as well. Results of studies derived from clinic-based populations cannot be generalized to the entire community of people with epilepsy. Thus, future researchers should make a concerted effort to seek individuals for their studies from the community at large, and in particular individuals who have limited contact with health care providers. These individuals are of the most interest because they can be expected to reveal the greatest diversity in self-management practices.

Epilepsy researchers have used different means of measuring compliance and different approaches to classifying patients as compliant or noncompliant. Such differences make it difficult to compare the results of studies and to be completely confident in drawing conclusions about the nature of epilepsy compliant behaviors. More research is required to evaluate and compare the different methods in order to obtain a reasonable and efficient method of assessment and classification. Consistency in measurement procedures among epilepsy researchers will strengthen conclusions drawn form their work. Likewise, additional work is necessary to develop and refine instruments to measure self-management practices other than medication compliance. Although the work by Di Iorio, Manteuffel, and Hennessy (1994) can serve as a beginning, as more self-management strategies are revealed, reliable and valid instruments must be constructed to measure them.

Longitudinal studies are needed to explore how self-management practices change over time and identify factors that initiate those changes. Likewise, well-designed clinical trials are required to explore more completely the usefulness of relaxation, biofeedback, and guided imagery as self-management strategies. Further, recent advances in statistical techniques help control for problems when quasi-experimental designs must be used and should be considered by researchers when a true experimental design is not possible. The statistical tests used for many of the medication compliance studies were limited to simple bivariate analyses such as correlations and *t*-tests, which can provide only a preliminary understanding of the nature of relationships. The disparate findings of many studies suggest that other explanatory variables may exist, but cannot be identified within the constraints of these simple statistical tests. At this point in the study of self-management practices, researchers should consider the use of multivariate statistics. These procedures allow for more powerful tests of the hypotheses and the discovery of mediating and moderating factors. Such information can lead to broader and deeper understanding of factors associated with self-management practices.

SUMMARY

The purpose of this chapter was to give an overview of the recent research related to epilepsy self-management. Most research has concentrated on medication compliance, and the results of this work have been fruitful, leading to changes in clinical practice. Spurred by the International Conference on Compliance in Epilepsy, researchers and clinicians are beginning to examine self-management practices other than medication compliance. Both current and future research will lead to a better understanding of factors associated with successful epilepsy self-management.

ACKNOWLEDGMENTS. The author acknowledges the financial support of the Epilepsy Foundation of America and wishes to thank Dr. Pete Link for his review of an earlier draft of the manuscript.

REFERENCES

Annegers, J. F. (1993). The epidemiology of epilepsy. In E. Wyllie (Ed.), *The treatment of epilepsy: Principles and practice* (pp. 157–164). Philadelphia: Lea & Febiger.

Bandura, A. (1986). *Social foundations of thought and action: A social cognitive theory*. Englewood Cliffs, NJ: Prentice-Hall.

Barry, E., & Hauser, W. A. (1994). Status epilepticus and antiepileptic medication levels. *Neurology, 44*, 47-50.

Becker, M. H., & Maiman, L. A. (1975). Sociobehavioral determinants of compliance with health and medical care recommendations. *Medical Care, 8*, 10-24.

Bryant, S. G., & Ereshefsky, L. (1981). Determinants of compliance in epileptic outpatients. *Drug Intelligence and Clinical Pharmacy, 15*, 572-577.

Cereghino, J. J., McNamara, J., Goldensohn, E. S., Porter, R., & Wannamaker, B. B. (1981). *How to recognize and classify seizures*. Landover, MD: Epilepsy Foundation of America.

Chandra, R. S., Dalvi, S. S., Karnad, P. D., Kshirsagar, N. A., & Shah, P. U. (1993). Compliance monitoring in epileptic patients. *Journal of the Association of Physicians in India, 41*, 431-432.

Cloyd, J. (1988). Pharmacokinetics and medication compliance. In D. Schmidt & I. E. Leppik (Eds.), *Compliance in epilepsy* (pp. 101-107). Amsterdam: Elsevier.

Commission for the Control of Epilepsy and Its Consequences. (1978). *Plan for nationwide action on epilepsy: Vols. 1 and 2*. DHEW Publication No. NIH 78-276. Washington, DC: U.S. Government Printing Office.

Cramer, J. A. (1991). Overview of methods to measure and enhance patient compliance. In J. A. Cramer & B. Spilker (Eds.), *Patient compliance in medical practice and clinical trials* (pp. 3-10). New York: Raven Press.

Cramer, J. A., & Mattson, R. H. (1991) Monitoring compliance with antiepileptic drug therapy. In J. A. Cramer & B. Spilker (Eds.), *Patient compliance in medical practice and clinical trials* (pp. 123-138). New York: Raven Press.

Cramer, J. A., Mattson, R. H., Prevey, M. L., Scheyer, R. D., & Ouellette, V. L. (1989). How often is medication taken as prescribed? *Journal of the American Medical Association, 261*, 3273-3277.

Cramer, J. A., Scheyer, R. D., & Mattson, R. H. (1990). Compliance declines between clinic visits. *Archives of Internal Medicine, 150*, 1509-1510.

Dawson, K. P., & Jamieson, A. (1971). Value of blood phenytoin estimation in management of childhood epilepsy. *Archives of Disease in Childhood, 46*, 386-388.

Di Iorio, C., Faherty, B., & Manteuffel, B. (1991). Cognitive-perceptual factors associated with antiepileptic medication compliance. *Research in Nursing and Health, 14*, 329-338.

Di Iorio, C., Faherty, B., & Manteuffel, B. (1992). Self-efficiency and social support in self-management of epilepsy. *Western Journal of Nursing Research, 14*, 292-307.

Di Iorio, C., Faherty, B., & Manteuffel, B. (1994). Epilepsy self-management: Partial replication and extension. *Research in Nursing and Health, 17*, 167-174.

Di Iorio, C., Hennessy, M., & Manteuffel, B. (1996). Epilepsy self-management: A test of a theoretical model. *Nursing Research, 45*, 211-217.

Dodrill, C. B., Batzel, L. W., Wilensky, A. J., & Yerby, M. S. (1987). The role of psychosocial and financial factors in medication noncompliance in epilepsy. *International Journal of Psychiatry in Medicine, 17*, 143-154.

Dowse, R., & Futter, W. T. (1991). Outpatient compliance with theophylline and phenytoin therapy. *South African Medical Journal, 80*, 550-553.

Dunbar, J. (1979). Issues in assessment. In S. J. Cohen (Ed.), *New directions in patient compliance*. Lexington, MA: Lexington Books and D. C. Heath.

Eisler, J., & Mattson, R. H. (1975). Compliance in anticonvulsant drug therapy. *Epilepsia, 16*, 203.

Ewart, C. K., Taylor, C. B., Reese, L. B., & DeBusk, R. F. (1983). Effects of early postmyocardial infarction exercise testing on self-perception and subsequent physical activity. *American Journal of Cardiology, 51*, 1076-1080.

Ferguson, K. J. (1982). Compliance with antiepileptic medication: A two-year follow-up study of adults with epilepsy. *Dissertation Abstracts International, 43*(06), 1804-B.

Friedman, I. M., Litt, I. F., King, D., Henson, R., Holtzman, D., Halverson, D., & Kraemer, H. (1986). Compliance with anticonvulsant therapy by epileptic youth. *Journal of Adolescent Health Care, 7*, 12-17.

Gibberd, F. B., Dunne, J. F., Handley, A. J., & Hazleman, B. L. (1970). Supervision of epileptic patients taking phenytoin. *British Medical Journal, 1*, 147-149.

Glasgow, R. E., Toobert, D. J., Riddle, M., Donnelly, J., Mitchell, D. L., & Calder, D. (1989). Diabetes-specific social learning variables and self-care behaviors among person with Type II diabetes. *Health Psychology, 8*, 285-303.

Godding, P. R., & Glasgow, R. E. (1985). Self-efficacy and outcome expectations as predictors of controlled smoking status. *Cognitive Therapy and Research, 9*, 583-590.

Gordis, L. (1976). Methodological issues in the measurement of patient compliance. In D. L. Sackett & R. B. Haynes (Eds.), *Compliance with therapeutic regimens* (pp. 51-66). Baltimore, MD: Johns Hopkins University Press.

Green, L. W., & Roter, D. (1978). The literature on patient compliance and implications for cost-effective patient education programs in epilepsy. In Commission for the Control of Epilepsy and Its Consequences, *Plan for nationwide action on epilepsy: Vol. II* (Part 1, pp. 391-417). DHEW Publication No. NIH 78-311. Washington, DC: U.S. Government Printing Office.

Green, L. W., & Simons-Morton, D. G. (1988). Denial, delay and disappointment: Discovering and overcoming the causes of drug errors and missed appointments. In D. Schmidt & I. E. Leppik (Eds.), *Compliance in epilepsy* (pp. 7-21). Amsterdam: Elsevier.

Hauser, W. A. (1993). The natural history of seizures. In E. Wyllie (Ed.), *The treatment of epilepsy: Principals and practice* (pp. 165-170). Philadelphia: Lea & Febiger.

Haynes, R. B. (1976). A critical review of the "determinants" of patient compliance with therapeutic regimens. In D. L. Sackett & R. B. Haynes (Eds.), *Compliance with therapeu-*

tic regimens (pp. 26-39). Baltimore, MD: Johns Hopkins University Press.

Hazzard, A., Hutchinson, S. J., & Krawiecki, N. (1990). Factors related to adherence to medication regimens in pediatric seizure patients. *Journal of Pediatric Psychology, 15*, 543-555.

Helgeson, D. C., Mittan, R., Tan, S. Y., & Chayasirisobhon, S. (1990). Sepulveda epilepsy education: The efficacy of a psychoeducational treatment program in treating medical and psychosocial aspects of epilepsy. *Epilepsia, 31*, 75-82.

Janz, N. K., & Becker, M. H. (1984). The health belief model: A decade later. *Health Education Quarterly, 11*, 1-47.

Jensen, M. P., Turner, J. A., & Romano, J. M. (1991). Self-efficacy and outcome expectancies: Relationship to chronic pain coping strategies and adjustment. *Pain, 44*, 263-269.

Kleinman, A. (1987). Anthropology and psychiatry: The role of culture in cross-cultural research on illness. *British Journal of Psychiatry, 151*, 447-454.

Kuhlman, W. N. (1978). EEG feedback training of epileptic patients: Clinical and electroencephalographic analysis. *Electroencephalography and Clinical Neurophysiology, 45*, 699-710.

Kurokawa, T., Minami, T., Kitamoto, I., Mizuno, Y., Maeda, Y., & Takaki, S. (1988). Compliance in epileptic children in Japan. In D. Schmidt & I. E. Leppik (Eds.), *Compliance in epilepsy* (pp. 147-151). Amsterdam: Elsevier.

Legion, V. (1991). Health education for self-management by people with epilepsy. *Journal of Neuroscience Nursing, 23*, 300-305.

Leppik, I. E., Cloyd, J. C., Sawchuk, R. J., & Pepin, S. M. (1979). Compliance and variability of plasma phenytoin levels in epileptic patients. *Therapeutic Drug Monitoring, 1*, 475-483.

Leppik, I. E., & Schmidt, D. (1988). Consensus statement on compliance in epilepsy. In D. Schmidt & I. E. Leppik (Eds.), *Compliance in epilepsy* (pp. 179-182). Amsterdam: Elsevier.

Loiseau, P., & Marchal, C. (1988). Determinants of compliance in epileptic patients. In D. Schmidt & I. E. Leppik (Eds.), *Compliance in epilepsy* (pp. 135-140). Amsterdam: Elsevier.

Lund, M. (1973). Failure to observe dosage instructions in patients with epilepsy. *Acta Neurologica Scandinavica, 49*, 295-306.

Lund, M., Jorgensen, R. S., & Kuhl, V. (1964). Serum diphenylhydantoin (phenytoin) in ambulant patients with epilepsy. *Epilepsia, 5*, 51-58.

Mattson, R. H., Cramer, J. A., Collins, J. F., & the Veterans Administration Epilepsy Cooperative Study Group. (1988). Aspects of compliance: Taking drugs and keeping clinic appointments. In D. Schmidt & I. E. Leppik (Eds.), *Compliance in epilepsy* (pp. 111-117). Amsterdam: Elsevier.

Nunnally, J. C., & Bernstein, I. H. (1994). *Psychometric theory* (3rd ed.). New York: McGraw-Hill.

O'Leary, A., Goodhart, F., Jemmott, L. S., & Boccher-Lattimore, D. (1992). Predictors of safer sexual behavior on the college campus: A social cognitive theory analysis. *Journal of American College Health, 40*, 254-263.

Parker, L. H., & Baer, G. R. (1986). Neurological and neuromuscular disorders. In K. A. Holroyd & T. L. Creer (Eds.), *Self-management of chronic disease: Handbook of clinical interventions and research* (pp. 415-440). Orlando, FL: Academic Press.

Peterson, G. M., McLean, S., & Millingen, K. S. (1982). Determinants of patient compliance with anticonvulsant therapy. *Epilepsia, 23*, 607-613.

Peterson, G. M., McLean, S., & Millingen, K. S. (1984). A randomized trial of strategies to improve patient compliance with anticonvulsant therapy. *Epilepsia, 25*, 412-417.

Rosenstock, I. M. (1966). Why people use health services. *Milbank Memorial Fund Quarterly, 44*, 94-127.

Sackett, D. L., & Haynes, R. B. (1976). Preface. In D. L. Sackett & R. B. Haynes (Eds.), *Compliance with therapeutic regimens* (pp. xi-xiv). Baltimore, MD: Johns Hopkins University Press.

Scheuer, M. L., & Cohen, J. (1993). Seizures and epilepsy in the elderly. In O. Devinsky (Ed.), *Neurological clinics in epilepsy I: Diagnosis and treatment* (pp. 787-804). Philadelphia: W. B. Saunders.

Schmidt, D., & Leppik, I. E. (1988). Compliance in epilepsy: Introduction. In D. Schmidt & I. E. Leppik (Eds.), *Compliance in epilepsy* (pp. 3-4). Amsterdam: Elsevier.

Shope, J. T. (1988). Compliance in children and adults: Review of studies. In D. Schmidt & I. E. Leppik (Eds.), *Compliance in epilepsy* (pp. 23-47). Amsterdam: Elsevier.

Stanaway, L., Lambie, D. G., & Johnson, R. H. (1985). Non-compliance with anticonvulsant therapy as a cause of seizures. *New Zealand Medical Journal, 98*, 150-152.

Takaki, S., Kurokawa, T., & Aoyama, T. (1985). Monitoring drug noncompliance in epileptic patients: Assessing phenobarbital plasma levels. *Therapeutic Drug Monitoring, 7*, 87-91.

Temkin, N. R., & Davis, G. R. (1984). Stress as a risk factor for seizures among adults with epilepsy. *Epilepsia, 25*, 450-456.

Trostle, J. (1988). Doctors' orders and patients' self-interest: Two views of medication usage? In D. Schmidt & I. E. Leppik (Eds.), *Compliance in epilepsy* (pp. 57-69). Amsterdam: Elsevier.

Trostle, J. A., Hauser, W. A., & Susser, I. S. (1983). The logic of noncompliance: Management of epilepsy from the patient's point of view. *Culture, Medicine and Psychiatry, 7*, 35-56.

Wannamaker, B. B., Dreifuss, F. E., Booker, H. E., & Willmore, L. J. (1984). *The comprehensive clinical management of the epilepsies*. Landover, MD: Epilepsy Foundation of America.

Wannamaker, B. B., Morton, W. A., Jr., Gross, A. J., & Saunders, S. (1980). Improvement in antiepileptic drug levels following reduction of intervals between clinic visits. *Epilepsia, 21*, 155-162.

12

Determinants of Regimen Adherence in Renal Dialysis

Alan J. Christensen, Eric G. Benotsch, and Timothy W. Smith

ADHERENCE IN RENAL DIALYSIS

Patient nonadherence with medical regimens is common in the treatment of many chronic diseases (Turk & Meichenbaum, 1991). For the over 165,000 end-stage renal disease patients in the United States, nonadherence is both pervasive and clinically significant. The goals of this chapter are to illustrate both the scope and the implications of nonadherence among ESRD patients, as well as to review the empirical literature aimed at identifying determinants of nonadherence. The chapter will also illustrate the assertion that adherence can be better understood by considering the interaction of patient individual differences with treatment and disease-related factors. Finally, the chapter discusses the implications of these issues for the design and implementation of related interventions.

Alan J. Christensen and Eric G. Benotsch • Department of Psychology, University of Iowa, Iowa City, Iowa 52242. **Timothy W. Smith** • Department of Psychology, University of Utah, Salt Lake City, Utah 84112.

Handbook of Health Behavior Research II: Provider Determinants, edited by David S. Gochman. Plenum Press, New York, 1997.

Overview of End-Stage Renal Disease (ESRD) and Renal Dialysis

End-stage renal disease (ESRD) is an incurable, chronic disease afflicting individuals of all ages, ethnic groups, and socioeconomic strata. From a policy standpoint, ESRD is unique. The Medicare ESRD entitlement program enacted in 1973 provides benefits to over 90% of individuals with chronic renal failure. In 1993, approximately \$5 billion in health care benefits were provided by Medicare for the treatment of ESRD (U.S. Renal Data System, 1993).

ESRD is most commonly due to the advanced complications of another medical condition (e.g., diabetes, hypertension). For other patients, the underlying etiology is specific to the renal system (e.g., glomerulonephritis, polycystic kidney disease). Of these conditions, complications of diabetes are the most common etiological factor, accounting for over one third of the new cases of ESRD (U.S. Renal Data System, 1993).

Whatever the cause of the disorder, all ESRD patients face a life-threatening loss of renal function. To compensate for the cessation of kidney function, ESRD patients must undergo renal replacement therapy to stay alive. Current treatments for ESRD include renal transplantation and several forms of renal dialysis. A successful renal transplant is thought to hold certain advantages in terms of patient quality of life (Christensen, Holman, Turner, Smith, & Grant, 1991). However, due to a perennial shortage of donor organs and a significant transplant rejection rate, the large majority of ESRD patients receive some form of renal dialysis. Currently, approximately 70% of the 165,000 ESRD patients in the United States are treated with one of two forms of renal dialysis (U.S. Renal Data System, 1993). These primary dialysis modalities are hemodialysis (either in-center or home administration) (80% of dialysis patients nationally) and continuous ambulatory peritoneal dialysis (CAPD) (15% of dialysis patients nationally).

The Renal Dialysis Treatment Context

There is an important difference in the roles taken by the patients who are undergoing the different forms of dialysis. The in-center hemodialysis patient is a passive recipient of treatment in the confines of a dialysis center. The dialysis procedure is performed three times a week by trained technicians in a hospital setting, requiring approximately 4 hours per session. The hemodialysis treatment is administered by way of a vascular connection made between the external, artificial kidney machine (the dialyzer) and the patient, usually through an arteriovenous fistula permanently placed in the patient's forearm. Little participation is allowed or required of the patient while undergoing dialysis. For a minority of patients, hemodialysis is carried out at home with assistance from a technician or caregiver. Although mechanically similar procedures are involved, home hemodialysis patients typically have the opportunity to be more actively involved in treatment delivery. However, the popularity of home hemodialysis administration has waned considerably in recent years. Currently, fewer than 1.5% of ESRD patients are undergoing this form of treatment.

In contrast to hemodialysis, CAPD treatment requires the patient to take an active role to ensure treatment success. For CAPD, a permanent catheter is surgically implanted in the patient's abdomen. CAPD is carried out manually by the patient, who uses a sterile tube to carefully connect the catheter to a bag of sterile dialysis solution (dialysate). The bag is elevated to allow the dialysate to flow into the peritoneal cavity. After this procedure is completed, the bag is tucked away under the patient's clothing. Over the next 4–6 hours (8 hours while sleeping), the patient remains ambulatory as continuous dialysis proceeds. During this time, blood filters through the peritoneal membrane, leaving toxins behind in the dialysate. After this "dwell time" is complete, the bag is lowered and the used solution is allowed to drain back into the bag, in which it is discarded, and the procedure begins again. Because of the intricacies of the procedures involved, the successful administration of CAPD is clearly dependent on the patient's taking a more active role in the treatment than does a patient undergoing hemodialysis. In contrast to the diminished use of home hemodialysis, the popularity of CAPD has steadily increased since the mid-1980s (U.S. Renal Data System, 1993).

The availability of different treatment modalities, each with its own unique characteristics and patient demands, makes the management of ESRD unique. Both hemodialysis and CAPD are medically acceptable treatment alternatives for the large majority of ESRD patients. As a result, provider and patient preferences play a key role in treatment assignment decisions, as do other nonmedical factors.

Overview of the Problem of Nonadherence

Patient nonadherence is an important clinical concern in all forms of renal dialysis treatment. In addition to undergoing the dialysis procedure itself, patients are required to follow a multifaceted treatment regimen. Both CAPD and hemodialysis patients are required to take regular doses of phosphate-binding medication as well as to modify their diet due to the body's inability to excrete phosphorus while undergoing treatment. For many patients, phosphate-binding medication is poorly tolerated by the digestive tract, leading to unpleasant gastrointestinal side effects. If the medication regimen is not followed, however, serum phosphorus (P) will rise and serious decreases in calcium and subsequent bone demineralization can occur (Lewis, 1987).

Hyperkalemia is also a clinically significant problem for all dialysis patients due to the body's inability to regulate serum potassium (K). As a result, patients are also required to follow strict dietary guidelines to maintain safe serum K levels (i.e., limited consumption of potassium-rich foods). If dietary guidelines are not followed, serum K will rise and can engender potentially life-threatening cardiovascular complications, such as cardiac arrhythmia (Wright, 1981).

Serum P and serum K levels are assessed approximately monthly as part of the routine biochemical monitoring of dialysis patients. Both higher serum P and higher serum K levels are typically interpreted as reflecting poorer adherence. In both cases, values above 5.5 meq/liter are generally considered indicative of problematic adherence (Wolcott, Maida, Diamond, & Nissenson, 1986).

In the case of hemodialysis treatment, there are also extreme limitations on the amount of fluid that can be safely consumed due to the intermittent nature of the fluid and waste clearance performed by the artificial kidney (Wright, 1981). Prolonged fluid overload is also a potentially life-endangering condition and is associated with congestive heart failure, hypertension, dizziness, shortness of breath, and severe muscle cramping. Previous reports have suggested that adhering to the fluid-intake restrictions may be the most challenging and stressful aspect of the hemodialysis regimen (Baldree, Murphy, & Powers, 1982; Rosenbaum & Ben-Ari Smira, 1986).

Interdialytic weight gain (IWG) is typically used to define adherence to the fluid-intake restrictions. IWG is determined by subtracting the postdialytic weight for the previous treatment session from the predialytic weight for the current session. The values resulting from this computation are believed to be a valid reflection of the amount of fluid that the patient ingests between dialysis sessions (Manley & Sweeney, 1986). Higher IWG values are interpreted as reflecting poorer patient adherence, with values over 2.5 kg (or over 4% of the patient's body weight) generally indicative of problematic adherence (Wolcott et al., 1986).

A past review of the compliance literature suggested that between 30% and 50% of dialysis patients do not adhere to diet, fluid-intake, and medication regimens (Wolcott et al., 1986). More recently published studies have reported similarly poor adherence in this population (Bame, Petersen, & Wray, 1993; Christensen et al., 1992; Schneider, Friend, Whitaker, & Wadhwa, 1991; Weed-Collins & Hogan, 1989). In general, these reports indicated that nonadherence is most common for fluid-intake and medication guidelines and somewhat less common for dietary restrictions. The high prevalence of nonadherence is particularly alarming, given the potential for serious medical complications and diminished life expectancy (De-Nour, 1981; Plough & Salem, 1982)

DETERMINANTS OF PATIENT ADHERENCE

Given the prevalence and clinical importance of nonadherence in all forms of renal dialysis therapy, it is not surprising that considerable empirical attention has been devoted to identifying factors related to adherence. Research has examined the relationship of a broad range of patients' individual differences and social context variables to renal dialysis regimen adherence. These variables compose four general categories: (1) demographic variables, (2) patient beliefs, (3) social resources, and (4) stylistic or personality influences. The typical approach in this research has involved examining the concurrent or, more rarely, the prospective association of these variables to one or more of the biochemical markers believed to reflect patient adherence. Studies involving each of these four categories of predictor variables are discussed below.

Demographic Variables

Despite considerable research, demographic variables have not been found to be consistently related to adherence among dialysis patients. There are isolated reports of more favorable medication, fluid-intake, and dietary regimen adherence for female hemodialysis patients (Boyer, Friend, Chlouverakis, & Kaloyanides, 1990; Morduchowicz et al., 1993), patients with a shorter disease duration (Boyer et al., 1990; Brown & Fitzpatrick, 1988), and diabetic as compared to nondiabetic CAPD and hemodialysis patients (Christensen, Benotsch, Wiebe, & Lawton, 1996). Patient age, however, appears to be the only demographic factor that has proven to be a replicable correlate of adherence. In a number of studies, younger patients have exhibited consistently poorer adherence to various aspects of the prescribed dialysis regimen when compared to older patients (Bame et al., 1993; Boyer et al., 1990; Christensen & Smith, 1995; Cummings, Becker, Kirscht, & Levin, 1982). A similar effect for age has been observed for other medical regimens, including diabetic control (e.g., Johnson, 1980) and prescription medication use (e.g., Bush & Osterweis, 1978).

Patient Beliefs

Since the formulation of the health belief model (HBM) (Rosenstock, 1966), individual differences in health-related cognitions have received considerable attention as determinants of patient adherence. The specific components of the HBM as applied to adherence behavior include a patient's perceived susceptibility to complications, perceived benefits of executing a prescribed behavior, perceived barriers to adherence, and an internal (e.g., perception of symptoms) or external (e.g., educational efforts) triggering stimulus (Becker & Maiman, 1975). These HBM variables have themselves received little empirical support as determinants of adherence among renal dialysis patients (Wolcott et al., 1986). One study reported that perceived barriers (e.g., "being away from home," "medication cost") were negatively related to phosphate-binding medication adherence among in-center hemodialysis patients (Weed-Collins & Hogan, 1989). With few exceptions, however, other cognitive factors composing the HBM have been found to be unrelated to adherence in this population (Cummings et al., 1982; Hartmann & Becker, 1978; Rosenbaum & Ben-Ari Smira, 1986). Rosenbaum and Ben-Ari Smira (1986) concluded that the failure of health beliefs (e.g., the perceived benefits of adhering) to predict adherence in a sample of hemodialysis patients was due to the difficulty of successfully executing the prescribed behavioral change (i.e., extreme fluid restriction). From this perspective, motivation or intention to adhere may not be closely linked to success in adhering to a regimen that is demanding or requires certain behavioral or self-control skills that some patients may not possess (e.g., the ability to delay gratification).

There is some evidence to suggest that behaviorally specific self-efficacy expectations are modestly related to fluid-intake adherence (Rosenbaum & Ben-Ari Smira, 1986; Schneider et al., 1991). Patients who believe that they are capable of performing compliance behaviors are more likely to do so. This association appeared to be due largely to patients' perceived success at adhering in the past and attributing that success to their own efforts. This interpretation suggests that the specific attributions patients make regarding their past adherence may play a role in mediating adherence.

Another cognitive construct that has been applied to the prediction of adherence behavior among dialysis patients involves individual differences in perceived control over health. The constructs of generalized (Rotter, 1966) and health-specific locus of control (Wallston, Wallston, &

DeVellis, 1978) have both received considerable attention in the adherence literature. Locus of control reflects the degree to which individuals believe that attaining a desired outcome (e.g., a positive health outcome) is contingent either upon their own behavior or upon some external influence. Several studies reported that hemodialysis patients with an internal locus of control exhibited more favorable adherence to dietary and fluid-intake aspects of the treatment regimen (Kaplan De-Nour and Czaczkes, 1972; Oldenburg, MacDonald, & Perkins, 1988; Poll and Kaplan De-Nour, 1980). Other research suggests, however, that control expectancies are not significantly related to hemodialysis regimen adherence. This lack of an association has been observed in studies employing both generalized locus of control measures (Schneider et al., 1991; Wittenberg et al., 1983) and measures of health-specific locus of control (Brown & Fitzpatrick, 1988).

Wallston and colleagues extended their work regarding health-related beliefs and health behavior with the introduction of a measure of "perceived health competence" (M. S. Smith, Wallston, & Smith, 1995). Perceived health competence (PHC) reflects an individual's perceived ability to influence personal health outcomes effectively. The broadly conceived PHC construct incorporates both behavioral or self-efficacy expectancies and outcome expectancies (Wallston, 1992). In contrast, health locus of control (HLC) reflects only individuals' expectancies regarding the *outcome* of health-related behavior, not their perceived ability to execute effectively the behaviors that may be necessary for a desired outcome to occur.

The newly introduced PHC measure has yet to be adequately examined as a determinant of adherence in any population. Early work with the measure suggests that PHC and HLC may be multiplicative determinants of adherence by dialysis patients (Christensen, Wiebe, Benotsch, & Lawton, 1996). In this study involving a mixed sample of 81 hemodialysis and CAPD patients, higher PHC was associated with more favorable medication regimen adherence only for those patients who believed strongly in provider control over health outcomes. This pattern suggested that a dialysis patient's perceived ability to manage health effectively (perceived health competence) is related to adherence only when the patient believes that positive health outcomes are contingent upon following the advice and actions of health care providers.

Social Resources

Considerable evidence suggests that the availability and perceived quality of social resources are important correlates of adherence across a wide range of preventive and chronic therapeutic domains (e.g., Kaplan & Hartwell, 1987; Ruggeiro, Spirito, Bond, Couston, & McGarvey, 1990; Zweig, LeFevre, & Kruse, 1988). Less research is available, however, regarding adherence among renal dialysis patients. Christensen et al. (1992) examined the effects of social support in the family with regard to patient adherence in a sample of 78 in-center and home hemodialysis patients. Results indicated that patients holding perceptions of a more supportive family environment, characterized by greater cohesion and expressiveness among family members and less intrafamily conflict, exhibited significantly more favorable adherence to fluid-intake restrictions than did patients reporting less family support. Family support, however, was not associated with adherence to dietary restrictions. In a similar vein, better communication within the family was found to be related to more favorable fluid-intake adherence among 40 home hemodialysis patients (Pentecost, Zwerenz, & Manuel, 1976). Two other studies reported that more favorable marital adjustment of the spouses of in-center hemodialysis patients was related to better fluid-intake adherence, but not to dietary adherence (Somer & Tucker, 1988, 1992).

Collectively, these studies reflect a relatively consistent association of family environment factors and patient adherence. The role of extrafamilial social resources, however, is less clear.

Hitchcock, Brantley, Jones, and McKnight (1992) reported that perceived satisfaction with social support was not significantly related to dietary adherence defined by serum K levels. Similarly, a composite measure of perceived support was not related to biochemical markers of fluid-intake or medication adherence (Boyer et al., 1990). Both of these studies examined samples of in-center hemodialysis patients.

Personality Influences

Efforts to identify stable personality characteristics that are predictive of adherence in this population are extremely limited. Rosenbaum and Ben-Ari Smira (1986) asserted that patient adherence outcomes can be explained in part by presumably stable individual differences in learned resourcefulness. This construct, measured by the Self-Control Schedule (SCS) of Rosenbaum (1980), is believed to reflect one's tendency to apply self-control skills in solving behavioral problems (e.g., use of strategies to delay gratification or tolerate frustration). These authors reported that lower SCS scores were related to poorer adherence with the fluid-intake regimen among 53 in-center hemodialysis patients. Adherence to other aspects of the dialysis regimen was not examined. A path-analytical model applied to their data indicated that greater resourcefulness was associated with stronger self-efficacy expectations and a tendency to attribute past adherence success to their own efforts. These cognitive factors were in turn significantly associated with patient adherence. Rosenbaum and Ben-Ari Smira (1986) interpreted this pattern as suggesting that the cognitive factors of self-efficacy expectations and attributions of success may mediate the association between the resourcefulness trait and adherence.

The view that individual differences in personality can be aggregated into five underlying traits has received considerable empirical and theoretical attention since the 1950s (see the review by Digman, 1990). Moreover, there is increasing recognition of the utility of a five-factor personality taxonomy in elucidating correlates of health-related outcomes, including patient adherence (T. W. Smith & Williams, 1992). A conceptual examination of the five-factor taxonomy suggests that Dimension III, labeled Conscientiousness by Costa and McCrae (1992), may be the most accurate trait descriptor of those qualities of the individual thought to be important in terms of adherence behavior. The Conscientiousness factor has been interpreted as "will to achieve," "dependability," and "self-control" by various five-factor theorists (Digman, 1990). There are currently few data to examine the potential relevance of conscientiousness to patient adherence in any population. In preliminary work with the construct, Christensen and Smith (1995) reported that conscientiousness scores from the NEO-Five Factor Inventory (Costa & McCrae, 1991) were a significant correlate of medication adherence among renal dialysis patients. Conscientiousness was not related, however, to serum K-defined dietary adherence. Additional research involving conscientiousness and other personality traits is clearly warranted.

THE PERSON BY CONTEXT INTERACTIVE FRAMEWORK

The limited and inconsistent effects of patient characteristics on adherence might reflect the fact that these associations vary across features of the disease or related treatments. That is, specific cognitive or social factors might be associated with better adherence only for some subgroups of patients, and the association might be absent (or even opposite) in other subgroups. Since the causes, consequences, and medical management of ESRD are quite varied, the influences on adherence might differ as a function of these contextual factors. The studies reviewed ignore such possible moderating factors, because they examine only the main effects of predictors in what are likely to be quite heterogeneous samples of patients. More specific effects on adherence might be obscured in the process.

To explore this possibility, an interactive approach is necessary. The basic assumption in this perspective is that relevant contextual or situational features should be explicitly assessed and the interaction of these factors with patient variables tested directly. This general person by context interaction perspective has a long history in personality and clinical psychology (e.g., Beutler, 1991; Dance & Neufeld, 1988; Magnusson & Endler, 1977). This perspective has also been explored in medical contexts. Perhaps the most common theme has involved tests of the hypothesis that the effectiveness of interventions intended to prepare patients for stressful medical procedures varies as a function of individual differences in coping style (Schultheis, Peterson, & Selby, 1987).

The interactive model and its potential benefits can be illustrated by some of our previous work on emotional adjustment in ESRD. Depression is common in ESRD populations (Christensen, Holman, Turner, & Slaughter, 1989; Craven, Rodin, & Johnson, 1987) and is associated with increased risk of premature mortality (Burton, Kline, Lindsay, & Heidenheim, 1986). Thus, factors that contribute to depression are potentially quite important in the clinical care of ESRD patients.

The association between internal health locus of control and depression was examined in a sample of 96 patients undergoing in-center hemodialysis (Christensen, Turner, Smith, Holman, & Gregory, 1991). It was hypothesized that this association would vary as a function of patients' treatment history and the severity of their disease. Specifically, an internal locus of control was anticipated to be associated with less depression for patients received their first course of dialysis, since a sense of control—even if illusory—should provide some protection against depression (Taylor & Brown, 1988). Patients returning to dialysis following a failed renal transplant, however, have experienced a clear demonstration that their treatment outcome is largely uncontrollable. This disconfirmation of control expectancies was expected to be associated with increased depression. Further, this interaction between locus of control and treatment history was expected to be apparent among patients experiencing the stress of more severe disease, but not among patients with less severe disease. This latter prediction is based on the assumption that some minimal level of disease-related stress is necessary for emergence of depression and its moderation by other factors. The Sickness Impact Profile (SIP) (Bergner, Bobbit, Carter, & Gilson, 1981), a behaviorally based measure of illness-related physical impairment, was used as the measure of disease severity. Depression was assessed through the use of the Beck Depression Inventory (BDI) (Beck, Ward, Mendelson, Mock, & Erbaugh, 1961).

The results closely matched the predicted pattern. For patients with low disease severity (as measured by the SIP), depression levels (as measured by the BDI) were generally low and unaffected by control expectations or treatment history. For patients with more severe disease, however, as depicted in Figure 1, an internal locus of control was associated with less depression if patients had not previously experienced a failed transplant. For patients who had suffered a failed transplant, an internal locus of control was associated with high levels of depression. Thus, this outcome appeared best explained by the

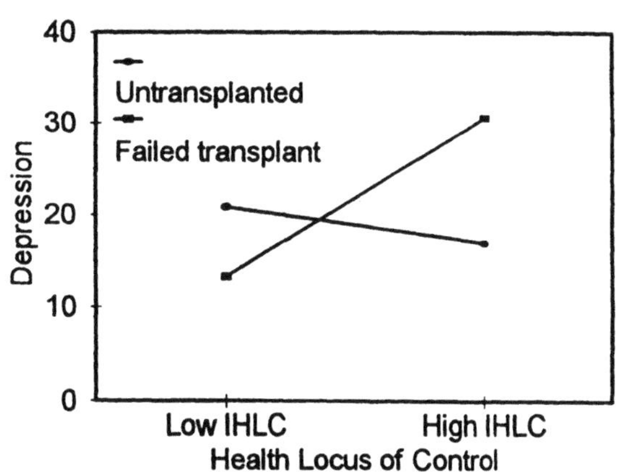

Figure 1. Effects of internal health locus of control and treatment status on adjusted Beck Depression Inventory scores for patients with severe disease. From Christensen, Turner, et al. (1991).

interactive effects of cognitive individual differences, treatment history, and the nature of the disease.

In other studies, the interactional framework has been used to explicate the determinants of adherence among renal dialysis patients. Medical patients vary widely in their preferred level of involvement in their own medical care. Some patients prefer a traditional, passive patient role; others prefer a more active collaborative involvement with their health care providers (Clymer, Baum, & Krantz, 1984). In study of in-center and home hemodialysis patients, adherence was predicted to be maximized in cases in which the patients' preferences matched the type of treatment they received (Christensen, Smith, Turner, Holman, & Gregory, 1990). As depicted in Figure 2, serum K levels suggested that this postulate was indeed valid. Among patients undergoing the more staff-directed in-center hemodialysis who nevertheless preferred active involvement in their own health care delivery, dietary adherence was worse. In contrast, among patients undergoing hemodialysis at home, where patient involvement and control are greater, patients with strong preferences for active involvement displayed better adherence. Moreover,

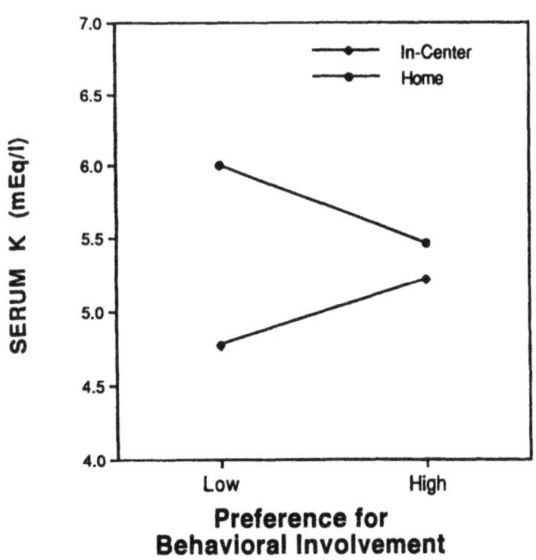

Figure 2. Effects of preference for behavioral involvement and mode of hemodialysis administration (i.e., in-center versus home) on serum K. From Christensen et al. (1990).

among the patients dialyzing at home, those with low preferences for involvement in their own care had higher, clinically elevated serum K levels. Thus, dietary adherence was best described as an interaction between patient preferences for involvement and the levels of involvement permitted or required by the particular treatment they received. A similar though weaker pattern was found for fluid-intake adherence. Once again, problematic adherence was more likely among "mismatched" patients.

One unresolved issue in this interactive perspective is the nature of the relevant individual difference dimension(s). As is obvious in this review of the relevant literature, many different individual differences have been assessed. To reduce this variety to its essential elements, two major constructs were identified underlying six of the scales commonly used in this area (Christensen, Smith, Turner, & Cundick, 1994). In confirmatory factor analyses, an Information Vigilance factor was assessed through scales measuring information seeking, internal health locus of control, and the monitoring of sensory information. This factor can be interpreted as reflecting the tendency or motivation to attend actively to threat-relevant information and sensory experiences related to health and treatment. A second higher-order factor—Active Coping—was assessed by preference for decision making in health care, preference for behavioral involvement, and the expectation that health care professionals can control one's health (inverse loading). This factor can be interpreted as reflecting the tendency or motivation to exercise personal control in health contexts. These two dimensions were only moderately correlated ($r = 0.26$) in our sample of 52 center hemodialysis and 34 CAPD patients.

As depicted in Figure 3, the Information Vigilance factor was positively associated with concurrent dietary adherence among CAPD patients, consistent with the increased demands for self-monitoring and self-care in this group. Among in-center hemodialysis patients, however, the opposite pattern emerged: Information Vigilance

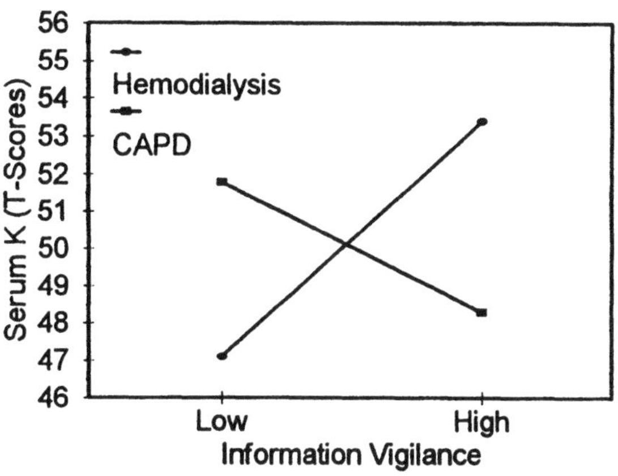

Figure 3. Effects of Information Vigilance and dialysis type (i.e., CAPD versus hemodialysis) on serum potassium. From Christensen et al. (1994).

was associated with worse adherence. It may be that vigilance without the opportunity for constructive involvement is not adaptive, perhaps because it impedes the use of coping strategies that are useful when confronting less modifiable stressors (e.g., distraction). In prospective analyses over a 6-month follow-up period, a similar though only marginally significant pattern emerged. Contrary to expectation, the Active Coping dimension did not interact with treatment modality to predict adherence, but this factor was prospectively associated with decreased depression. Thus, this study provides some additional support for the general view that adherence is an interactive function of aspects of the patient and features of the treatment context.

The general stress and coping paradigm (Lazarus, 1993) is the foundation of much of the clinical and research literature on emotional adjustment and adherence in chronic medical illness. An extension of the interactive model to this perspective would lead to the prediction that adjustment and adherence would be best when the coping strategies employed by patients were consistent with the demands of their illness and its treatment.

To address this hypothesis, 60 ESRD patients undergoing in-center hemodialysis were asked to complete two forms of the Ways of Coping Checklist (WOC) (Folkman, Lazarus, Dunkel-Schetter, DeLongis, & Gruen, 1986). Instructions given for the measure were modified in order to obtain a situation-specific assessment of coping with two distinct stressful encounters differing in terms of how amenable each was to patient control. Directions for the first form asked subjects to recall and describe "the last time you experienced a problem with the dialysis procedure itself" (a relatively uncontrollable situation). Subjects were then asked to respond to the WOC items on the basis of how they dealt with the specific problem they had just described. Directions for the second form asked subjects to recall "the last time you experienced a problem with your fluid intake or blood chemistries" (a relatively controllable situation). Subjects then completed another set of WOC items using this situation as the target encounter.

Consistent with the matching or interactional model, adherence to fluid-intake restrictions was best when patients employed planful problem solving when confronting potentially controllable stressors. In contrast, when dealing with less controllable stressors, coping through the use of emotional self-control was associated with better adherence. Thus, the benefits and liabilities of specific coping strategies depended on the specific problem or stressor (Christensen et al., 1996).

As a group, this set of studies underscores the potential importance of the interactive perspective. Results are not completely consistent across studies, and the more definitive prospective studies are still quite rare. Nonetheless, the available evidence suggests that a more contextual, interactive perspective could enhance our understanding of adherence in this population.

SUMMARY OF RESEARCH EXAMINING DETERMINANTS OF ADHERENCE

Research over two decades since the mid-1970s involving psychological and social factors and dialysis regimen adherence has produced few consistent trends. Several qualitative aspects of the patient's family environment have proven to be replicable correlates of adherence. In general, greater levels of family and marital support are associated with better adherence. The role of other social context factors is less clear. As is the case with many chronic diseases, the family of the renal dialysis patient faces considerable disease and treatment-related stress (Christensen, Turner, Slaughter, & Holman, 1989). Further, the chronic illness itself may contribute to an erosion of extrafamilial sources of support. For these reasons, the quality of the family environment may be a particularly important social factor to consider in understanding patient adjustment, including adherence to the dialysis regimen.

Research has had limited success identifying cognitive variables that are related to adherence. There is evidence of a modest relationship between self-efficacy expectations and future adherence. This association, however, appears to be largely due to a patient's perceived success at adhering in the past and the stability of that success over time (e.g., Rosenbaum & Ben-Ari Smira, 1986). Demonstrating that efficacy expectations are predictive of change in adherence requires further research.

Factors that compose the health belief model have not proven to be consistent predictors of adherence in this population. In contrast, assessments of patients' self-control skills reflect one of the more consistent determinants of adherence. This pattern suggests that nonadherence in this population may be more a function of coping efficacy and less one of motivation, knowledge, or intention. The role of other individual difference factors is less clear due either to inconsistent results across studies (e.g., health locus of control) or inadequate research (e.g., conscientiousness).

Other work (e.g., Christensen et al., 1990, 1994) suggests that the association of patients' individual differences with adherence is perhaps better understood from a perspective that also considers the contextual features of the patients' disease and treatment. The predictive utility of patients' individual differences is enhanced when the interactions of these factors with various features of the disease and related treatments are considered. Compliance is best when characteristics of the patient (e.g., coping styles) "fit" or "match" the adaptive demands inherent in the disease status or treatment. Further research using this interactive approach will help clarify what treatment is most adaptive for a particular patient.

Major Limitations in ESRD Adherence Research

A highly diverse range of psychosocial factors have been examined as potential correlates of adherence among renal dialysis patients. A pervasive methodological limitation of past research is the reliance on correlational, cross-sectional designs. Three studies have examined the association of patients' individual differences and future (as opposed to concurrent) adherence (Christensen et al., 1994; Rosenbaum & Ben-Ari Smira, 1986; Schneider et al., 1991). The latter two studies, however, failed to consider *change* in patient adherence as a criterion measure. While these studies speak to the stability of the observed associations, they fail to provide firm evidence of the causal ordering of the variables. A clearer demonstration of the predictive effect of psychosocial variables would involve predicting change in adherence outcomes over time. This strategy was used by Christensen et al. (1994) in a test of interactions between coping style and dialysis type. In this study, however, a statistically significant cross-sectional effect was only marginally significant when residualized change in adherence (i.e., follow-up adherence after controlling for baseline levels) was examined as the outcome variable, although the pattern of the coping style by dialysis type interaction was virtually identical.

One likely reason for the limited success of prospective research is that adherence behavior among renal dialysis patients is believed to be quite stable over time (Christensen et al., 1994; Rosenbaum & Ben-Ari Smira, 1986; Wolcott et al., 1986). For example, Rosenbaum and Ben-Ari Smira reported a 0.55 correlation between interdialytic weight gain (IWG) assessments conducted at 1-year intervals. This degree of stability increases the difficulty of predicting change in adherence outcomes when using nonexperimental, classificatory variables (e.g., personality factors) that are also presumed to be quite stable.

An alternative methodological strategy that has not yet been used involves obtaining an assessment of the hypothesized predictor variables before patients initiate the prescribed regimen (i.e., prior to dialysis therapy). For many patients, end-stage renal disease is a progressive condition that may not require renal replacement therapy for some time. Targeting future dialysis patients who are at an earlier stage of renal failure may provide a unique opportunity to predict adherence to a future regimen.

A common observation in the adherence literature involves poor correspondence between different aspects of a multifaceted treatment regimen (e.g., Glasgow, McCaul, & Schaefer, 1987; Orme & Binik, 1989). Further, different aspects of a given regimen appear to have distinct psychosocial correlates, as was clearly the case in the studies reviewed in this chapter. There was an almost universal lack of consistency in the findings reported across outcome measures for a given renal dialysis patient sample.

It is possible that patients' individual differences are more or less correlated with particular aspects of the regimen because of the distinct set of challenges posed by each prescribed activity. Another possibility is that the biochemical outcome criteria typically used in this research reflect differentially valid indicators of adherence behavior. For example, serum K is known to be influenced by factors other than patient dietary behavior (e.g., potassium concentrate in the dialysate, a variety of acute medical illnesses). Not surprisingly, serum K levels appear to be the outcome measure least consistently related to the hypothesized psychosocial predictor. In contrast, IWG is thought to be a more valid reflection of the patient's behavior between dialysis sessions. Nevertheless, all biochemical markers used in past research remain imperfect measures of patient adherence. To further improve the clarity of adherence outcome measurement, future research might consider employing multiple methods of adherence assessment (e.g., patient diaries, pill counts, behavioral observation) as an adjunct to the presumed "gold standard" physiological end points.

A final limitation evident in the studies reviewed herein is the failure to consider adherence in patients undergoing CAPD. Approximately 17,000 patients are undergoing this form of treatment in the United States (U.S. Renal Data System, 1993). Despite the rapidly increasing popularity of this relatively new modality, little is known about factors related to adherence among CAPD patients. As discussed above, this form of dialysis allows the patient more control over treatment administration. What is not yet clear from research is the influence of this greater patient involvement on adherence outcomes. The interactive framework proposed in this chapter suggests that this influence may depend upon patient individual differences (e.g., coping style). This possibility deserves further study.

Clinical Implications of Adherence Research

A more effective approach to understanding determinants of patient adherence might involve evaluating the effects of intervention strategies designed to manipulate those factors previously found to be associated with adherence (e.g., social support or behavioral coping skills interventions). This strategy would provide a methodological improvement as well as enhance the clinical utility of our knowledge regarding determinants of patient adherence. Unfortunately, there is little research evaluating the effect of intervention techniques.

There is modest evidence to suggest that behavioral strategies (e.g., behavioral contracting, positive reinforcement) are associated with improved adherence among hemodialysis patients (Barnes, 1976; Hart, 1979; Hegel, Ayllon, Thiel, & Oulton, 1992; Keane, Prue, & Collins, 1981). In general, these studies are limited to single-subject or small-group designs. The effect of other intervention techniques is even less clear. Findings involving the modification of health-related knowledge or beliefs are mixed (Cummings, Becker, Kirscht, & Levin, 1981; Hegel et al., 1992). The potential influence of modifying the patients' social environment has yet to be examined in this population. Research involving adherence in populations other than ESRD, however, has provided evidence that interventions aimed at increasing social support are associated with more favorable patient adherence (Levy, 1983).

The interactive approach illustrated herein may be useful in identifying the intervention strategies that are most adaptive for a particular patient given a certain set of contextual circumstances. For example, in treatment contexts demanding greater patient control (e.g., CAPD), interventions involving the promotion of patient self-management or instruction in problem-solving skills might be preferred. Alternatively, interventions directed toward emotional regulation or cognitive change might be most desirable for patients undergoing a less controllable form of dialysis. Although no studies to date have tested this hypothesis in ESRD, the results of related trait by treatment interaction studies in clinical and health psychology suggest that such efforts are likely to be useful (e.g., Dance & Neufeld, 1988; Schultheis et al., 1987).

CONCLUDING OBSERVATIONS

Though recent decades have seen important advances in the medical management of end-stage renal disease, patient nonadherence to the renal dialysis regimen continues to be a pervasive clinical problem impeding the benefits that might otherwise be derived from these technological advances. While descriptive research has been modestly successful in identifying determinants of adherence in this population, inconsistencies in the available findings and methodological limitations underscore the need for further research. This need is particularly great if empirical studies are to lead to changes in the clinical management of renal dialysis patients.

REFERENCES

Baldree, K. S., Murphy, S. P., & Powers, M. J. (1982). Stress identification and coping patterns in patients on hemodialysis. *Nursing Research, 31*, 107-112.

Bame, S. I., Petersen, N., & Wray, N. P. (1993). Variation in hemodialysis patient compliance according to demographic characteristics. *Social Science in Medicine, 37*, 1035-1043.

Barnes, M. R. (1976). Token economy control of fluid overload in a patient receiving hemodialysis. *Journal of Behavior Therapy and Experimental Psychiatry, 7*, 305-306.

Beck, A. T., Ward, C. H., Mendelson, M., Mock, J., & Erbaugh, J. (1961). An inventory for measuring depression. *Archives of General Psychiatry, 4*, 561-571.

Becker, M. H., & Maiman, L. A. (1975). Sociobehavioral determinants of compliance with health and medical care recommendations. *Medical Care, 13*, 10-24.

Bergner, M., Bobbit, R. A., Carter, W. B., & Gilson, B. S. (1981). The Sickness Impact Profile: Development and final revision of a health status measure. *Medical Care, 19*, 787-805.

Beutler, L. E. (1991). Have all won and all must have prizes? Revisiting Luborsky et al.'s verdict. *Journal of Consulting and Clinical Psychology, 59*(2), 226-232.

Boyer, C. B., Friend, R., Chlouverakis, G., & Kaloyanides, G. (1990). Social support and demographic factors influencing compliance of hemodialysis patients. *Journal of Applied Social Psychology, 20*, 1902-1918.

Brown, J., & Fitzpatrick, R. (1988). Factors influencing compliance with dietary restrictions in dialysis patients. *Journal of Psychosomatic Research, 32*, 191-196.

Burton, H. J., Kline, S. A., Lindsay, R. M., & Heidenheim, A. P. (1986). The relationship of depression to survival in chronic renal failure. *Psychosomatic Medicine, 48*, 261-269.

Bush, P. J., & Osterweis, M. (1978). Pathways to medicine use. *Journal of Health and Social Behavior, 19*, 179-189.

Christensen, A. J., Benotsch, E., Wiebe, J., & Lawton, W. J. (1996). Coping with illness-related stress: Effects on adherence among hemodialysis patients. *Journal of Consulting and Clinical Psychology, 63*, 454-459.

Christensen, A. J., Holman, J. M., Turner, C. W., & Slaughter, J. R. (1989). Quality of life in end-stage renal disease: Influence of renal transplantation. *Clinical Transplantation*, *3*, 46-53.

Christensen, A. J., Holman, J. M., Turner, C. W., Smith, T. W., & Grant, M. K. (1991). A prospective exmaination of quality of life in end-stage renal disease. *Clinical Transplantation*, *5*, 46-53.

Christensen, A. J., & Smith, T. W. (1995). Personality and patient adherence: Correlates of the five-factor model in renal dialysis. *Journal of Behavioral Medicine*, *18*, 305-313.

Christensen, A. J., Smith, T. W., Turner, C. W., & Cundick, K. E. (1994). Patient adjustment and adherence in renal dialysis: A person by treatment interactional approach. *Journal of Behavioral Medicine*, *17*, 549-566.

Christensen, A. J., Smith, T. W., Turner, C. W., Holman, J. M., & Gregory, M. C. (1990). Type of hemodialysis and preference for behavioral involvement: Interactive effects on adherence in end-stage renal disease. *Health Psychology*, *9*(2), 225-236.

Christensen, A. J., Smith, T. W., Turner, C. W., Holman, J. M., Gregory, M. C., & Rich, M. A. (1992). Family support, physical impairment, and adherence in hemodialysis: An investigation of main and buffering effects. *Journal of Behavioral Medicine*, *15*(4), 313-325.

Christensen, A. J., Turner, C. W., Slaughter, J. M., & Holman, J. M. (1989). Perceived family support as a moderator of psychological well-being in end-stage renal disease. *Journal of Behavioral Medicine*, *12*, 249-265.

Christensen, A. J., Turner, C. W., Smith, T. W., Holman, J. M., & Gregory, M. C. (1991). Health locus of control and depression in end-stage renal disease. *Journal of Consulting and Clinical Psychology*, *59*(3), 419-424.

Christensen, A. J., Wiebe, J. S., Benotsch, E. G., & Lawton, W. J. (1996). Perceived health competence, health locus of control, and patient adherence in renal dialysis. *Cognitive Therapy and Research*, *20*, 411-421.

Clymer, R., Baum, A., & Krantz, D. S. (1984). Preferences for self-care and involvement in health care. In A. Baum, S. E. Taylor, & J. E. Singer (Eds.), *Handbook of psychology and health: Vol. 4, Social psychological aspects of health* (pp. 149-166). Hillsdale, NJ: Erlbaum.

Costa, P. T., Jr., & McCrae, R. R. (1991). *The NEO Five-Factor Inventory*. Odessa, FL: Psychological Assessment Resources.

Costa, P. T., Jr., & McCrae, R. R. (1992). *The NEO Personality Inventory-R: Professional Manual*. Odessa, FL: Psychological Assessment Resources.

Craven, J. L., Rodin, G. M., & Johnson, L. (1987). The diagnosis of major depression in renal dialysis patients. *Psychosomatic Medicine*, *49*, 482-492.

Cummings, C. K., Becker, M. H., Kirscht, J. P., & Levin, N. W. (1981). Intervention strategies to improve compliance with medical regimens by ambulatory hemodialysis patients. *Journal of Behavioral Medicine*, *4*, 111-127.

Cummings, K. M., Becker, M. H., Kirscht, J. P., & Levin, N. W. (1982). Psychosocial factors affecting adherence to medical regimens in a group of hemodialysis patients. *Medical Care*, *20*, 567-580.

Dance, K. A., & Neufeld, R. W. J. (1988). Aptitude-treatment interaction research in the clinical setting: A review of attempts to dispel the "patient uniformity myth." *Psychological Bulletin*, *104*, 192-213.

De-Nour, A. K. (1981). Prediction of adjustment to chronic hemodialysis. In N. Levy (Ed.) *Psychonephrology: Vol. 1* (pp. 117-131). New York: Plenum Press.

Digman, J. M. (1990). Personality structure: Emergence of the five-factor model. *Annual Review of Psychology*, *41*, 417-440.

Folkman, S., Lazarus, R. S., Dunkel-Schetter, C., DeLongis, A., & Gruen, R. J. (1986). Dynamics of a stressful encounter: Cognitive appraisal, coping, and encounter outcomes. *Journal of Personality and Social Psychology*, *50*, 992-1003.

Glasgow, R. E., McCaul, K. D., & Schafer, L. C. (1987). Self-care behaviors and glycemic control in Type 1 diabetes. *Journal of Chronic Diseases*, *40*, 399-412.

Hart, R. (1979). Utilization of token economy within a chronic dialysis unit. *Journal of Consulting and Clinical Psychology*, *47*, 646-648.

Hartman, P. E., & Becker, M. H. (1978). Noncompliance with prescribed regimen among chronic hemodialysis patients: A method of prediction, education, and diagnosis. *Dialysis and Transplantation*, 7, 978-986.

Hegel, M. T., Ayllon, T., Thiel, G., & Oulton, B. (1992). Improving adherence to fluid-restrictions in male hemodialysis patients: A comparison of cognitive and behavioral approaches. *Health Psychology*, *11*, 324-330.

Hitchcock, P. B., Brantley, P. J., Jones, G. N., & McKnight, G. T. (1992). Stress and social support as predictors of dietary compliance in hemodialysis patients. *Behavioral Medicine*, *18*, 13-20.

Johnson, S. B. (1980). Psychosocial factors in juvenile diabetes: A review. *Journal of Behavioral Medicine*, *3*, 95-116.

Kaplan, R. M., & Hartwell, S. L. (1987). Differential effects of social support and social network on physiological and social outcomes in men and women with Type II diabetes mellitus. *Health Psychology*, *6*, 387-398.

Kaplan De-Nour, A., & Czaczkes, J. W. (1972). Personality factors in chronic hemodialysis patients causing noncompliance with medical regimen. *Psychosomatic Medicine*, *34*, 333-344.

Keane, T. M., Prue, D. M., & Collins, F. L. (1981). Behavioral contracting to improve dietary compliance in chronic renal dialysis patients. *Journal of Behavior Therapy and Experimental Psychiatry*, *12*, 63-67.

Lazarus, R. S. (1993). Coping theory and research: Past, present, and future. *Psychosomatic Medicine*, *55*, 234-247.

Levy, R. L. (1983). Social support and compliance: A selective review and critique of treatment integrity and outcome measurement. *Social Science in Medicine*, *17*, 1329-1338.

Lewis, S. C. (1987). Acute and chronic renal failure. In S. Lewis & I. Collier (Eds.), *Medical-surgical nursing assessment and management of clinical problems* (pp. 1198-1200). New York: McGraw-Hill.

Magnusson, D., & Endler, N. S. (1977). *Personality at the crossroads: Current issues in interactional psychology*. Hillsdale, NJ: Erlbaum.

Manley, M., & Sweeney, J. (1986). Assessment of compliance in hemodialysis adaptation. *Journal of Psychosomatic Research, 30*, 153-161.

Morduchowicz, G., Sulkes, J., Aizie, S., Gabbay, U., Winkler, J., & Boner, G. (1993). Compliance in hemodialysis patients: A multivariate regression analysis. *Nephron, 64*, 365-368.

Oldenburg, B., MacDonald, G. J., & Perkins, R. J. (1988). Factors influencing excessive thirst and fluid intake in dialysis patients. *Dialysis and Transplantation, 17*, 21-40.

Orme, C. M., & Binik, Y. M. (1989). Consistency of adherence across regimen demands. *Health Psychology, 8*, 27-43.

Pentecost, R. L., Zwerenz, B., & Manuel, J. W. (1976). Intrafamily identity and home dialysis success. *Nephron, 17*, 88-103.

Plough, A. L., & Salem, S. (1982). Social and contextual factors in the analyses of mortality in end-stage renal disease: Implications for health policy. *American Journal of Public Health, 72*, 1293-1295.

Poll, I. B., & Kaplan De-Nour, A. (1980). Locus of control and adjustment to chronic hemodialysis. *Psychological Medicine, 10*, 153-157.

Rosenbaum, M. (1980). A schedule for assessing self-control behaviors. *Behavior Therapy, 11*, 109-121.

Rosenbaum, M., & Ben-Ari Smira, K. (1986). Cognitive and personality factors in the delay of gratification in hemodialysis patients. *Journal of Personality and Social Psychology, 51*, 357-364.

Rosenstock, I. M. (1966). Why people use health services. *Milbank Memorial Fund Quarterly, 44*, 94-127.

Rotter, J. B. (1966). Generalized expectancies for internal versus external control of reinforcement. *Psychological Monographs, 80* (entire No. 609).

Ruggiero, L., Spirito, A., Bond, A., Coustan, D., & McGarvey, S. (1990). Impact of social support and stress on compliance in women with gestational diabetes. *Diabetes Care, 13*, 441-443.

Schneider, M. S., Friend, R., Whitaker, P., & Wadhwa, N. K. (1991). Fluid noncompliance and symptomatology in end-stage renal disease: Cognitive and emotional variables. *Health Psychology, 10*, 209-215.

Schultheis, K., Peterson, L., & Selby, V. (1987). Preparation for stressful medical procedures and person × treatment interactions. *Clinical Psychology Review, 7*, 329-352.

Smith, M. S., Wallston, K. A., & Smith, C. A. (1995). The development and validation of the perceived health competence scale. *Health Education Research: Theory and Practice, 10*, 51-64.

Smith, T. W., & Williams, P. G. (1992). Personality and health: Advantages and limitations of the five-factor model. *Journal of Personality, 60*, 395-423.

Somer, E., & Tucker, C. M. (1988). Patient life engagement, spouse marital adjustment, and dietary adherence of hemodialysis patients. *Journal of Compliance in Health Care, 3*, 57-65.

Somer, E., & Tucker, C. M. (1992). Spouse-marital adjustment and patient dietary adherence in chronic hemodialysis: A comparison of Afro-Americans and Caucasians. *Psychology and Health, 6*, 69-76.

Taylor, S. E., & Brown, J. D. (1988). Illusion and well-being: A social-psychological perspective on mental health. *Psychological Bulletin, 103*, 193-210.

Turk, D. C., & Meichenbaum, D. (1991). Adherence to self-care regimens: The patient's perspective. In J. J. Sweet, R. H. Rozensky, and S. M. Tovian (Eds.), *Handbook of clinical psychology in medical settings* (pp. 249-266). New York: Plenum Press.

U.S. Renal Data System. (1993). *USRDS Annual Report*. Bethesda, MD: National Institute of Diabetes and Digestive and Kidney Diseases, The National Institutes of Health.

Wallston, K. A. (1992). Hocus-pocus, the focus isn't strictly on locus: Rotter's social learning theory modified for health. *Cognitive Therapy and Research, 16*, 183-199.

Wallston, K. A., Wallston, B. S., & DeVellis, R. (1978). Development of the Multidimensional Health Locus of Control Scales. *Health Education Monographs, 6*, 160-170.

Weed-Collins, M., & Hogan, R. (1989). Knowledge and health beliefs regarding phosphate-binding medication in predicting compliance. *ANNA Journal, 16*, 278-283.

Wittenberg, S. H., Blanchard, E. B., Suls, J., Tennen, H., McCoy, G., & McGoldrick, M. D. (1983). Percpetions of control and causality as predictors of compliance and coping in hemodialysis. *Basic and Applied Social Psychology, 4*, 319-336.

Wolcott, D. W., Maida, C. A., Diamond, R., & Nissenson, A. R. (1986). Treatment compliance in end-stage renal disease patients on dialysis. *American Journal of Nephrology, 6*, 329-338.

Wright, L. F. (1981). *Maintenance hemodialysis*. Boston: G. K. Hall.

Zweig, S., LeFevre, M., & Kruse, J. (1988). The health belief model and attendance for prenatal care. *Family Practice Research Journal, 8*, 32-41.

13

Adherence to Mammography and Breast Self-Examination Regimens

Victoria L. Champion and Anna Miller

INTRODUCTION

Breast cancer strikes more women than any other cancer, both in Europe and in the Untied States (Packer, Tong, Bolden, & Wingo, 1996). The American Cancer Society estimates that 184,300 women will be diagnosed with breast cancer in 1996 and 44,300 will die from the disease. Currently, scientists are working on identifying factors that increase breast cancer risks and identifying, through genetic markers, women most susceptible to breast cancer. To date, however, efforts to control breast cancer rely to a large extent on screening for early detection. Current literature supports mammography, clinical breast examination, and breast self-examination for breast cancer screening.

Research related to the efficacy of breast cancer screening will first be presented. Second, literature related to adherence for mammography and breast self-examination, respectively, will be reviewed, with attention to both descriptive and intervention studies. Following the review of each topic, methodological and design problems, as well as future research issues, will be addressed. The major studies published from the early 1980s to the early '90s will be described; the plethora of studies generated for both mammography and breast self-examination, however, makes a comprehensive review of all published studies impossible.

Victoria L. Champion • School of Nursing, Indiana University, Indianapolis, Indiana 46202-5117. **Anna Miller** • School of Nursing, Ball State University, Muncie, Indiana 47306.

Handbook of Health Behavior Research II: Provider Determinants, edited by David S. Gochman. Plenum Press, New York, 1997.

EFFICACY OF BREAST CANCER SCREENING

Literature supports a three-pronged approach to breast cancer screening, including mammography, clinical breast exam (CBE), and breast self-examination (BSE). Studies since the early 1980s have demonstrated the beneficial effects of screening, particularly in the 50- to 65-year-old age group. Several prospective mortality-based intervention studies have provided the scientific rationale for mammography screening guidelines (Anderson et al., 1988; Roberts et al., 1990; Shapiro, Venet, Strax, Venet, & Roeser, 1982; Tabar et al.,

1985, 1992). For instance, the Health Insurance Plan (HIP) began in 1963 and enrolled over 60,000 women who were randomly assigned either to annual mammography and CBE or to a control group receiving only routine physical examination. Mortality differences emerged after 4 years, and after 7 years, the cumulative mortality rate from breast cancer was reduced by 35% in the screened group (Shapiro et al., 1982). Mortality differences between screened and nonscreened women in these prospective trials ranged from 20% to 35%. A 10-year update indicated a continued mortality benefit, with the screened group having a relative breast cancer mortality of 0.70 (Tabar et al., 1992). In addition to the prospective intervention studies, four nonexperimental studies have found a mortality benefit for mammography screening (Collete, Rombach, Day, & DeWaard, 1984; Miller; 1993; Verbeek, Hendriks, & Holland, 1985; Verbeek et al., 1984). Women who participated in screening experienced only 0.53-0.62 times the mortality of nonscreened women. Three of the aforementioned studies included CBE in the protocol. None tested the effect of CBE alone (Collette et al., 1984; Roberts et al., 1990; Shapiro et al. 1982). Results from a Canadian study, however, did not demonstrate mortality benefit to mammography screening either in women aged 40-49 or in women aged 50-59 (Mettlin & Smart, 1993; Miller, 1993), although criticisms such as outdated equipment were offered.

The efficacy of BSE alone also has been studied, although randomized prospective mortality data are not yet available. Prospective randomized mortality studies for BSE are under way, with preliminary results favoring BSE groups for detection of cancer and earlier stage of diagnosis (Koroltchouk, Stanley, & Stjensward, 1990; Semiglazov & Moiseenko, 1987). To date, retrospective studies have reported that the practice of BSE may result in an earlier stage, smaller tumor size, and/or decreased node involvement (Feldman, Carter, Nicastri, & Hosat, 1981; Greenwald et al., 1978; Mant, Vessey, Neil, McPherson, & Jones, 1986). Three studies have lent support to the relationship between BSE and survival, and a meta-analysis of past reports found a significant effect for the benefits of BSE (Foster & Costanza, 1984; Hill, 1988; Huguley, Brown, Greenberg, & Clark, 1988; Kuroishi et al., 1992). In one prospective trial, a significantly better actuarial survival for those who attended BSE instruction versus those in a control group was reported (Locker et al., 1989). Critics of BSE have suggested, however, that these reports are retrospective and prone to design problems and that other reports have not demonstrated BSE effect (Philip, Harris, Flaherty, Joslin, 1986; Senie, Rosen, Lesser, & Kinne, 1981; Smith & Burns, 1985). Newcomb et al. (1991) reported no difference in prior BSE frequency between patients with late-stage breast cancer and case control subjects, but found a 35% decrease in advanced-stage breast cancer when proficiency was analyzed separately, leading to the conclusion that BSE might be effective if practiced correctly (Newcomb et al., 1991). Most recently, Gastrin et al. (1994) reported significantly lower mortality (odds ratio = 0.71) for a population of 28,785 women who were enrolled in a BSE program compared to what was expected in the general Finnish population.

A further analysis suggests a mortality benefit for BSE even when mammography and CBE are completed. On the basis of mathematical models, Shwartz (1992) proposed that the high survival rate of women with interval tumors in the HIP and Breast Cancer Detection Demonstration Project (BCDDP) may be due to the practice of regular BSE by 85% of the women. Although mammography should be considered the primary screening modality, it is estimated that between 10% and 15% of tumors are not detectable by mammography, especially those concealed by dense parenchymal tissue. This circumstance provides a convincing argument for BSE, since many such lesions are palpable (Bassett & Butler, 1991).

Despite its apparent effectiveness, acceptance of breast cancer screening is not optimal. Although mammography utilization is reported to have dramatically increased in the last few years, rates for compliance with initial screening guidelines still are low (Breen & Kessler, 1994; Zapka & Berkowitz, 1992). Age differences are also evident, with older women being less likely to be screened (Costanza, Stoddard, Gaw, & Zapka, 1992). Similarly, BSE has been inadequate in terms of both frequency and proficiency (Champion & Scott, 1993; Newcomb et al., 1991; O'Malley, 1993). Newcomb et al. (1991) found that only 8% of women reported proficient practice.

DETERMINANTS OF MAMMOGRAPHY ADHERENCE

The literature on mammography is vast. An attempt was made to review major studies published since the mid-1980s. The section on descriptive studies considers separately those that used attitudinal theories such as the Health Belief Model (HBM), those that addressed knowledge, and those that identified barriers to practice. Additionally, studies addressing provider recommendation are discussed. The intervention section reviews, respectively, community-based studies, worksite studies, and, individually oriented interventions. Limitations and future research directions are finally addressed.

Descriptive Research

Attitudinal/Belief Variables

The HBM was used to identify health beliefs and modifying factors influencing mammography behavior, using a sample of 882 women (mean age: 49) who had been invited to participate in a low-cost breast cancer screening program for university and medical center employees (Rutledge, Hartmann, Kinman, & Winfield, 1988). Only 382 (22%) of 1700 eligible women participated in the screening. Perceived susceptibility and benefits were related to mammography screening, while perceived severity was not related. Primary influences on participation included low cost, convenience, age, knowledge, and value of mammography as a screening tool. Primary barriers for nonparticipants were cost and not having a physician recommend mammography.

Another study guided by the HBM involved a probability telephone survey of 852 women of age 40 years or older (Fulton et al., 1991). Using logistic regression, significant predictors for having biannual mammography included the modifying factors of receiving gynecological care in the past year, having a regular source for gynecological care, having had a diagnostic mammogram, receiving a physician recommendation for mammography, and having the perception that mammography was safe.

Montano and Taplin (1991) tested an expanded model of the Theory of Reasoned Action, adding the variables of affect (emotional reaction to mammography), past mammography behavior, and facilitating conditions (factors that make mammography easier or more difficult). The sample for this prospective study was 946 women 40 years of age or older enrolled in a health maintenance organization (HMO) who were invited to obtain free mammography. Using multiple regression analysis, the variables of attitude, subjective norm, and affect were significant predictors of both intention and behavior, with affect and attitude accounting for more variance than did subjective norm. Variables with bivariate significance, but not multivariate significance, included susceptibility, efficacy of mammography, income, and the health habits of exercise, seat belt use, and Pap test frequency.

Champion (1991, 1992a) combined the HBM and the Theory of Reasoned Action to examine both mammography use (compliance with American Cancer Society [ACS] guidelines) and intention in a randomly selected sample of 322 women of ages 35 and over. Knowledge, social influence, general health motivation, and control over getting breast cancer also were assessed. Barriers had the strongest bivariate correlation with intention, followed by control, and family history of breast cancer. Multiple regression identified family history of breast cancer, barriers, and control as significant predictors for intention. For actual compliance with guidelines, age had the strongest bivariate and multivariate correlation, with a negative relationship indicating that older women were less compliant with mammography guidelines. Other variables that distinguished compliant from noncompliant women included knowledge, socioeconomic status (SES), seriousness, susceptibility, benefits, control over getting breast cancer, physician recommendation for mammography, health motivation, and having breast cancer symptoms. Using similar measures, Hyman, Baker, Ephraim, Moadel, and Philip (1994) found that race, perceived benefits, and barriers, as well as family history, predicted breast cancer screening.

Stein, Fox, Murata, and Morisky (1992) assessed the influence of HBM variables on prior mammography use and future intention for mammography, using path analysis with SES as a background factor. In this cross-sectional study of 1057 randomly selected women over 35 years of age, physician influence was the most powerful predictor of prior mammography use, with perceived susceptibility and barriers also being significant. HBM variables combined with SES accounted for 47% of the variance for prior mammography and 27% for future intentions.

Rakowski et al. (1992) examined mammography stage-of-adoption and decisional balance constructs drawn from the Transtheoretical Model of Behavioral Change, using a convenience sample of 142 women of ages 40 and older at three worksites. Positive perceptions of mammography ("pro" scores) were significantly higher for women at the maintenance stage (had several prior mammograms and planning for more) than for women in both precontemplation (no prior mammography and no plans for same) and contemplation (one or no prior mammograms, but with plans for mammography). Barriers ("cons") were significantly fewer for women in the maintenance stage than for those in contemplation and precontemplation. In a later replication study of 676 randomly selected women of ages 40-79, Rakowski, Fulton, and Feldman (1993) added a fifth stage, that of relapse, and separated prior mammography behavior from future intentions, thus defining two separate stages of adoption. Analysis of covariance showed that regular prior mammography was related to a more favorable decisional balance, as was the combination of prior mammography and intention for future mammography. As anticipated, women in the relapse group had a negative decisional balance, similar to precontemplators.

Taplin and Montano (1993) compared beliefs about mammography and breast cancer between women of ages 40-64 years and women 65 and older. Women 65 and older were less likely to believe that mammography could find nonpalpable tumors, but were more likely to believe that mammography was important even when asymptomatic. Findings may be limited because the participants had high educational levels (65% had at least a college education) and were primarily Caucasian.

Knowledge

Several studies have identified a significant relationship between mammography use and knowledge about breast cancer and mammography guidelines. In a study of 234 women 65 or older, Rimer, Jones, Wilson, Bennett, and Engstrom (1983) found that older women had a serious lack of knowledge about cancer risk and treatment. Similarly, Fox, Klos, Tsou, and Baum (1987) found that while 58% of 257 women 20 and older knew the recommendation for baseline mammography, only 46% of women knew the frequency for women ages 40-49, and only 34% knew that annual mammography is recommended for women 50 years or older. In addition, age has been found to be universally related to knowledge (Rimer, Ross, Cristinzio, & King, 1992).

National Health Interview Survey (NHIS) data from 1987 and 1990 for women 40 years or older reflect similar knowledge deficits. In this analysis, the primary reason cited for not having mammography in the past 3 years was not knowing that asymptomatic mammography is needed (48% in 1987, 41% in 1990), followed by lack of physician recommendation (30% in both years)

(Breen & Kessler, 1994). Although cost concern rates remained low, they more than doubled from 1987 to 1990 (2.7% to 7.2%). Qualitative studies using focus groups support the quantitative finding (Rimer & King, 1992; Schechter, Vanchieri, & Crofton, 1990).

Barriers

Many studies have examined similar barriers to mammography (Champion, 1992b; Rimer, Keintz, Kessler, Engstrom, & Roson, 1989; Stein, Fox, & Murata, 1991; Zapka, Stoddard, Costanza, & Greene, 1989). Barriers have included lacks of perceived need, and time, inconvenience, fear of results or radiation, cost, pain, and lack of physician recommendation.

In the 1989 Wisconsin Behavioral Risk Factor Survey, no recommendation from a physician was one of the three most common reasons the 692 women cited for not having had a mammogram (Lantz, Remington, & Soref, 1990). Other studies confirm this barrier (Baines, To, & Wall, 1990; Lane, Polednak, & Burg, 1992; Lerman, Rimer, Trock, Balshem, & Engstrom, 1990; Rutledge et al., 1988). For women of ages 65-80 years, Rimer and King (1992) found that the most frequently cited reasons for not having a mammogram were that it was not necessary, no physician recommendation, had not thought about it, being asymptomatic, and being older.

Some studies identify cost as a barrier. In a naturalistic study made possible by changes in federal funding policies during an intervention project, Lane and Fine (1983) found a significantly higher rate of compliance with mammography screening for women whose mammograms were paid for by the project than among women who paid for mammography themselves. Several studies found that reduced fees increased mammography use (Kruse & Phillips, 1987; Rutledge et al., 1988; Tippy, Falvo, & Woehlke, 1989), as did HMO membership (Rimer, Resch, et al., 1992; Taplin, Anderman, & Grothaus, 1989). Two studies found increased mammography use related to willingness to pay more than $50 out of pocket for mammography (Miller & Champion, 1993; Rimer, Trock, Engstrom, Lerman, & King, 1991). Cost also has been cited as a major concern in other studies (Glockner, Hilton, Holden, & Norcross, 1992; Lantz et al., 1990; Stein et al., 1991). However, Rimer et al. (1989) found that cost was not a significant barrier for the 156 noncompliers in a group of 484 asymptomatic women who were offered free mammography; Zapka et al. (1989) did not find cost significantly related to utilization in a probability sample of 1185 women; and cost was not a significant barrier in early reports from the six National Cancer Institute Breast Cancer Screening Consortium (NCI BCSC) sites (NCI BCSC, 1990).

Kruse and Phillips (1987) studied barriers and influencing factors for 735 women 30 years of age and older who had mammograms at two rural hospitals over a 3-month period. During this time, the cost of mammography was reduced from $85 to $55 as part of a county-wide campaign to increase breast cancer screening. Factors influencing the mammography decision cited by 50-60% of all women were physician encouragement, print media, electronic media, and reduced cost of mammography. Both mammography use and perceived barriers varied according to education and income. Screened women had significantly more education and higher household incomes than women in the general population, and white women were more likely to be screened than black women. Women with less education and lower income were more likely to identify the importance of physician encouragement than were more affluent and educated women. More highly educated and affluent women were more likely to identify the influence of books, magazines, and newspapers, as well as reduced cost. Women with no prior mammography rated the reduced cost as a more important factor than did women with prior mammography. Like that of other studies, the generalizability of this study was limited by the primarily white population.

The health behavior of mammography tends not to occur in isolation from other health behaviors. Based on NHIS-Health Promotion Disease Prevention (NHIS-HPDP) data (N = 40,104), Rakowski, Rimer, and Bryant (1993) found that women were less likely to have ever had a mammogram if they smoked, reported no regular exercise, had had no recent CBE, did not know BSE, and had no regular source of care. Interestingly, complete abstinence from alcohol was associated with less likelihood of being screened with mammography. These authors conclude that the consistent significance of not smoking, regular exercise, and knowledge about BSE imply that mammography screening may be part of broader lifestyle patterns for some women and that more data about these health practices may help identify underutilizers. As with most studies, the authors express caution about self-reported data and problems of recall time frames. Rimer et al. (1991) found that nonsmoking and seeing a doctor regularly even when healthy had bivariate significance for both recent and repeat mammography.

Health Care Provider Recommendation

In addition to personal variables, mammography behavior and intention are strongly influenced by the behaviors of health care professionals, as has already been noted. Several studies found that physician recommendation varies according to specialty, with gynecologists most likely to recommend mammography, followed by internists, with family practice physicians least likely to make such a recommendation (Fulton et al., 1991; Weinberger et al., 1991; Zapka, Hosmer, Costanza, Harris, & Stoddard, 1992). Zapka et al. (1989) found that the difference in practice specialty did not hold for adherence over time and suggested that differential patterns of mammography according to physician specialty may be a reflection of care-seeking patterns in the United States. Family practice physicians may defer to a woman's gynecologist for mammography referral. Regardless of specialty, physicians with greater knowledge about breast cancer and screening guidelines and more positive perceptions of mammography efficacy are more likely to recommend mammography (Battista, Williams, & McFarlane, 1990; Weinberger et al., 1991).

As with physician recommendation, studies support a relationship between increased mammography utilization and HMO membership, with focus on early detection and prompt treatment. For example, in the RAND experiment comparing random assignment to an HMO versus a fee-for-service plan, more preventive care, including mammography, was provided in the HMO setting (Manning, Liebowitz, Goldberg, Rogers, & Newhouse, 1984). Differences in utilization rates also were found for CBE, Pap test, and colorectal screening. Likewise, Johnson and Murata (1991) found that in a group of 827 patients, women HMO members receiving care at a family health center were 2.5 times more likely to have screening mammography than women enrolled in fee-for-service plans, Medicare, or Medi-Cal. Rimer, Ross, et al. (1992) found that HMO membership appeared to reverse the usual age-related decline in mammography use for women more than 50 years old.

Independent of socioeconomic differences, there is some indication that convenient access to low-cost or free mammography removes utilization differences (Lane et al., 1992). Compared to community respondents, screening rates among women using a public health center but having an annual income below $15,000 were higher. Likewise, having health insurance increases mammography use (Fajardo, Saint-Germain, Meakem, Rose, & Hillman, 1992; Fox & Stein, 1991; Kirkman-Liff & Kronenfeld, 1992; Zapka, Stoddard, Maul, & Costanza, 1991; Zapka et al., 1992). Medicare coverage of biannual mammography may or may not increase utilization, depending in part on physician recommendation patterns for elderly women (Burg & Lane, 1992).

Analysis of NHIS data revealed no significant racial-ethnic differences in mammography utilization, after controlling for education and income (Breen & Kessler, 1994; Calle, Flanders, Thun, & Martin, 1993). Other studies indicate that screening for Hispanic women, particularly those with little English language skill, lags behind (NCI, 1993; Stein et al., 1991). Unfortunately, other than national sampling analysis, most studies had small numbers of nonwhite respondents, thus precluding separate analysis of racial-ethnic differences in predictors for mammography use.

Summary

Consistent and significant correlations have been found between utilization and the HBM variables of susceptibility, benefits, and barriers. Predictive relationships also have been identified for the Theory of Reasoned Action variables of subjective norm and the Transtheoretical Model variables of stages-of-adoption and decisional balance. The mammography decision, however, appears to be a complex process prompted by a combination of personal attitudes, knowledge, health habits, demographic data, and health care system influences. The strongest and most consistent predictors of mammography use are knowledge about guidelines, physician recommendation for mammography, age, educational status, income, and perceived barriers. Costs also appear to make a difference in mammography use for women of all economic levels.

Intervention Research

Community-Based Studies

In an attempt to achieve the goal of an 80% annual mammography rate for women 50 years of age and older, the National Cancer Institute (NCI) funded six regional population-based research projects across the country, beginning in 1987. Each project site conducted baseline surveys, community-based interventions, and follow-up evaluations. Each of the six completed projects succeeded in increasing mammography frequency in its intervention communities, using a wide variety of activities directed toward primary care physicians, community women, and radiologists (NCI, 1993).

At the Philadelphia site, the Fox Chase Cancer Center implemented an intervention program (US Healthcheck) for 50,000 women of ages 50-74 who were enrolled in an HMO between 1987 and 1992 (NCI, 1993). The program was designed to remove two significant barriers: lack of physician recommendation and cost. Annually, all women were sent packets of health education materials and a free mammography referral to a specific radiology site. If no mammography report was received within 45 days, reminder letters were sent. After 95 days with no report, women received one of three randomly selected interventions: (1) second reminder letter, (2) letter from the primary care physician recommending scheduling a preventive visit, or (3) telephone counseling from someone trained to help women overcome barriers to mammography (NCI, 1993). The HBM and Transtheoretical Model provided the conceptual bases for telephone counseling. Program evaluation showed that although the telephone counseling was the most expensive part of the reminder system ($4.92 per call), it also was the most effective. In the telephone interviews, counselors reviewed individual perceptions about susceptibility and perceived benefits of mammography and CBE, and then helped women overcome their personal barriers to taking action.

The Fox Chase site also included a physician intervention. Interventions directed toward physicians included a self-paced tutorial program about breast cancer and computer-generated comparisons of referral practices among physicians in the program. Analysis of tumor stage at diagnosis found that more than 90% of cancers were stage I or II, 5% were stage III, and none were stage IV.

The Awareness of Breast Cancer Screening Project at State University of New York at Stony Brook used different combinations of interventions in three towns, two of which had disproportionately high breast cancer mortality rates (NCI, 1993). A fourth community served as a control for this 1987-1991 study of women of ages 50-75. Low-cost mammography was provided in one community, and a new federal-state breast cancer program provided free mammography in a second community 1 year after project initiation. Other interventions included mass public information campaigns by mail and media, volunteers, speakers bureaus, and flyer distribution by local businesses. African-American and Hispanic advisory group members helped plan programs targeting minority women, such as a health and beauty program for Hispanic women and a gospel program at a black church. For group presentations, a game format helped women identify and discuss personal barriers to mammography. In 6- to 12-month follow-up surveys, more than half reported having mammography after group presentations, and more than half of those women believed that the presentations influenced their decision.

Physician participation in needs assessment and continuing medical education (CME) activities was facilitated by endorsement from physician organizations, key practitioners, hospital department heads, and the American Cancer Society (ACS). Outcome evaluation revealed a decrease from 44% to 24% of women who reported not having mammography because of no physician recommendation (NCI, 1993). In addition, statistically significant increases occurred in physician recommendations for asymptomatic mammography referral, annual and regular referral, and family practitioner referral rates, and there were statistically significant decreases in participants' concern about cost, radiation, and cost-effectiveness. Changes in the control community were not statistically significant.

A 4-year project involving an intervention and a comparison city was conducted at the University of Massachusetts (UMass) (NCI, 1993). Designed to increase and sustain mammography and CBE use by women of ages 50–75, interventions were first directed toward physician mammography referral behavior. Between 1987 and 1990, there was a 50% increase (from 46% to 91%) in the percentage of physicians who reported having recommended annual mammography in the intervention community. Primary care physician interventions included CME programming, grand rounds lectures, and office practice reminder system workshops. Educational and training sessions also were provided for radiologists and radiology technicians. Community interventions included mass media activities, targeted interventions in a family health center, a Breast Health Awareness Month, mammography-focused birthday cards, health fairs, community group educational efforts, and worksite educational materials distribution. Mammography utilization rates increased from 30% to 53%, although there was no significant difference between the intervention and comparison cities due to unanticipated activities introduced in the comparison city.

UMass staff also addressed health systems issues, including legislative efforts toward increased economic access and mammography facility quality control. Within a family health center clinic system, the project trained aides as patient health educators and instituted a physician referral reminder system, a postcard reminder system, and a system to track mammography from referral through radiology reports. Post-intervention screening rates increased from 14% to 56% for women of age 50 years or older (NCI, 1993).

The University of California at Los Angeles Community Mammography Program was targeted toward increasing age-specific adherence to mammography guidelines for women of ages 35–89 (NCI, 1993). Baseline data revealed that 79% of Hispanic women had never had mammography, compared with 52% and 51% of non-Hispanic white and black women, respectively (Fox & Stein, 1991). Only 14% of women choosing a Spanish interview had ever had mammography. Interventions included targeted media campaigns, community presentations, health fairs, volunteers, and a guide to radiology facilities. Patient education brochures and materials were based on the HBM, using focus groups to identify age-, education-, and culturally relevant materials. Outreach to Hispanic women was through a bilingual health education director, bilingual educational materials, church-based subsidized mobile van screenings, presentations at English as a Second Language (ESL) classes, and Spanish media inserts. Between 1988 and 1990, utilization (measured as mammography last year) more than doubled for Hispanics in the treatment community, compared to a control community, despite a significant increase in Spanish-speaking residents in the treatment community.

Following a needs assessment, a multidisciplinary CME program was designed to address cost-containment strategies for screening mammography, radiation risks, mammography efficacy, ACS guidelines, patient concerns, and breast cancer incidence and mortality rates. Gynecologists had the most significant increases in referral rates (NCI, 1993). Researchers suggested that targeted interventions may be needed to reach family practice and internal medicine physicians, and recommended working with respected community groups and physicians to lend medical credibility to intervention programs.

The New Hanover Breast Cancer Screening Program at the University of North Carolina (1987-1991) was designed to increase annual mammography use and physician referral rates among women 50 years of age and older (NCI, 1993). In addition to community interventions similar to these at other NCI sites, a gospel music festival and walk/run marathon were held, and project staff collaborated with a minority task force. Program interventions were based on emphasizing the woman's role in requesting mammography, as well as on providing free mammograms during a cancer screening week and a 6-month reduced-fee mammography program ($29) at a local hospital. Primary care physicians were reached through medical society activities, newsletters, and a large physician membership on the advisory board. In the intervention county, rates for having mammography in the preceding year increased from 35% to 55%, compared with an increase from 30%-40% in the control county. Total mammograms also increased significantly in the intervention county, with an 89% rise.

Despite vigorous minority-targeted public education, black women have continued to have lower mammography utilization, with 19% post-intervention rates for blacks compared to 40% for whites (NCI, 1993). Researchers found that many African-American women did not want to think about breast cancer, their fear of finding cancer outweighing mammography benefits. Harris (NCI, 1993) suggested that follow-up studies should be done to examine whether increased screening will continue after the project "cues to action" are finished.

The University of Washington Fred Hutchinson Cancer Research Center (FHCRC) project used a community organization model to support local initiatives and build local capacity for sustained screening beyond the project time frame. FHCRC staff planned a menu of activities that physician and community boards could select for their counties. Interventions incorporating predisposing, enabling, and reinforcing factors were directed toward increasing mammography and CBE use among women of ages 50-74. Activities unique to this project included rural breast cancer bingo games, urban fashion shows, a quilting contest, breast screening videotape, and physician office staff training. Project data analysis is incomplete. Evaluation will address whether the intensive community organization efforts produced long-term increased mammography utilization.

Mammography rates also increased significantly in five of the six NCI BCSC control communities, after adjusting for age, education, and income (Coleman, Feuer, & NCI BCSC, 1992). Expanded publicity in the lay and professional press may have contributed to this increase. In 1991, increased mammography use was significantly related to annual income greater than $15,000, personal history of benign breast disease, and CBE use. However, a disturbing trend was noted. Among women with mammography, the percentage of women who also had a CBE declined significantly between 1988 and 1991, raising the question of whether an increased focus on mammography may have overshadowed the need for regular CBE and BSE.

Worksite-Based Studies

Several studies have examined the effectiveness of workplace mammography. A 1988 study of one workplace program reported 22% overall participation (Rutledge et al., 1988). A more favorable result was reported by Bodner et al. (1992), when 53% of eligible women participated in an employer-sponsored mammography screening program at Dow Chemical Company. Screening participants were younger than nonparticipants, and more than half were less than 45 years old. For women over 55 years of age, the screening rate was 32%, and current employees were more likely to be screened than retirees (62% versus 20%). Interestingly, four times as many women chose screening with a mobile unit as opposed to a traditional hospital site.

Rimer, Resch, et al. (1992) conducted a study in which women of ages 65 and older ($N = 412$) in eight retirement communities were randomly assigned to control groups (cost subsidy for mammography) and experimental groups (cost subsidy, access to mobile mammography, and tailored health education interventions). Educational materials included a video, printed materials, group discussions, mailed announcements and reminders, and informational letters for women to give to their primary physician. Incentives for mobile mammography were provided. Women in the experimental groups were significantly more likely to have obtained mammography than were the control groups. Findings are limited, however, by small numbers of African-American women and significant differences between control and experimental groups for race, education, and physician recommendation for mammography.

Mayer et al. (1993) conducted a nonequivalent control group study of 1113 randomly selected women at two university campuses. Information about breast cancer screening and recent insurance coverage of mammography was provided through brochures, newsletters, workshops, and a lottery incentive. Although utilization rates increased in both the intervention group and the control group, differences were not significant. At the end of the first year, however, there was a significant increase in reported mammography use among women 50 years of age and older, (86% versus a baseline 67%). Other reports of increased acceptance of workplace screening did not include participation rates (Glanz, Rimer, Lerman, & Gorchov, 1992; Kessler, Rimer, Devine, Gatenby, & Engstrom, 1991).

In an attempt to reach poor African-Americans and Hispanics in Dade County, Florida, information was conveyed through community newspapers, churches, Head Start, various community groups, and minority radio station messages and interview call-in programs (Zavertnik, 1993). Mobile van mammography at community clinics provided cost-effective increased access. On the basis of comparisons with prior breast cancer treatment data, the program was estimated to have saved nearly $1 million dollars over 5 years through early detection and prompt treatment.

Individually Oriented Studies

McDonald et al. (1984) developed a computer medical record system to remind Midwestern general medicine clinic physicians in a university hospital that their patients were due for preventive care services. Patient participants were 65% African-American, and 60% were over 50 years old. Significant increases in mammography referral were identified when reminders were attached to patient charts. Referral patterns were predicted by the degree to which resident physicians read the reminders. Residents with positive attitudes toward computers were more likely to read the reports. In a similar practice setting in New York state, chart reminders were the most successful of strategies designed to increase mammography referrals (Nattinger, Panzer, & Janus, 1989). After 6 months, this prospective controlled study found that mammography referral rates were 54% when chart audits were used, 62% when patient handouts and radiology requisitions were attached to patient charts, and 36% when no interventions were used. No racial-ethnic differences were found.

Skinner, Strecher, and Hospers (1994) compared the effectiveness of standardized reminder letters and computer-generated individualized mailed messages tailored to address women's specific screening and risk status as well as perceptions of breast cancer and mammography. Study participants (N = 899) were randomly selected from two North Carolina family practice groups. After controlling for baseline status, letter type was not associated with stage of adoption in the total sample. Tailored letters, however, had a significant effect on both stage of adoption and mammography use for African-American and lower-income (<$26,000) women. In addition, women receiving tailored letters were more likely to remember and to have read the materials than those receiving standardized letters.

Sung et al. (1992) found that in-home educational interventions delivered to low-income, inner-city African-American women by lay health workers increased the women's mammography adherence, increased their knowledge, and changed their attitudes toward breast and cervical cancer. The women were recruited from community health clinics, door-to-door canvassing in public housing projects, and a community-based advocacy organization. Two educational programs addressed BSE and mammography through printed materials, demonstrations, and video presentations.

In a prospective randomized study, Champion (1994) tested the effect of a belief-oriented intervention as compared to an information intervention. A total of 301 randomly selected women were randomly assigned to one of four groups: (1) control group, (2) belief intervention group, (3) information group, (4) belief and information group. Results indicated that the group that received both the information and the belief intervention was significantly more compliant 1 year following intervention than the control group. In addition, the group receiving the belief intervention alone was significantly more compliant than the control group, although the effects were not as great as for the combined group. The belief intervention included counseling regarding HBM variables.

Methodological Problems

A variety of methodological issues were identified in a review of the mammography utilization literature. The most serious issue is the consistent undersampling of minority populations. Other than studies of national data sets such as the NHIS, only a handful of studies included more than 10% nonwhite women. Therefore, predictive findings and recommendations cannot be generalized for large segments of the population.

A second methodological issue relates to utilization measurement, particularly for adherence over time. Comparisons among studies is difficult because adherence is measured variably as following ACS guidelines for 5 years (Champion, 1992b), annual mammography for 2 years (Rakowski, Rimer, & Bryant, 1993), and repeat mammography with no time specified. Study comparisons also are difficult because populations vary greatly in age.

Measurement of attitude and knowledge also suffers from lack of consistent measurement scales. A few studies used scales that have been tested for reliability and validity, but no two researchers used the same scales to measure HBM variables. No consistent model was used to examine predictor variables, and therefore research studies did not examine a consistent set of variables, which limits the comparability of multivariate analyses.

The impact on utilization of cost, insurance coverage, and income was also difficult to evaluate. Income generally was regarded as a demographic variable and not included in multivariate analysis, because of missing data. Analysis of demographic and economic variables was complicated by inconsistent use of categories for age, education, insurance, and income. Acceptable out-of-pocket costs for mammography were not estimated.

Future Research Directions

Undoubtedly, one of the most critical research needs is to address mammography utilization by minority women, particularly African-American and Hispanic women. Longitudinal intervention studies involving primarily minority women are crucial to determine specific predictive variables. Furthermore, studies are needed that include both white and minority women, with sufficient numbers of minorities to make race- and ethnicity-specific predictive comparisons. Rural women of all socioeconomic levels are another undersampled group, although urban-rural differences in utilization are identified in large population-based data set analysis (Breen & Kessler, 1994; Calle et al., 1993). The more recent literature in this review revealed an increase in studies of older women, addressing a prior concern that older women were undersampled.

A second critical need is to address interval compliance. Most studies to date have addressed one-time mammography screening. Although one-time mammography rates doubled in the early 1990s (Breen & Kessler, 1994), interval compliance rates lagged behind. Mortality benefit for mammography screening will be realized only as women are screened at appropriate intervals. Studies to address development of this continued behavior are urgently needed.

Further research is needed to clarify the influence on the mammography decision of economic barriers such as cost and insurance coverage. Prospective longitudinal studies should address the impact of Medicare coverage on mammography use for older women. Research also needs to address possible interactions among variables, such as between HMO membership and beliefs, and between physician recommendation and beliefs.

Workplace research needs to examine site-specific predictors, such as organizational support for mammography and health promotion in general, as well as employee demographics and individual predisposing factors, such as beliefs, knowledge, health status, and health habits. Mobile van mammography use also needs further exploration to determine whether this screening approach can increase use consistently over time or whether it simplify increases one-time mammography. Mammography is most useful over time when comparisons can be made with prior films. Tracking issues also need to be addressed, so that when women receive mammography at different sites, those essential comparisons can be made.

The diversity of predictive variables suggests the use of a broad model to study utilization, such as addressing in more detail the entire HBM or using the Aday and Andersen Behavioral Model of Health Services Use. Further testing of the Theory of Reasoned Action and stages of adoption may provide clues to mammography use in hard-to-reach populations.

Longitudinal studies need to test adaptations of health promotion and health education efforts directed toward low-income, low-educational-level, and minority and rural women. Kruse and Phillips (1987) suggest that public education materials may be effective primarily for women with higher incomes and educational levels, and physicians may therefore need to spend more time discussing mammography with women who have lower incomes and less education. It is unlikely, however, that such extra attention is actually given to these women.

DETERMINANTS OF BREAST SELF-EXAMINATION ADHERENCE

Descriptive Research

Many descriptive studies have been reported that relate belief variables to BSE using the health belief model (HBM) (Becker, 1974) and the Theory of Reasoned Action (Ajzen & Fishbein, 1980). Alagna and Reddy (1984) used the HBM and the multidimensional health locus of control scale to predict proficient BSE technique and lesion detection for 73 women attending a health fair clinic. Perceptions of the efficacy of BSE was the strongest single predictor. Powerful others, health locus of control, knowledge of correct BSE behaviors, and chance locus of control contributed to the performance variance. Perceived barriers, susceptibility, and severity, and internal locus of control were not predictive, perhaps due to the small sample size.

In 1984, a random sample of women was surveyed ($N = 825$) to predict attendance or nonattendance at a BSE class and satisfactory versus nonsatisfactory BSE practice at a follow-up interview (Calnan & Moss, 1984). Perceived susceptibility and severity were significantly related to attending class. Beliefs concerning benefits and barriers were predictive of BSE practice 1 year after classes. Other variables predicting attendance included use of preventive health services, patterns of personal health behavior, past experience with breast cancer, and personal knowledge of women with breast cancer. At the same time, Calnan and Rutter (1986) reported significant correlations in studying women who were invited to attend BSE class in England (Calnan & Rutter, 1986). During this analysis, women were divided into three groups: attenders, nonattenders, and control. Predictions of behavior at time of initial BSE class and 1 year later were reported. For all three groups, perceived vulnerability was the best predictor of both frequency and technique, although perceived value of BSE was also a significant predictor.

Rutledge reported two studies in which beliefs as well as self-concept, age, and social network were related to BSE practice. In the first study (Rutledge, 1987), 103 women from nine women's groups were assessed using the HBM construct scales of Champion (1984) to measure perceived susceptibility, seriousness, benefits, and barriers. Benefits, barriers, and self-concept were found to be significantly related to frequency of BSE. In a later study (Rutledge & Davis, 1988), a self-report questionnaire was given to 248 women in an industrial college and a YWCA setting. Frequency was used to index BSE compliance. Variables related to BSE frequency included individual items measuring susceptibility, seriousness, benefits, barriers, and general health motivation, as well as confidence, active learning experience with BSE, physician inquiry, age, and encouragement from a health care provider.

Several authors have reported predictors of BSE among elderly women. In one study of 105 female subjects in a senior citizens center with the HBM theoretical framework, frequency and proficiency for BSE were studied (Lashley, 1987). Variables predictive of frequency were barriers, race, and age. Results were inconsistent with the HBM, with increased barriers related to more frequent BSE. BSE proficiency, however, was negatively related to barriers, as predicted. Caucasian and younger subjects reported fewer barriers and had higher technique scores. Williams (1988) assessed 253 women of ages 62–93 for frequency of BSE, health beliefs, health history, and knowledge. Health motivation, barriers, susceptibility, and benefits were found to predict frequency of BSE. In addition, women who had been taught by a nurse performed more frequently. Baulch, Larson, Dodd, and Deitrich (1992) reported on deficits such as visual acuity, tactile sensitivity, and mobility of older women. Limitations including range of motion and inability to use the hands correctly were identified in a significant number of women. Data suggested that when assessing compliance in older women, physical deficits may result in limitation of practice.

Lauver and Angerman (1988) assessed the reliability and validity of selected beliefs and attitudes and their relationship to BSE. Their sample included 64 women attending health programs in a community setting. Factors found to be related to frequency of BSE included self-reported confidence, being able to remember the BSE technique, and interference of BSE with daily activities.

In a series of studies, Champion (1987) assessed the relationship of selected variables to

BSE frequency and proficiency. Using a sample of 588 women with frequency as an outcome variable, barriers, knowledge, susceptibility, and seriousness were significantly related to performance (Champion, 1987). Educational level also was found to be related, with those of higher education having increased frequency. In a later study assessing both frequency and proficiency, past frequency, barriers, health motivation, control, confidence, benefits, and susceptibility were significantly related to current frequency (Champion, 1990). Having BSE checked by a physician and having been taught by a doctor were also related to total behavior.

Looking at validity and reliability of scales, Champion (1993) found significant relationships between BSE performance and susceptibility, seriousness, benefits, barriers, health motivation, and confidence, respectively. Assessing both direct and indirect relationships, Champion and Miller (1992) found that susceptibility, barriers, and health motivation were related to BSE behavior, and significant correlations also were present between perceived confidence and control and perceived control and health motivation.

Ronis and Kaiser (1989) assessed BSE behavior using LISREL analysis. Most predicted paths were supported with their study sample of 619 Detroit women. Beliefs related to benefits and barriers had direct effects on the practice of BSE. Susceptibility had direct effects on BSE, but did not interact with severity as hypothesized. Severity was related to benefits, with high severity of late-stage disease correlated with increased benefit and severity for early-stage disease correlated with decreased benefit.

Shepperd, Solomon, Atkins, Foster, and Frankowski (1990) compared two samples of women of childbearing age: those who had lower income and education and those who had higher income and education. Using regression analysis, forgetting, reliance on medical personnel, and low confidence in performing BSE were the best predictors of BSE frequency. When assessing quality of BSE practice, knowledge was the most significant predictor.

Wyper (1990) used variables from the HBM to study BSE performance using both frequency and thoroughness. A total of 200 women completed a self-administered questionnaire using items related to the HBM. Seriousness and susceptibility formed a threat index, and benefits were weighed against barriers to determine perceived efficacy of BSE. Perceived susceptibility was significantly related to thoroughness of practice, whereas benefits and barriers, both alone and in combination, were related to frequency and thoroughness of practice.

Fletcher, Morgan, O'Malley, Earp, and Degnan (1989) studied the relationship between attitudes, knowledge, and sociodemographic characteristics, respectively, and BSE in older women (Fletcher, Morgan, et al., 1989). Women 40-68 years of age were interviewed, with BSE sensitivity and specificity measured by observing their BSE performance using silicone breast models that contained a total of 18 lumps. Variables with significant univariate association were entered into multivariate analyses. Variables that best explained sensitivity included employment status, health interest, perceived vulnerability to breast cancer, information about health, and knowledge. Use of correct BSE method, knowledge, and self-confidence were related to frequency and intent. The lack of association between proficiency and frequency raises the question about appropriateness of studies measuring only BSE frequency (Fletcher, Morgan, et al., 1989).

Based on the Theory of Reasoned Action, personal normative influences on BSE in older women were examined (Lierman, Young, Kasprzyk, & Benoliel, 1990). The sample consisted of 93 volunteers whose age ranged from 52 to 90 years. Outcome measures included intention and BSE frequency. Intention was strongly correlated with BSE performance, as were attitude and social norms. An attitude score was obtained by questions asking about beliefs regarding the outcome of BSE performance multiplied by the evaluation of these outcomes. Affect was defined as a general feeling of favorableness or unfavorableness toward BSE performance. Social norms included items related to friends, family, regular doctor, husband, friends of family with cancer, daughter, sister, health insurance programs, magazines, newspapers, and advertisements. Social norms were again rated according to the respondent's perceptions of whether the person or group expected her to perform BSE and her motivation to comply. A global social norm measure used a single item asking if most people who were important to the respondent thought she should perform BSE. Using multiplicative scales for attitude and social norm, results support the Theory of Reasoned Action.

In summary, most studies have found significant though moderate correlations with the attitudinal variables specified by the Health Belief Model. The most consistent correlations have been between perceived barriers to practice and BSE frequency or proficiency. Less consistent but significant correlations have been found between perceived susceptibility and benefits, respectively, and the practice of BSE. The least significant variable has been that of perceived seriousness. For the studies that measured seriousness, low or nonsignificant correlations were found with BSE behavior. The reason for this finding may be that perceived seriousness demonstrated little variance, since most women consider breast cancer as very serious. With decreased variance, power is not available to detect significant correlations. In addition to the original Health Belief Model variables, the variable of self-reported confidence was significantly related to BSE proficiency, as was knowledge. Of particular note, two studies that used analyses allowing for the detection of indirect paths found increased effects for attitudes in predicting BSE.

Intervention Research

BSE behavior has been the subject of many intervention studies as well as descriptive studies. For this review, attention was paid to the studies conducted from the mid-1980s to the mid-1990s.

Mamon and Zapka (1985) reported on a randomized trial to improve frequency and proficiency for BSE using a sample of college-age women. Classrooms were randomly assigned to one of four subgroups. Using a Solomon 4-Group design, BSE performance was measured using a 19-item proficiency index. Follow-up response rates for 6-month interviews ranged from 76% to 91%. Subjects were randomly assigned to groups of between 328 and 342 members, allowing adequate sample size for power. Frequency of BSE increased by 26% and proficiency improved by 26%, indicating that the educational program had significant effects.

Calnan (1985) identified a random sample of women of ages 45–64 years from two health districts in the United Kingdom. In the experimental district (BSE district), women were invited to a class on BSE. The educational intervention included an instructional film, discussion, and lecture. Subjects were assessed at baseline and 1 year following the intervention program. Outcomes included assessment of beliefs, behavior, intention, frequency, and proficiency. Women in the district where BSE was offered had a significantly greater number of satisfactory BSE performance outcomes than women in control communities. In addition, women who attended class were significantly different from nonattenders. BSE proficiency, however, was measured by four questions that may not have been adequate for assessing this behavior.

Meyerowitz and Chaiken (1987) used a decision-making theory with "framing" to account for decision making under conditions of risk. Framing related to messages in which BSE was addressed with either positive or negative consequences. Study participants were 90 undergraduate females. Women were randomly assigned to one of four conditions: (1) a pamphlet emphasizing negative consequences of failing to perform BSE, (2) a pamphlet emphasizing positive consequences, (3) a pamphlet with no statements about importance of BSE, and (4) a no-pamphlet control. All pamphlets provided information about BSE. A follow-up telephone interview 4 months after the pamphlets were distributed assessed attitudes and intentions for BSE frequency.

The group that received the pamphlet emphasizing negative consequences of not performing BSE had higher frequency for BSE than other groups.

Baines, Krasowski, and Wall (1988) tested the effectiveness of reminder calendars in increasing BSE frequency and competence. Depending upon whether they were scheduled to return for annual screening in odd or even months, women either were assigned to a control group or received calendars to record the date of BSE. BSE frequency was assessed through questionnaires completed at annual screening and by nurse examiners who evaluated BSE proficiency. No significant difference was found between experimental and control groups. Lauver (1989) tested four informational interventions on frequency and proficiency for BSE. A total of 204 women were recruited from meetings and industrial sites. Interventions included: (1) taped information about BSE, a pamphlet, and a reminder calendar; (2) information packet plus tactile sensory information on texture of normal as opposed to abnormal tissue; (3) information packet plus instructions on coping with an abnormal finding; and (4) combination of groups (2) and (3). At 3 and 6 months post-intervention, frequency and proficiency of BSE were assessed by telephone interview. Although significant effects pre- to postintervention were realized, no differences among groups were found. An interaction between receiving sensory information and previous experience was observed at 3 months, indicating that women who had previously performed BSE and received sensory information increased scores more than those who received only information.

Assaf, Cummings, Graham, Metlin, and Marshall (1985) compared three methods of BSE training: (1) a pamphlet describing how to do BSE, (2) a videotaped demonstration of BSE plus pamphlet, and (3) training practice and feedback on a breast model plus a pamphlet. A total of 462 women from a cancer screening clinic were studied over a 3-month period. Women were scheduled for 3-month follow-up, with 84% completing the interview. Both BSE frequency and proficiency were tested as outcome measures, as was lump detection performance. Women who were trained on the breast model were significantly more likely to report monthly BSE practice, had higher levels of confidence, and demonstrated higher proficiency scores. BSE proficiency was most strongly associated with accuracy of lump detection.

Young and Marty (1985) completed an experimental intervention that included a lecture related to breast cancer and BSE as well as a film and examination of a breast model. Guided practice over clothing with instructor feedback was included. College women completed pre- and postintervention questionnaires assessing frequency, confidence, and BSE performance at baseline and 3½ months after intervention. Subjects in the experimental group had significantly higher reported frequency.

Carter, Feldman, Tiefer, and Hausdorff (1985) conducted a randomized trial in comparing three BSE experimental formats on improving BSE frequency and proficiency. A sample of 1733 women were randomly assigned to one of three experimental groups. One group received an educational session using a cognitive approach in which factual information was given. A second group received an affective approach in which feelings about breast cancer and BSE were addressed. A third experimental group received both types of material. Follow-up periods ranged from 3 to 24 months. Significant differences were not found between groups; however, frequency and proficiency improved in all groups. Of particular interest is that this study used both an observation checklist and lump detection on silicone models to assess outcomes.

Fletcher et al. (1990) assessed 300 women who were randomly assigned to one of three groups using the outcomes of BSE frequency and proficiency. Groups included: (1) a Mammacare group that received a 45-minute nurse instruction, stressing tactile skills; (2) a traditional group that received a 30-minute nurse instruction emphasizing circular technique; and (3) a control group. In addition, women in each group were split in terms of receiving or not receiving physician encouragement. The group that was taught using the Mammacare method had a breast model to practice technique at home. Both intervention groups had pamphlets and calendar reminders. Outcomes included sensitivity and specificity measurements on breast models, frequency of BSE, and observed proficiency. Physician encouragement had little or no effect on outcomes. The experimental group receiving Mammacare instruction had significant increases for identifying lumps in the manufactured model as compared to women in the traditional teaching or control group. Frequency improved in all groups. Mayer and Frederiksen (1986) randomly assigned faculty and staff to one of three groups: (1) phone prompt, (2) mail prompt, and (3) no-prompt control. A workshop included a lecture on breast cancer and BSE, a demonstration by the instructor, and a practice session on detecting lumps in a breast model. Subjects were randomly assigned to receive bimonthly mail or phone prompts or no prompts. A strength of this study was that the participants were matched prior to randomization with respect to previous BSE behavior, age, and educational level. Groups receiving both mail and phone prompts were more likely to have completed BSE at least once. Groups did not differ, however, regarding monthly practice.

In a carefully executed study, Grady (1988) tested rewards for increasing BSE compliance. Self-rewards included a list of 25 suggested rewards that were under the woman's control and included such things as reading a desired book. Women were recruited from a family practice and, using a factorial design, were assigned to either an external reward, a self-reward, or a no-reward group. The self-reward group included a self-management calendar with reminder stickers, and the external reward group received a lottery ticket or Susan B. Anthony dollar every time the investigators received a BSE record. In addition, for women in the self-reward group, self-reward items were suggested for use after doing BSE. Frequency for BSE was determined by the number of returned BSE record forms. Women in the external reward group reported significantly higher rates of BSE than those in the no-reward group.

Worden et al. (1990) tested a community-wide program of BSE training and maintenance. All women in each of four Vermont communities were assigned to one of the following groups: (1) BSE training plus maintenance, (2) training alone, (3) control with full measurement, or (4) control with low measurement. The BSE training program consisted of presentations by local health agency nurses to small groups of women in clubs and organizations. Presentations were approximately an hour in length and included films, discussion about barriers to BSE, guided practice, and a question-and-answer period. In addition, a calendar booklet to cue women to BSE was left with subjects. Activities designed to address barriers to adherence following initial BSE training were emphasized. Strategies focused on maintenance, confidence, and decreasing anxiety. Random digit dialing telephone surveys were conducted at baseline and at 1- and 2-year follow-up with all adult women in the first three communities, a total of 637 women. The low-measure control group received only baseline and 2-year follow-up surveys and included 238 women. Home interviews were completed to determine BSE palpation skills and lump detection in models and were done at both 1-year and 2-year follow-up surveys. Significant results surfaced for women receiving the training program as compared with the control group. Follow-up surveys indicated significant increases in BSE frequency, quality, and number of detected lumps. At 2-year follow-up, women in the community receiving maintenance showed greater improvement in quality of BSE and breast lump detection than women in other communities.

Champion and Scott (1993) used a prospective randomized approach to assess the effect of information belief strategies in increasing BSE frequency and proficiency. Using a 2 × 2 factorial design, 301 women were randomly assigned to one of four groups: (1) control, (2) belief intervention, (3) information intervention, or (4) belief/information intervention. Women in the belief group received counseling related to health beliefs about susceptibility, seriousness, benefits, barriers, health motivation, and control. Women in the information group received a standardized teaching approach using ACS guidelines. Women in the belief/information group received a combination of both belief and information interventions. Results indicated significant increases in proficiency in the group receiving the information intervention. An additional significant effect in lump detection was observed for women receiving both belief and information interventions. Outcome variables were measured by self-reported frequency and proficiency scales as well as nurse observation, checklists, and lump detection in synthetic models.

Most intervention studies found increased frequency or proficiency in BSE following interventions. One study found that information emphasizing the negative consequences of not performing BSE increased practice.

Most interventions reviewed in this section included demonstration with corrective feedback. This approach was successful in increasing both BSE frequency and proficiency. In addition, the studies that incorporated belief messages—such as addressing benefits or susceptibility, or discussion of barriers—increased one or more of BSE frequency, proficiency, and lump detection. Studies using lump detection as part of the outcome measures provided the most useful information about the impact of educational strategies. Finally, several studies tested the effects of prompts on BSE behavior. Although significant results were realized, this approach may be impractical to implement over time.

Methodological Problems

Many issues surfaced in the review of adherence literature related to BSE. This behavior was studied frequently during the decade in question using many descriptive and intervention approaches, but there were many measurement problems. Many studies attempted to link attitudinal variables from the HBM or Fishbein and Ajzen with BSE behavior. A variety of scales or single items were used to measure predictive constructs, usually with little or no attempt to address measurement issues. A few studies did use scales that have been developed and tested for validity and reliability (Rutledge, 1987; Champion, 1993; Lashley, 1987). The somewhat low correlations of attitude with behavior that were found may be related to measurement. If attitudinal or behavioral measures do indeed incorporate error, low correlations might be expected. It is only through using measurements that have been consistently tested and shown to be valid and reliable that true correlations can surface. With such a lack of consistency in measuring, comparisons among studies are difficult. Even more problematic, however, were measurements for BSE behavior. Fletcher, Morgan, et al. (1989) found no correlation between frequency and proficient practice, yet several studies used only self-reported frequency as an outcome measure. It is possible that frequency is overreported using self-report measures and that frequency may not relate to actual proficiency of BSE. Even the proficiency scales that were used in several studies are open to self-report bias. The best measure of BSE proficiency is ability to detect actual lumps in a synthetic model (Champion & Scott, 1993; Fletcher, O'Malley, Pilgrim, & Gonzalez, 1989; Worden et al., 1990).

Another issue related to measurement of constructs is that of adequate models to assess relationships. In most of the studies reviewed, relationships were tested using simple bivariate correlations or linear multiple regressions. Only two studies attempted to assess indirect relationships of BSE to practice. Using a LISREL approach, indirect influence of variables became apparent. Many studies were perhaps limited in findings because assessment of indirect paths was lacking.

Still another measurement issue concerns that of sampling. Many studies used convenience sampling, and several studies used college populations. Because frequency of breast cancer is so low in young women and because these samples may be very different from the general population, results cannot be generalized. Only a few studies used probability sampling, and even fewer attempted to assess culturally or generationally diverse populations. With these limitations, it is difficult to generalize findings to women most likely to benefit from BSE.

Still another concern is that of maintaining behavior over time. Many studies assesses behaviors at 3-6 months after intervention. Few studies assessed BSE over time, and those that did generally found a decrease in BSE frequency. Maintenance of BSE remains a problem. Many of the interventions did increase BSE proficiency and frequency at least temporarily, but how long this increase continued is not known. In one of the more thorough studies, Fletcher (1993) reported that after 1 year, only a small percentage of women could be classified as frequent and competent practitioners.

Future Research Directions

Future interventions must stress the positive aspects of BSE practice. Future work on BSE also must address several of the methodological issues presented herein. First, adequate measurement of BSE proficiency using synthetic models for lump detection must be used. Second, interventions need to be time-efficient and simple for delivery to large numbers of women. As reported by Baulch et al. (1992), BSE ability may be limited in older women who have limited range of motion. In addition, BSE maintenance may be a separate but just as important goal as initially attaining competence. Studies to assess competent practice must include longitudinal designs. Finally, the cost-effectiveness of interventions to increase BSE must be addressed. In today's health care arena, it is especially important to identify the cost of training women in BSE, and this issue has received little attention.

In summary, BSE may have unrealized potential to detect breast cancer even with periodic mammography. However, unless the methodological issues that have surfaced during past research are addressed, and women are trained to examine their breasts effectively, BSE efficacy may not be realized.

REFERENCES

Ajzen, I., & Fishbein, M. (1980). *Understanding attitudes and predicting behavior*. Englewood Cliffs, NJ: Prentice-Hall.

Alagna, S. W., & Reddy, D. M. (1984). Predictors of proficient technique and successful lesion detection in breast self-examination. *Health Psychology*, *3*(2), 113-127.

Anderson, I., Aspergren, K., Janzon, L., Landberg, T., Lindholm, K., Linell, F., Ljungberg, O., Ranstam, J., & Sigfusson, B. (1988). Mammographic screening and mortality from breast cancer: The Malmo mammographic screening trial. *British Medical Journal*, *297*, 342-348.

Assaf, A. R., Cummings, K. M., Graham, S., Mettlin, C., & Marshall, J. R. (1985). Comparison of three methods of teaching women how to perform breast self-examination. *Health Education Quarterly*, *12*(3), 259-272.

Baines, C. J., Krasowski, T. P., & Wall, C. (1988). Incentives for breast self-examination: Role of the calendar. *Cancer Detection and Prevention*, *13*, 109-114.

Baines, C. J., To, T., & Wall, C. (1990). Women's attitudes to screening after participation in the national breast screening study. *Cancer*, *65*, 1663-1669.

Bassett, L., & Butler, D. (1991). Mammography and early breast cancer detection. *American Family Physician*, *43*(2), 547-557.

Battista, R. N., Williams, J. I., & McFarlane, L. A. (1990). Determinants of preventive practices in fee-for-service primary care. *American Journal of Preventive Medicine*, *6*,(1), 6-11.

Baulch, Y. S., Larson, P. J., Dodd, M. J., & Deitrich, C. (1992). The relationship of visual acuity, tactile sensitivity, and mobility of the upper extremities to proficient breast self-examination in women 65 and older. *Oncology Nursing Forum*, *19*(9), 1367-1372.

Becker, M. H. (1974). *The health belief model and personal health behavior*. Thorofare, NJ: Charles B. Slack.

Bodner, K. M., Bond, G. G., Phillips, P. L., Bollinger, L. J., Lipps, T. E., & Cook, R. R. (1992). Preliminary evaluation of an employer-sponsored mammography screening program. *Journal of Occupational Medicine*, *34*, 793-796.

Breen, N., & Kessler, L. (1994). Changes in the use of screening mammography. Evidence from the 1987 and 1990 National Health Interview Surveys. *American Journal of Public Health*, *84*, 62-67.

Burg, M. A., & Lane, D. S. (1992). Mammography referrals for elderly women: Is Medicare reimbursement likely to make a difference? *Health Services Research*, *27*, 505-516.

Calle, E. E., Flanders, W. D., Thun, M. J., & Martin, L. M. (1993). Demographic predictors of mammography and Pap smear screening in US women. *American Journal of Public Health*, *83*, 53-60.

Calnan, M. (1985). An evaluation of the effectiveness of a class teaching breast self-examination. *British Journal of Medical Psychology*, *58*, 317-329.

Calnan, M. W., & Moss, S. (1984). The health belief model and compliance with education given at a class in breast self-examination. *Journal of Health and Social Behavior*, *25*, 198-210.

Calnan, M., & Rutter, D. R. (1986). Do health beliefs predict health behavior? An analysis of breast self-examination. *Social Science and Medicine*, *22*(6), 673-678.

Carter, A. C., Feldman, J. G., Tiefer, L., & Hausdorff, J. K. (1985). Methods of motivating the practice of breast self-examination: A randomized trial. *Preventive Medicine*, *14*, 555-572.

Champion, V. L. (1984). Instrument development for health belief model constructs. *Advances in Nursing Science*, *6*(3), 73-85.

Champion, V. L. (1987). The relationship of breast self-examination to health belief model variables. *Research in Nursing and Health*, *10*, 375-382.

Champion, V. L. (1990). Breast self-examination in women 35 and older: A prospective study. *Journal of Behavioral Medicine*, *13*(6), 523-528.

Champion, V. L. (1991). The relationship of selected variables to breast cancer detection behaviors in women 35 and older. *Oncology Nursing Forum*, *18*, 733-739.

Champion, V. L. (1992a). Breast self-examination in women 65 and older. *Journal of Gerontology*, *47*(Special Issue), 75-79.

Champion V. L. (1992b). Compliance with guidelines for mammography screening. *Cancer Detection and Prevention*, *16*, 253-258.

Champion V. L. (1993). Instrument refinement for breast cancer screening behaviors. *Nursing Research*, *42*, 139-143.

Champion V. L. (1994). Strategies to increase mammography utilization. *Medical Care*, *32*(2), 118-129.

Champion V. L., & Miller, T. K. (1992). Variables related to breast self-examination. *Psychology of Women Quarterly*, *16*, 81-96.

Champion V. L. & Scott, C. (1993). Effects of a procedural/belief intervention on breast self-examination performances. *Research in Nursing and Health*, *16*, 163-170.

Champion V. L., Skinner, C. S., Miller, A. M., Goulet, R. J., & Wagler, K. (in press). Factors influencing effect of mammography screening in a university workplace. *Cancer Detection and Prevention*.

Coleman, E. A., Feuer, E. J., & the NCI Breast Cancer Screening Consortium. (1992). Breast cancer screening among women from 65 to 74 years of age in 1987-88 and 1991. *Annals of Internal Medicine*, *117*, 961-966.

Collette, H. J. A., Rombach, J. J., Day, N. E., & DeWaard, F. (1984). Evaluation of screening for breast cancer in a non-randomized study (The Dom Project) by means of a case-control study. *Lancet*, Vol. 1 (8388), 1224-1226.

Costanza, M. E., Stoddard, A., Gaw, V. P., & Zapka, J. G. (1992). The risk factors of age and family history and their relationship to screening mammography utilization. *Journal of American Geriatric Society*, *40*(8), 774-778.

Degnan, D., Harris, R., Ranney, J., Quade, D., Earp, J. A., & Gonzalez, J. (1992). Measuring mammography: Two methods compared. *American Journal of Public Health*, *82*(10), 1385-1386.

Fajardo, L. L., Saint-Germain, M., Meakem, T. J., Rose, C., & Hillman, B. J. (1992). Factors influencing women to undergo screening mammography. *Radiology*, *184*, 59-63.

Feldman, J. G., Carter, A. C., Nicastri, A. D., & Hosat, S. T. (1981). Breast self-examination: Relationship to stage of breast cancer at diagnosis. *Cancer*, *47*, 2740-2745.

Fletcher, S. W. (1993). Board recommends changes of draft breast cancer screening guidelines. *Journal of the National Cancer Institute*, *85*(22), 1794-1795.

Fletcher, S. W., Morgan, T. M., O'Malley, M. S., Earp, J. A. L., & Degnan, D. (1989). Is breast self-examination predicted by knowledge, attitudes, beliefs, or sociodemographic characteristics? *American Journal of Preventive Medicine*, *5*(4), 207-215.

Fletcher, S. W., O'Malley, M. S., Earp, J. A. L., Morgan, T. M., Lin, S., & Degnan, D. (1990). How best to teach women breast self-examination. *Annals of Internal Medicine*, *112*, 772-779.

Fletcher, S., O'Malley, M., Pilgrim, C., & Gonzalez, J. (1989). How do women compare with internal medicine residents in breast lump detection? *Journal of General Internal Medicine*, *4*, 277-283.

Foster, R. S., & Costanza, M. C. (1984). Breast self-examination practices and breast cancer survival. *Cancer*, *53*(4), 999-1005.

Fox, S. A., Klos, D. S., Tsou, C. V., & Baum, J. K. (1987). Breast cancer screening recommendations: Current status of women's knowledge. *Family and Community Health*, *10*(3), 39-50.

Fox, S. A., & Stein, J. A. (1991). The effect of physician-patient communication on mammography utilization by different ethnic groups. *Medical Care*, *29*(11), 1065-1082.

Fulton, J. P., Buechner, J. S., Denman Scott, H., DeBuono, B. A., Feldman, J. P., Smith, R. A., & Kovenock, D. (1991). A study guided by the health belief model of the predictors of breast cancer screening of women ages 40 and older. *Public Health Reports*, *106*, 410-420.

Gastrin, G., Miller, A., To, T., Aronson, K., Wall, C., Hakana, M., Louhivuori, K., & Pukkala, E. (1994). Incidence and mortality from breast cancer in the Mama program for breast screening in Finland, 1973-1986. *Cancer*, *73*(8)1, 2168-2173.

Gallup Organization. (1988). *Women's attitudes regarding breast cancer*. Princeton, NJ: Gallup Organization.

Glanz, K., Rimer, B. K., Lerman, C., & Gorchov, P. McG. (1992). Factors influencing acceptance of mammography: Implications for enhancing worksite cancer control. *American Journal of Health Promotion*, 7, 28-36.

Glockner, S. M., Hilton, S. V. W., Holden, M. G., & Norcross, W. A. (1992). Women's attitudes toward screening mammography. *American Journal of Preventive Medicine*, *8*, 69-77.

Grady, K. E. (1988). The effect of reward on compliance with breast self-examination. *Journal of Behavioral Medicine*, *11*(1), 43-57.

Green, L., Kreuter, M., Deeds, S., & Partridge, K. (1980). *Health education planning: A diagnostic approach*. Palo Alto, CA: Mayfield.

Greenwald, P., Nasca, P., Lawrence, E., Norton, J., McGarrah, P., Gabride, T., & Carlton, K. (1978). Estimated effect of breast self-examination and routine physician examination on breast-cancer mortality. *New England Journal of Medicine*, *299*(6), 271-273.

Haughey, B. P., Marshall, J. R., Nemoto, T., Kroldart, K., Mettlin, C., & Swanson, M. (1988). Breast self-examination: Reported practices, proficiency, and stage of disease at diagnosis. *Oncology Nursing Forum*, *15*(3), 315-319.

Hill, D., White, V., Jolley, D., & Mapperson, K. (1988). Self-examination of the breasts: Is it beneficial? Meta-analyses of studies investigating BSF and extent of disease in patients with breast cancer. *British Medical Journal*, *297*, 271-273.

Huguley, C., Brown, R., Greenburg, R., & Clark, W. Breast self-examination and survival from breast cancer. *Cancer*, *62*, 1389-1396.

Hyman, R. B., Baker, S., Ephraim, R., Moadel, A., & Philip, J. (1994). *Journal of Behavioral Medicine*, *17*(4), 391-406.

Johnson, R., & Murata, P. (1988). Demographic, clinical, and financial factors relating to the completion rate of screening mammograph. *Cancer Detection and Prevention*, *11*, 259-266.

Kessler, H. B., Rimer, B. K., Devine, P. J., Gatenby, R. A., & Engstrom, P. F. (1991). Corporate-sponsored breast cancer screening at the work site: Results of a statewide program. *Radiology*, *179*, 107-110.

Kirkman-Liff, B., & Kronenfeld, J. (1992). Access to cancer screening services for women. *American Journal of Public Health*, *82*, 733-735.

Koroltchouk, V., Stanley, K., & Stjensward, J. (1990). The control of breast cancer: A World Health Organization perspective. *Cancer*, *65*(12), 2803-2810.

Kruse, J., & Phillips, D. M. (1987). Factors influencing women's decision to undergo mammography. *Obstetrics and Gynecology*, *70*, 744-748.

Kuroishi, T., Tominaga, S., Ota, J., Horino, T., Taguchi, T., Ishida, T., Yokoe, T., Izuo, M., Ogita, M., Ito, S., Abe, R., Yoshida, K., Morimoto, T., Enomoto, K., Tashiro, H., Kashiki, Y., Yamamoto, S., Kido, C., Honda, K., Sasakawa, M., Fukuda, M., & Watanabe, H. (1992). The effect of breast self-examination on early detection and survival. *Japanese Journal of Cancer Research*, *83*, 344-350.

Lane, D. S., & Fine, H. L. (1983). Compliance with mammography referrals. *New York State Journal of Medicine*, *83*, 173-176.

Lane, D. S., Polednak, A. P., & Burg, M. A. (1992). Breast cancer screening practices among users of county-funded health centers vs women in the entire community. *American Journal of Public Health*, *82*, 199-203.

Lantz, P. M., Remington, P. L., & Soref, M. (1990). Self-reported barriers to mammography: Implications for physicians. *Wisconsin Medical Journal*, *89*, 602-606.

Lashley, M. E. (1987). Predictors of breast self-examination practice among elderly women. *Advances in Nursing Science*, *9*(4), 25-34.

Lauver, D., (1989). Instructional information and breast self-examination practice. *Research in Nursing and Health*, *12*, 11-19.

Lauver, D., & Angerman, M. (1988). Development of a questionnaire to measure beliefs and attitudes about breast self-examination. *Cancer Nursing*, *11*(1), 51-57.

Lauver, D., & Angerman, M. (1989). Overadherence with breast self-examination recommendations. *IMAGE: Journal of Nursing Scholarship*, *22*(3), 148-152.

Lerman, C., Rimer, B., Trock, B., Balshem, A., & Engstrom, P. F. (1990). Factors associated with repeat adherence to breast cancer screening. *Preventive Medicine*, *19*, 279-290.

Lierman, L. M., Young, H. M., Kasprzyk, D., & Benoliel, J. Q. (1990). Predicting breast self-examination using the theory of reasoned action. *Nursing Research*, *39*(2), 97-101.

Locker, A. P., Casildine, J., Mitchell, A. K., Blamey, R. W., Roebuck, E. J., & Elston, C. W. (1989). Results from a seven-year programme of breast self-examination in 89,010 women. *British Journal of Cancer*, *60*(3), 401-405.

Mamon, J. A., & Zapka, J. G. (1985). Improving frequency and proficiency of breast self-examination: Effectiveness of an education program. *American Journal of Public Health*, *75*(6), 618-624.

Manning, W. G., Leibowitz, A., Goldberg, G. A., Rogers, W. H., & Newhouse, J. P. (1984). A controlled trial of the effect of a prepaid group practice on use of services. *New England Journal of Medicine*, *310*, 1505-1510.

Mant, D., Vessey, M. P., Neil, A., McPherson, K., & Jones, L. (1986). Breast self examination and breast cancer stage at diagnosis. *British Journal of Cancer*, *55*(2), 207-211.

Mayer, J. A., & Frederiksen, L. W. (1986). Encouraging long-term compliance with breast self-examination: The evaluation of prompting strategies. *Journal of Behavioral Medicine*, *9*(2), 179-189.

Mayer, J. A., Jones, J. J., Eckhardt, L. E., Haliday, J., Bartholomew, S., Slymen, D. J., & Hovell, M. F. (1993). *American Journal of Preventive Medicine*, *9*, 244-249.

McDonald, C. J., Hui, S. L., Smith, D. M., Tierney, W. M., Cohen, S. J., Weinberger, M., & McCabe, G. P. (1984). Reminders to physicians from an introspective computer medical record. *Annals of Internal Medicine*, *100*, 130-138.

Mettlin, C. J., & Smart, C. R. (1993). The Canadian National Breast Screening Study: An appraisal and implications for early detection policy. *Cancer*, *72*(4), 1461-1465.

Meyerowitz, B. E., & Chaiken, S. (1987). The effect of message framing on breast self-examination attitudes, intentions, and behavior. *Journal of Personality and Social Psychology*, *52*(3), 500-510.

Miller, A. B. (1993). Canadian National Breast Screening Study: Public health implications. *Canadian Journal of Public Health*, *84*(1), 14-16.

Miller, A., & Champion, V. L. (1993). Mammography in women 50 and Older. Predisposing and enabling characteristics. *Cancer Nursing*, *16*(4), 260-269.

Montano, D. E., & Taplin, S. H. (1991). A test of an expanded theory of reasoned action to predict mammography participation. *Social Science and Medicine*, *6*, 733-741.

Nattinger, A. B., Panzer, R. J., & Janus, J. (1989). Improving the utilization of screening mammography in primary care practices. *Archives of Internal Medicine*, *149*, 2087-2092.

NCI (1993). *The picture of health: How to increase breast cancer screening in your community*. Bethesda, MD: Author.

NCI Breast Cancer Screening Consortium. (1990). Screening mammography: A missed clinical opportunity? *Journal of the American Medical Association*, *264*, 54-58.

Newcomb, P. A., Weiss, N. S., Storer, B. E., Scholes, D., Young, B. E., & Voigt, L. F. (1991). Breast self-examination in relation to the occurrence of advanced breast cancer. *Journal of the National Cancer Institute*, *83*, 260-265.

O'Malley, M. (1993). Cost-effectiveness of two nurse-led programs to teach breast self-examination. *American Journal of Preventive Medicine*, *9*(3), 139-144.

Parker, S., Tong, T., Bolden, S., & Wingo, P. (1996). Cancer statistics. *CA—A Cancer Journal for Clincians*, *44*(1), 5-45.

Philip, J., Harris, G., Flaherty, C., & Joslin, C. A. F. (1986). Clinical measures to assess the practice and efficiency of breast self-examination. *Cancer*, *58*, 973-977.

Rakowski, W., Dube, C. E., Marcus, B. H., Prochaska, J. O., Velicer, W. F., & Abrams, D. B. (1992). Assessing elements of women's decisions about mammography. *Health Psychology*, *11*, 111-118.

Rakowski, W., Fulton, J. P., & Feldman, J. P. (1993). Women's decision making about mammography: A replication of the relationship between stages of adoption and decisional balance. *Health Psychology*, *12*, 209-214.

Rakowski, W., Rimer, B. K., & Bryant, S. A. (1993). Integrating behavior and intention regarding mammography by respondents in the 1990 National Health Interview Survey of Health Promotion and Disease Prevention. *Public Health Reports*, *108*, 605-624.

Rimer, B., Jones, W., Wilson, C., Bennett, D., & Engstrom P. (1983). Planning a cancer control program for older citizens. *Gerontologist*, *23*, 384-389.

Rimer, B. K., Keintz, K. M., Kessler, H. B., Engstrom, P. F., & Rason, J. R. (1989). Why women resist screening mammography: Patient-related barriers. *Radiology*, *172*, 243-246.

Rimer, B. K., & King, E. (1992). Why aren't older women getting mammograms and clinical breast exams? *Women's Health Institute*, *2*, 94-101.

Rimer, B. K., Resch, N., King, E., Ross, E., Lerman, C., Boyce, A., Kessler, H., & Engstrom, P. F. (1992). Multistrategy health education program to increase mammography use among women ages 65 and older. *Public Health Reports*, *107*, 369-380.

Rimer, B. K., Ross, E., Cristinzio, C. S., & King, E. (1992). Older women's participation in breast screening. *Journal of Gerontology*, *47*, 85-91.

Rimer, B. K., Trock, B., Engstrom, P. F., Lerman, C., & King, E. (1991). Why do some women get regular mammograms? *American Journal of Preventive Medicine*, *7*, 69-74.

Roberts, M. M., Alexander F. E., Anderson, T. J., Chetly, U., Donnan, P. T., Forrest, P., Hepburn, W., Huggins, A., Kirtpatrick, A. E., Lamb, J., Muir, B. B., & Prescott, R. J. (1990). Edinburgh trial of screening for breast cancer: Mortality at seven years. *Lancet*, *335*, 241-246.

Ronis, D. L., & Kaiser, M. K. (1989). Correlations of breast self-examination in a sample of college women: Analyses of linear structural relations. *Journal of Applied Social Psychology*, *19*, 1068-1084.

Rutledge, D. N. (1987). Factors related to women's practice of breast self-examination. *Nursing Research*, *36*(2), 117-121.

Rutledge, D. N., & Davis, G. T. (1988). Breast self-examination compliance and the health belief model. *Oncology Nursing Forum*, *15*(2), 175-179.

Rutledge, D. N., Hartmann, W. H., Kinman, P. O., & Winfield, A. C. (1988). Exploration of factors affecting mammography behaviors. *Preventive Medicine*, *17*, 412-422.

Schechter, C., Vanchieri, C. F., & Crofton, C. (1990). Evaluating women's attitudes and perceptions in developing mammography promotion messages. *Public Health Reports*, *105*, 253-257.

Semiglazov, V. F., & Moiseenko, V. M. (1987). Breast self-examination for the early detection of breast cancer: A USSR/WHO controlled trial in Leningrad. *Bulletin of the World Health Organization*, *65*(3), 391-396.

Senie, R. T., Rosen, P. P., Lesser, M. L., & Kinne, D. W. (1981). Breast self-examination and medical examination related to breast cancer stage. *American Journal of Public Health*, *71*(6), 583-590.

Shapiro, S., Venet, W., Strax, P., Venet, L., & Roeser, R. (1982). Ten- to fourteen-year effect of screening on breast cancer mortality. *Journal of the National Cancer Institute*, *69*(2), 349-355.

Shepperd, S. L., Solomon, L. J., Atkins, E., Foster, R. S., Jr., & Frankowski, B. (1990). Determinants of breast self-examination among women of lower income and lower education. *Journal of Behavioral Medicine*, *13*(4), 359-371.

Shwartz, M. (1992). Validation of a model of breast cancer screening: An outlier suggests the value of breast self-examination. *Medical Decision Making*, *12*, 222-228.

Skinner, C. S., Strecher, V. J., & Hospers, H. (1994). Physicians' recommendations for mammography: Do tailored messages make a difference? *American Journal of Public Health*, *84*, 43-49.

Smith, E. M., & Burns, T. L. (1985). The effects of breast self-examination in a population-based cancer registry. *Cancer, 55*, 432-437.

Stein, J. A., Fox, S. A., & Murata, P. J. (1991). The influence of ethnicity, socioeconomic status, and psychological barriers on use of mammography. *Journal of Health and Social Behavior, 32*, 101-113.

Stein, J. A., Fox, S. A., Murata, P. J., & Morisky, D. E. (1992). Mammography usage and health belief model. *Health Education Quarterly, 4*, 447-462.

Sung, J. F. C., Coates, R. J., Williams, J. E., Liff, J. M., Greenberg, R. S., McGrady, G. E., Avery, B. Y., & Blumenthal, D. S. (1992). Cancer screening intervention among black women in inner-city Atlanta—Design of a study. *Public Health Reports, 107*, 381-388.

Tabar, L., Fegerberg, G., Duffy, S., Day, N., Gad, A., & Grontoft, O. (1992). Update of the Swedish two-county program of mammographic screening for breast cancer. *Radiologic Clinics of North America, 30*, 187-209.

Tabar, L., Gad, A., Holmberg, L. H., Ljungquist, U., Fagerberg, C. J. G., Baldetorp, L., Grontoft, O., Lundstrom, B., & Manson, J. C. (1985). Reduction in mortality from breast cancer after mass screening with mammography. *Lancet, 1*, 829-832.

Taplin, S., Anderman, C., & Grothaus, L. (1989). Breast cancer risk and participation in mammographic screening. *American Journal of Public Health, 79*, 1494-1498.

Taplin, S. H., & Montano, D. E. (1993). Attitudes, age, and participation in mammographic screening: A prospective analysis. *Journal of the American Board of Family Practice, 6*, 13-23.

Tippy, P., Falvo, D. R., & Woehlke, P. (1989). Fee structure as a determinant of patient's choice to undergo mammography. *Family Practice Research Journal, 9*, 43-51.

Verbeek, A. L. M., Hendriks, J. H. C. L., & Holland, R. (1985). Mammographic screening and breast cancer mortality: Age specific effects in Nijmegen project, 1975-1982. *Lancet, 1*, 865-866.

Verbeek, A. L. M., Holland, R., Sturmans, F., Hendriks, J. H. C. L., Mravunac, M., & Day, N. E. (1984). Reduction of breast cancer mortality through mass screening with modern mammography. *Lancet, 1*, 1222-1223.

Weinberger, M., Saunders, A. F., Samsa, G. P., Bearon, L. B., Gold, D. T., Brown, T., Booher, P., & Loehrer, P. J., (1991). Breast cancer screening in older women: Practices and barriers reported by primary care physicians. *Journal of American Geriatric Society, 39*, 22-29.

Williams, R. D. (1988). Factors affecting the practice of breast self-examination in older women. *Oncology Nursing Forum, 15*(5), 611-616.

Worden, J. K., Solomon, L. J., Flynn, B. S., Costanza, M. C., Foster, R. S., Dorwaldt, M. A., & Weaver, S. O. (1990). A community-wide program in breast self-examination training and maintenance. *Preventive Medicine, 19*, 254-269.

Wyper, M. A. (1990). Breast self-examination and the health belief model: Variations on a theme. *Research in Nursing and Health, 13*, 421-428.

Young, M., & Marty, P. J. (1985). Improving the practice of breast self-examination through assessment of alternative teaching formats. *Patient Education and Counseling, 7*, 303-310.

Zapka, J. G., & Berkowitz, E. (1992). A qualitative study about breast cancer screening in older women: Implications for research. *Journal of Gerontology, 47*(Special Issue), 93-100.

Zapka, J., Hosmer, D., Costanza, M., Harris, D., & Stoddard, A. (1992). Changes in mammography use: Economic need and service factors. *American Journal of Public Health, 82*, 1345-1351.

Zapka, J. G., Stoddard, A. M., Costanza, M. E., & Greene, H. L. (1989). Breast cancer screening by mammography: Utilization and associated factors. *American Journal of Public Health, 79*, 1499-1502.

Zapka, J. G., Stoddard, A., Maul, L., & Costanza, M. E. (1991). Interval adherence to mammography screening guidelines. *Medical Care, 29*, 697-707.

Zavertnik, J. J. (1993). Strategies for reaching poor blacks and Hispanics in Dade County, Florida. *Cancer, 72*(Suppl.), 1088-1092.

14

Compliance with Antituberculosis Regimens and the Role of Behavioral Interventions

Donald E. Morisky and Daniel M. Cabrera

INTRODUCTION

The history of tuberculosis (TB) in the United States and its most recent resurgence beginning in 1985 has been well documented (Comstock, 1994). Incidence rates had been on the decline since 1950, with a low of 9.1 per 100,000 population during the early 1980s (Wilson, 1990). Between 1985 and 1992, however, the number of cases of TB in the United States increased by 20% (Johnson, 1994). Freudenberg (1994) further notes that as many as 19 million persons in the United States have latent TB that has the possibility of becoming active.

A detailed strategic plan to reduce the annual TB case rate in the United States to less than 1 case per million was published by the Centers for Disease Control and Prevention (CDC) in 1989 (CDC, 1989). Many factors, however, prevented this plan from becoming a reality. As noted by Frieden (1994), TB and its control are manifestations of social and economic development and would require a major public health commitment.

Sociopolitical factors cited as promoting the resurgence of TB include a deteriorating public health infrastructure (Bloom & Murray, 1982; Brudney & Dobkin, 1991; Etkind, Boutotte, Murray, et al., 1992; Reichman, 1991; Sbarbaro, 1990), the growing number of overcrowded and poorly ventilated homeless shelters, prisons that may not adequately screen their captive population (Braun et al., 1989; CDC, 1992; Snider & Hutton, 1989a), lack of substance abuse rehabilitation centers for drug-abusing TB-active patients (Gerstein & Harwood, 1990; White House, 1994), and individuals co-infected with TB and HIV (Braun, Cote, & Rabkin, 1993). According to Braun et al. (1993, p. 2865), "In 1990, more than half of the deaths with tuberculosis in persons 20-49 years of age occurred in persons who also had AIDS listed on their death certificate."

Also contributing to this resurgence in TB is

Donald E. Morisky and Daniel M. Cabrera • Department of Community Health Sciences, School of Public Health, University of California, Los Angeles, California 90095-1772.

Handbook of Health Behavior Research II: Provider Determinants, edited by David S. Gochman. Plenum Press, New York, 1997.

increased immigration from countries where TB is endemic (CDC, 1990). Recent proposed shifts in immigration-related policy restricting undocumented immigrants from receiving nonemergency medical care at public health clinics threaten to hasten the spread of TB even more because undocumented aliens may fear that seeking medical care would lead to deportation. Asch found that such a policy increases an individual's delay from first experiencing symptoms to actually seeking care (Asch, Leake, & Gelberg, 1994). The spread of TB would be facilitated by additional contacts infected by persons with active TB. Without the implementation of effective measures to address the social, economic, and political conditions facilitating the spread of TB, prospects for a reversal of this trend are unlikely.

HEALTH BEHAVIOR ISSUES IN THE MANAGEMENT AND CONTROL OF TUBERCULOSIS

Compliance

Once an individual seeks or initiates care, lack of compliance with an antituberculosis regimen may lengthen and complicate treatment, as well as promote the development of multidrug-resistant forms of TB (Fox, 1983; Kopanoff, Snider, & Johnson, 1988; Sbarbaro, 1985). As defined in the medical literature, *compliance* is the extent to which a patient's health behavior coincides with medical advice (Haynes et al., 1976; Hulka, 1979). Inherent in this perspective are certain assumptions: that the diagnosis and prescribed treatment are correct; that when patients have a good understanding of the information (i.e., nature of the illness and the importance of completing treatment) provided by the physician, patients will comply. This definition orients health behavior researchers to assess a patient's behaviors from the clinician's perspective. Conceptualizing health behaviors in this manner places the preponderance of responsibility for compliance on the patient's shoulders. It also encourages health care providers (and health behavior researchers) to attribute a failure of treatment to personality flaws of the *patient* (e.g., being poorly motivated, superstitious, irresponsible) and reduces the likelihood that providers will institute needed reform in the delivery of health care services (Sumartojo, 1993).

This perspective is challenged by proponents of an alternate viewpoint, who offer a less pejorative term, *adherence*. This perspective considers the impact of the sociocultural context in which patients must manage their treatment (Hunt, Jordan, Irwin, & Browner, 1989), as well as the importance of cooperation between patients and providers (Sumartojo, 1993).

Patients may need to sort through a variety of demands in daily life, most of which may not be medical in nature. Hunt et al. (1989) found that a major factor affecting levels of long-term compliance is how readily the treatment fits into the person's established lifestyle. Hunt et al. (1989) state that in order to understand health behavior, it is essential to examine how patients actively interpret their diagnosis and treatment. These researchers concluded that the issue in health behavior is *not* compliance, but controlling symptoms with treatments that patients can live with. Thus, proponents of the "adherence" perspective view the sociocultural context as an important area of study in both applied and behavioral research (Rubel & Moore, 1994).

Measurement Strategies

Strategies for measuring compliance in TB management range from direct measures (taking assays for the presence of antituberculosis drugs, chemical markers, pill counts) to indirect (eliciting self-reports from patients; monitoring health status, appointment keeping, and punctuality; and assessment from health care providers). The percentage of TB-active patients in the United States who complete their care ranges from 70% to 75% (Addington, 1979; Combs et al., 1987; Cross et al., 1980). The rates of completion for patients on preventive treatment are even worse, ranging from 5% to 22% (Comstock, 1983; Wobeser, & Hoeppner, 1989). In addition, 33% of persons prescribed preventive therapy in the United States fail to pick up medications needed to complete 6 months of continuous therapy (Snider & Hutton, 1989b).

In general, approximately one half of health care appointments are kept for chronic health conditions (DiMatteo & DiNicola, 1982). Appointment-keeping rates for patients returning for TB screening or who are asymptomatic and on preventive chemotherapy are considerably lower.

A Psychosocial Model of Compliance Behavioral Constructs

Conceptual Framework

Figure 1 presents a model that conceptualizes factors that are proposed to affect compliance behaviors. The factors are classified as cognitive (or intrapsychic), environmental, and reinforcing. This section describes a psychosocial model of compliance behavioral constructs that encompasses these factors.

Cognitive Factors

Cognitive factors that affect patient compliance include the level of TB-related knowledge (regarding the nature of disease and treatment), health beliefs (susceptibility to a disease, severity of disease, benefits of health action, perceived barriers, cues to action), health values (how much health is valued), and attitudes (toward the health care system and toward the disease itself). Figure 1 outlines the various factors that are conceptualized to significantly affect compliance-

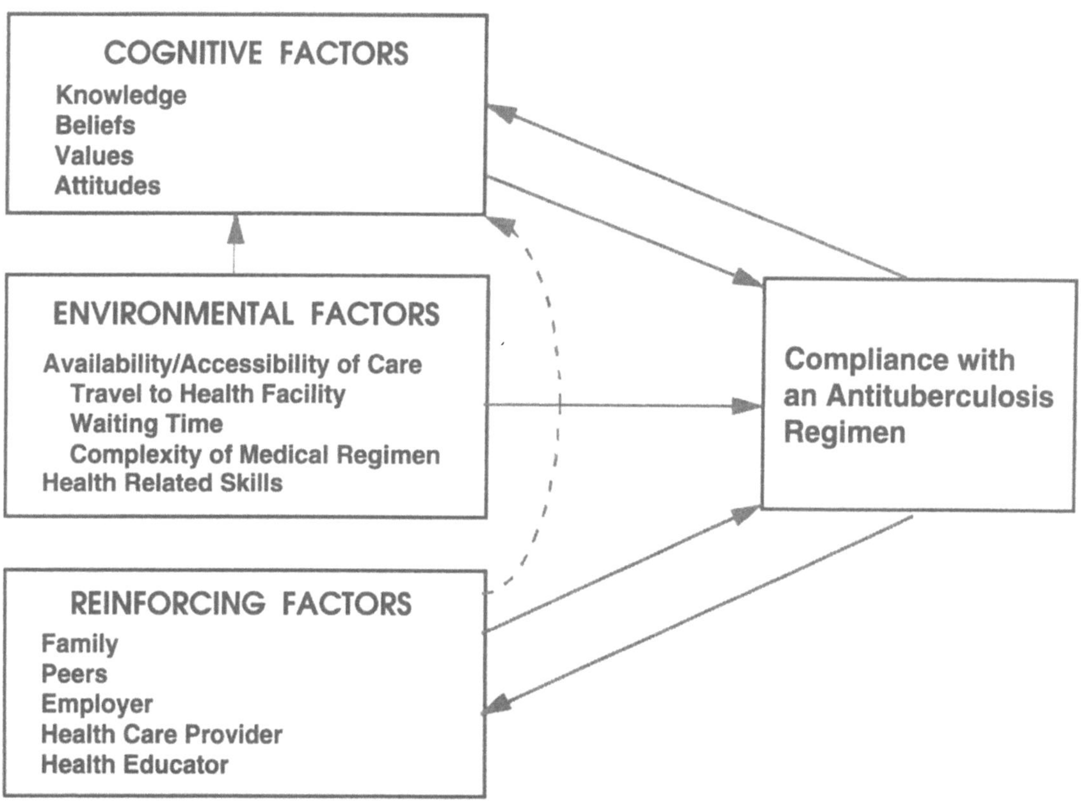

Figure 1. Three categories of factors that contribute to compliance with an antituberculosis regimen.

related behaviors including appointment keeping and medication taking.

TB-Related Knowledge. Compliance with a medical regimen is one of the most significant challenges for TB educators in most settings. Yet Johnson (1994) notes that the major limitation of current efforts to control TB is ineffective education due in part to a failure to set goals, determine priorities, and define approaches to TB education based on the needs of a specific target population. Such an approach requires soliciting advice from experts in TB control, universities, HIV/drug treatment programs, community organizations, and the target population itself. Community input and participation are essential to (1) ensure that the resulting intervention addresses appropriate areas and (2) promote a sense of program ownership by the community that will increase the likelihood of success.

Johnson (1994) recommends that each TB control program accommodate the varying needs of its particular patient population (e.g., homeless, undocumented alien) and develop appropriate health education goals. Before providers can educate, however, they need to become aware of barriers that prevent patients from fully participating in TB control activities. Barriers identified by Rubel and Moore (1994) include the perceived disappearance of tuberculosis as a public health problem, language barriers, poverty, mistrust, and myths about tuberculosis.

Individuals who are at risk for exposure to TB, are infected, or have active TB need to be educated about exposure, transmission, treatment, and control; attitudes related to illness; and the public health system (Johnson, 1994). Numerous studies have demonstrated the value of and need for this education. Asch et al. (1994) reported that 71% of patients interviewed ($N = 313$) said that their physician discovered their TB when they sought care for one of the classic symptoms of TB: coughing, fatigue, fever, swollen glands, or weight loss. Menzies, Rocher, and Vissandjee (1993) reported that 73% of patients who had a good understanding of their disease and treatment successfully completed their therapy, compared to 57% of patients who were judged to have fair or poor understanding.

However, while knowledge of a disease and its treatment has been said to be necessary for behavior change, it does not appear to be sufficient.

Health Beliefs. Health beliefs are other important cognitive factors that affect health-related behaviors. The health belief model (HBM) identifies several of these beliefs: susceptibility to the disease (i.e., perceived risk), perceived severity of the disease (i.e., if I get it, how serious is it?), perceived benefits of the health action (what is the efficacy of the treatment?), cues to action (i.e., what prompts the initiation of health behavior?), and perceived barriers to taking the action (what will it cost me in terms of money, time, other resources?) (Hochbaum, 1958). Additional components added to the original model include an individual's value of health and self-efficacy (Bandura, 1991).

However, while this model was originally designed to explain screening behaviors, Johnson (1994) notes that the HBM has been less predictive in more recent applications to health-seeking behaviors, attributing this failure to complex sociocultural and economic codeterminants that remain poorly defined.

Other beliefs can also influence the degree of patient compliance. A recent study among young, low-income Spanish-speaking clients of community clinics found that belief in the curability of a disease was found to be associated with appointment keeping (Hass, 1993). The value of this information lies in its utility to predict a likely response to a recommendation on preventive treatment. Identification and treatment of individuals at this early stage can significantly reduce the development of active TB and consequent additional infections.

Health Values

Individual behavior is motivated by a lifetime of experiences, which shape beliefs. Health beliefs, in turn, combine with cultural influences to shape each individual's values. Values are deep-seated, enduring orientations toward social goods and evils, right and wrong, and ethical and unethical behavior. An individual's value of health value is often measured by prioritizing health over travel, family, job, and money.

Attitudes toward the health care system/provider are another cognitive factor that affects compliance. If individuals have previously had negative experiences (e.g., limited access to health care, poor provider satisfaction), they may be less likely to seek treatment for symptoms or may prematurely terminate their treatment. A later section on provider-patient interaction will discuss this point in greater detail.

Environmental Factors: Availability and Accessibility of Care

Werhane, Snukst-Torbeck, and Schraufnagel (1989) suggest that a significant portion of the blame for compliance problems may rest with the health care system. Indeed, the crumbling infrastructure of public health programs adversely affects the efforts of TB control and management. Organizational problems and barriers within that system can hamper an individual's perception of availability of and accessibility to medical care (Rubel & Garro, 1992). Problems and barriers include compromised quality of care (i.e., an inadequate referral system, failure to provide appropriate follow-up services, incomplete and/or unavailable medical charts, changes in staff personnel leading to poor satisfaction with the provider, affordability, lack of a monthly follow-up for signs and symptoms and missed appointments), patients' perception of clinic facilities as being inhospitable, the distance to clinics and concomitant transportation problems, lengthy waiting times to see the provider, lack of flexible clinic hours (i.e., evening, weekends), a dearth of appropriate bilingual/bicultural staff, and restrictive policies targeting undocumented immigrants.

Since TB cases are disproportionately overrepresented among disenfranchised populations, barriers that reduce the availability and accessibility (perceived and actual) of health care may discourage or delay individuals' initially seeking care or, once in care, their continuing or completing their treatment. In addition, health-related skills that serve to facilitate or enable the health behavior change process will be discussed in the following section.

Availability of and Accessibility to Care

Quality of Care. A tacit assumption of the compliance literature is that the health care provider can correctly diagnose a medical condition and prescribe the appropriate treatment. A review by Reichman and Riegel (1994), however, found numerous instances documenting deficiencies in physician knowledge of TB. These deficiencies included: a failure to suspect TB and make diagnosis promptly, even when patients presented with clinical symptoms of TB (Bobrowitz, 1982; Counsell, Tan, & Dittus, 1990; Enarson, Grzybowski, & Dorken, 1978; Flora, Modilevsky, Antoniskis, & Barnes, 1990; Katz, Rosenthal, & Michaeli, 1985; Mathur et al., 1994; Page & Lunn, 1984); patients with active disease not being suspected of having TB after initial evaluation, thus leading to a significant delay in diagnosis and hospital room isolation and longer hospitalization (Counsell et al., 1990); delays in diagnoses and treatment resulting from atypical presentation, inadequate use of TB skin test, misinterpretation of chest X rays, and slow confirmation of TB by lab cultures (Mathur et al., 1994). Reichman and Riegel (1994) concluded that in most of the studies reviewed (Bobrowitz, 1982; Byrd et al., 1977; Counsell et al., 1990; Enarson et al., 1978; Flora et al., 1990; Glassroth, Hopewell, Baily, & Harden, 1990; Katz et al., 1985; Kissner, 1987; Kopanoff et al., 1988; Mahmoudi & Iseman, 1993; Mathur et al., 1994; Nolan, 1986; Page & Lunn, 1984), a large percentage of the physicians did not use recommended treatment regimens and information sources for TB.

Reichman and Riegel (1994) suggest that

these deficiencies stem in part from a shift in the responsibility for TB management to private practice physicians inexperienced with the disease. A proposed explanation for inadequate medical training in TB etiology and treatment is that it may be due to the relegation of TB to a minor area of medical school curricula (Huber & Miller, 1976; Reichman, 1994). This limited experience and knowledge may compromise TB control and management efforts and lead to both delays in diagnosis and errors in treatment (Bobrowitz, 1982; Byrd et al., 1977; Counsell et al., 1990; Enarson et al., 1978; Flora et al., 1990; Glassroth et al., 1990; Katz et al., 1985; Kissner, 1987; Kopanoff et al., 1988; Mahmoudi & Iseman, 1993; Mathur et al., 1994; Nolan, 1986; Page & Lunn, 1984).

Reichman and Riegel (1994) identify specific educational and behavioral objectives that physicians must meet in order to adequately manage TB in high-risk areas. Physicians should be willing to participate; be capable and engaged in screening, diagnosing, treating, and counseling; be engaged in contact tracing for TB; and finally recognize and refer multidrug-resistant TB cases.

Physician Attitudes. In addition to a lack of experience with TB, a suggested problem in physician attitudes toward TB management is that some who themselves have either latent or active TB may be poor compliers. For instance, physician noncompliance has been observed for TB screening (Geiseler, Nelson, & Crispen, 1987), failure to follow up with prophylaxis therapy after testing positive (Fraser, Kilo, Bailey, Medoff, & Dunagan, 1994), and failure to take medication after receiving a diagnosis of active TB (Geiseler et al., 1987).

Geiseler et al. (1987) suggested that physicians who are themselves noncompliant might demonstrate reduced enthusiasm to ensure compliance by their own TB patients. Reichman and Riegel (1994) suggest that such lack of enthusiasm might in fact contribute to the problem of patient noncompliance.

Thus, Reichman and Riegel propose that TB interventions might target physicians' attitudes to increase their willingness to expand and maintain TB-related knowledge and implement recommended practices.

Follow-Up Services/Referral System. Organizational problems in providing follow-up services or adequate referrals as well as organizational barriers to obtaining the services needed for the diagnosis and treatment of TB adversely affect patient compliance. Etkind (1994) suggests an absence of technical directives or a failure to distribute patients to the appropriate health care providers as possible organizational problems. Freudenberg (1994) notes how the poor support structure for social and health-related agencies that address patients with other medical conditions can adversely affect the spread of TB. Citing an example, Freudenberg (1994) notes that the single greatest obstacle faced by persons with active TB who are also drug or alcohol abusers is lack of drug treatment services and options. Since these services can function as sources of referral to TB clinics, TB-active individuals may continue to go unexamined and untreated and continue to needlessly infect possibly many more individuals.

HIV-positive individuals (possibly co-infected with TB) who receive inadequate care due to a slow response from an overburdened health and social service system may also not be referred to an appropriate clinic. Etkind (1994) suggests that obstacles to treatment may also be a result of overall poor program management, poor referral services, and lack of a supportive environment.

Cost. While provision of reduced or cost-free care may remove some of the barriers to seeking and initiating care, an additional hidden cost may result from having to take time off work from a job in which the employer does not provide sick time. For individuals living near the poverty line, this necessity sets up a conflict in terms of what the patients value more, health or income. In addition, the increasing cost of antituberculosis medication must be absorbed by an already overburdened TB program budget.

Influence of Health Culture on Compliance. As mentioned previously, a major consideration in understanding compliance with a lengthy treatment period is the need to view a medical regimen within a patient's sociocultural context. For high-risk individuals, this context might include conditions of homelessness, poverty, unemployment, undocumented immigration status, fear of the United States health care system, language barriers, and substance abuse, as well as competing medical conditions.

An additional environmental factor that influences compliance is "health culture." Freudenberg (1994) notes that patients with alternate views of health and disease may not understand or accept the rationale for the TB treatment. Individuals become socialized into a particular "health culture" through observing the perceptions of their relatives, friends, and workmates regarding the nature, cause, and implications of a health problem. In the case of TB, the implications could include a delay in seeking care, varying responses to results of a TB skin test, and decisions to continue with care. The "health culture" is invoked by ill people to determine whether their symptoms are worthy of seeking care, the degree of severity, whom to seek out, and the length of treatment (Rubel & Moore, 1994).

The limitation of applying a value expectancy model such as the HBM (the validation of which has been carried out almost entirely in North America) in a cross-cultural setting is the model's failure to consider how the *nature* of an illness might affect health beliefs (Rubel & Garro, 1992). These authors note that the process of self-diagnosis and self-initiated efforts to seek care begins in the community, not in the medical setting. They further suggest that in order to facilitate the early removal of active disease from community settings, it is essential to comprehend in depth the perceptions and knowledge with which ordinary people attempt to manage symptoms that, although discomforting, or even impairing, may not be considered either as communicable or as serious threats to health (Mechanic, 1982).

Social Stigmatization by Provider, Family, and Friends. According to Goffman (1963), the original Greek meaning of the term *stigma* referred to bodily signs designed to expose something unusual and bad about the moral status of the person bearing the signs, which were tattooed. Quam (1990) notes that although today stigma is applied more to the disgrace itself than to the bodily evidence of it, the ascription of stigma to any condition arises out of the symbol system within a culture and, like other symbolic acts, follows a logic within which relationships are more emotional than rational.

In many cultures, the stigmatization ascribed to TB discourages individuals from discussing their illness with family or friends, delays them from seeking care (Zola, 1973), and discourages patients from completing care. This antipathy is in part due to the contagious nature of TB, which can inspire avoidance of victims rather than generate sympathy (Langeal et al., 1986). A review of the literature indicates that the degree and nature of this social stigma vary by culture and level of acculturation (Rubel & Garro, 1992). Sumartojo (1993) cites an unpublished study by Robinson and Eisenman (1982) reporting substantial differences in perceived stigma by level of acculturation: Spanish-speaking Latinos exhibited higher levels of stigma from TB compared to English-speaking Latinos.

Freudenberg (1994) notes that proposed legislation to restrict medical and social benefits to undocumented immigrants facilitates the perception of stigma by further isolating this disenfranchised group. Freudenberg (1994) further states that health care providers may not feel obliged to provide the same level of care to patients who are not United States citizens. This climate of distrust is counterproductive to TB control efforts in such areas as the identification of the contacts of TB-active patients and the implementation of worksite screening (Johnson, 1994).

The review by Ruble and Garro (1992) of the anthropological literature documents numerous cases of how individuals with TB can be highly stigmatized. In one case, a medical explanation, based on the germ theory, identifying a TB sufferer as an index case who could spread the disease to many others was akin to identifying that person as a sorcerer, since individuals in the community who were able to do so were considered to have negative supernatural powers. Another study demonstrates how delays in seeking care and failure to complete treatment are a result of the association of TB symptoms with witchcraft in East Africa (Ndeti, 1972). Yet another study (in Mexico City) reported on the effects of stigma on familial relations of hospitalized TB patients (Herrera, Senties, Esquivel, & Armas, 1971). Approximately 25% of those who dropped out of treatment did not inform their families of their TB diagnosis. Moysen and Arroyo Acevedo (1984) described these patients' fears as alienation from society and loss of home and familial affection. The findings of Mata (1985) from a focus group interview in Honduras revealed that some TB patients preferred death to social rejection.

In citing an unpublished study among Mexican immigrants in California, Rubel and Garro (1992) reported that the fear of social stigma strongly predicted patients' perceptions of their illness and its implications. Many patients had not mentioned the nature of their illness to household members, others had curtailed contacts with family and friends with whom they had enjoyed extensive relationships, and still others expressed fear that a spouse would discover their illness, refuse to eat or sleep with them, and even discontinue the relationship. One of the most striking features of these interviews was the systematic avoidance by respondents of the term "tuberculosis," an illness label familiar to the patients and consistently used by the county nurses and physicians who managed their treatment. The social stigma may well explain why so few of these patients would suggest to a coworker or acquaintance displaying the same symptoms that that person might also be suffering from TB.

Health-Related Skills

Health-related skills refer to a person's ability to perform the tasks that constitute a health-related behavior. These skills facilitate the accomplishment of the desired behavioral outcome. Examples of these skills include the ability to resist peer pressure (communication skills), monitoring of one's blood pressure, weight, and diet, as well as medication-taking skills.

Cues to action are signals that may prompt or initiate health behaviors. Cues to action may differ according to the specific health behavior involved. Experiencing symptoms of TB might be a cue to seek treatment. Conversely, patients who become asymptomatic as a result of taking their prescribed antituberculosis medication may prematurely terminate their medication because they feel they have been cured. Indeed, numerous studies have documented that levels of compliance are reduced with treatment for asymptomatic conditions (Cuneo & Snider, 1989; Fox, 1983; Haynes, 1976; Reichman, 1987). Findings by Langeal, Ulmer, and Weiss (1986) revealed a disturbing pattern of dropping out after only a short period of time among asymptomatic patients with inactive TB on preventive chemotherapy.

Patient's daily activities have been successfully incorporated as cues for taking medication. The effect comes from associating the new behavior (taking medicine) with an established activity (eating meals, brushing teeth, watching favorite daily news program). Telephone reminders to patients from clinic administrative staff the day before a scheduled appointment would be a cue to action for keeping an appointment (Tanke & Leirer, 1994).

Reinforcing Factors

Social support (emotional, tangible, informational) from family, peers, and employers and encouragement from health care providers and health educators (Buri et al., 1985; Miles & Maat, 1984; Yeager & Medinger, 1986) are factors that appear to reinforce compliance behaviors. Another strategy that has been successfully employed is the use of incentives. To determine whether noncompliance with appointment keeping could be reduced, Rice and Lutzker (1984) found a 50% increase in clinic visits and "better rates of compliance" among TB patients who were provided with direct incentives of reduced-rate or free follow-up care. To test their hypothesis of improving appointment-keeping behavior through an incentive scheme, patients were assigned to four groups: nontreatment control, modified appointment care, reduced-rate follow-up, and free follow-up care. Results indicated a significant increase in follow-up appointment keeping using both incentive schemes, whereas the modified appointment care was ineffective. A cost analysis showed that the no-treatment control and modified appointment care groups were the least expensive, but also the least effective. Although the incentive conditions were more expensive, they were more cost-effective and generated the most net revenue. Morisky et al. (1990) found improved rates of appointment-keeping behavior and adherence to the medical regimen for patients assigned to an educational intervention group. This group was assigned to a combined educational counseling session plus a reward scheme. Although the educational program was found to be extremely successful, the study design did not permit the assessment of separate and combined effects. An ongoing investigation by some members of the proposed research group is seeking to tease out the separate effects of these strategies with adult patients with active TB. While this study is also examining cost-effectiveness, additional research must still be conducted to provide scientific evidence as to the relative cost-effectiveness of various educational approaches that are geared toward adolescents.

Barry, Shirley, and Grady (1990) demonstrated the cost-effectiveness of a school-based TB screening program at the junior high level, which resulted in a net savings of $113,919. This savings was based on finding a significant percentage rate of tuberculin positivity among tenth and seventh graders (8.9% and 5.1%, respectively). These rates reflect the composition of the particular student population of that school (minorities, refugees, immigrants, or children of indigent parents), which had higher TB rates than the general population.

Provider-Patient Interaction. Provider encouragement that is perceived by patients to be sincere can be both a cause and an effect of a strong provider-patient relationship (Burl et al., 1985; Kearns, Cole, et al., 1985; Kilpatrick, 1987; McDonald, Mermon, & Reichman, 1982; Reichman, 1987; Sbarbaro, 1985; Snukst-Torbeck, Werhane, & Schreufnagel, 1987). Developing this relationship requires cultivating a sense of trust based on strong communicating skills, an ability to identify early in treatment a patient who may be a compliance risk, and a willingness to take appropriate action (Menzies et al., 1993). In an ideal world, health care providers and patients are partners in the successful choice and implementation of treatment delivery (Etkind, 1994). Achieving this end involves having providers ask patients about their TB-related attitudes and beliefs early on in treatment (Werhane et al., 1989), which would facilitate better understanding of noncompliant behavior.

Health care providers in general and physicians in particular need to ensure that patients have the information and required skills to successfully complete treatment. Providers should also be vigilant for indications of compliance problems by identifying and addressing barriers. Specific behavioral objectives for providers might include these (Snider & Hutton, 1989b)

1. Being specific about the behavior expected.
2. Discussing desired behaviors first.
3. Eliciting feedback and questions.
4. Providing written instructions.

The anti-immigration legislation limiting access to medical care might also damage the bond of trust that providers have spent a great deal of time cultivating. As noted, according to Asch et al. (1994), undocumented immigrants might fear that contact with the medical establishment will lead to deportation.

Adequate communication implies exchange of information between provider and patient in both directions, so that barriers are identified and addressed, knowledge is increased, skills are learned, and, if necessary, attitudes are changed. Successful communication is thus providing "content" within a "context" so that appropriate and targeted information is both accessible and intelligible to patients. In order to do so, providers need to have a knowledge and awareness of common behavioral patterns, problems, and shared concerns of their patients (Selwyn & O'Conner, 1992). Providers who demonstrate understanding, express care and concern, and provide information in a clear and concise manner (Barnhoorn & Adriaanse, 1992; Eisenberg, 1977; Pozsik, 1993) are more likely to satisfy their patients. For instance, Menzies et al. (1993) found that good communication with better patient understanding at the initiation of therapy enhanced compliance. Tanke and Leirer (1994) also found that patients (active and on preventive chemotherapy) who had already established a relationship with clinic staff were more likely to come to appointments than patients coming in for screening who had not previously attended a clinic.

A barrier to successful communication might include the physician's attitude/perception as to what constitutes "sufficient" communication skills. Some clinicians may define successful communication as simply spending additional time explaining treatments. However, physicians overestimate the time they spend encouraging patients to discuss psychological and social problems they encounter in trying to complete their treatment (Roter, 1977, 1994; Waitzkin, 1991). Rubel and Moore (1994) note the importance of information exchange in both TB prevention and treatment settings as supported by recent research in sociolinguistics.

Providers may feel that their patients should exert greater control over their own behavior and accept increased responsibility for their health (Knowles, 1977). The tacit assumption made is that patients have certain levels of resources available (education, income, high self-esteem). However, the majority of the disenfranchised population most likely to be affected by TB do not have such resources.

Directly Observed Therapy. According to Menzies et al. (1993), directly observed therapy (DOT) is utilized for selected patients with active disease who would not otherwise take their medication properly. This coercive strategy is employed to ensure that treatment is completed and decrease the chance that the patient will develop multidrug-resistant (MDR) TB. Factors that clinicians use to identify patients at risk include the following: a previous history of failure to take prescribed antituberculosis medication, homelessness, severe mental illness, use of injectable drugs. While DOT is labor-intensive, the cost to implement it is considerably less than the cost incurred with noncompliant patients who may be hospitalized or who develop MDR TB, as well as less than the cost of treating additional individuals exposed to TB.

Patients on DOT return to the chest clinic to take medication up to five times a week. However, outreach workers are also dispatched to the field when appropriate (e.g., patient lacks transportation or is incapacitated).

Social Support. Social support refers to a range of interpersonal exchanges that include not only the provision of physical, social, and emotional assistance, but also the subjective consequences of making individuals feel that they are the object of enduring concern by others (Pilisuk & Parks, 1981).

Numerous studies have demonstrated how social support has improved patient compliance with an antituberculosis treatment. Hass (1993) found that Spanish-speaking patients who were offered instrumental social support from family or friends (e.g., transportation to clinic or child care) were more likely to make a follow-up appointment. Sumartojo (1993) found that patients who received emotional support from family members (e.g., positive attitude about patient taking medicine) were more likely to be adherent (56% versus 28%). In addition, patients who felt supported by their physicians were also more likely to be adherent (83% versus 58%). Barnhoorn and Adriaanse (1991) found similar results with patients in India. Patients who felt rejected by others and who separated themselves were less likely to complete their treatment.

METHODOLOGICAL ISSUES

As with other health behavior research, studies in TB control reveal numerous methodological issues. Three of these issues will be briefly discussed.

The first issue is more conceptual than methodological in nature, but is included in this discussion because of its methodological implications. The basic issue is the tendency for investigators of compliance behaviors to focus their examination on the patient. Johnson (1994) suggests that a failure to recognize the multicausal nature of the problem is brought on by an emphasis on biomedical rather than behavioral interventions as contributing to this situation. Research focused solely on the patient makes it less likely that behavioral researchers will consider the adverse effects of a deteriorating public health infrastructure on TB control interventions.

A second methodological issue arises from difficulties in comparing studies that use different measures of compliance (i.e., pill counts, urine assays, appointment keeping, self-reports, and physician assessment). Besides measuring different aspects of compliance, each measure differs in its degree of validity and reliability. The validity of patient self-reports may be threatened by (1) social desirability (not wanting to appear as irresponsible if medicine was not taken) or (2) the culturally sensitive nature of certain topics (social stigma). Physician assessment of patient compliance may be an unreliable predictor of completion of care. Menzies et al. (1993) notes that clinic attendance is not equivalent to medication taking. Even if clinic attendance is regular, urine assay used to detect the presence of rifampin and isoniazid can be influenced by the patient's rate of metabolism of the drug or subverted by the patient's occasional refusal to provide urine samples for testing (Burkhardt & Nel, 1980; Sumartojo, 1993). Review of medical charts is hampered by missing or inaccurate data. Furthermore, there are generally no standardized procedures for entering compliance information on patients.

A related issue is the possibility that patients may not be equally compliant on all measures. Sumartojo (1993) notes that patients may keep all their appointments but fail to have drug metabolites in their urine assay. This variability makes interpretation of results very complex. Despite methodological limitations, however, inclusion of multiple measures of compliance is recommended.

A third methodological issue concerns the selection bias found in many studies: Patients who are studied are those who sought or received care; those not included are individuals unable to overcome barriers to care. Thus, the patient population is not representative of all individuals with active TB. Appropriate research questions to address this issue might include the following:

- If individuals who seek treatment are different from those who do not, how might those differences influence later compliance behaviors?
- Are those individuals who seek care only those who are experiencing symptoms?
- If so, in what ways are individuals who experience symptoms but do not seek care different?

Before issues of selection bias can be resolved, examinations of these research questions should proceed.

A SYSTEMS APPROACH TO THE CONTROL OF TUBERCULOSIS IN THE COMMUNITY

Clinic Care Approaches

A systems approach is recommended for the control of TB in the community in general and of TB treatment delivery in particular. Because the approach requires health care providers (physicians, nurses, outreach workers) to work as a team, it is essential that programmatic goals and objective be clearly stated and agreed upon and adequately communicated and that a mechanism to continually monitor progress be in place. Conditions preventing the implementation of such a system include a deteriorating public health infrastructure brought about by decreased funding and shifting priorities.

Etkind (1994) views overall poor program management as another obstacle to providing adequate treatment. Examples include a lack of clear programmatic directives or a failure in communicating them to clinicians.

Implementation of a systems approach assumes that barriers in the health care delivery system are identified, addressed, and resolved in order to ensure successful completion of care. Etkind (1994) identifies a number of such barriers, including access to health care (cost, distance, flexible hours), inappropriately trained staff, inadequate support services (pharmacy, social services), and failure to include patients as active participants in their care.

A systems approach also requires health care providers to view TB within its social context. Doing so requires assessment of both medical and nonmedical issues that may adversely affect a patient's treatment regimen. Medical issues include competing treatment(s) for other illness(es) that may increase the complexity of a patient's daily medical regimen. Nonmedical issues include housing problems, substance abuse, domestic violence, and mistrust and alienation from the health care system. While it may appear that these issues go beyond the purview of the clinic care setting, it should be recognized that support services provide a foundation for TB treatment. Hence, even though individuals enroll in a TB program, other survival needs may take priority, setting the groundwork for noncompliance. Thus, a systems approach should contain a medical component as well as a referral component that directs patients to agencies that address substance abuse, public assistance, housing, and entitlements.

Health Education Policy

Health education policy should reflect and support the systems approach. Although the content should continue to address traditional education areas (nature of TB, transmission, and treatment), culturally appropriate and sensitive materials should also be integrated into the curriculum (i.e., effects of social stigma, practical suggestions for managing medication taking, and incorporation of social support into the treatment regimen).

Presentation of the content is an essential component of the health education experience. The messenger should therefore understand the needs and concerns of the targeted population and be able to communicate effectively in order to be seen as a credible source of information. In certain communities, it might be necessary for health educators to be bilingual and bicultural; in another setting, well-trained peer educators might be a more effective strategy.

Staff Training

Medical staff training should include a component dealing with both clinic- and patient-based factors that affect patient compliance. Staff assessment procedures regarding a patient's likelihood of completing treatment should reflect an awareness of these factors. In addition, Rubel and Garro (1992) suggest that when a patient is informed of the definite diagnosis of TB, the patient's own view of the problem should be ascertained, along with its causes, implications, and expectations for treatment. This process facilitates the establishment of a treatment plan suited to the patient's particular needs and concerns.

Outreach

TB control efforts might be expanded by utilizing outreach strategies, particularly through the indigenous channels of communication. Specific activities include street outreach, providing funding to community organizations for education and services, creation of community and regional coalitions for advocacy and planning (Freudenberg, 1994), and establishing cooperative efforts with community leaders and groups by engaging them in educational development. Johnson (1994) suggests that the educational initiative should be dictated by the opinions expressed by the group targeted for education. Ultimately, the gap between the "underserved" and the health care delivery system should be bridged.

CONCLUSION

This chapter addressed major areas of concern in the management and control of tuberculosis and the role of behavioral interventions. As presented, the problem of non-adherence to medical recommendations can be significantly reduced through appropriate interventions. These interventions entail improved provider-patient interaction, patient activation, and follow-up services. Implemented in a systematic manner, these approaches can improve compliance behavior, resulting in a higher proportion of patients completing antituberculosis therapy.

REFERENCES

Addington, W. W. (1979). Patient compliance: The most serious remaining problem in the control of tuberculosis in the United States. *Chest*, *76*, 741-743.

Asch, S., Leake, B., & Gelberg, L. (1994). Does fear of immigration authorities deter tuberculosis patients from seeking care? *Western Journal of Medicine*, *161*, 373-376.

Bandura, A. (1991). Self-efficacy mechanism in physiological activation and health promoting behavior. In J. Madden, IV, S. Matthysse, & J. Barchas (Eds.), *Neurobiology of learning, emotion and affect* (pp. 229-269). New York: Raven Press.

Barnhoorn, F., & Adriaanse, H. (1992). In search of factors responsible for noncompliance among tuberculosis patients in Wardha District, India. *Social Science and Medicine*, *34*, 291-306.

Barry, M. A., Shirley, L., Grady, M. T., Etkind, S. W., Almeida, C., Bernardo, J., & Lamb, G. A. (1990). Tuberculosis infection in urban adolescents: Results of a school-based testing program. *American Journal of Public Health*, *80*, 439-441.

Bloom, B. R., & Murray, C. J. L. (1982). Tuberculosis undiagnosed until autopsy. *American Journal of Medicine*, *72*, 850-858.

Bobrowitz, I. D. (1982). Active tuberculosis undiagnosed until autopsy. *American Journal of Medicine*, *72*, 650-658.

Braun, M. M., Cote, T. R., & Rabkin, C. S. (1993). Trends in death with tuberculosis during the AIDS era. *Journal of the American Medical Association*, *269*, 2865-2868.

Braun, M. M., Truman, B. I., Magurie, B., DiFerdinando, G. T., Jr., Wormaer, G., Broaddue, R., & Morse, D. L. (1989). Increasing incidence of tuberculosis in a prison inmate population: Association with HIV infection. *Journal of the American Medical Association*, *261*, 393-397.

Brudney, K., & Dobkin, J. (1991). Resurgent tuberculosis in New York City: HIV, homelessness, and the decline of TB control programs. *American Review of Respiratory Disease*, *144*, 745-749.

Burkhardt, K. R., & Nel, E. E. (1980). Monitoring regularity of drug intake in tuberculosis patients by means of simple urine tests. *South African Medical Journal*, *57*, 981-985.

Buri, P. S., Vathesatogkit, P., Charoenpan, P., Kiatboonsri, S., & Buranaratchada, S. A. (1985). A clinic model for better tuberculosis treatment outcome and factors including compliance. *Journal of the Medical Association of Thailand*, *68*, 358-360.

Byrd, R. B., Horn, B. R., Solomon, D. A., Griggs, G. A., & Wilder, N. J. (1977). Treatment of tuberculosis of the nonpulmonary physician. *Annals of Internal Medicine*, *86*, 799-802.

Centers for Disease Control and Prevention. (1989). A strategic plan for the elimination of tuberculosis in the United States. *Morbidity and Mortality Weekly Report*, *38*(Suppl. 5-3), 1-25.

Centers for Disease Control and Prevention. (1990). Tuberculosis among foreign-born persons entering the United States: Recommendations of the Advisory Council for the Elimination of Tuberculosis. *Morbidity and Mortality Weekly Report*, *39*(Suppl. R-18), 1-23.

Centers for Disease Control and Prevention. (1992). Prevention and control of tuberculosis among homeless persons: Recommendations of the Advisory Council for the Elimination of Tuberculosis. *Morbidity and Mortality Weekly Report, 41*(RR-5), 13-22.

Combs, D. L., O'Brian, R. J., Geiter, L. J., & Snider, D. E. (1987). Compliance with tuberculosis regimes: Results from USPHS therapy trial 21. *American Review of Respiratory Disease, 135*, A138.

Comstock, G. W. (1983). New data on preventive treatment with isoniazid. *Annals of Internal Medicine, 98*, 663-665.

Comstock, G. W. (1994). Tuberculosis: Is the past once again prologue? *American Journal of Public Health, 84*, 1729-1731.

Counsell, S. R., Tan, J. S., & Dittus, R. S. (1990). Unsuspected pulmonary tuberculosis is not prevented. *American Review of Respiratory Disease, 141/123*, 6-40.

Cross, F. S., Long, M. W., Banner, A. S., & Snider, D. E. (1980). Rifampin-Isoniazid therapy of alcoholic and non-alcoholic tuberculosis patients in a US Public Health Service cooperative trial. *American Review of Respiratory Disease, 122*, 349-353.

Cuneo, W., & Snider, D. E. (1989). Enhancing patient compliance with tuberculosis therapy. *Clinics in Chest Medicine, 3*, 375-379.

DiMatteo, M. R., & DiNicola, D. D. (1982). *Achieving patient compliance: The psychology of the medical practitioner's role*. New York: Pergamon Press.

Eisenberg, L. (1977). The search for care. *Daedalus (Winter)*, 235-246.

Enarson, D. A., Grzybowski, S., & Dorken, E. (1978). Failure of diagnosis as a factor in tuberculosis mortality. *Canadian Medical Association Journal, 118*, 1520-1522.

Etkind, S. (1994). *Quality of services workgroup paper*. Working paper.

Etkind, S., Boutotte, J., Murray, C., & Nardell, E. (1992). Tuberculosis nurse elimination: Implications for future TB control in the United States. *American Review of Respiratory Disease, 145*(4), A222 (abstr. suppl.).

Flora, G. S., Modilevsky, T., Antoniskis, D., & Barnes, P. (1990). The undiagnosed tuberculosis in patients with human immunodeficiency virus infection. *Chest, 98*, 1056-1059.

Fox, W. (1983). Compliance of patients and physicians: Experience and lessons from tuberculosis. *British Medical Journal, 287*, 33-35.

Fraser, V. J., Kilo, C. M., Bailey, T. C., Medoff, G., & Dunagan, W. C. (1994). Screening of physicians for tuberculosis. *Infection Control and Hospital Epidemiology, 15*, 95-100.

Freudenberg, N. (1994). *Tuberculosis control for vulnerable populations*. Working paper.

Frieden, T. R. (1994). Tuberculosis control and social change. *American Journal of Public Health, 84*, 1721-1723.

Geiseler, P. J., Nelson, K. E., & Crispen, R. G. (1987). Tuberculosis in physicians: Compliance with preventive measures. *American Review of Respiratory Disease, 135*, 3-9.

Gerstein, D., & Harwood, H. (1990). *Treatment of drug abuse*. Washington, DC: National Academy of Sciences.

Glassroth, J. B., Hopewell, P. C., Baily, W. C., & Harden, J. (1990). Why tuberculosis is not prevented. *Review of Respiratory Disease, 141/123*, 6-40.

Goffman, E. (1963). *Stigma: Notes on the management of spoiled identity*. Englewood Cliffs, NJ: Prentice-Hall.

Hass, M. R. (1993). *Health seeking and patient adherence: Tuberculosis screening and Latino immigrants*. Ph.D. dissertation. University of California at Irvine.

Haynes, R. B. (1976). A critical review of the "determinants" of patient compliance with therapeutic regimens. In D. L. Sackett & R. B. Haynes (Eds.), *Compliance with therapeutic regimens* (pp. 26-39). Baltimore, MD: Johns Hopkins University Press.

Haynes, R. B. (1979). Determinants of compliance: The disease and the mechanics of treatment. In B. Haynes, D. W. Tayler, & D. Sackett (Eds.), *Compliance in health care* (pp. 49-62). Baltimore, MD: Johns Hopkins University Press.

Herrera, M., Senties, R., Esquivel, E., & Armas, J. (1971). Problematica sociologica del enfermo tuberculoso internando en hospitales de estancia prolongada. *Salud Publica de Mexico, 13*, 749-762.

Hochbaum, G. M. (1958). *Public participation in medical science programs: A sociopsychological study*. PHS Publication No. 572. Washington, DC: United States Government Printing Office.

Huber, G. L., & Miller, R. D. (1976). Training of undergraduate medical school students in pulmonary diseases: A regional analysis of New England medical schools. *Chest, 70*, 267-273.

Hulka, B. (1979). Patient-clinician interactions and compliance. In B. Haynes, D. W. Tayler, & D. Sackett (Eds.), *Compliance in health care* (pp. 63-77). Baltimore, MD: Johns Hopkins University Press.

Hunt, L. M., Jordan, B., Irwin, S., & Browner, C. H. (1989). Compliance and the patient's perspective: Controlling symptoms in everyday life. *Culture, Medicine and Psychiatry, 13*, 315-334.

Johnson, M. P. (1994). *Public education for Tuberculosis and Behavior Conference*. Working paper for Tuberculosis and Behavior Conference.

Katz, I., Rosenthal, T., & Michaeli, D. (1985). Undiagnosed tuberculosis in hospitalized patients. *Chest, 87*, 770-774.

Kearns, T. J., Cole, C. H., Farer, L. S., Leff, A. R., Reza, R. J., Sbarbaro, J. A., & Stead, W. W. (1985). Public health issues in control of tuberculosis. *Chest, 87*(Suppl.), 1355-1375.

Kilpatrick, G. S. (1987). Compliance in relation to tuberculosis. *Tubercule, 68*(Suppl.), 31-32.

Kissner, D. G. (1987). Tuberculosis: Missed opportunities. *Archives of Internal Medicine, 147*, 2037-2040.

Knowles, J. H. (1977). The responsibility of the individual. *Daedalus (Winter)*, 57-80.

Kopanoff, D. E., Snider, D. E., Jr., & Johnson, M. (1988). Recurrent tuberculosis: Why do patients develop disease again? A United States Public Health Service cooperative survey. *American Journal of Public Health, 78*, 30-33.

Langeal, R. A., Ulmer, R. A., & Weiss, D. J. (1986). An intervention to improve the compliance to year-long isoniazid (INH) therapy for tuberculosis. *Journal of Compliance in Health Care* 1(1), 47-54.

Mahmoudi, A., & Iseman, M. D. (1993). Pitfalls in the care of patients with tuberculosis. *Journal of the American Medical Association*, *270*, 65.

Mata, J. I. (1985). Integrating the client's perspective in planning a tuberculosis education and treatment program in Honduras. *Medical Anthropology (Winter)*, 57-64.

Mathur, P., Sacks, L., Auten, G., Sall, R., Levy, C., & Gordin, F. (1994). Delayed diagnosis of pulmonary tuberculosis in city hospitals. *Archives of Internal Medicine*, *154*, 306-310.

McDonald, R. J., Mermon, A. M., & Reichman, L. B. (1982). Successful supervised ambulatory management of tuberculosis treatment failures. *Annals of Internal Medicine*, *96*, 297-302.

Mechanic, D. (1982). The epidemiology of illness behavior and its relationship to physical and psychological distress. In D. Mechanic (Ed.), *Symptoms, illness behavior, and help-seeking* (pp. 1-24). New York: Prodist.

Menzies, R., Rocher, I., & Vissandjee, B. (1993). Factors associated with compliance in treatment of tuberculosis. *Tubercule and Lung Disease*, *74*, 32-37.

Miles, S. H., & Maat, R. B. (1984). A successful supervised outpatient short-course tuberculosis treatment program in an open refugee camp on the Thai-Cambodian border. *American Review of Respiratory Disease*, *130*, 827-830.

Morisky, D. E., Malotte, C. K., Choi, P., Davidson, P., Rigler, S., Sugland, B., & Langer, M. (1990). A patient education program to improve adherence rate with antituberculosis drug regimens. *Health Education Quarterly*, *17*, 253-267.

Moysen, J. S., & Arroyo Acevedo, A. P. (1984). Critique of the validity of methods for detection and confirmation of pulmonary tuberculosis as a problem of public health [Critica de la validez de los metodos de detección y confirmación de la tuberculosis pulmonar como un probema de salud publica]. *Salud Publica de Mexico*, *26*, 546-555.

Ndeti, K. (1972). Sociocultural aspects of tuberculosis defaultation: A case study. *Social Science and Medicine*, *6*, 397-412.

Nolan, R. J., Jr. (1986). Childhood tuberculosis in North Carolina: A study of opportunities for intervention in the transmission of tuberculosis in children. *American Journal of Public Health*, *76*, 26-30.

Page, M. I., & Lunn, J. S. (1984). Experience with tuberculosis in a public teaching hospital. *American Journal of Medicine*, *77*, 667-670.

Pilisuk, M., & Parks, S. (1981). The place of networks analysis in the study of supportive social associations. *Basic and Applied Social Psychology*, *2*, 121-135.

Pozsik, C. J. (1993). Compliance with tuberculosis therapy. *Medical Clinics of North America*, *77*(6), 1289-1301.

Quam, M. D. (1990). The sick role, stigma, and pollution: The case of AIDS. In D. A. Feldman (Ed.), *Culture and AIDS* (pp. 29-44). New York: Praeger.

Reichman, L. B. (1987). Compliance in developed nations. *Tubercule*, *68*, 25-29.

Reichman, L. B. (1991). The U-shaped curve of concern. *American Review of Respiratory Disease*, *144*, 741-742.

Reichman, L. B. (1994). Multidrug-resistant tuberculosis: Meeting the challenge. *Hospital Practice*, *29*(5), 85-96.

Reichman, L. B., & Riegel, L. (1994). *Physician knowledge and practices of tuberculosis management: Problem definition*. Working paper.

Rice, J. M., & Lutzker, J. R. (1984). Reducing non-compliance to follow-up appointment keeping at a family practice center. *Journal of Applied Behavior Analysis*, *17*, 303-311.

Robinson, J., & Eisenman, S. (1982). *Hispanic perceptions and beliefs toward tuberculosis: A pilot study*. Unpublished manuscript.

Roter, D. L. (1977). Patient participation in the patient-provider interaction: The effects of patient question asking on the quality of interaction, satisfaction and compliance. *Health Education Monographs (Winter)*, 281-315.

Roter, D. L. (1994). *Doctors talking with patients/patients talking with doctors*. Westport, CT: Auburn House.

Rubel, A. J., & Garro, L. C. (1992). Social and cultural factors in the successful control of tuberculosis. *Public Health Reports*, *107*(6), 626-638.

Rubel, A. J., & Moore, C. C. (1994). *Recommended sociobehavioral research for more successful tuberculosis control*. Working paper.

Sbarbaro, J. A. (1985). Strategies to improve compliance with therapy. *American Journal of Medicine*, *79*(Suppl. 6A), 34-37.

Sbarbaro, J. A. (1990). Elimination: Of tuberculosis or of tuberculosis control programs. *Bulletin of the International Union Against Tuberculosis and Lung Disease*, *65*(2-3), 47-48.

Selwyn, P. A., Hartel, D., Lewis, V. A., Schoenbaum, E. E., Vermund, S. H., Klein, R. S., Walker, A. T., & Friedland, G. H. (1989). A prospective study of the risk of tuberculosis among intravenous drug users with human immunodeficiency virus infection. *New England Journal of Medicine*, *320*(9), 545-550.

Selwyn, P. A., & O'Conner, P. G. (1992). Diagnosis and treatment of substance users with HIV infection. *Primary Care Clinic in Office Practice*, *19*(1), 19-56.

Snider, D. E., Jr., Anders, H. M., & Pozsik, C. J. (1986). Incentives to take up health services [letter]. *Lancet*, *2*(8510), 812.

Snider, D. E., & Hutton, M. D. (1989a). Tuberculosis in correctional institutions. *Journal of the American Medical Association*, *261*, 436-437.

Snider, D. E., & Hutton, M. D. (1989b). *Improving patient compliance in tuberculosis treatment programs*. Atlanta, GA: CDC, Public Health Service, U.S. Department of Health and Human Services.

Snukst-Torbeck, G., Werhane, M. J., & Schreufnagel, D. (1987). Treatment of tuberculosis in a nurse-managed clinic. *Heart and Lung*, *16*, 30-33.

Sumartojo, E. (1993). When tuberculosis treatment fails: A social behavioral account of patient adherence. *American Review of Respiratory Disease*, *147*, 1311-1320.

Tanke, E. D., & Leirer, V. O. (1994). Automated telephone reminders in tuberculosis care. *Medical Care*, *32*(4), 380-389.

Waitzkin, H. (1991). *The politics of medical encounters: How patients and doctors deal with social problems*. New Haven, CT: Yale University Press.

Werhane, M. J., Snukst-Torbeck, G., & Schraufnagel, D. E. (1989). The tuberculosis clinic. *Chest*, *96*(4), 815-818.

White House. (1994). *National drug control strategy: Reclaiming our communities from drugs and violence*. Washington, DC: Government Printing Office.

Wilson, L. (1990). The historical decline of tuberculosis in Europe and America: Its cause and significance. *Journal of the History of Medicine and Allied Sciences*, *45*, 366-396.

Wobeser, B., & Hoeppner, V. (1989). The outcome of chemoprophylaxis on tuberculosis prevention in the Canadian Plains Indians. *Clinical and Investigative Medicine*, *12*, 149-153.

Yeager, H., & Medinger, A. E. (1986). Tuberculosis long term care beds: Have we thrown the baby out with the bathwater? *Chest*, *90*, 732-753.

Zola, I. K. (1973). Pathways to the doctor—from person to patient. *Social Science and Medicine*, 7, 677-689.

15

Acceptance of Cancer Screening

Barbara K. Rimer, Wendy Demark-Wahnefried, and Jennifer R. Egert

INTRODUCTION

The purpose of cancer screening is to detect cancer in its preclinical phase when the disease is most likely to be curable (Hennekens & Buring, 1987) and thereby enable achievement of the ultimate goal of screening—a reduction in morbidity and mortality from cancer. To be appropriate for screening, a disease should have high prevalence in the population (e.g., hypertension or breast cancer) and must have serious consequences, and there should be an effective screening intervention. The test should be sensitive and specific and have high predictive validity. The definition of effective is often a matter of debate, but the gold standard for determining effectiveness is usually a randomized clinical trial with a statistically significant reduction in mortality. The screening characteristics will be described in more detail, but even if a test were 100% sensitive and specific, the benefits would be achieved only to the degree to which everyone at risk received the test. This is the issue of compliance with or adherence to cancer screening.

Adherence means that a person follows recommended screening procedures. This chapter will provide an overview of adherence to screening for breast, cervical, skin, prostate, colorectal, and testicular cancer. For breast cancer and cervical cancer, unlike many other cancers, such as lung cancer, there are proven, acceptable, and cost-effective techniques for reducing cancer mortality through screening. In the case of colorectal cancer and skin cancer, there is good reason to believe that mortality can be reduced through screening. The jury is still out on prostate cancer screening, although it is recommended by the American Cancer Society and many other organizations. There are no randomized clinical trial data on testicular cancer, but screening has been recommended by some organizations.

For reasons due to people themselves, providers, and the health care system, cancer screening falls short of the ideal. Nonadherence reduces

Barbara K. Rimer • Duke Comprehensive Cancer Center, Duke University Medical Center, Durham, North Carolina 27710. **Wendy Demark-Wahnefried** • Sarah Stedman Center for Nutritional Studies, Duke University Medical Center, Durham, North Carolina 27710. **Jennier R. Egert** • Department of Psychology, Social, and Health Sciences, Duke University, Durham, North Carolina 27710.

Handbook of Health Behavior Research II: Provider Determinants, edited by David S. Gochman. Plenum Press, New York, 1997.

the potential of screening to lower the risk of death and disability from these diseases. The success of public health initiatives has directed our attention to the need to incorporate compliance-enhancing strategies into the constellation of behavioral, social, and community factors that affect individuals. This chapter will provide an overview of contemporary issues in cancer screening adherence, with special attention to several cancers that have been inadequately studied—colorectal, skin, prostate, and testicular cancers—and briefer discussions of breast and cervical cancers. Breast cancer screening is discussed in Chapter 13. This chapter does not include studies that focus on follow-up to abnormal screening exams or studies that are directed primarily at health providers.

CANCERS APPROPRIATE FOR SCREENING

Although there are more than 100 different cancers, most of them lack proven screening interventions. Only cancers of the breast, cervix, skin, colon-rectum, prostate, and testes have widely accepted screening interventions. Furthermore, not all have been proven by randomized clinical trials (RCTs) to reduce mortality, and different organizations have different recommendations regarding the tests. Although no RCT was ever conducted to prove the efficacy of the Pap test, there are excellent case-control and population data available to show that the Pap test saves lives. The efficacy of breast cancer screening has been proven for women aged 50-69, but not for women in their 40s (Fletcher, Black, Harris, Rimer, & Shapiro, 1993). Although the evidence for skin cancer screening has not been proven in an RCT, there are good circumstantial data to support the value of screening. There are now several strong but rather small studies to support colorectal screening using a fecal occult blood test in normal adults over age 50 and sigmoidoscopy every 5 years for those over age 50 (Mandelblatt, 1989).

There are no RCT data to support screening for two important male cancers: cancers of the prostate and testes. The latter, however, involves tests (self-exam and exam by a health professional) that are relatively simple and possibly cost-effective, while the former is dependent on tests, such as prostate specific antigen (PSA) testing, that have the potential for significant numbers of false positives.

THEORETICAL APPROACHES TO CANCER SCREENING

As will be discussed in the sections on cancers in specific sites, a variety of theories and models have been used in designing interventions to enhance acceptance of cancer screening. For many years, especially in breast cancer screening, where the largest body of work has been conducted, the health belief model (HBM) (Rosenstock, 1990) was the predominant theoretical model. It was thought that for a person to engage in cancer screening, the person had to feel susceptible to cancer, believe the disease would be serious, believe in the benefits, overcome barriers, and receive a cue to action. Self-efficacy also has been added to the model.

The HBM has been the most widely used theoretical model and has made major contributions to understanding the motivations for breast cancer screening (Bloom, 1994). For example, it led researchers to identify the central barriers to and facilitators of participation in screening (Rimer, Keintz, Kessler, Engstrom, & Rosan, 1989). This knowledge has guided the development of many interventions (e.g., Champion, 1994). According to Bloom (1994), the HBM has been predictive of screening behaviors for getting a mammogram and for screening for colorectal cancer.

Other theoretical models also have been used. Several researchers have been guided by the theory of reasoned action (Montano & Taplin, 1991). They have focused their inquiries on attitudes, beliefs, intentions, and behaviors. Social learning theory provides a rich source of behavioral techniques that can be applied to public health efforts to promote compliance. This model suggests that behavior is influenced by the reciprocal interplay of three primary influences: environmental events, reinforcement, and cognitive mediation (Bandura, 1986). Educational information, advice, modeling, and reminders are all examples of environmental actions that have been used to alter smoking and other behaviors in populations (Lichtenstein & Glasgow, 1992) and to promote compliance with antihypertensive medications (Morisky, 1986). Interventions that heighten feelings of personal efficacy and expectations for success are likely to be most effective in promoting health behavior change (Strecher, DeVellis, Becker, & Rosenstock, 1986).

Social learning theory (Perry, Baranowski, & Parcel, 1990) has played an important role in the development of cancer screening interventions for both health professionals and the public (Amezcua, McAlister, Ramirez, & Espinoza, 1990). Many of these interventions have used modeling techniques. Social learning theory also has been employed to promote physicians' involvement in public health efforts. For example, educating physicians and cueing them with chart reminders have been shown to increase their performance of cancer screening in clinical practice (Cohen, Halvorson, & Gosselink, 1994).

More recently, the transtheoretical model, also referred to as the stages of change model, has come to serve as a major theoretical foundation for cancer screening studies. Originally developed to alter addictive behaviors (Prochaska & DiClemente, 1985), such as smoking, it was extended by Rakowski, Rimer, and Bryant (1993) to the study of mammography. The transtheoretical model assumes that changing of behavior stages is a process that involves progression from precontemplation to contemplation, action, and maintenance, with the possibility of relapse at any point. The transtheoretical model is especially useful because it can be used to develop stage-based interventions (Rimer, 1995).

Several other theories have been used to explain cancer screening behaviors or to develop interventions or both. These include attribution theory (Rothman, Salovey, Turvey, & Fishkin, 1993), social network theory (Kang & Bloom, 1993), and health locus of control. In addition, a number of community organization models also have been employed.

The optimal approach to theory, however, is probably to use a mix of theories, depending on the level of intervention (Rimer, 1995). For example, the transtheoretical model might be used to develop cancer screening interventions for individuals at risk for the disease, while social learning theory might guide the development of interventions for health professionals.

ADHERENCE TO CERVICAL CANCER SCREENING

Cervical Cancer Screening Guidelines

All major medical organizations agree that regular Pap testing from the onset of sexual activity until about age 65 reduces death from cervical cancer. This view is accepted although there never has been an RCT to evaluate the Pap test, and precise estimates of sensitivity and specificity are not known (Wong & Feussner, 1993a). In fact, cervical cancer is considered almost totally avoidable through regular Pap tests. In 1993, 13,500 women were told they had cervical cancer, and 4400 died of the disease (American Cancer Society, 1993). Some populations, such as Alaskan natives, are especially at risk for cervical caner. There are fewer comprehensive current data on the use of cervical screening among women in the United States than there are on breast cancer screening. According to the 1987 National Health Interview Survey, about 11% of women overall reported never having had a Pap test: 10% of white women, 11.9% of black women, and 24.7% of Hispanic women. As age increased, the proportion of women who reported having had a Pap test declined (U.S. Department of Health and Human Services, Public Health Service, 1991). Black women were more likely to be screened regularly from ages 30 to 49, but in women age 70 and over, white women were more likely to have had a Pap test in the last 3 years. Pap test use is negatively related to age and positively associated with income (Mayer, Clapp, Bartholomew, & Elder, 1993).

Barriers to Adherence to Cervical Cancer Screening

The barriers to cervical cancer screening are very similar to those for breast cancer, i.e., lack of a provider recommendation, not knowing the importance of screening, and not getting regular preventive health care. Most women who have not had Pap tests have had contact with the health care system, indicating that, as for mammography, the failure of women to receive Pap tests reflects a missed clinical opportunity (Harlan, Bernstein, & Kessler, 1991). There is some evidence that embarrassment is a special problem for minority women (Richardson, 1987). Both procrastination and being too busy also are cited as barriers (Cockburn, Hirst, Hill, & Marks, 1990; Harlan et al., 1991). While expense is not the main barrier, it is noted by some women (Carney, Dietrich, & Freeman, 1992).

As with breast cancer, physician recommendation is an essential first step in use of the Pap test. Knowledge of screening guidelines also is important. In addition, Cockburn et al. (1990) showed that women who believed that healthy women do not need Pap tests were less likely to have had them. Older, unmarried, and Hispanic women are at risk for underusing Pap tests (Calle, Flanders, Thun, & Martin, 1993). Nationally, black women are screened at rates similar to or slightly higher than those for whites (Harlan et al., 1991). Some regional studies, however, have found Hispanic women more likely to be screened than black women (Berman, Bastani, Nisenbaum, Henneman, & Marcus, 1994). Women who lack a regular health care provider are least likely to be screened (Berman et al., 1994).

Interventions to Increase Acceptance of Cervical Cancer Screening

Outreach strategies have been used in many studies to increase use of cervical screening. Such an approach may be especially helpful in reaching low-income minority women. Lacey et al. (1993) sent volunteers to low-income housing projects as part of their research strategy. These programs resulted in significant increases in use of Pap tests.

Because most women are getting regular Pap tests, mass efforts to reach the small proportion of women in the United States who are underutilizers may not be efficient. Inreach strategies may be most effective. These are strategies aimed at women already in the health care system, e.g., women making visits to the emergency room of a hospital. Organizational and provider barriers must be addressed, because they are likely to be among the most salient. Attempts to streamline the process of appointments and waiting time seem to contribute to improved adherence (Harris et al., 1991). Invitations from providers also enhance cervical cancer screening (Creighton & Evans, 1992). The combination of health education and the immediate offer of a Pap test also increased screening in one study (Cockburn et al., 1991).

Inreach strategies that offer cervical screening to patients who are already in the health care system but have not been screened may be especially effective when combined with provider and organizational strategies (Celentano, Shapiro, & Weisman, 1982). Moreover, nurses can play a valuable role in facilitating cervical cancer screening, as Mandelblatt (1989) has shown. Prompting systems (Carney, Dietrich, & Freeman, 1992) may improve cervical cancer screening as well as breast cancer screening, and there is some evidence that screening of emergency hospital patients can be a useful component of case finding (Marcus et al., 1990). Ward compared a minimal intervention (suggest that woman make an appointment for a Pap test) to maximal intervention (counsel woman, trying to overcome barriers). The study involved 17 male practitioners. Both interventions increased the proportion of women who accepted opportunistic screening, and there were no differences between them. Overall, 61% of the women who were approached went on to have Pap tests.

One of the most carefully developed studies aimed at increasing use of Pap tests was conducted by Dignan et al. (1990) and directed at 25,000 women who lived in Forsyth County, North Carolina. The interventions included mass media, direct education workshops, and provision of education on cervical cancer screening to health care providers (Dignan, Michielutte, Wells, & Bahnson, 1994). Results of a quasi-experimental design evaluation found little change among the general population. However, high-risk women (older, low socioeconomic status [SES], those who do not receive regular care) showed a trend toward increased Pap testing.

Several studies have used nurses to deliver cervical cancer screening interventions (Ansell, Lacey, Whitman, Chen, & Phillips, 1994). This strategy appears especially effective. Particularly noteworthy was an 18-month intervention to increase breast and cervical screening among low-income African-American women in Chicago. Nurse clinicians and public health workers were used to promote screening and increase access. There were significant increases in knowledge and rates of Pap screening.

Because Pap testing is under the direct control of health providers, adherence-enhancing interventions should be directed at providers or at changing aspects of the health care delivery system. But interventions also have been, and must continue to be, directed at underutilizing women to overcome their barriers, which include lack of knowledge about the screening interval and the need for Pap tests in the absence of symptoms. Norman, Talbott, Kuller, Krampe, and Stolley (1991) argued that interventions should be tailored to sociodemographic, psychosocial, and motivational factors.

ADHERENCE TO COLORECTAL CANCER SCREENING

Background and Colorectal Cancer Screening Guidelines

Colorectal cancer is one of the leading causes of mortality in the Western world (Solomon & McLeod, 1993). Of Americans reaching the age of 50, 5% will develop this disease by age 80; 2.5% will die from it (Wont & Feussner, 1993b). Well-established risk factors for colorectal cancer include: familial polyposis syndromes, Crohn's disease, ulcerative colitis, age, family history, previous history of cancer (endometrial, ovarian, or breast), and Ashkenazi Jewish lineage (Oldenski & Flareau, 1992). Other risk factors, such as residence in the northeastern United States and obesity, also have been proposed (Ross, 1988).

Recent studies suggest a downward trend in colorectal mortality and a steady decline in distant disease incidence. Increased awareness and compliance with colorectal screening have been cited as reasons for this stage shift (Chu, Tarone, Chow, Hankey, & Gloecker Ries, 1994).

Colorectal Cancer Screening Modalities and Guidelines

Currently, there are three major screening modalities for colorectal cancer: the digital rectal exam (DRE), the fecal occult blood test (FOBT), and sigmoidoscopy. Screening guidelines for the general population vary considerably between major health organizations. The American College of Physicians, the U.S. Preventive Services Task Force, and the Canadian Task Force concluded that there is insufficient evidence at this time to warrant screening in the general population. Conversely, the National Cancer Institute, the World Health Organization, and the American Cancer Society favor annual DRE and FOBT for persons 50 years of age or older and recommend sigmoidoscopy every 3-5 years. Support for such recommendations has been accruing from five controlled clinical trials in the United States, Denmark, Sweden, and England. Although the results of all trials are still pending, those completed indicate that annual stool guiaic with follow-up sigmoidoscopy can reduce colorectal cancer mortality by one third. This accumulating evidence caused the U.S. Preventive Services Task Force (1996) to upgrade the evidence for colorectal screening in 1996. They now recommend FOBTS and sigmoidoscopy, interval unspecified.

Barriers to Adherence to Colorectal Cancer Screening

Issues of compliance and barriers to screening are reported for all colorectal screening modalities. Numerous surveys conducted in a variety of populations report the DRE as "embarrassing" and associated with "discomfort"; the FOBT, because it requires dietary modification (reduction of dietary peroxidases by exclusion of red meat and raw vegetables) and stool collection over the course of several days, as "inconvenient," "messy," and "disgusting"; and sigmoidoscopy, which requires the insertion of a fiber-optic probe/camera at least 35 cm into the rectum, as "painful" and "embarrassing" (McCarthy & Moskowitz, 1993; Myers et al., 1990). On the other hand, pre- and postsurveys conducted by McCarthy and Moskowitz (1993) suggest that although embarrassment, discomfort, and pain are significant barriers prior to testing, these objections are significantly reduced after people undergo sigmoidoscopy. Regarding FOBT, Myers, Balshem, Wolf, Ross, and Millner (1993) found that past screening history was positively related to future screening behavior. The exception to this finding was in persons found as false positives, who reported that they were less likely to participate in future FOBT screening. A number of general barriers, that are not test-specific have also been reported, including a disbelief that the test is important (Price, 1993) and a perception that colorectal cancer is incurable (Myers et al., 1990; Neale, Demers, & Herman, 1989; Price, 1993) and a lack of transportation (Price, 1993).

A number of facilitators for adherence to screening also have been identified. Research by Myers et al.1 (1991, 1993) suggests that physician recommendation exerts a strong influence on colorectal screening. Blalock, DeVellis, Afifi, and Sandler (1990) and Hunter et al. (1990) also found that personal experience with cancers of relatives or friends increases participation in screening by FOBT and sigmoidoscopy. In addition, increasing age, not smoking, and higher education levels in populations who believe that cancer is curable are likely to be associated with greater participation in colorectal screening activities (Myers et al., 1990). Good success also has been demonstrated by Neale et al. (1989) in conducting screening activities in the workplace.

Interventions to Increase Use of Colorectal Cancer Screening

Reminder letters, postcards, and telephone calls have proven effective in increasing compliance with FOBT screening in a number of studies (Thompson, Michnich, Gray, Friedlander, & Gilson, 1986). These interventions capitalize on the influence of the physician recommendation in promoting screening. Interactive discussion between the nurse or doctor and the patient or a reminder call with a review of testing procedures also improves on observed compliance with cued reminders (Myers et al., 1991). The review of test procedures, while increasing compliance, also may serve to reinforce the need for dietary restriction and thus reduce false-positive testing (Mitchell-Beren, Dodds, Choi, & Waskerwitz, 1989). Finally, a study conducted by Weinrich, Weinrich, Stronborg, Boyd, and Weiss (1993) that compared elderly education method (social learning-based program delivered by older, peer facilitators) was more effective in increasing knowledge of colorectal cancer and compliance with FOBT screening than programs that were more traditionally based.

Interventions directed toward the physician also are necessary if colorectal screening is to prove of optimal benefit. Physician surveys conducted by Costanza, Hoople, Gaw, and Stoddard (1993) suggest that physicians feel they lack the training and are hesitant to recommend sigmoidoscopy unless patient-initiated, since it is costly, time-consuming, and uncomfortable. Limited studies to increase colorectal screening behavior among primary care physicians using in-house colorectal educational sessions and chart prompts have shown modest success (Litzelman, Dittus, Miller, & Tierney, 1993). It appears that efforts to increase the primary care physician's knowledge and awareness with regard to colorectal screening and encourage mastery with regard to proctoscopic exams are necessary if colorectal screening is indeed to achieve success.

Summary

Colorectal cancer represents a major threat to the health of many Americans. With recent evidence that screening can reduce mortality, there is promise that deaths due to colorectal cancer can be reduced. The challenge, however, is to overcome the significant barriers associated with screening tests among both patients and physicians.

ADHERENCE TO SKIN CANCER SCREENING

Background

The incidence of skin cancer has increased worldwide, with United States incidence data mirroring this trend (Burton et al., 1993; D. L. Miller & Weinstock, 1994). In the United States, there has been a 120% increase in male melanoma cases since 1958 and a 48% increase in women (American Cancer Society, 1994). It is unclear whether this increase is due to actual changes in prevalence or is a function of increased awareness with subsequent diagnosis and/or improved reporting by tumor registries (Elwood, 1993). In 1996, it was expected that 36,000 new cases of melanoma would be diagnosed and 8300 deaths attributed to melanoma. Each year, there are also 700,000 nonmelanoma skin cancers diagnosed (American Cancer Society, 1996). The United States lags behind many other countries in the creative application of interventions to reduce the incidence of and mortality from melanoma and other skin cancers. Australia, which has the highest reported incidence of melanoma anywhere, has mounted successful population-based programs that have had dramatic effects (Marks & McCarthy, 1990).

Skin cancer screening consists of a medical history and a whole-body examination under strong lighting (Emmett, 1986). The whole-body examination includes systematic observation and palpation of the scalp, head and neck including the oral cavity, arms, interdigital spaces, palms, fingernails, trunk, genitalia, skin folds, feet, plantar surfaces, toenails, and interdigital webs (Mihm & Fitzpatrick, 1976). A skin self-examination (SSE), like breast self-examination for breast cancer detection, is a method by which individuals can monitor their own skin for potential malignancies. SSE involves undressing completely and with a full-length and hand-held mirror systematically examining the total body surface (R. J. Friedman, Rigel, & Kopf, 1985).

To identify these skin cancers, patients can familiarize themselves with the ABCDEs of melanoma: *A*symmetry, *B*order irregularity, *C*olor variegation, *D*iameter enlargement, and *E*levation (Emmett, 1986). They can also be taught to recognize basal cell carcinomas, which are characterized by small translucent papules that slowly expand, found mostly on the head and neck areas, and squamous cell carcinoma, which presents as a crusted, nonhealing area found mostly on sites chronically exposed to the sun (Mackie, 1992).

Rationale for Skin Cancer Screening

Screening for skin cancer is quick, painless, and inexpensive, and requires no special technology. Thus, it should be acceptable to most patients and clinicians. Because skin cancer screening is not technology-requisite, it can be done almost anywhere. Programs have been successfully conducted at churches, health fairs, and county fairs, and in mobile settings (Koh, Mackie, & Reintgen, 1993).

While no randomized trials proving the impact of skin cancer screening have been performed to date, research results suggest that skin cancer screening may lower mortality from skin cancer, and especially melanoma, by improving rates of early detection (Koh, Caruso, & Gage, 1990). Koh et al. (1993) found that melanoma survival rates compared to a national cancer database were higher in Florida, where a number of universities participated in an intensive public skin cancer screening program that included education programs for medical providers. Koh et al. (1991) found that screening programs attracted individuals more likely to have risk factors for melanoma as compared to the general population, thus maximizing the yield of the programs.

Skin Cancer Screening Guidelines

Experts have not agreed on screening guidelines for skin cancer. The U.S. Preventive Services Task Force recommends "routine screening for individuals at high risk" (e.g. those having a family or personal history of skin cancer, clinical evidence of precursor lesions, and increased exposure to sunlight). The task force does not define what is meant by "routine" screening, nor does it report specific recommendations for SSE. The American Cancer Society (1980) recommends a cancer-related checkup, including a skin examination, ever 3 years for the general population over the age of 20 years and "more frequently" for persons at risk. The National Cancer Institute (1994) also recognizes the benefits of skin cancer screening, but offers no specific guidelines for such screening. Other experts recommend yearly skin cancer screenings (R. J. Friedman et al., 1985), regular screening for the elderly (Beers, Fink, & Beck, 1991), and skin cancer screening for every new patient seen by a dermatologist (Howell, 1986).

Barriers to Skin Cancer Screening

Unlike the research for breast and cervical cancer, relatively few studies have focused on evaluating barriers to dermatological screening. Being young, female, educated, of a higher SES, having a suspicious lesion, and being at high risk or believing one is at high risk have been identified as facilitators to skin cancer screening (Girgis, Campbell, Redman, & Sanson-Fisher, 1991; Weinstock, 1990). Convenience in terms of the screening location has also been identified as a factor for participation (Rampen, Berretty, Van Huystee, Kiemeney, & Nijs, 1993). Most studies show that people who participate in free skin cancer screening often are concerned about symptoms (Girasek, 1986; Koh et al., 1991).

Girgis et al. (1991) identified additional predictors. In their study, 1344 randomly selected individuals were asked about their skin cancer screening habits. Men and people of lower occupational status, and individuals who were unemployed or too ill to work, or who did not have health insurance, were less likely to have been screened. People at high risk, who believed that it was likely that they would develop melanoma in their lifetime and who believed in the benefits of early detection for melanoma, were more likely to have been screened. Perhaps the most important finding from this study was that when a physician advocated it, 73% of patients performed SSE, compared to only 31% who did not receive such instruction. This last point highlights the potential influence general practitioners can have on improving adherence to skin cancer screening and is consistent with the strong impact that a physician's recommendation has in other studies. This study was conducted in Australia, where the prevalence of melanoma and nonmelanoma skin cancer is disproportionately high (Armstrong, 1988; Giles, Marks, & Foley, 1988) and intensive efforts have been implemented to educate and screen the public.

In a study aimed at assessing the predictors for SSE for skin cancer (L. C. Friedman, Bruce, Webb, Weinberg, & Cooper, 1993), 2213 individuals at high or moderate risk for skin cancer were offered the opportunity to participate in a free skin cancer screening program. Of this group, 384 opted to accept the invitation. Knowledge about SSE was associated with increased self-efficacy and also SSE frequency, a result the authors suggest highlights the importance of educating individuals about performing SSE.

Interventions to Promote Adherence to Skin Cancer Screening

Most skin cancer interventions have focused on educating the public regarding the risks for skin cancer and the importance of sunscreen use and other sun-blocking behaviors for the prevention of skin cancer. Studies attempting to improve preventive measures have focused on populations at risk, such as outdoor workers (Girgis, Sanson-Fisher, & Watson, 1994), families of melanoma patients (Masri et al., 1990), and the general population in Australia, where melanoma prevalence is unusually high (Hill, White, Marks, & Borland, 1993). Additionally, since early sun exposure is a risk factor, interventions have been instituted in school systems to educate children and their parents about the risk of sun exposure and sunburn (Girgis, Sanson-Fisher, Tripodi, & Golding, 1993). All of these interventions have shared varying degrees of success in increasing sun-protective behaviors.

Interventions as simple as distributing a large number of pamphlets encouraging SSE and illustrating the features of melanoma have been shown to increase the number of melanomas diagnosed at an early stage (3% preintervention to 21% postintervention) and to reduce the number of advanced lesions diagnosed in a community (60% preintervention to 14% postintervention) (Christofolini, Zumiani, Boi, & Piscoli, 1986). More extensive interventions aimed at educating the public as well as health care professionals and cosmetologists through statewide publicity and workshops also have improved public knowledge about melanoma and skin cancer and have increased screening behaviors and sun-protective measures (Ramsdell, Kelly, Coody, & Dany, 1991).

Summary

The literature on skin cancer screening suggests that education about the risks for skin cancer and the benefits of early diagnosis for survival remains the best method for encouraging skin cancer screening and regular self-examination. The availability of a prevention strategy (e.g., use of sunscreens and limiting sun exposure) means it must be a major feature of education programs. More research is needed to evaluate the effects of various interventions. Additionally, educational programs need to be focused not only on the general public and high-risk individuals, but also toward physicians to encourage recommendation for screening.

ADHERENCE TO PROSTATE CANCER SCREENING

Background

One out of 11 American men will develop prostate cancer during their lifetime, making it the most prevalent cancer among males in the United States. Approximately one fourth of these men will die from the disease, making it the second leading cause of male cancer-related death. In 1996, it is projected that 200,000 men were diagnosed with prostate cancer and 40,000 will die from it (American Cancer Society, 1996). Increases in both incidence and mortality are forecast. By the year 2000, it is estimated, "our country will see a 37% increase in prostate cancer deaths and a whopping 90% increase in new cases per year" (Carter & Coffey, 1990).

Rationale for Prostate Cancer Screening

Screening for prostate cancer has been advocated by some groups, such as the American Cancer Society and the American Urological Association, to promote earlier diagnosis and reduce mortality for prostate cancer.

For many years, screening for prostate cancer centered around the digital rectal exam (DRE). DREs are conducted by health care professionals who insert a gloved finger into the rectum and palpate the prostate gland through the rectal wall. The DRE has been criticized, however, for its lack of sensitivity.

A serological test with markedly improved sensitivity was developed by Wang et al. (1981). Prostate-specific antigen (PSA), a protease secreted exclusively by the prostatic epithelial cells, was identified as a tumor marker (Haas, Montie, & Pontes, 1993). Although the sensitivity and specificity of PSA testing are highly dependent on the threshold value used, a standard cutoff of 4 mg/ml (Hybritech assay) has a sensitivity of 57-81%. The fact that many benign conditions increase PSA results in a positive predictive value of only 35% (Garnick, 1993). While screening strategies for prostate cancer exist, screening is controversial for the following reasons: (1) It has a low positive predictive value, resulting in many false positives; (2) the science does not yet exist to distinguish virulent versus indolent disease, therefore clouding the benefit of treatment; (3) treatment is associated with significant morbidity (i.e., impotence, urinary incontinence); and (4) the value of screening in preventing mortality has not yet been proven.

The controversy surrounding prostate cancer screening has polarized recommendations for screening by authoritative agencies. The American Cancer Society and the American Urological Association currently endorse annual DRE and PSA testing in men over the age of 50 or age 40 for men at higher risk (i.e., African-Americans or men with a family history of prostate cancer). Screening is not recommended past the age of 70, since the advantage of screening may prove beneficial only in men who have at least a 10-year life expectancy. Conversely, the U.S. Preventive Services Task Force, the Canadian Task Force, and the American College of Physicians totally oppose prostate cancer screening. The National Cancer Institute recommends only annual DRE for the detection of both colorectal and prostate cancer. This recommendation is made for males over the age of 50, or for males over the age of 40 in high-risk groups. Faced with the controversy of prostate cancer screening, Chodak (1993) appealed for patient education, stating that "until proper studies are completed, patients may benefit most from an understanding of potential risks and benefits involved, allowing them to ultimately decide for themselves. Biased recommendations, either for or against screening, are probably not in the public's best interest."

Barriers to Adherence to Prostate Cancer Screening

A study by Demark-Wahnefried, Catoe, Paskett, Robertson, and Rimer (1993) of 1700 men participating in prostate cancer screening events supports the finding that mass screenings primarily attract white males, a number of whom have been previously screened for prostate cancer. They suggest that innovative strategies to reach populations currently underserved and at risk are necessary if optimal benefit is sought through mass prostate cancer screening. One such strategy is to offer screening at facilities within the African-American community or elicit the support of important community leaders and institutions within this subpopulation (e.g., black churches). Other reported barriers that must be overcome are cost, concern about physical discomfort and embarrassment associated with the DRE, and worry related to an abnormal exam (Demark-Wahnefried et al., 1993).

Summary

If men are to make an optimal informed decision regarding screening, decisions should be made, not en masse, but individually in consultation with one's primary care provider. The issues surrounding prostate cancer screening, however, are "complex ... difficult for physicians to give and even more difficult for patients to absorb" (Marshall, 1993). Currently, a minority of older men report that their physicians discuss prostate cancer or prostate cancer screening with them (Demark-Wahnefried et al., 1993). Until results of the Prostate, Lung, Colorectal, and Ovarian trial are available, men will be asked to decide for themselves regarding screening. Efforts directed toward easing the decision-making process and guiding physicians toward appropriate counseling are necessary if men are to make the best decisions related to screening in the future (Fleming, Wasson, Albertsen, Barry, & Wennberg, 1993).

The authors found no published reports of intervention studies designed to assess strategies to increase participation in prostate cancer screening.

ADHERENCE TO TESTICULAR CANCER SCREENING

Background

The incidence of testicular cancer has increased significantly since the mid-1950s, doubling in the past two decades (Giwercman, von er Maase, & Skakkebaek, 1993). Approximately 6100 cases of testicular cancer were reported in recent years, with most cases being white and of upper SES (Frame & Carlson, 1975). Age-specific incidence is bimodal, with the major peak occurring between the ages of 20 and 35 years and the lesser peak after age 70 (Sladden & Dickinson, 1993). Disease in older men is often the result of secondary tumors associated with lymphoma and brings low rates of mortality. Germ cell tumors, on the other hand, are most common in younger men, and the disease is more virulent (Vogt & McHale, 1992).

With 5-year survival rates greater than 90%, testicular cancer is the most curable solid tumor in men (Iammarino & Scardino, 1991). Screening in younger men has been proposed because of high cure rates and the influence of cure in reducing the loss of the most productive years of life (Raina et al., 1993). Screening for testicular cancer, however, remains controversial, and no RCTs have been conducted.

Rationale for Testicular Cancer Screening

With testicular cancer often presenting as a painless swelling or lump, proponents of screening argue that rates of cure could be enhanced and morbidity reduced if men received regular clinical testicular examination (CTE) by their primary care providers and learned how to perform routine testicular self-examination (TSE) (Giwercman et al., 1993). Educational efforts targeted toward both patients and physicians might reduce the lag time that often occurs, first, because of patient delay due to lack of knowledge, guilt, and embarrassment and, second, because of misdiagnosis (Iammarino & Scardino, 1991). A survey of 335 men diagnosed with testicular cancer suggests that patient delay in seeking care after the onset of symptoms ranges from 2 months to 3 years (Bosl et al., 1981).

Conversely, opponents of screening argue that the histology of the disease makes a larger contribution to mortality than stage (Frame & Carlson, 1975). They contend that the benefit of TSE is unproven, much as the value of BSE remains unproven, and that the disease is sufficiently rare in the general population to make palpation of the testes by the primary care physician unjustified (Frame & Carlson, 1975). It is acknowledged, however, that screening may be beneficial in high-risk subgroups, i.e., those diagnosed with cryptorchidism, gonadal dysgenesis, inguinal hernia, hydrocele, Klinefelter's syndrome, infertility, or mumps orchitis, or men with a previous or family history of testicular cancer (Giwercman et al., 1993).

Testicular Cancer Screening Guidelines

Current testicular cancer screening guidelines for the general population are varied. The American Cancer Society (ACS) takes the most proactive stance and supports the practice of CTE in periodic health examinations of all males over the age of 15. Additionally, the ACS recommends monthly TSE for all postpubertal males (U.S. Preventive Services Task Force [USPSTF], 1989). These guidelines are reiterated in the ACS's published plan for youth education, along with the goal of educating 80% of 18-year-old males on the process of TSE by the year 2000. Conversely, the USPSTF does not support efforts toward screening in the general population and recommends screening only for males at highest risk, i.e., those with histories of cryptorchidism, orchiopexy, or testicular atrophy (USPSTF, 1989). Guidelines of the Canadian Task Force parallel United States guidelines; screening is recommended only in males with histories of cryptorchidism, testicular atrophy, or ambiguous sex (hermaphroditism) (USPSTF, 1989). The National Cancer Institute has recently adopted the USPSTF recommendations, after many years of supporting early detection efforts for both men (monthly TSE) and health care providers (CTE).

Barriers to Adherence to Testicular Cancer Screening

If secondary prevention of testicular cancer is recommended, a number of barriers must be overcome. The first is the lack of awareness of testicular cancer and means of early detection. Research conducted in several male populations since 1980 suggests that 31-87% of men do not know that the testis can be affected by cancer. Knowledge among older professional men appears to be greater than that reported for college students and certain subgroups, i.e., African-Americans (Underwood-Millon & Sanders, 1991).

Studies conducted in a variety of male populations (e.g., high school and college students, men enlisted in the military, and male athletes) indicate that only 12-40% have ever heard of TSE and only 2-10% report conducting TSE on a regular basis (Wardle et al., 1994). Furthermore, studies conducted in high school and college males indicate that although males report routine TSE, few or none are able to correctly describe the procedure (Murphy & Brubaker, 1990; Reno, 1988; Sheley, Kinchen, Morgan, & Gordon, 1991; Vaz, Best, Davis, & Kaiser, 1989).

Research indicates that the lack of knowledge related to testicular cancer and TSE is a major deterrent for early detection efforts (Bell, 1990; Underwood-Millon & Sanders, 1991). A small number of studies have been undertaken to assess the impact of educational programs designed to increase the awareness of testicular carcinoma and the appropriate technique for TSE. Although some programs were not theory-driven or did not report theories underlying their development, frameworks established by the PRECEDE and health belief models, as well as Orem's self-care framework (e.g., Orem, 1985) and the theory of planned behavior (e.g., Ajzen and Fishbein, 1980), were used to develop interventions in a few studies (Martin, 1990; Murphy & Brubaker, 1990; Ostwald & Rothenberger, 1985; Rudolph & Quinn, 1988). Despite the diversity, all programs reported significant increases in knowledge regarding testicular cancer, and many had a significant impact on TSE.

Interventions to Increase Adherence to Testicular Self-Examination

The research of Brubaker and Wickersham (1990) suggests that college-age males were more likely to report TSE 6 weeks after participating in an educational session in which persuasive messages were used to challenge unfavorable views toward TSE than were males who attended traditional educational sessions (Brubaker & Wickersham, 1990).

A male cancer education program (prostate and testicular cancer) developed around a health behavior model and targeting intervention strategies toward predisposing, enabling, and reinforcing factors was pre- and posttested by Martin (1990) on 448 male employees in a large electrical power plant in the Southwest. Although the program was well received and was effective in increasing knowledge and changing beliefs, its efficacy was not tested against other programs, nor was its impact on TSE measured. A study conducted by Marty and McDermott (1985) incorporated elements of the health belief model in testing the impact of two testicular cancer educational programs on 128 college men, one delivered by a health professional and the other delivered by a college-age male who disclosed that he had testicular cancer. Although the men to whom the patient delivered the program were more likely to view the program as valuable and left the program with greater feelings of susceptibility ($p < 0.05$), there were no differences in resulting knowledge, and this study also did not measure the impact of educational programs on TSE. Since TSE is a primary end point of educational sessions, measurement of pre- and post-TSE behavior is vital if programs are to be thoroughly evaluated. Ideally, not only should the impact of educational sessions on TSE-related behavior be measured in the short term (i.e., 1 month to 6 weeks after the program), but also long-term changes in behavior should be monitored. To date, only one study has employed postprogram surveys to evaluate long-term changes in TSE-related behavior. The evaluation of a program developed by Ostwald and Rothenberger (1985) suggested that testicular cancer education programs can significantly increase the adoption of TSE by high school and college students ($N = 577$), both in the short term (1 month postprogram) and in the long term (1-2 years postprogram).

Finally, if programs for early detection of testicular cancer are to be implemented, it will be necessary for health care providers to educate men to practice TSE, to conduct CTE on their patients, and to handle suspicious cases both expediently and effectively. Two surveys conducted by Ogle, Snellman, and Henry (1988) and Sayger, Fortenberry, and Beckman (1988) suggest that although CTE is usually incorporated into clinical exams, few physicians instruct their patients on how to conduct TSE (17.5-29%). With findings of Sayger et al. (1988) indicating that 82% of physicians either are unfamiliar with TSE or never thought about including it in routine exams, there are obvious barriers that must be addressed. Sheley et al. (1991) contend that one barrier is the perception among health care providers that TSE is so easy that it requires no discussion (Sheley et al., 1991). If early detection efforts related to testicular cancer are to succeed, development of patient education programs and materials for physician use appears necessary in order to promote physician comfort in providing instruction and to do so in a time-efficient manner.

Summary

Testicular cancer is a highly curable malignancy that affects males primarily during puberty and early adulthood. Screening, which includes clinical testicle examination (CTE) during routine physical examinations and testicular self-examination (TSE), has been proposed in efforts to detect disease at an earlier stage when treatment is more efficacious and results in less morbidity. Surveys conducted since 1980 suggest that a lack of awareness of testicular cancer and TSE represent primary barriers to screening by both patient and provider. Educational programs, however, are effective in increasing both awareness and practice of TSE. Although screening guidelines currently vary, with the ACS and the NCI endorsing CTE during periodic medical exams and monthly TSE in postpubertal males, and the USPSTF recommending screening only in populations at highest risk (e.g., males having cryptorchidism, orchiopexy, or testicular atrophy), if indeed screening is to be promoted in the general population, significant barriers related to knowledge and awareness will have to be overcome in both patients and providers. Additional barriers will also have to be explored.

THE POTENTIAL IMPACT OF GENETIC ADVANCES ON CANCER GENETIC SCREENING

A revolution in molecular genetics means that within the next few years, there will most likely be a variety of blood tests that can be used to identify people at high risk for cancer. It is likely that melanoma and lung, breast, colorectal, kidney, prostate, and ovarian cancers all include some cases that are due to cancer susceptibility genes. Perhaps up to 10% of any of these cancers are the result of these genes. Most recently, the BRCA1 and 2 genes for breast cancer were identified. As blood tests are developed to identify people with genetic mutations, the public, or at least potentially high-risk persons (due to a strong family history), will be offered genetic testing for cancer. Data discussed by Lerman, Audrain, and Croyle (1994) suggest that there will be great interest in genetic testing. The majority of individuals from high-risk families surveyed by Lerman said they would want to be tested. Once people with cancer susceptibility genes have been identified, they can be targeted for surveillance programs.

Genetic counseling programs should be an integral component of genetic screening for cancer (Lerman et al., 1994). Careful attention should be paid to educating people about what genetic testing means and how to communicate results.

As Lerman et al. (1994) suggested, one of the greatest potential benefits of genetic testing will be the opportunity to reduce morbidity and mortality from cancer by motivating changes in personal risk and cancer screening behaviors. But unlike other areas of genetic screening, e.g., screening for cystic fibrosis or Huntington's disease, a negative result on a genetic screen is no guarantee that the person will not get cancer. Most cancers are due to a combination of genetic and other factors. In communicating test results, behavioral scientists will have to communicate that message along with appropriate behavior change and surveillance recommendations.

CONCLUSION

Adherence to cancer screening is affected by diverse factors related to individuals, their providers, and the health care system. All of these determinants must be understood before appropriate interventions can be devised. For example, although women should be knowledgeable about Pap tests, much of the decision making is in the domain of providers. In colorectal screening, a range of barriers exist, including patient, provider, and system factors. For some cancers, such as prostate, colorectal, breast, and cervical, concerns about pain and discomfort may be significant barriers. For others, such as testicular and skin cancer, knowledge factors may dominate. When the wrong target of intervention is selected, programs may be neither effective nor cost-effective. Multiple levels of intervention are needed to affect adherence, with interventions directed at patients, providers, and the health care system. It is important to tailor print, audiovisual, and interpersonal interventions to the sociocultural needs of target populations. Materials produced for community health research can be used in conjunction with health professional counseling protocols to encourage patient compliance. Public health programs also can use outreach advocacy methods to underserved populations and to make programs more accessible. Likewise, changes in clinic structures and reminders can enhance adherence because they affect the determinants of adherence.

The strongest public health initiatives embody an ecological approach with interventions directed not only at individuals, but also toward the groups to which they belong, workplaces, and governments (McLeroy, Bibeau, Steckler, & Glanz, 1988). Community-level prevention efforts should involve a wide variety of experts in developing and implementing health promotion programs. Thus, in the ideal scenario, individual behavior change should be supported in medical care, in the family, at work, and in the community.

In some areas of cancer screening, e.g., prostate and testicular, there are still controversies regarding whether screening is indicated. In almost all areas of cancer screening, there is a considerable distance to go before the majority of age-eligible people are getting screened on the recommended schedule. Behavioral interventions can effect a dramatic improvement in compliance with screening. Caution, however, is in order. Behavioral scientists must carefully evaluate efficacy data before they promote cancer screening tests. Interventions should be based not only on sound behavioral science but also on a solid foundation of epidemiological and medical science.

REFERENCES

Ajzen, I. G., & Fishbein, M. (1980). *Understanding attitudes and predicting social behavior*. Englewood Cliffs, NJ: Prentice-Hall.

American Cancer Society (1980). Cancer-related checkups: If you're between 20 and 40, if you're 40 and over.

American Cancer Society (1993). *Cancer facts & figures—1993*. Atlanta, GA: American Cancer Society.

American Cancer Society (1996). *Cancer facts & figures—1996*. Atlanta, GA: American Cancer Society.

Amezcua, C., McAlister, A., Ramirez A., & Espinoza, R. (1990). A su salud: Health promotion in a Mexican-American border community. In N. Bracht (Ed.), *Health promotion at the community level* (pp. 257-277). London: Sage.

Ansell, D., Lacey, L., Whitman, S., Chen, E., & Phillips, C. (1994). A nurse-delivered intervention to reduce barriers to breast and cervical cancer screening in Chicago inner city clinics. *Public Health Reports, 109*, 104-111.

Armstrong, B. K. (1988). The epidemiology and prevention of cancer in Australia. *Australian and New Zealand Journal of Surgery, 58*, 179-187.

Bandura, A. (1986). *Social foundations of thought and action*. Englewood Cliffs, NJ: Prentice-Hall.

Beers, M. H., Fink, A., & Beck, J. C. (1991). Screening recommendations for the elderly. *American Journal of Public Health, 81*(9), 1131-1140.

Bell, I. (1990). Testicular self examination. *Nursing Times, 86*(9), 38-39.

Berman, B. A., Bastani, R., Nisenbaum, R., Henneman, C. A., & Marcus, A. C. (1994). Cervical cancer screening among a low-income multiethnic population of women. *Journal of Women's Health, 3*(1), 33-43.

Blalock, S. J., DeVellis, B. M., Afifi, R. A., & Sandler, R. S. (1990). Risk perceptions and participation in colorectal cancer screening. *Health Psychology, 9*(6), 792-806.

Bloom, J. (1994). Guidelines for early detection of cancer. *Cancer, 4*(5), 1465.

Bosl, G. J., Vogelzang, N. J., Goldman, A., Fraley, E. E., Lange, P. H., Levitt, S. H., & Kennedy, B. J. (1981). Impact of delay in diagnosis on clinical stage of testicular cancer. *Lancet, 2*(8253), 970-973.

Brubaker, R. G., & Wickersham, D. (1990). Encouraging the practice of testicular self-examination: A field application of the theory of reasoned action. *Health Psychology, 9*, 154-163.

Burton, R. C., Coates, M. S., Hersey, P., Roberts, G., Chetty, M. P., Chan, S., Hayes, M. H., Howe, C. G., & Armstrong, B. K. (1993). An analysis of a melanoma epidemic. *International Journal of Cancer, 55*, 765-770.

Calle, E., Flanders, W., Thun, M., & Martin, L. (1993). Demographic predictors of mammography and Pap smear screening in U.S. women. *American Journal of Public Health, 33*(1), 51-60.

Carney, P., Dietrich, A. J., & Freeman, D. H. (1992). Improving future preventive care through educational efforts at a women's community screening program. *Journal of Community Health, 17*(3), 167-174.

Carter, H. B., & Coffey, D. S. (1990). The prostate: An increasing medical problem. *Prostate, 16*, 39-48.

Celentano, D. D., Shapiro, S., & Weisman, C. S. (1982). Cancer preventive screening behavior among elderly women. *Preventive Medicine, 11*, 454-463.

Champion, V. L. (1994). Strategies to increase mammography utilization. *Medical Care, 32*(2), 118-129.

Chodak, G. W. (1993). Screening for prostate cancer. *European Urology, 24*(Suppl. 2), 3-5.

Christofolini, M., Zumiani, G., Boi, S., & Piscioli, F. (1986). Community detection of early melanoma. *Lancet*, 156.

Chu, K. C., Tarone, R. E., Chow, W. H., Hankey, B. F., & Gloeckler Ries, L. A. (1994). Temporal patterns in colorectal cancer incidence, survival, and mortality from 1950 through 1990. *Journal of the National Cancer Institute, 86*(13), 997-1006.

Cockburn, J., Hirst, S., Hill, D., & Marks, R. (1991). Increasing cervical screening in women of more than 40 years of age: An intervention in general practice. *Medical Journal of Australia, 152*(4), 190-194.

Cohen, S. J., Halvorson, H. W., Gosselink, C. A. (1994). Changing physician behavior to improve disease prevention. *Preventive Medicine, 23*, 284-291.

Costanza, M. E., Hoople, N. E., Gaw, V. P., & Stoddard, A. M. (1993). Cancer prevention practices and continuing education needs of primary care physicians. *American Journal of Preventive Medicine, 9*(2), 107-112.

Craun, S. M., & Deffenbacher, J. L. (1981). Cancer knowledge and examination frequency in college students. *Journal of American College Health, 31*(12), 123-126.

Crawford, E. D., & DeAntoni, E. P. (1993). PSA as a screening test for prostate cancer. *Urologic Clinics of North America, 20*(4), 637-646.

Creighton, P. A., & Evans, A. M. (1992). Audit of practice based cervical smear programme: Completion of the cycle. *British Medical Journal, 304*(6832), 932-936.

Demark-Wahnefried, W., Catoe, K., Paskett, E., Robertson, C. N., & Rimer, B. K. (1993). Characteristics of men reporting for prostate cancer screening. *Urology, 42*(3), 269-275.

Dignan, M. B., Beal, P. E., Michielutte, R., Sharp, P. C., Daniels, L. A., & Young, L. D. (1990). Development of a direct education workshop for cervical cancer prevention in high risk women: The Forsyth County project. *Journal of Cancer Education, 5*(4), 217-223.

Dignan, M., Michielutte, R., Wells, H. B., & Bahnson, J. (1994). The Forsyth County cervical cancer prevention project: Cervical cancer screening for black women. *Health Education & Research, 9*(4), 411-420.

Elwood, J. M. (1993). Recent developments in melanoma epidemiology. *Melanoma Research, 3*, 149-156.

Emmett, E. A. (1986). Dermatological screening. *Journal of Occupational Medicine*, 28(10), 1045-1050.

Fleming, C., Wasson, J. H., Albertsen, P. C., Barry, M. J., & Wennberg, J. E. (1993). A decision analysis of alternative treatment strategies for clinically localized prostate cancer: Prostate patient outcomes research team. *Journal of the American Medical Association*, *269*, 2650-2658.

Fletcher, S., Black, W., Harris, R., Rimer, B., & Shapiro, S. (1993). Special Article: Report of the international workshop on screening for breast cancer. *Journal of the National Cancer Institute*, *85*, 1644-1656.

Frame, P. S., & Carlson, S. J. (1975). A critical review of periodic health screening using specific screening criteria: Selected diseases of the genitourinary system. *Journal of Family Practice*, *2*(3), 189-194.

Friedman, L. C., Bruce, S., Webb, J. A., Weinberg, A. D., & Cooper, H. P. (1993). Skin self-examination in a population at increased risk for skin cancer. *American Journal of Preventative Medicine*, *9*(6), 359-364.

Friedman, R. J., Rigel, D. S., & Kopf, A. W. (1985). Early detection of malignant melanoma: The role of physician examination and self-examination of the skin. *CA—A Cancer Journal for Clinicians*, *35*(3), 130-151.

Garnick, M. B. (1993). Prostate cancer: Screening, diagnosis, and management. *Annals of Internal Medicine*, *118*, 804-818.

Giles, G. G., Marks, R., & Foley, P. (1988). Incidence of nonmelanocytic skin cancer treated in Australia *British Medical Journal*, *296*, 13-17.

Girasek, D. C. (1986). Motivating the public to take advantage of skin cancer screening. *Journal of the American Academy of Dermatology*, *15*(2), 309-315.

Girgis, A., Campbell, E. M., Redman, S., & Sanson-Fisher, R. W. (1991). Screening for melanoma: A community survey of prevalence and predictors. *Medical Journal of Australia*, *154*, 338-343.

Girgis, A., Sanson-Fisher, R. W., Tripodi, D. A., & Golding, T. (1993). Evaluation of interventions to improve solar protection in primary schools. *Health Education Quarterly*, *20*(2), 275-287.

Girgis, A., Sanson-Fisher, R. W., and Watson, A. (1994). A workplace intervention for increasing outdoor workers' use of solar protection. *American Journal of Public Health*, *84*(1), 77-81.

Giwercman, A., von er Maase, H., & Skakkebaek, N. E. (1993). Epidemiological and clinical aspects of carcinoma in situ of the testis. Session 4: Carcinoma in situ of the testes—screening and management. *European Urology*, *23*, 104-114.

Haas, G. P., Montie, J. E., & Pontes, J. E. (1993). The state of prostate cancer screening in the United States. *European Urology*, *23*, 337-347.

Harlan, L. C., Bernstein, A. B., & Kessler, L. G. (1991). Cervical cancer screening: Who is not screened and why? *American Journal of Public Health*, *81*, 885-891.

Harris, R. P., Fletcher, S. W., Gonzalez, J. J., Lannin, D. R., Degnan, D., Earp, J. A., & Clark, R. (1990). Mammography and age: Are we targeting the wrong women? A community survey of women and physicians. *Cancer*, *67*, 2010-2014.

Hennekens, C. H., & Buring, J. E. (1987). *Epidemiology in medicine 1987*. Boston/Toronto: Little, Brown.

Hill, D., White, V., Marks, R., & Borland, R. (1993). Changes in sun-related attitudes and behaviors and reduced sunburn prevalence in a population at high risk of melanoma. *European Journal of Cancer Prevention*, *2*, 447-456.

Howell, J. B. (1986). Spotting sinister spots: A challenge to dermatologists to examine every new patient at increased risk for signs of early melanoma. *Journal of the American Academy of Dermatology*, *15*(4), 722-726.

Hunter, W., Farmer, A., Mant, D., Verne, J., Northover, J., & Fitzpatrick, R. (1990). The effect of self-administered fecal occult blood tests on compliance with screening for colorectal cancer: Result of a survey of those invited. *Family Practice*, *8*, 367-372.

Iammarino, N. J., & Scardino, P. T. (1991). Testicular cancer: The role of the primary care physician in prevention and early detection. *Journal of Texas Medicine*, *87*(5), 66-71.

Kang, S. H., & Bloom, J. R. (1993). Social support and cancer screening among older black Americans. *Journal of the National Cancer Institute*, *85*, 737-742.

Koh, H. K., Caruso, A., & Gage I. (1990). Evaluation of melanoma/skin cancer screening in Massachusetts: Preliminary results. *Cancer*, *65*, 375-379.

Koh, H. K., Geller, A. C., Miller, D. R., Caruso, A., Gage, I., & Lew, R. A. (1991). Who is being screened for melanoma/skin cancer: Characteristics of persons screened in Massachusetts. *Journal of the American Academy of Dermatology*, *24*(2), 271-277.

Koh, H. K., Mackie, R. M., & Reintgen, D. S. (1993). The prevention and early detection of melanoma: Screening for melanoma. *Cancer Screening*, *18*, 72-76.

Lacey, L. P., Phillips, C. W., Ansell, D., Whitman, S., Ebie, N., & Chen, E. (1989). An urban community-based cancer prevention screening and health education intervention in Chicago. *Public Health Report*, *104*(6), 536-541.

Lacey, L., Whitfield, J., DeWhite, W., Ansell, D., Whitman, S., Chen, E., & Phillips, C. (1993). Referral adherence in an inner city breast and cervical cancer screening program. *Cancer*, *72*, 950-955.

Lerman, C., Audrain, J., & Croyle, R. T. (1994). DNA-testing for heritable breast cancer risks: Lessons from traditional genetic counseling. *Annals of Behavioral Medicine*, *16*(4), 327-333.

Lerman, C., Trock, B., Rimer, B. K., Boyce, A., Jepson, C., & Engstrom, P. F. (1991). Psychological and behavioral implications of abnormal mammograms. *Annals of Internal Medicine*, *114*, 657.

Lichtenstein, E., & Glasgow, R. E. (1992). Smoking cessation: What have we learned over the past decade? *Journal of Consulting and Clinical Psychology*, *60*(4), 518-527.

Litzelman, D. K., Dittus, R. S., Miller, M. E., & Tierney, W. M. (1993). Requiring physicians to respond to computerized reminders improves their compliance with preventive care protocols. *Journal of General Internal Medicine, 8*(6), 311-317.

Mackie, R. (1992). Screening for skin cancer. *Occupational Health (London), 44*(7), 202-206.

Mandelblatt, J. (1989). Cervical cancer screening in primary care: Issues and recommendations. *Primary Care, 16*(1), 133-155.

Marcus, A. C., Crane, L. A., Kaplan, C. P., Goodman, K. J., Savage, E., & Gunning, J. (1990). Screening for cervical cancer in emergency centers and sexually transmitted disease clinics. *Obstetrics and Gynecology, 75*(3), 453-455.

Marks, R., & McCarthy, W. (1990). Skin cancer: Increasing incidence and public awareness. *Medical Journal of Australia, 153*, 505-506.

Marshall, K. G. (1993). Screening for prostate cancer: How can patients give informed consent? *Canadian Family Physician, 39*, 2385-2390.

Martin, J. P. (1990). Male cancer awareness: Impact of an employee education program. *Oncology Nursing Forum, 17*(1), 59-64.

Marty, P. J., & McDermott, R. J. (1985). Effects of two testicular cancer education programs on self examination knowledge and attitudes among college-aged men. *Health Education, 16*(3), 33-35.

Masri, G. D., Clark, W. H., Guerry, D., Halpern, A., Thompson, C. J., & Elder, D. E. (1990). Screening and surveillance of patients at high risk for malignant melanoma result in detection of earlier disease. *Journal of the American Academy of Dermatology, 22*(6), 1042-1048.

Mayer, J. A., Clapp, E. J., Bartholomew, S., & Elder, J. (1993). Facility-based in-reach strategies to promote annual mammograms. Presented at the 14th Annual Meeting of the Society of Behavioral Medicine, March, San Francisco.

McCarthy, B. D., & Moskowitz, M. A. (1993). Screening flexible sigmoidoscopy. Patient attitudes and compliance. *Journal of General Internal Medicine, 8*, 120-125.

McLeroy, K. R., Bibeau, D., Steckler, A., & Glanz, K. (1988). An ecologial perspective on health promotion programs. *Health Education Quarterly, 15*, 351-377.

Mihm, M. C., & Fitzpatrick, T. B. (1976). Early detection of malignant melanoma. *Cancer, 37*(Suppl.), 597-603.

Miller, D. L., & Weinstock, M. A. (1994). Non-melanoma skin cancer in the United States: Incidence. *Journal of the American Academy of Dermatology, 30*(5), 774-778.

Millon-Underwood, S., & Sanders, E. (1991). Testicular self-examination among African-American men. *Journal of the National Black Nurses Association, 5*(1), 18-28.

Mitchell-Beren, M. E., Dodds, M. E., Choi, K. L., & Waskerwitz, T. R. (1989). A colorectal cancer prevention, screening, and evaluation program in community black churches. *CA—A Cancer Journal for Clinicians, 39*(2), 115-118.

Montano, D. E., & Taplin, S. H. (1991). A test of an expanded theory of reasoned action to predict mammography participation. *Social Science and Medicine, 32*, 733-741.

Morisky, D. E. (1986). Nonadherence to medical recommendations for hypertensive patients: Problems and potential solutions. *Journal of Compliance in Health Care, 1*, 5-20.

Murphy, W. G., & Brubaker, R. G. (1990). Effects of a brief theory-based intervention on the practice of testicular self-examination by high school males. *Journal of School Health, 60*(9), 459-462.

Myers, R. E., Balshem, A. M., Wolf, T. A., Ross, E. A., & Millner, L. (1993). Adherence to continuous screening for colorectal neoplasia. *Medical Care, 31*, 508-519.

Myers, R. E., Ross, E. A., Wolf, T. A., Balshem, A., Jepson, C., & Millner, L. (1991). Behavioral interventions to increase adherence in colorectal cancer screening. *Medical Care, 29*, 1039-1050.

Myers, R. E., Trock, B. J., Lerman, C., Wolf, T., Ross, E., & Engstrom, P. F. (1990). Adherence to colorectal cancer screening in an HMO population. *Preventive Medicine, 19*, 502-514.

National Cancer Institute. (1994). *PDQ cancer screening/prevention summary: Skin cancer screening*. Bethesda, MD: National Cancer Institute.

Neale, A. V., Demers, R. Y., & Herman, S. (1989). Compliance with colorectal cancer screening in a high-risk occupational group. *Journal of Occupational Medicine, 31*(12), 1007-1012.

Norman, S. A., Talbott, E. O., Kuller, L. H., Krampe, B. R., & Stolley, P. D. (1991). Demographic, psychosocial, and medical correlates of Pap testing: A literature review. *American Journal of Preventive Medicine, 7*, 219-226.

Ogle, K. S., Snellman, L. A., & Henry, R. C. (1988). Breast and testicular examination in primary care. *American Journal of Preventive Medicine, 4*(1), 11-13.

Oldenski, R. J., & Flareau, B. J. (1992). Colorectal cancer screening. *Cancer Epidemiology, Prevention, and Screening, 19*(3), 621-635.

Orem, D. E. (1985). *Nursing concepts of practice* (p. 31). New York: McGraw-Hill.

Ostwald, S. K., & Rothenberger, J. L. (1985). Development of a testicular self-examination program for college men. *Journal of American College Health, 33*(6), 234-239.

Peeters, P. H., Verbeek, A. L. M., & Straatman, H. (1989). Evaluation of overdiagnosis of breast cancer in screening with mammography: Results of the Nijmegen programme. *International Journal of Epidemiology, 18*, 295.

Perry, C. L., Baranowski, T., & Parcel, G. S. (1990). How individuals, environments, and health behavior interact: Social learning theory. *Health behavior and health education* (pp. 161-186). San Francisco: Jossey-Bass.

Price, J. A. (1993). Perceptions of colorectal cancer in a socioeconomically disadvantaged population. *Journal of Community Health, 18*(6), 347-363.

Prochaska, J., & DiClemente, C. (1985). Common processes of self-change in smoking, weight control, and psychological distress. In S. Shiffman & T. Willis (Eds.), *Coping and substance use* (pp. 345-364). Orlando, FL: Academic Press.

Raina, V., Shukla, N. K., Rath, G. K., Gupta, N. P., Mishra, M. C., Chaterjee, T. K., & Kripalani, A. K. (1993). Clinical profile and problems of management of 108 cases of germ cell tumours of testis at Institute Rotary Cancer Hospital, All India Institute of Medical Sciences, New Delhi 1985-1990. *British Journal of Cancer*, *67*, 573-577.

Rakowski, W., Rimer, B., & Bryant, S. (1993). Integrating behavior and intention regarding mammography by respondents in the 1990 National Health Interview Survey of health promotion and disease prevention. *Public Health Reports*, *108*, 605.

Rampen, F. H. J., Berretty, P. J. M., Van Huystee, B. E. W. L., Kiemeney, L. A. L. M., & Nijs, H. H. M. (1993). Lack of selective attendance of participants at skin cancer/melanoma screening clinics. *Journal of the American Academy of Dermatology*, *29*(3), 423-427.

Ramsdell, W. M., Kelly, P., Coody, D., & Dany, M. (1991). The Texas skin cancer/melanoma project. *Texas Medicine*, *87*(10), 70-73.

Reno, D. R. (1988). Men's knowledge and health beliefs about testicular cancer and testicular self-examination. *Cancer Nursing*, *11*(2), 112-117.

Richardson, J. L. (1987). Frequency and adequacy of breast cancer screening among elderly Hispanic women. *Preventive Medicine*, *16*, 761-774.

Rimer, B. K. (1995). Audiences and messages for breast and cervical cancer screening. *Wellness Perspectives: Research, Theory and Practice*, *11*(2), 13-39.

Rimer, B. K., Keintz, M. K., Kessler, H. B., Engstrom, P. F., & Rosan, J. R. (1989). Why women resist screening mammography: Patient-related barriers. *Radiology*, *172*, 243-246.

Rosenstock, I. M. (1990). The health belief model. In K. Glanz, F. Lewis, & B. Rimer (Eds.), *Health education theory research and practice* (pp. 32-59). San Francisco: Jossey Bass.

Ross, C. C. (1988). Screening for colorectal cancer. *Australian Family Physician*, *38*(6), 105-114.

Rothman, A. J., Salovey, P., Turvey, C., & Fishkin, S. A. (1993). Attributions of responsibility and persuasion: Increasing mammography utilization among women over 40 with an internally oriented message. *Health Psychology*, *12*, 209.

Rudolf, V. M., & Quinn, K. L. M. (1988). The practices of TSE among college men: Effectiveness of an educational program. *Oncology Nursing Forum*, *15*(1), 45-48.

Sayger, S. A., Fortenberry, J. D., & Beckman, R. J. (1988). Practice patterns of teaching testicular self-examination to adolescent patients. *Journal of Adolescent Health Care*, *9*(5), 441-442.

Sheley, J. F., Kinchen, B. A., Morgan, M. A., & Gordon, D. F. (1991). Limited impact of testicular self-examination promotion. *Journal of Community Health*, *16*(2), 117-124.

Sladden, M., & Dickinson, J. (1993). Testicular cancer: How effective is screening? *Australian Family Physician*, *22*(8), 1350-1356.

Solomon, M. J., & McLeod, R. S. (1993). Screening strategies for colorectal cancer. *Colorectal Cancer*, *73*(1), 31-45.

Strecher, V. J., DeVellis, B. M., Becker, M. H., & Rosenstock, I. M. (1986). The role of self-efficacy in achieving health behavior change. *Health Education Quarterly*, *13*, 73-92.

Thompson, R. S., Michnich, M. E., Gray, J., Friedlander, L., & Gilson, B. (1986). Maximizing compliance with hemoccult screening for colon cancer in clinical practice. *Medical Care*, *24*(10), 904-914.

U.S. Department of Health and Human Services, Public Health Service. (1991). *Healthy People 2000*. Washington, DC: U.S. Government Printing Office.

U.S. Preventive Services Task Force. (1996). Screening for testicular cancer. *Guide to Clinical Preventive Services*, 52-54. Philadelphia: Williams & Wilkins.

Vaz, R. M., Best, D. L., Davis, S. W., & Kaiser, M. (1989). Evaluation of a testicular cancer curriculum for adolescents. *Journal of Pediatrics*, *114*, 150-153.

Vogt, H. B., & McHale, M. S. (1992). Testicular cancer: Role of primary care physicians in screening and education. *Postgraduate Medicine*, *92*(1), 93-101.

Wang, M. C., Papsidero, L. D., Kuriyama, M., Valenzuela, L. A., Murphy, G. P., & Chu, T. M. (1981). Prostate antigen: A new potential marker for prostatic cancer. *Prostate*, *2*, 89-96.

Wardle, J., Skoptok, A., Burckhardt, R., Vogele, C., Vilda, J., & Zarczynski, Z. (1994). Testicular self-examination: Attitudes and practices among young men in Europe. *Preventive Medicine*, *23*, 206-209.

Weinrich, S. P., Weinrich, M. C., Stronborg, M. F., Boyd, M. D., & Weiss, H. L. (1993). Using elderly educators to increase colorectal cancer screening. *Gerontologist*, *33*(4), 491-496.

Weinstock, M. A. (1990). Prevalence of the early warning signs of melanoma among participants in the 1989 Rhode Island skin cancer screening. *Journal of the American Academy of Dermatology*, *23*(3), 516-518.

Wong, J. G., & Feussner, J. R. (1993a). Screening for cervical cancer: Pap smears can save lives. *North Carolina Medical Journal*, *54*(7), 342-345.

Wong, J. G., & Feussner, J. R. (1993b). Screening for colon cancer: Is it worth the expense? *North Carolina Medical Journal*, *54*(12), 634-638.

16

Adherence to Dental Regimens

Kevin D. McCaul

DENTAL REGIMEN ADHERENCE AS HABIT

This chapter will cover some of what is known about adherence to dental regimens. Dental regimens are similar to other health-protective regimens that demand habitual behavior change. However, unlike the once-a-year mammogram, or the need to take medicine daily until a 3-week supply is exhausted, dental regimens typically require daily behavior change that may last a lifetime. Thus, dental regimens could have much in common with regimens such as those intended to control glucose levels and reduce complications from diabetes, to change diet and reduce obesity, or to increase exercise and lower high blood pressure. In a sense, when one intervenes to produce adherence to a dental regimen, one tries to *create* a habit.

Habit creation promises to be difficult for the kinds of health-protective behaviors just described, including dental regimen behaviors. Ronis, Yates, and Kirscht (1989) enumerated several reasons that it may be hard for persons to create a habit, especially on their own. Ronis and colleagues note that many people will never think about the need to perform such behaviors, others may decide against the action because it is difficult to do or unpleasant, those persons who do try to change their behavior will often forget to do so, and people may eventually become frustrated with trying to create a habit and abandon the attempt altogether.

The problems that confront persons making various kinds of lifestyle changes also must be overcome by those trying to protect their dental health. Consider the use of dental floss to prevent periodontal (gum) disease. Despite frequent advertising in the private sector (and perhaps because of occasional sarcastic comments by humorists), many persons fail to acknowledge that flossing has benefits for dental health. Moreover, even those who wish to begin a flossing regimen report many difficulties (O'Neill, Sandgren, McCaul, & Glasgow, 1987). Supporting the speculation of Ronis et al. (1989), beginning flossers argue that flossing is difficult to perform correctly and that it is hard to remember to floss. After many lapses, most people quit.

Although creating a flossing *habit* is difficult, initial attempts to increase flossing frequency meet with great success (McCaul, Glasgow, & O'Neill, 1992). Thus, the chief problem with this kind of dental regimen—as with so

Kevin D. McCaul • Department of Psychology, North Dakota State University, Fargo, North Dakota 58105.

Handbook of Health Behavior Research II: Provider Determinants, edited by David S. Gochman. Plenum Press, New York, 1997.

many other behavior change regimens—is relapse. To deal at length with this most important issue, the chapter is divided into two roughly equal sections. The first section describes the relapse problem, presenting previously unpublished data concerning the "relapse curve" in the dental area and specifying some variables that may predict relapse. The section concludes with ideas about the implications of relapse data for treatment programs.

The second section describes experiments conducted to improve adherence to plaque-control regimens. Most of the studies fail to examine adherence closely over a time sufficiently long to know about relapse. Still, some interventions show promise, and the section goes on to address two related questions: (1) What methodological issues surround studies intended to test effectiveness? (2) Are the benefits of treatment worth the cost?

Most of the chapter focuses on dental regimens for plaque control—regular, skilled, brushing and flossing. The ultimate purpose of plaque control is either to prevent gum disease or to maintain gum health following surgery. Focusing on this topic does mean that other important topics in dental regimens will be missed altogether, including cooperation in orthodontic treatment (Albino, Lawrence, Lopes, Nash, & Tedesco, 1991) and dental health professionals' own protective health behaviors (cf. McCaul, Bakdash, Geboy, Gerbert, Tedesco, 1990). The focus on plaque-control regimens was chosen in part because such regimens bear more than a superficial resemblance to other types of self-protective health regimens. Thus, the research process in behavioral dentistry can profit from what is known of other regimens, and perhaps researchers in other areas may be able to learn from findings in the dental area.

THE RELAPSE CURVE

A behavioral regimen can be effective in either preventing gum disease (Abdellatif & Burt, 1987; Axelsson & Lindhe, 1981; Lobene, Soparkar, & Newman, 1982) or relieving existing gum disease (Cercek, Kiger, Garrett, & Egelberg, 1983). The regimen includes thorough brushing and flossing to remove plaque. Performing these behaviors at least once every 24 hours appears to be sufficient as a protective regimen. Do people routinely engage in these behaviors on their own? National data suggest that most do not (Chen & Rubinson, 1982; Gift, 1986). Gift (1986), for example, summarized nearly 50 studies surveying plaque-control behaviors. She concluded that most people brush their teeth, but probably not in a way that reduces plaque effectively. Probably less than 10% of the population uses floss daily.

Investigators have tried many different tacks to encourage adherence. Most attempts, however, will prove successful only in the short run; people are less likely to become habitually adherent (Heasman, Jacobs, & Chapple, 1989). Three different studies examining adherence to a dental regimen of once-a-day plaque removal tested the power of different manipulations to improve maintenance, including social support, frequent patient contact, and flexible goal setting (McCaul et al., 1992). In each case, the intervention produced immediate changes that persisted at a reasonable level while the study was ongoing. Across the three studies, adherence rates to a once-a-day regimen averaged better than 70% for as long as 3½ months. In each of the three experiments, however, two other results were observed. First, the *control* conditions, which typically included skills training in the regimen and health education, produced adherence equal to that of the treatment conditions. Second, the changes produced in both intervention and control conditions routinely vanished during different follow-up periods, usually shortly after formal participation in the study ended.

Given the difficulty in producing lasting behavior change, it was decided that it would be useful to study the natural course of relapse for this regimen and to look for possible predictors of whether or not people would relapse. Thus, a study was designed in which participants at risk for gum disease went through a cognitive-behavioral treatment to promote plaque removal, followed by periodic assessments for 1 year. The measures and results of that unpublished study (McCaul, Thiesse-Duffy, O'Neill, Gravely, & Suda, 1993) are described here.

Possible Predictors of Relapse

Three different theoretical approaches to self-protective health behaviors were used to generate possible predictors of relapse. Social cognitive theory (Bandura, 1986) is, of course, a theoretical approach that has been applied broadly to human behavior. The theory suggests that expectations about performing a behavior such as flossing will be important, as will having the skill to perform the behavior and environmental support and reinforcement for performing the behavior. Four variables derived from this theory were gathered in the study. First, self-efficacy expectations have been shown to have strong predictive power for varied regimen behaviors (DiClemente, 1986; McCaul, Glasgow, & Schafer, 1987), including maintenance in the dental area (McCaul, Glasgow, & Gustafson, 1985; Tedesco, Keffer, Davis, & Christersson, 1993). Second, outcome expectations about the likely results of flossing were measured. Third, observations of plaque removal *skill* were gathered. Finally, one type of contextual factor—social support—was measured.

A second theoretical approach used to generate predictors was the Fishbein and Ajzen (1975) theory of reasoned action. Similar to social cognitive theory, the theory of reasoned action emphasizes cognitive variables, but it specifies different measurement operations. Attitude toward flossing was measured, for example. Attitude in the theory is predicted by beliefs, which would be similar to Bandura's conception of outcome expectations. But attitude, as measured in the theory of reasoned action, is defined as one's affective response toward the behavior. The theory also specifies that the immediate determinant of behavior is one's intentions, and so intent to perform plaque removal behaviors was measured.

The final theoretical approach was Leventhal's conception of illness representations (Leventhal, Zimmerman, & Gutmann, 1984). Leventhal argues that how an individual thinks about ("represents") illness can have powerful implications for regimen behavior. Some of the beliefs derived from this model would not be routinely measured from the perspective of either social cognitive theory or the theory of reasoned action. The beliefs measured in this study included beliefs about symptoms associated with poor plaque control, about reported symptom levels, and about the causes of gum disease.

It should be noted that the purpose of this study was not to test the three theoretical approaches against one another. Such a competitive test is difficult because some of the variables drawn from the different theories are difficult to distinguish conceptually. All three theories, for example, would include some version of beliefs about outcomes. Instead of whole theoretical approaches being tested, then, all variables generated by the three theoretical approaches were tested for their value as bivariate predictors of adherence.

Method

Participants

Participants included 65 men and 53 women at risk for developing gum disease. To identify possible participants, 349 individuals were screened at the campus dental office at North Dakota State University. Eligible participants ($N = 171$) showed bleeding upon probing in at least two of six examined sites, indicating at least a low level of existing gum disease (gingivitis). In addition, potential participants reported flossing less often than every other day. Eligible people were called, told that they were at risk of developing gum disease, and invited to take part in the study. Approximately 69% agreed. The mean age of participants was 23.7 years, and there were no significant differences on the screening criteria or other demographic variables between those who chose to participate and those who did not.

Procedure

Participants were randomly assigned to one of six conditions, formed by a 2 (type of treatment) × 3 (contact frequency) factorial design. The basic treatment for all subjects took place during three sessions in the dental office. At Session 1, all participants watched a 10-minute health education videotape describing the causes and prevention of gum disease. They learned how to brush and floss to control plaque, were asked to perform these behaviors thoroughly once each day, and were provided with self-monitoring booklets to record their behaviors each day during the first week.

The second session took place a week later, after subjects had some practice with daily self-monitoring and performing their new regimen behaviors. First, self-monitoring problems and plaque-removal skills were corrected for everyone. Then, participants were randomly assigned to one of two treatments. *Brief treatment* subjects received instructions for using disclosing tablets to note where plaque remained after initial brushing and flossing and were provided with new packets of floss. They were then excused. *Standard treatment* subjects received a dental exam to display how the first week of regimen activity reduced the plaque in their mouths. Because nearly all subject show plaque reductions, this feedback was expected to be highly reinforcing for subjects' initial attempts to produce a daily regimen. Standard treatment participants also received a 2-week self-monitoring booklet so that they could continue to self-monitor (brief treatment participants did not continue to self-monitor).

At the third treatment session, two weeks after Session 2, *brief treatment* subjects simply completed a variety of measures and were paid for participating. They were told that "the project is essentially over but we may be calling you to see how things are going." *Standard treatment* subjects received feedback on self-monitoring, corrective feedback on brushing and flossing techniques, praise for adherence, and information about "habit development." One aspect of habit development was to select a particular time every day to remove plaque, and participants each indicated the approximate time that they would perform their regimen. Finally, the experimenter identified possible barriers to adherence (e.g., lack of time, forgetting) and presented 12 possible solutions. Participants each selected two solutions that they would carry out.

Follow-up procedures differed according to three randomly assigned conditions that varied in the frequency of follow-up contacts. This aspect of the design was added because of the possibility that frequent calls would be reactive and would produce higher adherence. *Frequent contact* subjects were called every week for a month and then every other week for two additional months. *Infrequent contact* subjects were called once every 2-3 weeks after Session 3 and twice more during two subsequent months. *No contact* subjects received only a single phone call 10-12 weeks following Session 3. Regardless of condition, an interview was scheduled immediately whenever phone contacts indicated relapse. Then, all subjects were interviewed—whether they had relapsed or not—3 months following Session 3. Phone call follow-ups were completed 6 months and 1 year following Session 3.

Measures

From social cognitive theory, *self-efficacy expectations* were measured by asking participants to rate their certainty that they could floss frequently, floss on atypical days (e.g., a holiday), and floss with the correct skill. Scores were summed across these three areas (alpha = 0.71). *Outcome expectancies* for flossing were derived by summing responses to four questions about the consequences of removing plaque thoroughly or failing to do so (alpha = 0.61). For example, one item read: "If I don't remove plaque thoroughly, there is a good chance that I will experience gum disease during the next year." A behavioral observation measure of *plaque-removal skill* was created in which dental hygienists watched participants after they were given instructions to "floss as you think you *should*." The observers scored the participants' flossing skills according to whether they would effectively remove plaque (interrater reliability = 0.86). Finally, *social support* for regimen adherence was measured by the frequency with which persons who lived with the participant flossed their teeth. Nides et al. (1995) used a similar definition of social support to predict relapse following smoking by measuring whether their participants lived with others who were smokers.

From the theory of reasoned action (Fishbein & Ajzen, 1975), two measures were developed. *Attitudes* toward plaque removal were measured using five 7-point semantic-differential scales with end points such as "good" versus "bad" (alpha = 0.64). *Intention* to floss and remove plaque in the future was measured using two items that asked about participants' intention to floss daily (alpha = 0.91).

From perspectives concerning illness representations, subjects' *beliefs about symptoms* were computed by summing their beliefs about the symptoms that are actually associated with gum disease (e.g., bleeding gums). *Reported symptom levels* were measured by asking participants to rate the level of bleeding gums that they reported experiencing during the previous week. *Beliefs about the causes of gum disease* came from a single item that asked participants whether gum disease was caused more by personal ("1") or more by external ("7") factors.

Finally, several background variables were collected both to describe the sample and to establish a context for the operation of the theoretical predictors. Demographic measures were taken (e.g., age, gender), as were measures of participants' previous dental experiences (e.g., frequency of visiting the dentist). In addition, previous experience with plaque-removal behaviors was measured by asking about the frequency of brushing and flossing during an "average week."

Results

Group Differences

Preliminary relapse analyses included type of treatment and contact frequency as variables. The difference in treatment intensity had no significant effect. Overall, 50% of the standard treatment subjects had relapsed at 6 months compared to 62% of the brief treatment subjects, χ^2 (2) = 1.47, $p = 0.23$. Measurement frequency also did not affect reported relapse: frequent measurement = 52%, infrequent measurement = 65%, no contact = 53%, χ^2 (2) = 1.01, $p = 0.60$. It is an important finding that more frequent assessments had little influence on adherence. It is an even more important finding that brief treatment was essentially as effective in maintaining adherence as more intense treatment. These findings were similar to findings reported before (McCaul et al., 1992). Because the condition assignment did not produce meaningful relapse differences, group assignment was ignored in the data presented below.

The Relapse Curve

Relapse was defined as adherence of less than 43% (fewer than 3 days during the previous week) to the regimen of once-a-day plaque removal. This definition of relapse relies solely on participants' self-reports of regimen behaviors. Three arguments can be made, however, for the validity of the self-reports. First, in previous research, more objective data have been gathered that correlate with self-reports. McCaul et al. (1985), for example, measured the floss remaining in containers and found good correspondence between self-report of flossing frequency and this more objective measure. Second, subjects *do* seem to report relapse willingly; failure to engage in these behaviors probably does not carry the same social sanctions as some others (e.g., smoking). Finally, "honesty" estimates were made on the basis of inspection of the self-monitoring booklets (e.g., using different writing instruments, crumpled pages). No correlation was found between such estimates and subjects' relapse reports.

It is also important to note that defining relapse by using a level of 43%, which is somewhat arbitrary, does have a practical rationale. It is possible that every-other-day plaque removal may be sufficient to prevent gum disease (Gift, 1988). In the analyses described below, only subjects who reported being adherent at the end of treatment were included ($N = 110$, or 93% of the original sample). Figure 1 shows the cumulative percentage of the sample who lapsed into nonadherence during the year following treatment initiation.

As Figure 1 shows, most relapse took place rapidly after treatment, and then the relapse curve decelerated through the rest of the year. Half (52%) of all those persons who relapsed some time during the year actually did so within 1 month following treatment. Such data have been obtained before, of course, though for very different behaviors (e.g., for smoking [see Baer, Kamarck, Lichtenstein, & Ransom, 1989]). At 3 months, approximately half of the total sample had relapsed (47%), and this value increased only by 10% at the 6-month follow-up. At 1 year, 61% of the total sample had relapsed. It is important to note that 90% of the participants who were adherent for as long as 6 months continued to report being adherent at 1 year.

Maintenance in this study was significantly better than the levels observed in other studies. McCaul et al. (1992), for example, obtained 6-month adherence rates of around 25%. In contrast to earlier research, however, this study was conducted with participants identified by a dentist as at risk, and it was performed entirely within the context of dental visits. It is conceivable that this study portrays a more realistic adherence rate than the rates observed in earlier research.

Predicting Relapse

The 6-month data were used to define whether participants had relapsed, because that

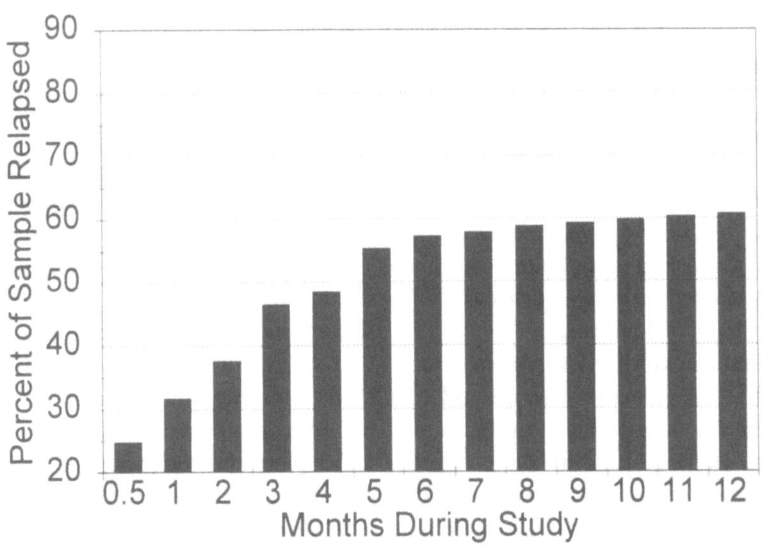

Figure 1. Cumulative percentage of the total sample defined as having relapsed during the 12 months posttreatment.

period provided reasonable sample sizes of relapsed ($N = 57$) and nonrelapsed ($N = 44$) people. (Seventeen fewer subjects were available for this analysis than at the outset of the study. As noted earlier, 8 subjects were nonadherent during treatment, and another 9 dropped out of the study before the 6-month follow-up.) Differences were examined between these two groups on the demographic variables described earlier. None of the demographic variables, including age, gender, and several dental health measures (e.g., frequency of dental visits, disease status), discriminated successful from nonsuccessful adherers. However, a measure of prior *regimen* behavior did predict relapse. Persons who maintained their performance had been flossing more frequently at pretest (see Table 1).

Table 1 shows the means for the theoretically derived predictors of relapse, which were all measured at the end of treatment. Social learning theory produced two variables that were related to relapse. Self-efficacy was a strong predictor, with those persons who maintained their behavior having stronger expectations that they would be able to do so. In addition, maintainers were somewhat more skilled at plaque removal than those persons who relapsed. The other two social learning theory variables—outcome expectations and social support—were unrelated to relapse. It is important to note that the outcome expectancy measure was limited in this study to expectations about disease. Other outcomes are possible (e.g., costs associated with flossing) and may be related to relapse.

Both variables drawn from the theory of reasoned action differentiated persons who relapsed from those who did not, although the effects were not large. Persons with a more favorable attitude toward flossing and those who intended to floss more frequently were less likely to relapse.

In contrast to the other two theoretical approaches, the variables drawn from conceptions about illness representation were unimportant; indeed, the means for reported symptoms were opposite to what might have been expected.

Table 1. Differences on Theoretical Variables between Participants Who Did and Did Not Relapse

	Means for groups		
Theory and variables	Did not relapse ($N = 44$)	Relapsed ($N = 57$)	p^a
Social learning			
Self-efficacy for flossing	379.50	334.57	0.002
Outcome expectancy	28.25	28.14	0.91
Flossing skills	15.23	14.46	0.08
Social support	1.81	1.35	0.38
Reasoned action			
Attitudes—removed plaque	6.54	6.34	0.07
Intention—floss	6.26	5.71	0.02
Illness representation			
Responsibility for gum disease	4.30	4.26	0.76
Reported symptoms—bleeding	1.59	1.78	0.16
Identify correct symptoms	4.23	4.18	0.71
Prior behavior			
Flossing at pretest	1.95	.93	0.01
Flossing at posttest	6.32	5.66	0.004

[a] p was derived from t-test results (2-tailed).

Persons who relapsed also reported having more bleeding, though not significantly so; it had been expected that persons reporting bleeding would be *less* likely to relapse.

The significant predictors of relapse are interesting because they all seem related to participants' own predictions about their likely success. Participants who maintained their regimen behaviors, for example, were performing those behaviors at a higher level both at pretest and at the end of the treatment (p's < 001). This more frequent performance may account for the slightly higher flossing skills of persons who maintained their regimen. Maintainers also had more positive attitudes toward removing plaque and intended to floss more frequently. Finally, those who managed to stay adherent were more likely to believe initially that they *could* do so—they reported a higher level of self-efficacy.

Other Predictors

At 3 months after treatment ended, all participants were interviewed, and almost half were still adherent then. Most of the interview measures failed to distinguish between those who were and were not adherent, with two potentially important exceptions. First, participants were asked whether they ever *thought* about gum disease, and approximately two thirds of the participants in each group said that they did. Then, those persons were asked whether they ever *worried* about gum disease. Of those still adherent, 63% worried, while of those who had relapsed, only 35% worried, χ^2 (1) = 4.85, p = 0.028. It may be that worry about disease contributes to continued adherence.

The notion of worry and disease is related to a second piece of data gathered in the interviews. Participants were asked whether they had kept their goal of daily plaque removal after the end of treatment or whether they had reduced their goal. Not surprisingly, fewer of the relapsed subjects (49%) had maintained the more stringent goal than those subjects who were still adherent (83%). More interestingly, however, subjects were asked whether they would reinstate their goal of once-daily plaque removal if they noticed signs of gum disease. Remarkably, 56 of the 57 non-adherent subjects reported that they would do so. This proportion (98.2%) was significantly larger than was observed in the adherent subjects [37 of 42, 88%; χ^2 (1) = 4.38, p = 0.036].

Discussion

What do people who relapsed "look like"? First, they were not doing much at all in terms of plaque removal when the study began, flossing on average less than once per week. People who were *already* engaging in the regimen to some extent were more likely to maintain the behavior. It is unclear whether this difference was due to differences in motivation or whether it was simply easier for persons who were more familiar with the regimen initially to adopt the behavior. The skill levels of those persons who maintained adherence also tended to be higher than those of persons who relapsed, suggesting that a reduction in barriers may be the important distinction here. These findings suggest that identifying which persons are "ready" to change would be as important for dental regimens as it is for other behaviors (Prochaska & DiClemente, 1983). On the other hand, the data could also be interpreted to suggest that, as in areas such as smoking, multiple attempts to adhere may eventually be successful. That is, it may be helpful to get people *started* in the regimen, even if they later "fail," because partial successes may increase the chances of success on the next attempt.

After the 3-week treatment, persons who relapsed looked different in several ways from those who eventually were more successful adherers. For example, they had been less adherent during the 3-week treatment, and they tended to have more negative attitudes about removing plaque. In a sense, they seemed to be *telling* the researchers that they were likely to relapse, because their intentions to floss and their self-efficacy for flossing were lower than those exhibited by nonrelapsed individuals. Dental professionals might best be able to identify likely candidates for relapse simply by asking patients whether they feel that they can maintain a plaque-removal program. This suggestion turns one's attention to the literature on patient-practitioner interaction. In dentistry, as in other health fields, communication between patient and practioner may be a crucial variable for improving adherence (DiNicola & DeMatteo, 1984).

Besides this "picture" of the person who relapses, the data have two additional implications, one pragmatic and one more theoretical. The practical lesson is that it could be argued that the treatment was a "success." Defining success is, of course, a matter of some subjectivity. But approximately one third of the participants were engaging in at least every-other-day plaque removal *one year after treatment*. Clearly, the treatment had some beneficial effects in motivating some persons to engage in some reasonable level of adherence. Imagine a similar treatment that could keep one third of high blood pressure patients exercising over a 1-year period or one third of persons with Type I diabetes sticking to a rigorous diet for a year.

Thus, if one shares this definition of success, the data suggest that dental professionals *can* make a difference. But do they? It turns out that, similar to other health professionals (Allen & Allen, 1986), dental professionals typically invest little effort in behavior change activities. Part of the problem may be that dental professionals view success from an individual rather than from a public health perspective. Thus, if the professional encourages three patients with beginning gum disease to change their behavior, and if only one of those individuals maintains the behavior change, the professional may feel that encouraging behavior change "doesn't work." In fact, dental professionals believe that they are successful with "only" about 50% of their patients (Milgrom, Weinstein, Chapko, Grembowski, & Spadafora, 1988), an estimate that probably overstates their actual success (Milgrom, Weinstein, Melnick, Beach, & Spadafora, 1989a). From a public health perspective, however, one might argue that a relatively small investment has led to a better than 25% payoff—an important success. It may be necessary to change the way in which such outcomes are framed in order to get professionals to do what they are capable of doing—producing behavior change among a minority of their patients.

The theoretical implications spring from two novel predictors of relapse that were identified. First, a significant proportion of subjects who maintained their regimen behaviors *worried* about disease. Second, nearly all of those who relapsed said that there was one thing that could prompt renewed adherence efforts: signs of disease. These data fit well with notions about illness representations and their relationship to regimen behaviors, and these ideas will be used in the next section in discussing treatments for increasing adherence.

INCREASING ADHERENCE

The data from McCaul et al. (1993) suggest that relatively brief treatments should work to promote initial success in changing plaque-control behavior. Indeed, one could argue that almost any kind of intervention will do. Thus, rewards will be effective (Iwata & Becksfort, 1981), as will other strategies typically associated with behavioral treatments (Stewart et al., 1991). Feedback and self-monitoring, for example, also seem to be effective (Baab & Weinstein, 1983; Glavind, Zeuner, & Attstrom, 1981). The data suggest that any reasonable educational treatment may boost adherence while a study is ongoing—perhaps for as long as 6 months (McCaul et al., 1992, Experiment 2).

That a variety of behavioral strategies such as monitoring increase adherence, even if only for a time, should not be seen as a trivial finding, especially in the dental area. Dental health professionals would typically like to meet with patients at least annually and often more frequently than that. Thus, *professionals* can maintain contact and monitoring; when adherence declines, the dental professional can probably reinstate the behavior with reminders, encouragement, reinforcement, or admonitions about disease. Self-care may then only have to bridge the gap between monitoring visits. Wolff et al. (1989) reported a study that supports this notion. Better than two thirds of their participants reported adherence to plaque control behaviors *4 years* after the study began. During those 4 years, however, the participants met with dental professionals a minimum of 14 times—at least every 4 months. Ockene and Camic (1985) have made the point that health professionals are effective behavior change agents generally; this effectiveness may be even more true of dental professionals, given their recall procedures. The reader should be reminded, however, that a significant proportion of the population never sees a dental professional, and many persons go infrequently, lessening the strength of this argument (Gallagher & Moody, 1981).

Despite the possibility that professionals can extend the adherence of some persons, it would still be important to look for strategies that might produce long-term maintenance. Dental care is costly; self-care would be cost-effective. The remainder of this chapter briefly presents four kinds of interventions that have shown the possibility of causing longer-term benefits. First, it considers several isolated reports of some insufficiently studied strategies. Then, it considers more traditional though intense cognitive behavior therapy. Finally, it turns to two types of what might be characterized as cognitive-emotional interventions.

Insufficiently Studied Strategies

An interesting report of the effectiveness of hypnosis was described by Kelly, McKinty, and Carr (1988), who assigned a sample of 96 dental patients to either an experimental group or a control group. Both groups received health education about flossing, including suggestions concerning the value of performing this behavior daily. The experimental group, however, received these suggestions under hypnosis. All patients were recalled 8 months later—a long follow-up period, given that they received no contact during those 8 months. The hypnosis group showed improved gingival health compared to patients in the control condition. The authors reported a perfect correspondence between gingival improvement and daily flossing, which is unusual. Indeed, researchers have generally failed to devote sufficient attention to the precise relationship between plaque-removal behaviors and dental health. Unfortunately, the authors did not present any data to explain *why* hypnosis might have long-term effects. Nevertheless, this approach is one of the very few to produce maintenance and, as such, might prompt further study.

Two other reports of long-term success originated in Europe. From Paris comes a report by Alcouffe (1988) of a study of 26 French periodontal patients who had been unresponsive to standard oral hygiene instructions. Half of these patients met with a psychologist, and half served as control participants. The experimental participants met in a single interview session, lasting an average of an hour, in which the psychologist and patient discussed problems concerning the oral hygiene treatment. Those patients who met with the psychologist exhibited improvement in plaque scores *2 years later*, whereas control participants showed no improvement. Alcouffe (1988) did not describe the content of the session with the psychologist in any depth, which is unfortunate, because these are striking differences to observe 2 years after treatment. Schou (1985) reported similarly amazing results in a study in which experimental participants met in therapy groups (there were no control participants in this study). It should be noted that all three studies in this section are included more for the sake of completeness than because the interventions are necessarily valid. In particular, neither Alcouffe nor Schou reported the kinds of details needed to understand their interventions. Still, two aspects of their procedures—meeting with a psychologist and group therapy—were used in one of the behavioral interventions considered in the next section.

Behavioral Interventions

Few researchers using behavioral interventions have included sufficiently long follow-up periods. When they have, they have typically reported poor maintenance (e.g., Weinstein, Milgrom, Melnick, Beach, & Spadafora, 1989). A similar conclusion could be drawn from a series of studies intended to promote the use of fluoride rinse among schoolchildren. Kegeles and Lund (1984) (cf. Lund & Kegeles, 1981) developed an innovative research program testing a fluoride mouth-rinsing intervention intended to prevent dental caries ("cavities"). A novel aspect of the program was that it included an excellent objective measure of adherence—a bottle containing rinse that the schoolchildren had to use on a schedule. Initial studies showed that rewards (i.e., prizes contingent on adherence) worked effectively and had a powerful impact on increasing use of the fluoride rinse (Kegeles, Lund, & Weisenberg, 1978).

Later, however, Kegeles and colleagues began to investigate maintenance, and they discovered that it was quite low. After rewards were terminated, adherence rates quickly plummeted to a level of approximately 10% of the children who continued to participate (Lund & Kegeles, 1982). These authors became sufficiently pessimistic about long-term behavior change to conclude that "it is clear that we do not currently know how to achieve it, notwithstanding expressions of confidence in the power of psychological knowledge" (Lund & Kegeles, 1984, p. 366).

With adults, such pessimism may be somewhat overstated. An intense behavioral intervention was constructed and recently tested by a group at the University of Washington. Hollis et al. (1994) administered a plaque-control program in five 90-minute sessions to small groups of older patients (aged 50–70) with moderate periodontal disease. The sessions were led by psychologists and included traditional behavioral training in skills acquisition, self-monitoring, and goal setting. They also included feedback about bleeding and, because the sessions were conducted in small groups, group influence in the form of norm setting and social support.

This intensive intervention produced strong effects on both behavior and clinical outcomes, which included plaque levels, gingival inflammation, and pocket depth. Moreover, the positive effects were maintained over at least 6 months. These data suggest that a strong, multicomponent, and lengthy cognitive-behavioral program *can* work over a longer period. It will be interesting to see whether most of these persons develop a "habit," i.e., maintain their behavior with little monitoring over longer times.

Cognitive Restructuring

Tedesco, Keffer, Davis, and Christersson (1992) added a neat twist to the behavioral treatments more typically constructed. They worked with over 150 adults with moderate periodontal disease. Participants attended four treatment sessions that included oral health education, skills training, and feedback. In addition, experimental participants underwent "cognitive restructuring." In particular, these subjects received vivid feedback about their performance accomplishments through "phase-contrast microscopy," a technique in which they viewed a slide of the microorganisms inhabiting their gums. Then they underwent tooth cleaning and had the opportunity to view a new slide that dramatically showed the reduction in bacteria. This process was repeated at each of the four sessions, which were separated by 1 month.

The experimental treatment failed to reveal any behavioral advantage for experimental subjects over the control treatment; experimental subjects reported the same level of brushing and flossing at follow-up as control participants. On the other hand, participants who returned for treatment maintained both behavior and dental health outcomes over a 9-month interval. The dropout rate was nearly 50%, though, and the authors noted that dental health was poorer among dropouts. Still, the authors suggested that "these data support the influence of scheduled visits on oral hygiene practices."

Illness Cognition Interventions

Although the focus on disease introduced by Tedesco et al. (1992) was novel, it is not the kind of treatment that the data presented here suggest might work. Specifically, the microscopic view of "organisms" may be too removed from one's experience with gum disease. The McCaul et al. (1993) data suggest that a focus on observable *symptoms* may remind patients of disease and prompt both worry and increased adherence behavior. Such an approach fits neatly with theories that emphasize the importance of how persons represent illness, suggesting that symptoms and labels (among other things) are each important (Leventhal, Diefenbach, & Leventhal, 1992). Researchers and professionals have probably underemphasized teaching about symptoms, especially because there is an obvious symptom that suggests at least risk of disease: bleeding from the gums. Professionals should be able to emphasize this highly visible symptom as an indicator of gum disease.

Bleeding can serve both as a cue toward action and, perhaps more important, as an emotional reminder of the value of performing the protective behavior. Noticing bleeding may prompt one to worry about gum disease, which in turn motivates the protective behavior. Easterling and Leventhal (1989) reported a similar sequence in a study of ex-cancer patients. Worry about cancer was determined both by beliefs in one's personal vulnerability and by the detection of symptoms interpreted as possibly indicating cancer. Easterling and Leventhal (1989) suggested that somatic cues could be used to prompt self-protective behavior, but they also pointed out that such cues will be important only if the "individual acknowledges that the target health risk is personally significant" (p. 795). The latter caveat again reinforces the important role of provider-patient interaction. The dental health professional would have to remind the patient of the consequences of gum disease to prompt personal significance while simultaneously describing the cue—gum bleeding—to prompt worry and subsequent adherence.

Only a few published studies have examined whether a focus on bleeding can help to maintain adherence. Walsh, Heckman, and Moreau-Diettinger (1985) reported a study in which 36 adults were randomly assigned to one of two treatments or a no-treatment control condition. The treatments added interproximal (between-teeth) cleaning with a toothpick to a standard plaque control regimen. Further, in one treatment, the researchers taught the group to use bleeding as a clue to interpret their gingival health. They were taught that the absence of bleeding should be taken as a positive sign of "health," whereas the return of bleeding should be perceived as a sign to use the toothpick more diligently. After 3 months, both treatment groups showed improved gingival health compared to the control condition, and the group taught to use bleeding as a cue was dramatically more likely to comply with instructions to return their "self-report compliance cards" (Walsh et al., 1985, p. 133). Of course, returning the cards does not necessarily mean that adherence to the behavioral regimen was higher. In addition, as has been noted, 3 months is not long enough to draw conclusions about *maintenance*. Nevertheless, these data support the hypothesized value of emphasizing bleeding in treatment.

So too do data briefly reported by Kallio and Ainamo (1986), although this study also suffers from the lack of behavioral measurement and a lengthy follow-up. The authors randomly assigned 66 army conscripts to an experimental group or a control condition. Treatment subjects received a self-assessment manual designed to focus their attention on bleeding as a sign of disease. Draftees in both groups received dental hygiene materials (e.g., floss). At 1 month later, participants returned, and those who had focused on their bleeding showed a meaningful reduction in gingival health, whereas control participants did not.

One other piece of data could be used to support the importance of symptoms. Specifically, it is likely that persons who have actually experienced and been treated for gum disease would be more likely to know about symptoms such as bleeding and therefore should also be more likely to follow plaque-control instructions. Some data suggest that this is indeed the case (Gift, 1988).

FUTURE RESEARCH

Methodological Issues

Future research regarding health-protective dental behaviors must focus on long-term behavior change, placing equal emphasis on measurement of behavior and health outcomes. This statement has two important methodological implications, and each is discussed in turn.

Long-Term Behavior Change

Given the emphasis on maintenance of behavior throughout this chapter, it may be overkill to stress the importance of studying behavior change over longer periods. But one might ask what "long-term" means. Although researchers could safely use a period such as 1 year, the important variable might be not so much the absolute length of time as how long contact is continued in the study. The relapse data show that when treatment ends, most people who are going to quit careful brushing and flossing do so quickly. If participants know that they are still being "studied," however, they may continue to adhere for longer periods (McCaul et al., 1992). This general phenomenon has been observed with other health behaviors as well, including smoking (Brandon, Zelman, & Baker, 1987). When the "treatment" ends, researchers who wish to know whether behavior change lasts should inform participants that the study itself is *over*. They should then be able to study relapse within a month or two.

Behavior and Dental Health

Many researchers, including behavioral psychologists, sometimes lose sight of the first purpose of behavioral interventions: to change *behavior* (Leventhal et al., 1984). Of course, thorough brushing and flossing behaviors are ultimately important because of their health-protective function—preventing or reducing gum disease. Interventions can have such effects, however, only *through* behavior change. Some dental researchers tend to define compliance as Kuhner and Raetzke (1989) did in a recent article: "Compliance was defined analytically as improvement in oral hygiene on baseline values" (p. 52). Researchers must at minimum report behavioral results, because behavior change and dental outcomes are imperfectly related. Indeed, the precise relationships between dental behavior and plaque and between plaque and disease are unclear (Newman, 1990). Kaplan (1990) has made a similar point regarding health behaviors across the spectrum; there is a need to focus on changing behavior but also to *measure* both behavior and health outcomes. Thus, it is crucial to consider how behavior is changed and what the benefits of such change are for dental health outcomes (i.e., plaque levels, gingival disease). Studies that neglect either of these two outcomes fail to contribute to knowledge in important ways. Moreover, it is only when the effects of behavior change on disease are known that one can speculate further about the costs and benefits of treatment.

Cost-Benefit Analysis

Dental disease is costly. It causes such outcomes as discomfort and pain, time lost from work, and expensive treatment. Estimates in 1985 were that treatment costs associated with periodontal disease were approximately $1.5 billion (Polson & Goodson, 1985), a figure that presumably jumped dramatically in the next decade as the population grew and aged and as health care costs climbed (Tedesco, Keffer, & Davis,

1991). Moreover, dental disease is pervasive. In the United States, as much as three fourths of the population may have some form of inflammatory periodontal disease (Jeffcoat, 1994; Polson & Goodson, 1985).

But such statistics reveal nothing of the psychological costs and benefits of the sorts of treatments described in this chapter. Is it worth five 90-minute group visits with a psychologist to create a plaque-removal habit? Although nearly everyone will have at least minor periodontal disease (Sheiham & Croog, 1981), far fewer will experience the more problematic negative effects of tooth loss or surgery to correct periodontal problems (Burt, 1988; National Institute of Dental Research, 1990). It is conceivable that, for most people, treatment of minor periodontal disease can be effective even if it consists only of low-intensity dental care and instruction in home care (Frandsen, 1986). More extensive time may be necessary only for a small subgroup of persons who experience more severe disease and a lowered quality of life (Kaplan, 1990). Interestingly, dentists typically do just the opposite: They spend more time with those patients who are *least* at risk for severe outcomes (Milgrom, Weinstein, Melnick, Beach, & Spadafora, 1989b).

It seems reasonable to reserve the "best" therapies only for those who are truly suffering from lowered quality of life due to periodontal disease. Such individuals should be highly motivated to seek treatment, and it will be worth spending the time to help them create a habit. For others, who will probably be most persons, dental health professionals should be encouraged and perhaps pushed to keep monitoring and to keep talking. Unfortunately, very few data are available to help determine which persons would benefit most from concerted effort, in part because the dental regimen literature has focused so exclusively on dental *disease*. Quality of life issues, and connections of dental disease to health perceptions, have been insufficiently studied (Coulter, Marcus, & Atchison, 1994).

SUMMARY AND IMPLICATIONS

This chapter has introduced a number of themes concerning what has been learned to date about adherence to dental regimens and the most efficient way to learn more in the future. The most important implications for dental health professionals, for researchers, and for both groups are discussed in this section.

For Dental Health Professionals

A number of theoretically derived predictors of relapse "work," and most are related to subjects' beliefs about whether they can maintain behavior—most important, self-efficacy expectations. Thus, patients seem to "know" whether they are likely to relapse, and professionals can rely on patients' wisdom to make treatment decisions. The data also suggest, however, that persons who have performed the regimen at least at some level are less likely to relapse. Because continual attempts to prompt adherence will probably increase the odds of eventually being successful, professionals should not abandon their attempts to encourage adherence and teach skills even to difficult patients; regimen advice may eventually "take." It is also clear that close monitoring serves to maintain adherence. Health professionals could use relatively inexpensive techniques (e.g., a tailored message via postcard) to remind patients about adherence *between* their more formal contacts. Finally, it may be most efficient for health professionals to select at-risk patients and to emphasize bleeding as a cue to action.

For Researchers

The chapter has indicated three important suggestions for researchers. First, those who are interested in self-protective dental *behavior* must include measures of behavior *and* dental health outcomes. Further, they should report the relationship between these measures. Second, researchers should begin to include quality of life measures in their work, and they should address the cost-effectiveness of treatment. Such measures may help to describe the importance of dental outcomes in the larger health milieu. Finally, any study dealing with adherence should deal with maintenance, whether maintenance is defined as what happens soon after contact ends or as adherence over a long time period.

For Professionals and Researchers

Given the difficulty of establishing habits, more effort should be spent on persons who are most at risk for disease and a poorer quality of life. Finally, it may be necessary to redefine what is meant by a successful treatment. Influencing some people some of the time may be a reasonable payoff on efforts intended to maintain a difficult-to-perform, lifetime habit.

ACKNOWLEDGMENTS. I wish to acknowledge the many persons who helped on the "dental grants," but especially Lynne Olsen, D.D.S.; Paula Wilson, Project Hygienist; Ellen Thiesse-Duffy, Project Director; Kit O'Neill, Ph.D.; and Russ Glasgow, co-PI. The National Institutes of Dental Research funded the original research reported in this paper (Grant DE06656).

REFERENCES

Abdellatif, H. M., & Burt, B. A. (1987). An epidemiological investigation into the relative importance of age and oral hygiene status as determinants of periodontitis. *Journal of Dental Research, 66*, 13-18.

Albino, J. E. N., Lawrence, S. D., Lopes, C. E., Nash, L. B., & Tedesco, L. A. (1991). Cooperation of adolescents in orthodontic treatment. *Journal of Behavioral Medicine, 14*, 53-70.

Alcouffe, F. (1988). Improvement of oral hygiene habits: A psychological approach. *Journal of Clinical Periodontology, 15*, 616-620.

Allen, J., & Allen, R. F. (1986). From short term compliance to long term freedom: Culture-based health promotion by health professionals. *American Journal of Health Promotion* (Fall) 39-47.

Axelsson, P., & Lindhe, J. (1981). Effect of controlled oral hygiene procedures on caries and periodontal disease in adults: Results after 6 years. *Journal of Clinical Periodontology, 8*, 228-239.

Baab, D., & Weinstein, P. (1983). Oral hygiene instruction using a self-inspection index. *Community Dentistry and Oral Epidemiology, 11*, 174-179.

Baer, J. S., Kamarck, T., Lichtenstein, E., & Ransom, C. C., Jr. (1989). Prediction of smoking relapse: Analyses of temptations and transgressions after initial cessation. *Journal of Consulting and Clinical Psychology, 57*, 623-627.

Bandura, A. (1986). *Social foundations of thought and action*. Englewood Cliffs, NJ: Prentice-Hall.

Brandon, T. H., Zelman, D. C., & Baker, T. B. (1987). Effects of maintenance sessions on smoking relapse: Delaying the inevitable. *Journal of Consulting and Clinical Psychology, 55*, 780-782.

Burt, B. A. (1988). Public health implications of recent research in periodontal diseases. *Journal of Public Health in Dentistry, 48*, 252-256.

Cercek, J. F., Kiger, R. D., Garrett, S., & Egelberg, J. (1983). Relative effects of plaque control and instrumentation on the clinical parameters of human periodontal disease. *Journal of Clinical Periodontology, 10*, 46-56.

Chen, M.-S., & Rubinson, L. (1982). Preventive dental behavior in families: A national survey. *Journal of the American Dental Association, 105*, 43-46.

Coulter, I. D., Marcus, M., & Atchison, K. A. (1994). Measuring oral health status: Theoretical and methodological challenges. *Social Science and Medicine, 38*, 1531-1541.

DiClemente, C. C. (1986). Self-efficacy and the addictive behaviors. *Journal of Social and Clinical Psychology, 4*, 302-315.

DiNicola, D. D., & DiMatteo, M. R. (1984). Practitioners, patients, and compliance with medical regimens: A social psychological perspective. In A. Baum, S. E. Taylor, & J. E. Singer (Eds.), *Handbook of psychology and health: Vol. IV, Social psychological aspects of health* (pp. 55-84). Hillsdale, NJ: Erlbaum.

Easterling, D. V., & Leventhal, H. (1989). Contribution of concrete cognition to emotion: Neutral symptoms as elicitors of worry about cancer. *Journal of Applied Psychology, 74*, 787-796.

Fishbein, M., & Ajzen, I. (1975). *Belief, attitude, intention, and behavior: An introduction to theory and research*. Reading, MA: Addison-Wesley.

Frandsen, A. (1986). Mechanical oral hygiene practices. In H. Loe & D. V. Kleinman (Eds.), *Dental plaque control measures and oral hygiene practices* (pp. 93-116). Oxford, England: IRL Press.

Gallagher, E. B., & Moody, P. M. (1981). Dentists and the oral health behavior of patients: A sociological perspective. *Journal of Behavioral Medicine, 4*, 283-296.

Gift, H. C. (1986). Current utilization patterns of oral hygiene practices. In H. Loe & D. V. Kleinman (Eds.), *Dental plaque control measures and oral hygiene practices* (pp. 39-71). Oxford, England: IRL Press.

Gift, H. C. (1988). Awareness and assessment of periodontal problems among dentists and the public. *International Dental Journal, 38*, 147-153.

Glavind, L., Zeuner, E., & Attstrom, R. (1981). Oral hygiene instruction of adults by means of a self-instructional manual. *Journal of Clinical Periodontology, 8*, 165-176.

Heasman, P. A., Jacobs, D. J., & Chapple, I. A. (1989). An evaluation of the effectiveness and patient compliance with plaque control methods in the prevention of periodontal disease. *Clinical Preventive Dentistry, 11*, 24-28.

Hollis, P., Little, S. J., Stevens, V. J., Mullooly, J., Johnson, B., & Adams, R. A. (1994). *Behavioral interventions for older periodontal patients*. Paper presented at the International Association of Dental Research.

Iwata, B. A., & Becksfort, C. M. (1981). Behavioral research in preventive dentistry: Educational and contingency management approaches to the problem of patient compliance. *Journal of Applied Behavior Analysis, 14*, 111-120.

Jeffcoat, M. K. (1994). Prevention of periodontal diseases in adults: Strategies for the future. *Preventive Medicine, 23*, 704-708.

Kallio, P., & Ainamo, J. (1986). Use of gingival bleeding self-assessment in reinforcement of oral health care. *Journal of Dental Research, 65*, 830.

Kaplan, R. M. (1990). Behavior as the central outcome in health care. *American Psychologist, 45*, 1211-1220.

Kegeles, S. S., & Lund, A. K. (1984). Adolescents' acceptance of caries-preventive procedures. In J. D. Matarazzo, S. M. Weiss, J. A. Herd, N. E. Miller, & S. M. Weiss (Eds.), *Behavioral health: A handbook of health enhancement and disease prevention* (pp. 895-909). New York: John Wiley & Sons.

Kegeles, S. S., Lund, A. K., & Weisenberg, M. (1978). Acceptance by students of a daily home mouthrinse program. *Social Science and Medicine, 12*, 199-210.

Kelly, M. A., McKinty, H. R., & Carr, R. (1988). Utilization of hypnosis to promote compliance with routine dental flossing. *American Journal of Clinical Hypnosis, 31*, 57-60.

Kuhner, M. K., & Raetzke, P. B. (1989). The effect of health beliefs on the compliance of periodontal patients with oral hygiene instructions. *Journal of Periodontology, 60*, 51-56.

Leventhal, H., Diefenbach, M., & Leventhal, E. A. (1992). Illness cognition: Using common sense to understand treatment adherence and affect cognition interactions. *Cognitive Therapy and Research, 16*, 143-163.

Leventhal, H., Zimmerman, R., & Gutmann, M. (1984). Compliance: A self-regulatory perspective. In D. Gentry (Ed.), *Handbook of behavioral medicine* (pp. 326-368). New York: Guilford Press.

Lobene, R. R., Soparkar, P. M., & Newman, M. B. (1982). Use of dental floss: Effect on plaque and gingivitis. *Clinical Preventive Dentistry, 4*, 5-8.

Lund, A. K., & Kegeles, S. S. (1981). Behavior modification of oral hygiene habits. In J. J. Hefferen, W. A. Ayer, & H. M. Koehler (Eds.), *Foods, nutrition and dental health: Vol. 3* (pp. 207-222).

Lund, A. K., & Kegeles, S. S. (1982). Increasing adolescents' acceptance of long-term personal health behavior. *Health Psychology, 1*, 27-43.

Lund, A. K., & Kegeles, S. S. (1984). Rewards and adolescent health behavior. *Health Psychology, 3*, 351-369.

McCaul, K. D., Bakdash, M. B., Geboy, M. J., Gerbert, B., & Tedesco, L. A. (1990). Promoting self-protective health behaviors in dentistry. *Annals of Behavioral Medicine, 12*, 156-160.

McCaul, K. D., Glasgow, R. E., & Gustafson, C. (1985). Predicting levels of preventive dental behaviors. *Journal of the American Dental Association, 111*, 601-605.

McCaul, K. D., Glasgow, R. E., & O'Neill, H. K. (1992). The problem of creating habits: Establishing health-protective dental behaviors. *Health Psychology, 11*, 101-110.

McCaul, K. D., Glasgow, R. E., & Schafer, L. C. (1987). Diabetes regimen behaviors: Predicting adherence. *Medical Care, 25*, 1-14.

McCaul, K. D., Thiesse-Duffy, E., O'Neill, H. K., Gravely, J. E., & Suda, K. T. (1993). Factors associated with relapse following dental treatment. Unpublished data. North Dakota State University, Fargo.

Milgrom, P., Weinstein, P., Chapko, M., Grembowski, D., & Spadafora, A. (1988). Dentists' attitudes and behaviors in counseling patients about oral self care. *Journal of the American College of Dentistry, 55*, 48-53.

Milgrom, P., Weinstein, P., Melnick, S., Beach, B., & Spadafora, A. (1989a). How effective is oral hygiene instruction? Results after 6 and 24 weeks. *Journal of Public Health Dentistry, 49*, 32-37.

Milgrom, P., Weinstein, P., Melnick, S., Beach, B., & Spadafora, A. (1989b). Oral hygiene instruction and health risk assessment in dental practice. *Journal of Public Health Dentistry, 49*, 24-31.

National Institute of Dental Research. (1990). Periodontal status of American adults. *NIDR Research Digest* (December), 1-2.

Newman, H. N. (1990). Plaque and chronic inflammatory periodontal disease. *Journal of Clinical Periodontology, 17*, 533-541.

Nides, M. A., Rakos, R. F., Gonzales, D., Murray, R. P., Tashkin, D. P., Bjornson-Benson, W. M., Lindgren, P., & Connett, J. E. (1995). Predictors of initial smoking cessation and relapse thru the first 2 years of the lung health study. *Journal of Consulting and Clinical Psychology, 63*, 60-69.

Ockene, J. K., & Camic, P. M. (1985). Public health approaches to cigarette smoking. *Annals of Behavioral Medicine, 7*, 14-86.

O'Neill, H. K., Sandgren, A. K., McCaul, K. D., & Glasgow, R. E. (1987). Self-control strategies and maintenance of a dental hygiene regimen. *Journal of Compliance in Health Care, 2*, 85-89.

Polson, A. M., & Goodson, J. M. (1985). Periodontal diagnosis: Current status and future needs. *Journal of Periodontology, 56*, 25-34.

Prochaska, J. O., & DiClemente, C. C. (1983). Stages and processes of self-change of smoking: Toward an integrative model. *Journal of Consulting and Clinical Psychology, 51*, 390-395.

Ronis, D. L., Yates, J. F., & Kirscht, J. P. (1989). Attitudes, decisions, and habits as determinants of repeated behavior. In A. R. Pratkanis, S. J. Breckler, & A. G. Greenwald (Eds.), *Attitude structure and function* (pp. 213-329). Hillsdale, NJ: Erlbaum.

Schou, I. (1985). Active-involvement principle in dental health education. *Community Dentistry and Oral Epidemiology, 13*, 128-132.

Sheiham, A., & Croog, S. H. (1981). The psychosocial impact of dental diseases on individuals and communities. *Journal of Behavioral Medicine, 4*, 257-272.

Stewart, J. E., Jacobs-Schoen, M., Padilla, M. R., Maeder, L. A., Wolfe, G. R., & Hartz, G. W. (1991). The effect of a cognitive behavioral intervention on oral hygiene. Journal of Clinical Periodontology *18*, 219-222.

Tedesco, L. A., Keffer, M. A., & Davis, E. L. (1991). Social cognitive theory and relapse prevention: Reframing patient compliance. *Journal of Dental Education, 55*, 575-585.

Tedesco, L. A., Keffer, M. A., Davis, E. L., & Christersson, L. A. (1992). Effect of a social cognitive intervention on oral health status, behavior reports, and cognitions. *Journal of Periodontology, 63*, 567-575.

Tedesco, L. A., Keffer, M. A., Davis, E. L., & Christersson, L. A. (1993). Self-efficacy and reasoned action: Predicting oral health status and behaviour at one, three, and six month intervals. *Psychology and Health, 8*, 105-121.

Walsh, M. M., Heckman, B. H., & Moreau-Diettinger, R. (1985). Use of gingival bleeding for reinforcement of oral home care behavior. *Community Dentistry and Oral Epidemiology, 13*, 133-135.

Weinstein, P., Milgrom, P., Melnick, S., Beach, B., & Spadafora, A. (1989). A study of relapse in plaque control programs: Results at 24 weeks. *Journal of Public Health Dentistry, 49*, 32-38.

Wolff, L. F., Pihlstrom, B. L., Bakdash, M. B., Schaffer, E. M., Aeppli, D. M., & Bandt, C. L. (1989). Four-year investigation of salt and peroxide regimen compared with conventional oral hygiene. *Journal of the American Dental Association, 118*, 67-72.

C. LIFESTYLE REGIMENS

ADHERENCE TO LIFESTYLE REGIMENS

The introductory material for Sections IIIA and IIIB is equally suitable as a context for this section. The issues identified and the analysis of the concepts of compliance, adherence, and acceptance are equally applicable for discussions of lifestyle regimens.

In Chapter 17, on weight loss and nutritional regimens, Chrisler places adherence within a context of sociocultural, gender, and age-related issues. In Chapter 18, Marcus, Bock, and Pinto provide a comprehensive discussion of a number of barriers to participation in exercise programs, and also emphasize the need for community and worksite programs.

In Chapter 19, Glasgow and Orleans discuss issues in adherence to smoking cessation programs within a context of the transtheoretical (or stages of change) model. At the same time, they emphasize the importance of a range of community-wide and specifically tailored intervention strategies and the role of facilitative environments.

Finally, in Chapter 20, Cohen and Colligan move the focus of adherence away from a strictly medical conception of health toward a broader view that encompasses engaging in safety behavior in occupation settings, stressing the importance of training and of environmental and organizational norms.

17

Adherence to Weight Loss and Nutritional Regimens

Joan C. Chrisler

INTRODUCTION

THE KING: You have a physician. What does he do?
MOLIÈRE: Sire, we converse. He gives me advice, which I do not follow, and then I get better.
—Treue (1958) (cited in Taylor, 1991, p. 312)

As long as there have been health "experts" to give advice, there have been patients who do not or cannot adhere to that advice. Molière, the witty 17th-century playwright, may be more honest than most about the extent of his adherence, but modern health care practitioners will surely recognize his attitude. Practitioners list adherence to treatment regimens among their greatest concerns and believe it to be a major cause of treatment failure (Meichenbaum & Turk, 1987). Adherence to lifestyle changes such as diet is much more difficult for most patients than adherence to "medical" tasks such as taking medication and keeping clinic appointments (Taylor, 1991).

Adherence may be defined as the extent to which the patient's behavior matches medical advice (Meichenbaum & Turk, 1987). The term *adherence* connotes active, voluntary behavior designed to produce a therapeutic effect. It is preferred to the older term *compliance*, which suggests passive obedience to a doctor's orders. Patients who are termed *noncompliant* are evaluated negatively by health care practitioners and are often assumed to be irresponsible (Meichenbaum & Turk, 1987), when in fact, as will be shown later in this chapter, they may be unable to adhere for many other reasons.

The words professionals choose to use are important clues to their attitudes, beliefs, definitions of problems, and potential solutions. If "compliance" is the problem, then one would look for ways to enforce obedience. If "adherence" is the problem, then one would look for ways to design treatment regimens that patients are able to follow. Another interesting semantic issue is the different terms in which practitioners and patients describe nonadherence to diets. What practitioners refer to as "dietary indiscretions" or "lapses," patients refer to as "cheating" (J. E. Antisdel, personal communication, March 1994).

Practitioners and patients may not agree on

Joan C. Chrisler • Department of Psychology, Connecticut College, New London, Connecticut 06320.

Handbook of Health Behavior Research II: Provider Determinants, edited by David S. Gochman. Plenum Press, New York, 1997.

which factors are most important in determining adherence. A survey of diabetic patients and their physicians by House, Pendleton, and Parker (1986) revealed that the patients most often mentioned environmental causes for dietary lapses, whereas the physicians perceived motivational problems as the primary cause. More surprising than the difference in perceptions was the authors' conclusion that physicians who want to increase their patients' adherence rates "must be aware that patients have a strong tendency to disclaim personal responsibility for failure to comply" (House et al., 1986, p. 434).

Clearly, it is easier to give dietary advice than to follow it. Practitioners' understanding of the difficulties patients face and their sensitivity to patients' complaints about dietary regimens might be increased if the practitioners themselves attempted to adhere to the diet in order to see what it is like to do so. Several investigators have attempted to alter the attitudes of dietitians by examining how well they adhered to the National Cancer Institute's nutritional guidelines (Wilson, Stitt, Bonner, & Balentine, 1990) or by placing them on a low-sodium, low-cholesterol diet, or a diabetic diet, for a week (Cotugna & Vickery, 1989, 1990). Although dietitians can be expected to be highly motivated to follow nutritional guidelines, they did not find it easy to adhere to the diets. The diabetic diet was particularly difficult. One student dietitian found it "absolutely impossible to fit [the] diet into [her] clinic and class schedule" (Cotugna & Vickery, 1989; p. 1301).

The Extent of the Problem

A literature search located many studies of dietary adherence, most of which support the conclusion that it is difficult to change one's eating habits. Studies of patients on diabetic diets reported rates of "good" adherence that varied from 20% (Irvine, 1989) to 73% (R. M. Anderson, Fitzgerald, & Oh, 1993). In a National Health Survey (Holland, 1968) of 1957 people with diabetes, 53% of the respondents reported that they adhered to their diet; 22% said they had never been given any dietary advice. Dietary adherence rates for patients on hemodialysis have been found to vary from 39% (Procci, 1978) to 42% (Brown & Fitzpatrick, 1988). In one study, 52% of breast cancer patients were able to maintain a low-fat diet for 2 years (Holm, Nordevang, Ikkala, Hallstrom, & Callmer, 1990); in another study, however, only 30% of people with high cholesterol were able to adhere to a low-cholesterol diet for 3 months (Kushner, 1993). Still another study found that only 20% of people on a very low-calorie weight-loss diet were able to adhere to it for 2 weeks (Heller & Edelmann, 1991). Dropout rates from commercial weight-loss programs range from 20% to 80% (J. W. Anderson & Gustafson, 1989).

Methodological Issues

It is difficult to compare the result of one study with another or to know how reliable the adherence rates are. Methods of assessing adherence vary from study to study, and they are not necessarily described in detail (Wing, Epstein, & Norwalk, 1984). Many reseachers ask participants in their studies to keep food diaries, but they may choose to analyze them daily or simply to take several random days for analysis. Some take physiological measurements, i.e., blood levels of glucose or cholesterol, as indicators of adherence. Others rely on retrospective questionnaires to ask about food intake over various periods (from a week to a year) or simply ask participants how well they would say that they adhere to their diets. Some longitudinal studies report that adherence got better after an intervention or worse over time without indicating how good it was in the beginning. Retrospective self-reports are probably the most undependable, particularly when patients must rely on their memory for food consumption over a long period. The reliability of physiological measurements, however, must also be questioned; diet does not account for all the variance in blood glucose levels.

WHY IS IT SO DIFFICULT TO ADHERE TO A DIET?

I can resist everything except temptation.
—OSCAR WILDE (1915)

Everyone has to eat, and in wealthy countries such as the United States, the variety of food choices available is dazzling. Temptations are everywhere, and people are constantly subjected to advertisements that encourage them to "give in." American culture sends mixed messages about eating. Dieting has become a $30 billion a year industry (Stoffel, 1989), and people are told by medical, fashion, and social "authorities" that it is important to be thin. Yet the commercial media also tell people that food preferences, like fashion preferences, define our personal style, that people deserve to indulge themselves with the finest (i.e., the sweetest, the fattiest) foods, that food is an expression of love, that it can serve as a reward, that it is essential for holiday celebrations. Furthermore, there is evidence (Logue, 1986) that attraction to calorie-dense foods (e.g., sweets) is biologically "wired-in." The natural preference for such foods dates from a time when they were far less available than they are today and when the sweetest foods were also high in vitamins and fiber (e.g., berries, carrots).

Given the cultural and personal importance of certain foods and their perceived relevance to quality of life, practitioners must determine whether the diet is acceptable to the patient. If it is not, it is doomed to failure. Lifestyle changes are difficult to make, particularly in the presence of variable social support and conflicting cultural messages. To be successful, patients need more than the usual "talking to" and list of dietary restrictions from a physician or nurse. They need education and supervision by a dietitian, which is generally not covered by health insurance (Henkin, Garber, Osterlund, & Darnell, 1992), and behavioral advice and psychological support from a psychotherapist as well.

Sociocultural Issues in Diet Adherence

Food habits vary considerably among ethnic groups, and in order for a diet to be successful, it must be culturally acceptable (Berg & Berg, 1989; Kittler & Sucher, 1990). It is important to begin the process of dietary modification by inquiring what patients typically eat and what they are willing to eat. Changes in food consumption are made with the most difficulty in core foods (those eaten frequently, which form the foundation of the cuisine), more easily in secondary core foods (eaten widely, but not daily), and most easily in peripheral foods (Kittler & Sucher, 1990). Patients often report that it is easier to change their eating patterns at breakfast and lunch than at dinner (Kittler & Sucher, 1990), which more often consists of traditional foods and involves family interactions. Immigrants may prefer traditional foods more strongly when they are ill or under stress (Kittler & Sucher, 1990), which can work against adherence to medical advice.

Religious dictates may interfere with dietary adherence, and practitioners should also inquire about them. Some religions (e.g., Judaism, Hinduism, and Mormonism) have many dietary guidelines, whereas others (e.g., Catholicism, Buddhism) have few (Kittler & Sucher, 1990). Knowing patients' religious affiliations may not be sufficient to understand how they affect their food choices because people vary considerably in how closely they adhere to religious guidelines. Some would never consider deviating from the guidelines, whereas others adhere to them only at certain times of the year (e.g., Passover, Lent, Ramadan). Patients should not have to "cheat" or feel that they have disappointed their doctors or "ruined" their diets because they ate a food associated with a religious holiday as part of a family celebration.

The patient's socioeconomic status must

also be taken into account when planning a diet. If the recommended foods are not available or are too expensive to purchase, the diet is certain to fail. Fresh foods are more easily available to rural than to urban poor people. Patients on economic assistance programs may be limited in the types of foods they can purchase (Kittler & Sucher, 1990), or they may have to buy cheaper, less healthful foods in order to manage to feed their families.

Age-Related Issues in Diet Adherence

Children may be placed on restricted diets for medical conditions such as diabetes, phenylketonuria, or food allergies or sensitivities, or in an attempt to control behavior disorders such as hyperactivity. Practitioners may assume that because children do not prepare their own food adherence is not as much a problem as it is with adults. Adults must be properly educated and motivated, however, so that they can encourage their children to stay on their diets. Children must also be educated, motivated, and supervised. They have many opportunities to accept food from others (e.g., at school, at friends' homes), and they must be able to discriminate between appropriate and inappropriate foods and to explain their reason for refusal to others. Food fads are common among children, generally for the newest type of candy or breakfast cereal, and it is at least as difficult for children as it is for adults to restrict consumption of foods associated with celebrations and holidays (e.g., birthday cakes, Halloween candy). Thus, children and their parents need specialized counseling and assistance in order to promote adherence.

That maturity increases from childhood to adolescence may suggest that adolescents would be more adherent to diets, but the increasing need for peer approval may work against their doing so. Teenagers also have food fads, and they are known to have unusual eating habits (Logue, 1986). Binge eating is common among adolescents (Logue, 1986), especially when engaged in activities with friends such as watching football games or attending slumber parties. Moreover, the preferred foods for bingeing are sweets, alcohol, or snacks high in salt or fat. Dieting for weight loss or gain is also common among teenagers. It is not unusual for adolescent girls to skip meals or insist upon eating only certain kinds of foods (e.g., salads, cottage cheese, diet soda). Student athletes may be encouraged by their coaches or teammates to engage in purging behaviors or to eat certain types of food in order to "bulk up" (Hudson, Pope, & Katz, 1993; Szymanski & Chrisler, 1991). Although generally unhealthful, these behaviors can be particularly dangerous for those with diabetes. One study (Jacobson et al., 1990) found that adolescent diabetics were more adherent to their medical regimens if they were preadolescent when diagnosed, and several studies have found evidence of clinical or subclinical disordered eating (including the manipulation of insulin dosages) among teenage girls with diabetes (Antisdel & Chrisler, 1994; Hilliard & Hilliard, 1984; LaGreca, Schwartz, & Satin, 1987).

Incidence of chronic illness increases with age, and the elderly are the population most likely to be given a restricted diet. In fact, many older people have more than one chronic illness, and they may be given more than one type of diet to follow, which can lead to confusion about conflicting advice or to a decision to ignore their diets because it seems that nothing they enjoy is recommended by their doctors. Quality of life may be more important than length of life (Shifflett, 1987), so some older people may prefer to maintain their present habits rather than attempt to change them. Some may reject certain foods as being age-inappropriate, believing, for example, that milk is for children (Kittler & Sucher, 1990), or they may refuse to accept the idea that foods they were once told were "good" for them (e.g., butter, eggs) are now "bad" for them. In addition, age-related physiological changes may interfere with diet adherence. Older people have fewer taste buds than young people (Logue, 1986), and so they may add more salt to their foods than they used to do in order to taste the same flavor. This practice may cause problems for those on low-salt diets, who may judge to be "not very" salty a dish that a dietitian would judge "extremely" salty.

Gender-Related Issues in Diet Adherence

Several studies (Chaiken & Pliner, 1987; Mori, Pliner, & Chaiken, 1987) have found that eating small amounts of food is associated with feminity, which is not surprising given the estimates that 80% of women in the United States are on weight-loss diets (Steiner-Adair, 1988) and 9 out of 10 participants in weight-loss programs are women (Freedman, 1986). Food preparation, knowledge of nutrition, and dieting behavior are all considered to be in women's sphere, and many practitioners have found that men on low-salt or "healthy heart" diets adhere better when they have wives to prepare their meals and monitor their eating behavior. The fact that many foods are gender-related (e.g., salads are for women, red meat is for men) may also affect people's willingness to adhere to their diets.

Women's greater experience with dieting does not result in better adherence. Most weight-loss diets fail, and women's previous experience with failure may make them less optimistic than men about their ability to adhere to a diet. Talk about "cheating" and eating "bad" foods is common among women, who often encourage each other to do it. Lapses in adherence to a weight-loss diet have less serious consequences than lapses in adherence to a diabetic diet, yet the women may be so accustomed to this cycle of "good" and "bad" eating that they do not discriminate between the types of diets.

Furthermore, weight-loss diets may interfere with women's ability to adhere to other nutritional regimens, as in the case of adolescent diabetics with disordered eating. Recommended foods may be perceived as too high in calories or may not be compatible with the latest fad diet recommended by the supermarket tabloids. Many periodicals aimed at women feature a new weight-loss strategy each month—usually proclaimed as a major scientific breakthrough and often nutritionally inadequate. That women would want to try these fad diets should not be surprising given the importance of attractiveness for women's social success (e.g., Saltzberg & Chrisler, 1995; Freedman, 1986).

Predictors of Adherence to Diets

Aspects of the patient's medical condition predict adherence. The more serious the illness for which the diet was recommended, the better the adherence will be (DiMatteo et al., 1993). Patients who are asymptomatic generally have lower adherence (Carmody, Fey, Pierce, Connor, & Matarazzo, 1982), and those who believe their health is poor (Irvine, 1989) or who have multiple chronic illnesses (B. V. Reid, 1992) generally try harder to adhere. Hemodialysis decreases patients' preference for salt, which makes it easier for them to stay on a low-salt diet, but it makes them thirstier, which makes it more difficult to adhere to recommendations for reduced fluid intake (Shepherd, Farleigh, Atkinson, & Pryor, 1987).

Aspects of the diets also predict adherence. Unpleasant side effects, e.g., constipation from increased use of calcium tablets (Johnston, 1989) or flatuence from high-fiber diets, can reduce adherence. One study (Ho, Lee, & Meyskens, 1991) found that elderly people were more likely to modify their eating habits if the recommended foods aided in digestion or bowel functioning. If the foods are readily available (Baranowski et al., 1993) and if the patients like the foods (Baranowski et al., 1993; Barnes & Terry, 1991; Heiby, Gafarian, & McCann, 1989), the dietary modification will be more successful. The more control patients have over the selection and preparation of food, the better their adherence will be (Schmid, Jeffery, Onstad, & Corrigan, 1991). The more expensive the foods and the longer it takes to prepare them, the harder it will be to adhere to the diet (Urban, White, Anderson, Curry, & Kristal, 1992). Finally, the easier a diet is to understand, the easier it is to adhere to it (Shifflett, 1987).

Practitioners' attitudes and behaviors also affect adherence rates. If practitioners have low expectations for adherence, their patients' adherence is generally poor (Secker-Walker, Morrow, Kresnow, Flynn, & Hocheiser, 1991). Patients whose physicians ordered more medical tests during the screening visit had better adherence (DiMatteo et al., 1993), as did those who were enrolled in ongoing treatment sessions to educate them and supervise their behavior (Miller, Wikoff, Garrett, McMahon, & Smith, 1990; Morisky, DeMuth, Field-Fass, Green, & Levine, 1985; Schmid et al., 1991). Patients of endocrinologists adhered to their diets better than patients of other specialists (DiMatteo et al., 1993), perhaps because the disorders treated by endocrinologists are seen by patients as more serious or as requiring more dietary modification. It appears that those patients who are more involved in their treatment are also more adherent to their diets (Tucker et al., 1987).

Patients' attitudes and personal characteristics also predict adherence. Those who are pessimistic (Shifflett, 1987), stressed, socially isolated (Carmody et al., 1982), depressed (Carmody et al., 1982; Morley & Perry, 1991; Tracy, Green, & McClearly, 1987), helpless, and negative (Holm et al., 1990) generally show poor adherence to diets. So do those with external locus of control (Holm et al., 1990), high panic-fear scores on the Minnesota Multiphasic Personality Inventory (Flanagan & Wagner, 1991), low frustration tolerance, inability to delay gratification, excessive dependency needs, hostility, and a tendency to deny their illness (Stewart, 1983). Married, skilled professionals with a "high self-concept" were found to be most adherent to a hemodialysis diet (Hoover, 1989). Those with a positive attitude toward the diet (Barnes & Terry, 1991), good problem-solving skills (Fehrenbach & Peterson, 1989), and the ability to generate strategies for coping with temptations (Hanna, Ewart, & Kwiterovich, 1990), and those who felt susceptible to a shortened life span (Harris, Skyler, Linn, Pollack, & Tewksbury, 1982) tended to have better adherence.

Children with lower socioeconomic status and poor knowledge of diabetes show lower adherence to their diet (Chazan et al., 1982), and children's satisfaction with their diets has been linked to their parents' attempts to involve them in meal planning and food choice (Hanna et al., 1982). Parents' attitudes and behaviors have been correlated with children's adherence to their diets, and one study (Becker, Maiman, Kirscht, Haefner, & Drachman, 1977) found that a high fear message to mothers predicted children's weight loss.

The attitudes and behaviors of family members are important to adults as well as to children. In fact, one study (Shenkel, Rogers, Perfetto, & Levin, 1985-1986) reported that the importance to significant others of following the diet was a better predictor of adherence than the patients' own beliefs. Lack of support from family members has been correlated with low adherence, and patients have complained about the difficulty of having to cook separate meals for self and others when the family refuses to accept the dietary modifications (Holm et al., 1990). Families associated with good adherence have been described (Sherwood, 1983) as understanding, supportive, organized, and neither overly involved nor disengaged.

Other factors that have been found to influence adherence include time and place of eating. Patients find it easiest to adhere to their diets at home and most difficult to adhere at work (Miller, Wikoff, Keen, & Norton, 1987). The day of the week also affects adherence; it is easier to adhere to the diet on weekdays, hardest on weekends and holidays (Cotugna & Vickery, 1990). Several studies (e.g., Brown & Fitzpatrick, 1988; DiMatteo et al., 1993) have reported that adherence declines over time; the longer the patient has been following the diet, the more dietary lapses there will be.

Finally, as might be expected from these accumulated findings, Fishbein's model of reasoned action (Miller, Wikoff, & Hiatt, 1992), the health belief model, social learning theory, and models of consumer information processing

(Rimer, Glanz, & Lerman, 1991) all predict to some degree successful adherence to dietary and nutritional regimens.

HOW CAN ADHERENCE TO DIETS BE INCREASED?

It is important for practitioners to view lifestyle changes as "a negotiated agreement rather than a coercive obedience" to "doctor's orders" (Cotugna & Vickery, 1990, p. 123). Practitioners should be flexible when engaged in diet planning, become familiar with unusual foods, and realize that people have different schedules on weekends and holidays than on weekdays (Cotugna & Vickery, 1990). Patients, especially African-Americans, prefer physician communication that is high in both affectivity and information (O'Hair, O'Hair, Southward, & Krayer, 1987). Both patient satisfaction and physician communication have been found to predict adherence (O'Hair et al., 1987), so practitioners should attempt to be warm, caring, empathic, cooperative, and receptive (Cotugna & Vickery, 1990) to patients' involvement in treatment planning.

Information about medical conditions and education about the diets are essential, although not sufficient, for good adherence. J. W. Anderson and Gustafson (1989) advise practitioners to simplify the diet, give specific advice in basic vocabulary, present dietary advice in order of importance, and use repetition. It may be helpful to introduce dietary modifications one at a time and make certain that the patient understands and can implement each before trying the next (Hoover, 1989). Diets should be presented to patients in written form as well as described orally. It is especially necessary to do so for anxious patients or those with poor memories. It may also be helpful when educating patients about good nutrition to stress its importance to stamina and attractiveness, particularly when working with women and adolescents (Ausenhus, 1988).

Patients also need skills training if they are going to succeed with their diets. Cooking demonstrations (Rimer et al., 1991) and practice in such skills as calculating portion size may be particularly useful. Giving patients spice packets to make bland foods more appealing (Lewis, Robinson, & Robinson, 1990) or referring them to cookbooks with recipes specific to their needs (e.g., low-fat, low-salt) may also help to increase adherence. Teaching consumer skills, e.g., how to read labels and look for the "healthy heart" options on menus, has been found to increase self-efficacy and adherence (Rimer et al., 1991). Patients might like to attend occasional group meetings with other people on a similar diet in order to share cooking and consumer tips. Many patients will also need assertiveness training to help them refuse food pressed on them by others or to persist in their inquiries (e.g., to waiters) about ingredients.

Behavior therapy techniques such as modeling and contingency contracting have been found to increase adherence (McCann, Retzlaff, Dowdy, Walden, & Knopp, 1990; Morgan & Littell, 1988; Rimer et al., 1991). Dietary changes should be gradual, goals should be reasonable, progress should be monitored, and successes should be rewarded. For children, one can develop token economies in which points toward preferred activities are awarded for adherence (P. Reid & Appleton, 1991). Patients should be helped to anticipate difficulties (e.g., holidays, travel) in order to plan in advance how to deal with them (J. W. Anderson & Gustafson, 1989). Memory aids can be developed for patients who need them (e.g., children, the elderly). For example, Epstein, et al. (1981) have described for young diabetics the traffic light diet, which divides foods into red (stop/avoid), yellow (caution/moderation), and green (go/no restriction) categories.

Because social support is positively associated with adherence (Ruggiero, Spirito, Bond, Coustan, & McGarvey, 1990), many researchers recommend involving significant others in treatment planning and diet monitoring. Patients may be more likely to adhere to their diets if the whole family eats the same food (Missiou-Tsagaraki,

Soulpi, & Loumakou, 1988). It may be helpful to have family or friends present while patients are learning about their diets (Cohen et al., 1991), and family members involved in cooking and food shopping should be invited to call on practitioners whenever they have questions about the diet. Family members can play important roles by encouraging patients to adhere to their diets and rewarding them for their successes. They can also provide feedback to practitioners about patients' progress. They should be encouraged to see themselves as "supporters," however, rather than as "enforcers." For example, parents should avoid putting their children in a position of having to lie about dietary adherence (Gross, 1990).

Realistic planning should also include acknowledgment that there will be times when patients will not be able to adhere to their diets. Dietary lapses should be seen as "slips" or "mistakes," not as "failures." Patients need relapse training so they will be able to anticipate making mistakes, know in advance how to deal with them, and then get back on track. Negative emotions are associated with relapse (Brownell, Marlatt, Lichtenstein, & Wilson, 1986), so it will be particularly important that patients learn techniques for moderating emotional reactions. Thought stopping and reframing will help patients to avoid labeling themselves as failures who have "blown" their diet. Long-term follow-up appointments or group sessions can provide necessary support for patients struggling with relapse.

CONCLUSION

Although there has been considerable research on adherence to weight loss and nutritional regimens, more carefully conducted studies are needed in which the manipulation of treatment variables can be reliably addressed. Chubon (1989) has suggested that researchers have often asked the wrong question: Instead of focusing on why patients don't do what they are told, researchers ought to be asking them why they do what they do. Better insight into patients' motivations and their experience of environmental and psychological barriers to adherence would be helpful to practitioners who are trying to design more realistic diets.

Patients would be better helped and more securely supported in their efforts to adjust to dietary modifications if health care practitioners worked in interdisciplinary teams. Work on adherence to diets is being carried out by dietitians, nutritionists, psychologists, social workers, anthropologists, public health experts, epidemiologists, nurses, and physicians in various specialties. These professionals work together only in limited ways, and they probably do not regularly read each other's journals. To be properly cared for in the ways suggested in the literature on good adherence, patients will need medical, nutritional, psychological, and behavioral advice to take them from diagnosis to dietary education to long-term follow-up.

Finally, practitioners must realize that the sociocultural milieu influences their patients' ability to adhere to treatment regimens. Dieting is now a "cultural requirement" for women (Herman & Polivy, 1983) and weight a "normative discontent" (Rodin, Silberstein, & Striegel-Moore, 1985). Because most weight-loss diets fail, most women (and many men) have experience with diets to which they could not adhere or with regaining weight after a diet to which they had adhered successfully. These experiences undoubtedly interfere with people's expectations for adherence to nutritional regimens and may also cause them to doubt that their adherence or lack of it will have any real effect on their medical conditions.

It is also necessary that professionals take responsibility for their role in promoting unnecessary dieting. They should not recommend weight-loss diets for those who are only mildly or moderately "overweight" (cf. Chrisler, 1993, 1994). Successful dietary modification is difficult to achieve; professionals should be saving their serious sermons and their best efforts to encourage and support those changes they are confident can be made and will produce effects that promote their patients' health.

REFERENCES

Anderson, J. W. & Gustafson, N. J. (1989). Adherence to high carbohydrate, high fiber diets. *Diabetes Educator, 15,* 429-434.

Anderson, R. M., Fitzgerald, J. T., & Oh, M. S. (1993). The relationship between diabetes-related attitudes and patients' self-reported adherence. *Diabetes Educator, 19,* 287-292.

Antisdel, J. E., & Chrisler, J. C. (1994). *Disordered eating among adolescent and young adult women with diabetes and phenylketonuria.* Manuscript under review.

Ausenhus, M. K. (1988). Osteoporosis: Prevention during the adolescent and young adult years. *Nurse Practitioner, 13*(9), 44-48.

Baranowski, T., Domel, S., Gould, R., Baranowski, J., Leonard, S., Treiber, F., & Mullis, R. (1993). Increasing fruit and vegetable consumption among 4th and 5th grade students: Results from focus groups using reciprocal determinism. *Journal of Nutrition Education, 25,* 114-120.

Barnes, M. S., & Terry, R. D. (1991). Adherence to the cardiac diet: Attitudes of patients after myocardial infarction. *Journal of the American Dietetic Association, 91,* 1435-1437.

Becker, M. H., Maiman, L. A., Kirscht, J. P., Haefner, D. P., & Drachman, R. H. (1977). The health belief model and prediction of dietary compliance: A field experiment. *Journal of Health and Social Behavior, 18,* 348-366.

Berg, J., & Berg, B. L. (1989). Compliance, diet, and cultural factors among black Americans with end-stage renal disease. *Journal of the National Black Nurses Association, 3*(2), 16-28.

Brown, J., & Fitzpatrick, R. (1988). Factors influencing compliance with dietary restrictions in dialysis patients. *Journal of Psychosomatic Research, 32,* 191-196.

Brownell, K. D., Marlatt, G. A., Lichtenstein, E., & Wilson, G. T. (1986). Understanding and preventing relapse. *American Psychologist, 41,* 765-782.

Carmody, T. P., Fey, S. G., Pierce, D. K., Connor, W. E., & Martarazzo, J. D. (1982). Behavioral treatment of hyperlipidimia: Techniques, results, and future directions. *Journal of Behavioral Medicine, 5,* 91-116.

Chaiken, S., & Pliner, P. (1987). Women, but not men, are what they eat: The effect of meal size and gender on perceived masculinity and femininity. *Personality and Social Psychology Bulletin, 13,* 166-176.

Chazan, B. I., MacLaren, A., Shetty, Y. P., Tooley, E., Moore, A., & Wilkinson, E. (1982). The effect of locus of control and socio-economic status on control of diabetes in adolescents. *Pediatric and Adolescent Endocrinology, 10,* 39-42.

Chrisler, J. C. (1993). Feminist perspectives on weight loss therapy. *Journal of Training and Practice in Professional Psychology, 7,* 35-48.

Chrisler, J. C. (1994). Reframing women's weight: Does thin equal healthy? In A. Dan (Ed.), *Reframing women's health: Multidisciplinary research and practice* (pp. 330-338). Thousand Oaks, CA: Sage.

Chubon, S. J. (1989). Personal descriptions of compliance by rural southern blacks: An exploratory study. *Journal of Compliance in Health Care, 4*(1), 23-38.

Cohen, S. J., Weinberger, M. H., Fineberg, N. S., Miller, J. Z., Grim, C. E., & Luft, F. C. (1991). The effect of a household partner and home urine monitoring on adherence to a sodium restricted diet. *Social Science and Medicine, 32,* 1057-1061.

Cotugna, N., & Vickery, C. E. (1989). Student dietitians' experiences with dietary compliance. *Journal of the American Dietetic Association, 89,* 1301-1303.

Cotugna, N., & Vickery, C. E. (1990). Diabetic diet compliance: Student dietitians reverse roles. *Diabetes Educator, 16,* 123-126.

DiMatteo, M. R., Sherbourne, C. D., Hays, R. D., Ordway, L., Kravitz, R. L., McGlynn, E. A., Kaplan, S., & Rogers, W. H. (1993). Physicians' characteristics influence patients' adherence to medical treatment: Results from the medical outcomes study. *Health Psychology, 12,* 93-102.

Epstein, L. H., Beck, S., Figueroa, J., Farkas, G., Kazdin, A. E., Daneman, D., & Becker, D. (1981). The effects of targeting improvements in urine glucose on metabolic control. *Journal of Applied Behavioral Analysis, 14,* 365-375.

Fehrenbach, A. M., & Peterson, L. (1989). Parental problem-solving skills, stress, and dietary compliance in phenylketonuria. *Journal of Consulting and Clinical Psychology, 57,* 237-241.

Flanagan, D. A., & Wagner, H. L. (1991). Expressed emotion and panic-fear in the prediction of diet treatment compliance. *British Journal of Clinical Psychology, 30,* 231-240.

Freedman, R. (1986). *Beauty bound.* Lexington, MA: Lexington Books.

Gross, A. M. (1990). Behavioral management of the child with diabetes. In A. M. Gross & R. S. Drabman (Eds.), *Handbook of clinical behavioral pediatrics* (pp. 147-163). New York: Plenum Press.

Hanna, K. J., Ewart, C. K., & Kwiterovich, P. O., Jr. (1990). Child problem solving competence, behavioral adjustment, and adherence to lipid-lowering diet. *Patient Education Counseling, 16,* 119-131.

Harris, R., Skyler, J. S., Linn, M. W., Pollack, L., & Tewksbury, D. (1982). Psychological factors affecting diabetes control. *Pediatric and Adolescent Endocrinology, 10,* 123-132.

Heiby, E. M., Gafarian, C. T., & McCann, S. C. (1989). Situational and behavioral correlates of compliance to a diabetic regimen. *Journal of Compliance in Health Care, 4,* 101-116.

Heller, J., & Edelmann, R. J. (1991). Compliance with a low

calorie diet for two weeks and concurrent and subsequent mood changes. *Appetite, 17*, 23-28.

Henkin, Y., Garber, D. W., Osterlund, L. C., & Darnell, B. E. (1992). Saturated fats, cholesterol, and dietary compliance. *Archives of Internal Medicine, 152*, 1167-1174.

Herman, P., & Polivy, J. (1983). *Breaking the diet habit*. New York: Basic Books.

Hilliard, J. R., & Hilliard, P. J. (1984). Bulimia, anorexia nervosa, and diabetes: Deadly combinations. *Psychiatric Clinics of North America, 7*, 367-379.

Ho, E. E., Lee, F. C., & Meyskens, F. L., Jr. (1991). An exploratory study of attitudes, beliefs, and practices related to the interim dietary guidelines for reducing cancer in the elderly. *Journal of Nutrition for the Elderly, 10*(4), 31-49.

Holland, W. H. (1968). The diabetes supplement of the National Health Survey. *Journal of the American Dietetic Association, 52*, 387-390.

Holm, L. E., Nordevang, E., Ikkala, E., Hallstrom, L., & Callmer, E. (1990). Dietary intervention as adjuvant therapy in breast cancer patients: A feasibility study. *Breast Cancer Research and Treatment, 16*, 103-109.

Hoover, H. (1989). Compliance in hemodialysis patients: A review of the literature. *Journal of the American Dietetic Association, 89*, 957-959.

House, W. C., Pendleton, L., & Parker, L. (1986). Patients' versus physicians' attributions of reasons for diabetic patients' noncompliance with diet. *Diabetes Care, 9*, 434.

Hudson, J., Pope, H., & Katz, D. (1983). Anorexia and "reverse anorexia" among 108 male body builders. *Comprehensive Psychiatry, 34*, 406-409.

Irvine, A. A. (1989). Self care behaviors in a rural population with diabetes. *Patient Education and Counseling, 13*, 3-13.

Jacobson, A. M., Hauser, S. T., Lavori, P., Wolfsdorf, J. I., Hersokowitz, R. D., Milley, J. E., Bliss, R., Gelfand, E., & Wertlieb, D. (1990). Adherence among children and adolescents with insulin-dependent diabetes mellitus over a four-year longitudinal follow-up: I. The influence of patient coping and adjustment. *Journal of Pediatric Psychology, 15*, 511-526.

Johnston, J. E. (1989). Prevention of osteoporosis: The calcium controversy. *Journal of the American Academy of Nurse Practitioners, 1*(4), 126-131.

Kittler, P. G., & Sucher, K. P. (1990). Diet counseling in a multicultural society. *Diabetes Educator, 26*, 127-131.

Kushner, R. F. (1993). Long-term compliance with a lipid-lowering diet. *Nutrition Reviews, 51*, 16-23.

LaGreca, A. M., Schwartz, L. T., & Satin, W. (1987). Eating patterns in young women with IDDM: Another look. *Diabetes Care, 10*, 657-660.

Lewis, D. J., Robinson, J. A., & Robinson, K. (1990). Spice of life: A strategy to enhance dietary compliance. *American Nephrology Nurses Association Journal, 17*, 387-389, 401.

Logue, A. W. (1986). *The psychology of eating and drinking*. New York: Freeman.

McCann, B. S., Retzlaff, B. M., Dowdy, A. A., Walden, C. E., & Knopp, R. H. (1990). Promoting adherence to low fat, low cholesterol diets: Review and recommendations. *Journal of the American Dietetic Association, 90*, 1408-1417.

Meichenbaum, D., & Turk, D. C. (1987). *Facilitating treatment adherence: A practitioner's guidebook*. New York: Plenum Press.

Miller, P., Wikoff, R., Garrett, M. J., McMahon, M., & Smith, T. (1990). Regimen compliance two years after myocardial infarction. *Nursing Research, 39*, 333-336.

Miller, P., Wikoff, R., & Hiatt, A. (1992). Fishbein's model of reasoned action and compliance behavior of hypertensive patients. *Nursing Research, 41*, 104-109.

Miller, P., Wikoff, R., Keen, O., & Norton, J. (1987). Health beliefs and regimen adherence of the American Indian diabetic. *American Indian and Alaska Native Mental Health Research, 1*(1), 27-39.

Missiou-Tsagaraki, S., Soulpi, K., & Loumakou, M. (1988). Phenylketonuria in Greece: 12 years experience. *Journal of Mental Deficiency Research, 32*, 271-287.

Morgan, B. S., & Littell, D. H. (1988). A closer look at teaching and contingency contracting with Type II diabetes. *Patient Education and Counseling, 12*, 145-158.

Mori, D., Pliner, P., & Chaiken, S. (1987). "Eating lightly" and the self-presentation of femininity. *Journal of Personality and Social Psychology, 53*, 693-702.

Morisky, D. E., DeMuth, N. M., Field-Fass, M., Green, L. W., & Levine, D. M. (1985). Evaluation of family health education to build social support for long-term control of high blood pressure. *Health Education Quarterly, 12*, 35-50.

Morley, J. E., & Perry, H. M., III. (1991). The management of diabetes mellitus in older individuals. *Drugs, 41*, 548-565.

O'Hair, D., O'Hair, M. J., Southward, G. M., & Krayer, K. J. (1987). Physician communication and patient compliance. *Journal of Compliance in Health Care, 2*, 125-129.

Procci, W. R. (1978). Dietary abuse in hemodialysis patients. *Psychosomatics, 19*, 16-24.

Reid, B. V. (1992). "It's like you're down on a bed of affliction": Aging and diabetes among black Americans. *Social Science and Medicine, 34*, 1317-1323.

Reid, P., & Appleton, P. (1991). Insulin dependent diabetes mellitus: Regimen adherence in children and young people. *Irish Journal of Psychology, 12*, 17-32.

Rimer, B. K., Glanz, K., & Lerman, C. (1991). Contributions of public health to patient compliance. *Journal of Community Health, 16*, 225-240.

Rodin, J., Silberstein, L., & Striegel-Moore, R. (1985). Women and weight: A normative discontent. In T. B. Sonderegger (Ed.), *Nebraska symposium on motivation: Psychology and gender* (pp. 267-304). Lincoln: University of Nebraska Press.

Ruggiero, L., Spirito, A., Bond, A., Coustan, D., & McGarvey, S. (1990). Impact of social support and stress on compliance in women with gestational diabetes. *Diabetes Care*, *13*, 441-443.

Saltzberg, E. A., & Chrisler, J. C. (1995). Beauty is the beast: Psychological effects of the pursuit of the perfect female body. In J. Freeman (Ed.), *Women: A feminist perspective* (5th ed.) (pp. 306-315). Mountain View, CA: Mayfield.

Schmid, T. L., Jeffery, R. W., Onstad, L., & Corrigan, S. A. (1991). Demographic, knowledge, physiological, and behavioral variables as predictors of compliance with dietary treatment goals in hypertension. *Addictive Behaviors*, *16*, 151-160.

Secker-Walker, R. H., Morrow, A. L., Kresnow, M. J., Flynn, B. S., & Hochheiser, L. I. (1991). Family physicians' attitudes about dietary advice. *Family Practice Research Journal*, *11*, 161-170.

Shenkel, R. J., Rogers, J. P., Perfetto, G., & Levin, R. A. (1985/1986). Importance of "significant others" in predicting cooperation with diabetic regimen. *International Journal of Psychiatry in Medicine*, *15*, 149-155.

Shepherd, R., Farleigh, C. A., Atkinson, C., & Pryor, J. S. (1987). Effects of hemodialysis on taste and thirst. *Appetite*, *9*, 79-88.

Sherwood, R. J. (1983). Compliance behavior of hemodialysis patients and the role of the family. *Family Systems Medicine*, *1*, 60-72.

Shifflett, P. A. (1987). Future time perspective, past experiences, and negotiation of food use patterns among the aged. *Gerontologist*, *27*, 611-615.

Steiner-Adair, C. (1988). *Tyranny of weightism: A mandate for change*. Paper presented at the annual Anorexia Bulimia Care Conference, Boston, April.

Stewart, R. S. (1983). Psychiatric issues in renal dialysis and transplantation. *Hospital and Community Psychiatry*, *34*, 623-628.

Stoffel, J. (1989). What's new in weight control: A market mushrooms as motivations change. *New York Times*, Nov. 26, C17.

Szymanski, L., & Chrisler, J. C. (1991). Eating disorders, gender role, and athletic activity. *Psychology*, *28*(1), 20-29.

Taylor, S. E. (1991). *Health psychology* (2nd ed.). New York: McGraw-Hill.

Tracy, H. M., Green, C., & McCleary, J. (1987). Noncompliance in hemodialysis patients as measured with the MBHI. *Psychology and Health*, *1*, 411-423.

Tucker, C. M., Ziller, R. C., Chennault, S. A., Somer, E., Schwartz, M. G. Swanson, L. L., Blake, H. A., & Finlayson, G. C. (1987). Adjustment to hemodialysis treatment through behavioral controls. *Journal of Psychopathology and Behavioral Assessment*, *9*, 219-227.

Urban, N., White, E., Anderson, G. L.,Curry, S., & Kristal, A. R. (1992). Correlates of maintenance of a low-fat diet among women in the Women's Health Trial. *Preventive Medicine*, *21*, 279-291.

Wilde, O. (1915). *Lady Windermere's fan: A play about a good woman*. London: Methuen.

Wilson, G. D., Stitt, K. R., Bonner, J. L., & Balentine, M. (1990). Dietary guidelines: Compliance and attitudes of a selected group of registered dietitians. *Journal of the American Dietetic Association*, *90*, 572-574.

Wing, R. R., Epstein, L. H., & Norwalk, M. P. (1984). Dietary adherence in patients with diabetes. *Behavioral Medicine Update*, *6*, 17-21.

18

Initiation and Maintenance of Exercise Behavior

Bess H. Marcus, Beth C. Bock, and Bernardine M. Pinto

INTRODUCTION

New guidelines developed by the United States Centers for Disease Control and Prevention and the American College of Sports Medicine state that significant health benefits can be gained by participating in daily bouts of moderate-intensity physical activity (Pate et al., 1995). Many of the things people already do, such as brisk walking, heavy housework, or climbing stairs, can produce health benefits if performed for a sufficient duration. Many people, however, think of physical activity and exercise as being different. For many, "exercise" is a vigorous, structured activity performed in a gym or in a class or an activity that requires an exercise machine. On the other hand, overuse of the phrase "physical activity" can mislead people into believing that any activity, including casual strolling or light housework, counts. It is the aim of this chapter to encourage a broad understanding that health benefits can be obtained by both vigorous exercise and moderate-intensity physical activity. In this chapter, therefore, the terms *physical activity* and *exercise* are used interchangeably.

Physical activity has been identified as a health behavior with potential benefits for improved physical and psychological health in men and women of all ages. While inactivity has been established as a risk factor for coronary heart disease, increased physical activity is significantly correlated with changes in other major cardiovascular risk factors such as high-density lipoprotein cholesterol and body mass index (Bovens et al., 1993). Epidemiological studies suggest that increased activity, in addition to providing protection against coronary heart disease, appears to provide protective benefits against colon cancer in men (e.g., Kohl, LaPorte, & Blair, 1988) and against breast cancer (Bernstein, Henderson, Hanisch, Sullivan-Halley, & Ross, 1994) and certain reproductive cancers in women (see the review by Pinto & Marcus, 1994). Exercise is recommended as an adjunctive treatment to diet for control of non-insulin-dependent diabetes mellitus and facilitates weight maintenance in men (King, Frey-Hewitt, Dreon, & Wood, 1989)

Bess H. Marcus, Beth C. Bock, and Bernardine M. Pinto • Miriam Hospital and Brown University School of Medicine, Providence, Rhode Island 02906.

Handbook of Health Behavior Research II: Provider Determinants, edited by David S. Gochman. Plenum Press, New York, 1997.

and women (Craighead & Blum, 1989). Physical activity can also help prevent other chronic diseases such as osteoporosis in postmenopausal women (R. Marcus et al., 1992). Finally, there is evidence that participation in resistance exercise training can counteract muscle weakness and frailty in nursing home residents (Fiatarone et al., 1994).

Exercise is believed to offer psychological benefits for adults that include improvements in anxiety, depression and self-concept. It appears that acute physical activity is followed by transitory reductions in anxiety that last for about 2-5 hours following the activity (Raglin, 1990). With adoption of regular exercise regimens, significant improvements in anxiety, depression, and self-esteem have been found with clinical samples (e.g., Pappas, Golin, & Meyer, 1990) and retirees (King, Taylor, & Haskell, 1993), but such significant changes have not always been reported for individuals within the normal range on these dimensions (Hughes, 1984).

In sum, physical activity offers a number of important health benefits for the prevention and treatment of chronic diseases. Evidence for the psychological benefits of exercise is less clear. There is a consensus, however, that mood improvement and tension reduction are associated with participation in regular exercise.

PREVALENCE OF PARTICIPATION

The United States Centers for Disease Control and Prevention (USCDCP) and the American College of Sports Medicine (ACSM) (Pate et al., 1995) have recommended that every American adult engage in at least 30 minutes of moderate physical activity (e.g., brisk walking, gardening) on most, and ideally all, days of the week. Despite increasing evidence of the benefits of physical activity, data from the Behavioral Risk Factor Surveillance System showed that 58% of the United States population are sedentary (irregular or no leisure time activity) (USCDCP, 1993). These data suggest that the prevalence of sedentary lifestyle does not differ by sex; however, sedentary behavior is more characteristic of minorities (64%) than of non-Hispanic whites (57%). Income and education appear to be inversely related to sedentary lifestyle. Of those earning less than $15,000, 65% are inactive, versus 48% of those earning more than $50,000. Of those with less than high school education, 72% are sedentary, versus 50% of college-educated individuals (USCDCP, 1993).

Beyond adolescence and early adulthood, both national samples and community studies reveal a decrease in participation in regular activity (Schoenborn, 1986). Even among adults who take up exercise, 50% of men and women are likely to drop out within 6 months (Dishman, 1990; Sallis et al., 1986). Limited data on older adults suggest that this decline continues through age 80, with progressively larger proportions of men and women reporting that they get no leisure time physical activity (Caspersen & DiPietro, 1991; Caspersen, Merritt, Heath, & Yeager, 1990). The decline in activity with age is particularly disappointing, given the evidence suggesting that people who increase their activity during adulthood can reduce their risk for cardiovascular disease to the level of those who have been active for many years (Paffenbarger et al., 1993).

When type of activity is examined, there is a trend for women to report lower participation in vigorous activity compared to men (Sallis et al., 1986). In a community sample of California adults, Sallis et al. (1986) found that 5% of women adopted vigorous activity versus 11% of men, but 34% of women adopted moderate activity versus 26% of men. When the intensity of the activity is standardized for declining cardiovascular fitness, the proportion of men reporting regular and intense activity increases around retirement and remains relatively stable through age 80 (Caspersen et al., 1990). In contrast, the proportion of women reporting regular and intense activity continues to decline in older age groups. The USCDCP reports that 65% of older women are sedentary versus 59% of older men (USCDCP, 1993). Hence, although participation in regular activity could improve cardiovascular status among older women, this group is less likely to be active.

DETERMINANTS OF PHYSICAL ACTIVITY

In the exercise literature, the task of identifying the determinants of physical activity has been complicated by varying operational definitions of terms such as *exercise* and *physical activity*. Determinants also appear to vary across phases of activity such as adoption, maintenance, relapse, and resumption of regular activity. Further, the determinants associated with regular participation in activity also vary across the type of activity being considered (e.g., vigorous exercise, moderate exercise, structured exercise classes, home exercise). In general, the factors associated with physical activity participation have been classified into three groups: personal characteristics (e.g., demographics), psychological variables (e.g., self-efficacy), and environmental factors (e.g., type of exercise program, accessibility of exercise facilities). This chapter will briefly highlight some of these determinant factors (see the detailed review by King et al., 1992).

Personal Characteristics

Reviews on determinants of exercise participation reveal that African-American women, the less educated, overweight individuals, and the elderly are more likely to be inactive (King et al., 1992). The role of demographic factors appears to vary according to the type of physical activity being assessed. For example, women and the elderly are less likely to endorse participation in vigorous exercise, but may report participation in household activity (B. H. Marcus, Pinto, Simkin, Audrain, & Taylor, 1994). Similarly, white collar workers may be more likely to engage in leisure time recreational activities than blue collar workers (King, Carl, Birkell, & Haskell, 1988). Data from cross-sectional studies suggest that participating in organized sports in youth is related to activity in later years, but this relationship does not appear to hold after controlling for confounding factors such as fitness and cardiovascular health (Dishman & Dunn, 1988).

Although the relationship between regular activity and the practice of other healthful behaviors appears to be modest at best (Blair, Jacobs, & Powell, 1985), negative health status variables appear to predict inactivity. For example, some studies have shown that smokers are less likely to report regular exercise (Emmons, Marcus, Linnan, Rossi, & Abrams, 1994), and being overweight appears to be negatively related to adherence to cardiac rehabilitation programs (e.g., Oldridge, Donner, Buck, & Jones, 1983). Knowledge of one's health status may prompt adoption of activity, but it does not appear to facilitate maintenance of activity (Godin, Desharnis, Jobin, & Cook, 1987).

Psychological Characteristics

Among the psychological factors that have been examined, the confidence to perform a specific activity (self-efficacy), self-motivation, belief in the health benefits of exercise, perceptions of being in good health, and perceived exercise enjoyment have been associated with higher levels of physical activity in men and women (King et al., 1992). Self-efficacy appears to be related to the adoption of vigorous activity in men and to the adoption and maintenance of moderate activity among men and women in both structured and at-home exercise (Sallis et al., 1986). It has also been found to predict compliance in cardiac rehabilitation programs (Ewart, Stewart, Gillilan, & Kelemen, 1986). Self-efficacy is likely to interact with an individual's exercise history and associated success. Indeed, a history of successfully engaging in leisure time physical activity and the development of self-regulatory skills such as goal setting, self-reinforcement, and self-monitoring have also been found to predict exercise participation (Dishman, Sallis, & Orenstein, 1985; Martin & Dubbert, 1982).

Environmental and Program Characteristics

Environmental cues or prompts have been found to facilitate adoption and maintenance of physical activity (e.g., Brownell, Stunkard, Albaum, 1980). As with other health behaviors, educators and researchers have begun to examine the role of social support (parents, friends, exercise staff) in exercise behavior. Family social support has been identified as a strong predictor of exercise maintenance for women (Dubbert, Stetson, & Corrigan, 1991), and recent studies have shown that individuals who exercise with their spouses have higher rates of exercise adherence than those who exercise alone (Raglin & Wallace, 1993).

The type, complexity, convenience, and costs of physical activity programs, such as location and intensity, also influence exercise participation and maintenance. Sallis et al. (1986) found a 50% dropout rate from vigorous activity (e.g., running) and a dropout rate of 25-35% from moderate activity (e.g., walking) over a 1-year follow-up in a community sample. Moderate-intensity home-based exercise programs have been found to have higher adherence rates and at the same time to produce fitness and psychological benefits among retirees comparable to those produced by higher-intensity group programs (e.g., King, Haskell, Taylor, Kraemer, & DeBusk, 1991; King et al., 1993). Such studies have led to the recent USCDCP and ACSM recommendation for the promotion of moderate exercise in the United States population (Pate et al., 1995).

BARRIERS TO PARTICIPATION

Barriers to participation in physical activity may be broadly conceived of in terms of environmental, cognitive, and perceived or actual factors. In general, environmental barriers represent practical factors such as the convenience of facilities, financial considerations, and both work and childcare schedules. Although environmental barriers frequently interfere with participation in physical activity among men (Sallis, Hovell, & Hofstetter, 1992a), these barriers tend to have greater effect among women and low-income individuals (Etkin, 1994; Verhoef, Hamm, & Love, 1993; Zakarian, Hovell, Hofstetter, Sallis, & Keating, 1994).

Cognitive barriers are essentially attitudes and beliefs that can interfere with an individual's participation in physical activity. Cognitive barriers involve societal expectations and norms and the individual's stage of readiness for exercise, self-efficacy beliefs, and decision-making processes. Although both men and women tend to be equally influenced by cognitive barriers, women and older individuals may be especially affected due to societal expectations that they will be less active (Lee, 1993).

Both actual and perceived barriers consistently predict the amount of participation in vigorous activity in men and women (Sallis et al., 1989; Sallis et al., 1992a). Conversely, failure to overcome existing barriers may account for the high relapse rate observed among many intervention studies (King et al., 1992).

Environmental Issues

Elements in both the physical and the social environment can promote or discourage exercise participation and physical activity. Receiving support from others in one's social group seems particularly important for women. Prospective studies have demonstrated that family participation in exercise and receiving support from family and friends are strong predictors of exercise maintenance among women, but not among men (Dubbert et al., 1991). Although the degree to which parents are physically active appears to affect their children's physical activity levels (McMurray et al., 1993; Stucky-Ropp & DiLorenzo, 1993), the extent to which children's activity influences parents' is unclear (Sallis et al., 1992b).

Factors in the physical environment, such as

the availability and proximity of community facilities and safe environments that are conducive to physical activity, have an important influence on exercise participation. Convenient access to facilities has consistently emerged as a predictor of exercise participation in community-based samples (Sallis et al., 1989; 1990). Most adults believe that greater availability of exercise facilities, such as bicycle trails, swimming pools, tennis courts, playing fields, and community recreation centers, would help them become more involved in regular exercise (Harris, Caspersen, DeFriese, & Estes, 1989). Prospective studies are needed, however, to determine the most effective ways of using such community resources to enhance regular participation. Worksite-based exercise programs and flexible work schedules to permit exercise participation have resulted in increased rates of exercise participation among employees (King et al., 1992; Shephard, 1992). Prompts or cues in the physical environment can also increase physical activity, particularly when placed at strategic choice points. For example, a sign promoting stair climbing placed near an escalator increased the likelihood that people would choose to use the stairs (Brownell et al., 1980). Factors related to neighborhood safety are likely influences on physical activity, but have received minimal attention.

Limited access to training and information about physical activity can also act as a barrier to participation in exercise. People may depend on medical personnel for advice about exercise (Godin & Shephard, 1990; Wallace, Brennan, & Haines, 1987); however, few physicians routinely give advice about physical activity (King et al., 1992). The popular media often serve, by default, as an important source of information about physical activity and health (Worsley, 1989). Television and magazines have increasingly featured information about physical activity (Weston & Ruggiero, 1985-1986; Wiseman, Gray, Mosimann, & Ahrens, 1992). Unfortunately, other media, such as newspapers, may provide little support for women's physical activity (Theberge, 1991).

Cognitive Barriers

What individuals believe about themselves and their ability to be physically active can serve either to encourage or to discourage exercise participation. One cognitive factor that has received much attention is self-efficacy. Self-efficacy is a central concept within social learning theory (Bandura, 1977, 1986). Self-efficacy involves the degree of confidence individuals have that they can participate in a healthful behavior across a broad range of specific, salient situations. Self-efficacy remains an important determinant of physical activity even in the presence of other factors such as gender and past performance/exercise history, which are known to affect exercise participation. Among male and female adolescents, for example, self-efficacy is an important predictor of participation in vigorous physical activity, even after adjusting for the presence of other variables such as gender, age, and whether physical education was required in school (Zakarian et al., 1994). These findings are consistent with results showing that self-efficacy beliefs are strong predictors of participation in physical activity among adults (Armstrong, Sallis, Hovell, & Hofstetter, 1993; B. H. Marcus, Eaton, Rossi, & Harlow, 1994; Reynolds et al., 1990; Sallis et al., 1986; Sallis, Pinski, Patterson, & Nader, 1988; Sallis et al., 1992a).

Decision-making constructs, such as decisional balance, have been shown to be important determinants of participation in physical activity. Decisional balance is based on the theoretical model of decision making developed by Janis and Mann (1977). It involves a comparison of the perceived positive aspects (pros) and negative aspects (cons) of a behavior. Several procedures have been developed to help individuals understand how they are making decisions about exercise. These procedures were first developed to help individuals attempting to change health-related behaviors such as smoking (Marlatt & Gordon, 1985; Velicer, Clemente, Prochaska, Brandenburg, 1985). For example, in one such procedure, clients generate responses to both short-

and long-term consequences of making a behavioral change and of failing to achieve the desired behavior. This procedure can be used to discuss the content of these responses and devise ways to avoid or cope with the negative consequences of the behavior change. B. H. Marcus, Rakowski, and Rossi (1992) adopted and applied these decision-making procedures to exercise adoption using a decisional balance questionnaire.

The use of a decisional balance sheet procedure, in which the individual writes down anticipated consequences of exercise participation in terms of gains and losses to self and to others and approval or disapproval from others and from self, may promote an awareness of the benefits and costs of exercise participation that are salient to the individual (Hoyt & Janis, 1975; Wankel, 1984). Individuals with a positive decisional balance, who see more benefits to physical activity or who value the benefits of physical activity above the costs, are more likely to participate in physical activity (B. H. Marcus & Owen, 1992; B. H. Marcus, Rakowski, & Rossi, 1992).

Another cognitive factor that is often overlooked is an individual's readiness to become physically active. Most exercise interventions have been designed for persons who are ready to take action to become more physically active. Unfortunately, only about 10% of the population are ready to do so (B. H. Marcus, Rossi, Selby, Niaura, & Abram 1992). Programs designed to increase physical activity have not historically targeted people who are not yet ready to launch into a regular exercise program, a failure that perhaps accounts for the 50% dropout rate from exercise programs (Dishman, 1990). Ironically, in addition to comprising a majority of the population, those who are not yet so ready are also the segment who would benefit the most from interventions tailored to their stage of preparedness (or unpreparedness) for exercise.

Barriers Specific to Women

A number of factors that affect participation in physical activity seem to influence women more than men (B. H. Marcus, Dubbert, King, & Pinto, 1995). Certain developmental milestones, such as adolescence or becoming a parent, can have significant impact on participation in physical activity. For example, although preadolescent girls are as active as boys, girls experience a substantial reduction in physical activity during adolescence (Alpert et al., 1982; Fitness Profile in American Youth, 1983). The factors that influence participation in physical activity during adolescence differ between boys and girls. Among adolescent girls, prior levels of physical activity, intentions to exercise, lower stress levels, and having family and friends who exercise are important influences on physical activity levels (Reynolds et al., 1990). Social support and social attitudes also play a significant role in adult women's participation in physical activity. Numerous reports have documented that receiving support from family and friends is a strong predictor of women's participation in exercise (Sallis et al., 1992a; Lee, 1993). Most women, however, do not have peer role models for appropriate kinds and levels of physical activity (Theberge, 1991). While many women's magazines now feature photographs and stories about health and physical activity, many health club employees are not professionally trained and may not be sensitive to issues specifically relevant to women's exercise (Etkin, 1994).

Being married and having children can have a significant impact on women's activity levels. Unmarried women report participation in significantly more vigorous activity than married women (Verhoef & Love, 1992). The responsibilities incurred by having multiple roles, such as parent, employee, and spouse, can limit the time available to engage in exercise programs. Childcare responsibilities can present a major barrier to women's participation in exercise. For example, in cross-sectional studies of women, significantly fewer women who exercised regularly had young children living at home (B. H. Marcus, Pinto, et al., 1994). Family responsibilities may leave women with less discretionary time available for exercise, even when such programs are otherwise convenient. Worksite exercise programs tend to be used by women who are already physically active, suggesting that current workplace exercise programs do not serve the needs of women who may need such programs the most (Verhoef et al., 1993).

Although lack of time and inconvenient schedules are the most prevalent and frequently cited reasons for nonparticipation in worksite programs (Dishman, 1982; King et al., 1992), it remains unclear to what extent lack of time is truly a barrier to physical activity or an excuse indicative of a lack of interest. Population surveys indicate that regular exercisers are just as likely as sedentary individuals to view time as an activity barrier (Dishman et al., 1985). Nonetheless, recent research continues to show that age, having children, lack of time and energy, and lack of social support are significant barriers to women's participation in exercise (Sallis et al., 1992a; Verhoef et al., 1993).

Barriers Related to Aging

Physical activity has consistently been found to decrease with age after late adolescence or early adulthood in both national samples (Gartside, Khoury, & Glueck, 1984; Schoenborn, 1986) and community studies (Ballard-Barbash et al., 1990; Folsom et al., 1985). Data on older adults suggest that this decline continues after age 50 (Feather, 1982), with progressively larger proportions of men and women reporting that they get no leisure time physical activity through age 80 (Caspersen & DiPietro, 1991; Caspersen et al., 1990). These findings are particularly distressing, because some researchers have suggested that as much as half of the physical decline associated with aging is preventable through improved lifestyle habits, such as participation in regular exercise (Astrand, 1992; Rogers, Meyer, & Martel, 1990). Much of what is known about the effects of aging is confounded with the effects of prolonged disuse. As more information comes to light regarding the modifying effects of diet, exercise, personal habits, and psychosocial factors on the aging process, it will be easier to determine which effects of aging are truly intrinsic and which are extrinsic and due to the influence of these moderating factors (Rowe & Kahn, 1987).

Barriers That Affect Underserved Populations

Economic opportunity can have a significant impact on exercise participation and choice of exercise activity. Data suggest that low-income and minority individuals engage in less leisure time physical activity than the general population (B. S. Lewis & Lynch, 1993). Poverty is a barrier to participation in many subtle as well as obvious ways. Those with limited financial resources may find club memberships and the purchase of exercise bicycles or other home exercise equipment prohibitively expensive (Etkin, 1994). The fitness industry can create significant barriers to participation among people with limited income. Participation in many activities, such as jogging, skating, and aerobics, can be quite low in cost; fitness institutions, however, can create an atmosphere in which people with little money to spend on fashion may feel out of place at these activities (Etkin, 1994). Simple programs to improve fitness, such as walking, are rarely offered in courses, yet these may be the types of programs more suitable for low-income people, after safety issues have been given due consideration.

Summary

A number of environmental and cognitive barriers have been identified that are associated with participation in physical activity. Environmental barriers include the availability of safe and convenient facilities, childcare responsibilities, and economic considerations. Cognitive barriers include self-efficacy, decision-making processes, and stage of readiness for behavior change. Interventions designed to increase individual participation in exercise will need to address these barriers. Additional work is needed to determine which barriers are amenable to intervention and which are resistant to change. Some barriers may function as a method of defending current behavioral practices and therefore may not be amenable to treatment. The use of decisional balance procedures may prove useful in clarifying which factors are "excuses" and which are true barriers to exercise participation.

APPLICATION OF THEORETICAL MODELS

Stages of Change Model

The transtheoretical model that has been used in the study of addictions is now being applied to exercise adoption and is helping to change the way professionals think about designing exercise interventions (e.g., Armstrong et al., 1993; Barke & Nicholas, 1990; Booth et al., 1993; Lee, 1993; B. H. Marcus, Banspach, et al., 1992; Sonstroem, 1987). The transtheoretical model integrates current behavioral status with a person's intention to maintain or change a pattern of behavior (DiClemente et al., 1991; Prochaska & DiClemente, 1983). As applied to physical activity, precontemplation includes individuals who engage in no physical activity and do not intend to start. People in the contemplation stage do not participate in physical activity, but intend to start. Those in preparation participate in some physical activity, but not regularly. Regular activity is defined as at least 3 times per week for at least 20 minutes each time (ACSM, 1990) or engaging in a total of at least 30 minutes of physical activity on most days of the week (Pate et al., 1995). The action stage includes subjects who currently participate in regular activity but have done so for less than 6 months; the maintenance stage entails participation in regular physical activity for 6 months or longer (B. H. Marcus, Rossi, Selby, Niaura, & Abrams, 1992).

The transtheoretical model incorporates three other important constructs in addition to stage of change: (1) decisional balance (B. H. Marcus, Rakowski, & Rossi, 1992; Velicer et al., 1985) and (2) self-efficacy (DiClemente, Prochaska, & Gibertini, 1985; B. H. Marcus, Selby, Niaura, & Rossi, 1992), both of which have been described previously, and (3) processes of behavior change (B. H. Marcus, Rossi, et al., 1992; Prochaska, Velicer, DiClemente, & Fava, 1988). The processes of change are covert or overt activities that individuals use to modify a particular behavior. The ten processes most commonly studied include consciousness raising, dramatic relief, environmental reevaluation, self-reevaluation, social reevaluation, social liberation, helping relationships, counterconditioning, reinforcement management, and stimulus control. These processes have their roots in a variety of therapy systems.

Measures have been developed to assess the stages and processes of change (B. H. Marcus, Rossi, et al., 1992; B. H. Marcus & Simkin, 1993) as well as self-efficacy (B. H. Marcus, Selby, et al., 1992) and decision-making (B. H. Marcus, Rakowski, & Rossi, 1992) for physical activity. B. H. Marcus, Selby, et al. (1992) demonstrated adequate test-retest reliability for the stages of exercise adoption instrument over a 2-week period (kappa = 0.78). Concurrent validity for the instrument was demonstrated by its significant association with the Seven Day Physical Activity Recall Questionnaire (Blair, 1984) in a sample of employees (B. H. Marcus & Simkin, 1993).

Interventions based on the transtheoretical model utilize the concept of matching treatment to the individual's stage of readiness for change. For example, a stage-matched exercise-promotion intervention for individuals in the early stages of change (precontemplation and contemplation) would focus on increasing awareness of the benefits of exercise and would encourage thinking about becoming active. Materials designed for individuals in the later stages would focus more on getting the individual to begin exercising and on strategies for maintaining an active lifestyle.

The transtheoretical model was used to design an intervention to increase the adoption of physical activity among community volunteers (B. H. Marcus, Banspach, et al., 1992). The program delivered a 6-week stage-matched intervention without concurrent control consisting of self-help materials, a resource manual, and organized physical activity. Following the intervention, 30% of those in Contemplation at baseline and 61% of those in Preparation at baseline progressed to Action, and an additional 31% in Contemplation progressed to Preparation, demonstrating that the subjects had become significantly more active.

These findings were replicated in a randomized controlled trial of a stage-matched physical activity intervention at the workplace (B. H. Marcus et al., 1994). In this second study, employees were randomized to a stage-matched self-help intervention or a standard care self-help intervention. The interventions consisted of printed materials delivered at baseline and again at 1 month. A chi-square analysis was conducted to examine the relative efficacy of the interventions in enhancing the adoption and maintenance of exercise among employees. Comparison of the results from baseline to the 3-month follow-up revealed that more subjects in the stage-matched group demonstrated stage progression; in contrast, more subjects in the standard self-help group displayed stage stability or stage regression [$\chi^2(2) = 10.69$ $p \leqslant .001$].

Relapse-Prevention Model

The relapse-prevention (RP) model of Marlatt and Gordon (1985) was utilized in four studies of exercise behavior (Belisle, Roskies, & Levesque, 1987; King & Frederiksen, 1984; B. H. Marcus & Stanton, 1993; Martin et al., 1984). The RP model is derived from social learning theory and has been used mostly to understand relapse behavior in regard to addictive habits (e.g., smoking, drinking). The basic concepts of the RP model, however, may apply equally well to an understanding of relapse from positive behaviors, such as participation in physical activity. The goal of RP is to help people who are attempting to modify their behavior to learn to anticipate, avoid, and, if necessary, cope with situations that may lead to a return to the problem behavior.

Of the four studies that used RP, two demonstrated significant increases in both exercise program attendance and short-term maintenance (Belisle et al., 1987; King & Frederiksen, 1984), whereas two yielded no significant effects (B. H. Marcus & Stanton, 1993; Martin et al., 1984). Flaws in these studies included conducting follow-ups only on program adherers (B. H. Marcus & Stanton, 1993), presentation of RP at only one session (King & Frederiksen, 1984), nonrandom assignment of subjects to treatments (Belisle et al., 1987), and confounding treatment groups and leaders (Martin et al., 1984).

It is of interest that neither the B. H. Marcus and Stanton (1993) study nor the Martin et al. (1984) study showed significant benefits of participation in an RP program. These two studies included a planned relapse as a primary component of treatment, while the other two studies (Belisle et al., 1987; King & Frederiksen, 1984) did not. It seems possible that this particular aspect of the RP model is ineffective with acquisition behaviors such as exercise. Participation in physical activity should be performed on a daily basis to obtain maximal benefits. It may be that requiring subjects to take 7-10 days off from exercise while the habit is developing serves to decrease the strength of the overall RP program.

Social Learning and Social Cognitive Theories

Social learning (Bandura, 1977) and social cognitive theories (Bandura, 1986) focus on the importance of an individual's ability to control behavior. Key strategies that are used include goal setting, self-monitoring, and modeling.

This model has been one of the best-researched models in regard to the study of exercise behavior. Intervention studies have focused on goal setting, feedback, problem solving, self-monitoring, and self-reinforcement (Dishman, 1991; King et al., 1991; Knapp, 1988; Martin & Dubbert, 1982; Martin et al., 1984; Oldridge & Jones, 1983). For example, a cross-sectional investigation suggests that behavioral skills, combined with self-motivation, can explain a significant amount of the variance in activity behavior (Heiby, Onorato, & Sato, 1987). Numerous studies have documented that self-efficacy beliefs are potent predictors of participation in physical activity (e.g., Armstrong et al., 1993; Sallis et al., 1986, 1988, 1992a).

Self-efficacy is believed to be the key mediator that determines which behaviors an individual attempts to change and how successful that attempt will be. Self-efficacy theory posits that one's personal experience, vicarious experience, and physiological state (e.g., health status) are major components of how one's efficacy expectations are formed and later modified. Most of the studies that have been conducted using self-efficacy theory have yielded positive findings in predicting present and future exercise behavior in a variety of populations (e.g., Desharnais, Bouillon, & Godin, 1986; Ewart, Taylor, Reese, & DeBusk, 1983; Sallis et al., 1992a).

Summary

It appears that applying theoretical models to the design and conduct of exercise programs is useful. The studies reviewed indicate that utilizing psychological models and theories enhances both the assessment and the treatment process for individuals striving to initiate, adopt, and maintain physical activity behavior. Theoretically grounded and psychometrically sound assessment instruments seem critical to helping in the development of effective treatment programs. Much more work remains to more fully apply the models reviewed herein as well as the other models that have been applied to exercise behavior (King et al., 1992).

INTERVENTION STUDIES

Community-Based Interventions

Community-wide interventions can be an effective method for reaching large numbers of people. Community approaches to health promotion can have dramatic effects on lifestyle change and physical fitness levels within targeted communities (Abbott & Raeburn, 1989; King et al., 1991). For community interventions to be comprehensive, however, the type of exercise behaviors desired, the current status of these behaviors in the community, and the factors that influence these behaviors need to be understood (Simons-Morton, O'Hara, & Simons-Morton, 1986). For example, participation in regular physical activity depends in part on the availability and proximity of exercise facilities and environments conducive to physical activity. Most adults report that greater availability of exercise facilities would help them exercise more regularly (Harris et al., 1989). In addition to the availability of safe and appropriate facilities and resources within the community, the use of environmental prompts can promote increased activity (Mayer & Geller, 1982-1983).

More directive interventions that provide resource manuals describing activity options in the community and offer no-cost organized activities, such as fun walks or activity nights, can also increase exercise participation within a community (B. H. Marcus, Banspach, et al., 1992). Not all community-based interventions need to take place in group settings, however. In fact, most Americans prefer to engage in physical activity on their own, outside a formal group setting (King, 1991). Community-wide interventions using individually tailored, home-based exercise prescriptions have proven effective in increasing fitness levels (King et al., 1991).

As with other types of exercise interventions, community-based interventions need to consider that people within the community will represent a variety of stages of readiness for exercise. In addition, community-based interventions do not necessarily need to target only exercise behavior to have effects. Some community-wide interventions, such as the Stanford Five-City Project, have produced increases in physical activity participation as part of a multiple-risk-factor intervention program (Farquhar et al., 1990).

Physician Training

Physicians offer an attractive vehicle for effecting change in the activity habits of individuals, since a majority of people, especially older people, visit physicians several times each year (Cohen & MacWilliam, 1995). Physicians are being urged to help reduce the prevalence of sedentary lifestyles by counseling their patients to exercise (Harris et al., 1989; U.S. Preventive Services Task Force, 1989). However, while most patients state that they believe their physician thinks exercise is important, and would welcome relevant counseling from their doctors, the available data indicate that most physicians do not discuss exercise with their patients (Henry, Ogle, & Snellman, 1987; Rosen, Logson, & Demak, 1984; Wechsler, Levine, Idelson, Rohman, & Taylor, 1983). Only a minority of physicians perceive exercise as very important for the average person (Wechsler et al., 1983), and fewer than 50% routinely ask patients about their exercise habits (Henry et al., 1987). Physicians who do provide exercise counseling tend to do so only for patients who are at high risk for disease (Rosen et al., 1984; Wells, Lewis, Leake, Schleiter, & Brook, 1986).

Important barriers to exercise counseling by physicians include perceived lack of counseling skills, lack of confidence in counseling ability, perceived ineffectiveness of counseling, lack of organizational support, little or no reimbursement for preventive counseling, and limited availability of materials to aid both the patient and the physician (Kottke, Brekke, Solberg, & Hughes, 1989; C. E. Lewis, Clancy, Leake, & Schwartz, 1991; C. E. Lewis, Wells, & Ware, 1986; Orleans, George, Houpt, & Brodie, 1985; Rosen et al., 1984; Wells, Lewis, Leake, & Ware, 1984). Improvement is also needed in physicians' understanding of the need for physical activity among persons with disabilities. While most healthy adults feel that their physician wants them to exercise, many disabled men and women who are motivated to exercise feel that their physician is opposed to their doing so (Godin & Shephard, 1990).

Although the number of studies of physician-based exercise interventions is limited, the data indicate that physician-delivered counseling can increase patient activity levels (e.g., Lewis & Lynch, 1993; Logsdon, Lazaro, & Meier, 1989). Logsdon et al. (1989), in a multisite, multibehavior intervention by primary care physicians, found that significantly more patients who received physician counseling reported starting to exercise compared to control subjects seen by the same physicians but not given exercise counseling (33.8% versus 24.1%). This greater rate of exercise adoption in the intervention group was achieved despite the complex nature of the multiple-risk-factor intervention offered to study patients and the very limited training and support provided to physicians.

Even extremely brief interventions by physicians can be quite effective. In a recent study, family practice physicians were trained to give brief exercise advice to their adult patients (Lewis & Lynch, 1993). At the 1-month follow-up, there was a significant increase in exercise participation among patients who were advised to exercise. Physician interventions may be particularly effective when matched to the individual patient's stage of readiness for exercise adoption (e.g., Calfas, Long, Sallis, Patrick, & Campbell, 1994; Goldstein et al., 1994).

Interventions in the Workplace

One promising approach to increasing levels of physical activity is worksite-based interventions (Blair, Piserchia, Wilbur, & Crowder, 1986; Fielding, 1984; Godin & Shepard, 1990). The rising cost of providing health insurance for employees, and the increased number of health insurance programs that offer incentives for reducing health risk behaviors, have increased companies' interest in worksite-based exercise programs. Companies sponsoring these programs may reduce costs to their business, such as costs associated with health insurance and absenteeism (Shephard, 1988, 1992). Worksite health promotion and education campaigns have been successfully used to increase exercise adoption among employees (Blair et al., 1986; Brill et al., 1991; King et al., 1988). Employee participation can be maximized through offering a variety of physical activities, maximizing convenience, and permitting employees to exercise on company time or allowing flexible time schedules to use facilities (Brill et al., 1991; Iverson, Fielding, Crown, & Christenson, 1985). While educational campaigns can aid recruitment, employee involvement in program setup and administration may also be important to program success (King et al., 1988). Incentives and awards for regular participation have also been used to enhance continued participation (USDHHS, 1990).

As with community-based interventions, worksite programs need to accommodate the current needs of workers and the factors that affect physical activity. The needs of male and female workers may be different in both these respects (Teufel, 1992). Interventions should be developed with clear goals in mind. Educational interventions work well to increase an individual's knowledge base regarding physical activity. If the goal is to increase physical activity behaviors, however, behaviorally tailored interventions are more effective (Gomel, Oldenburg, Simpson, & Owen, 1993). Additionally, worksite surveys indicate that only 10% of workers are ready to take action to change their activity patterns (B. H. Marcus, Rossi, et al., 1992). Designing separate interventions to specifically meet the needs of individuals at each stage may be a more effective way to help people change sedentary lifestyles (B. H. Marcus, Banspach, et al., 1992; B. H. Marcus, Emmons, et al., 1994).

Summary

Interventions to increase physical activity have successfully been applied to worksite, community, and physician's office settings. Each setting has special demands, however, and interventions will need to take into account those factors that can constitute barriers within the targeted setting. Additional work is needed to determine the most effective methods for increasing physical activity among workers and community residents. Thus far, the majority of studies in these settings have enrolled self-selected samples of people who volunteer to participate in a physical activity program. This practice does not reach the majority of individuals who are most sedentary and would stand to benefit most from these interventions. While interventions in physicians' offices avoid the problem of self-selection, additional support is needed for such interventions.

FUTURE RESEARCH AND METHODOLOGICAL ISSUES

Earlier sections of this chapter have highlighted issues that merit further investigation. There are, however, some broader challenges that confront the researcher and health educator working toward exercise promotion. More work needs to be conducted examining both the determinants of physical activity participation and methods of increasing individual patterns of physical activity. Work focusing on frequency, intensity, and units of time is particularly needed, since individuals want to know more about minimal and optimal doses of physical activity. The new CDC/ACSM recommendations (Pate et al., 1995) on light versus moderate versus vigorous exercise, and on continuous versus intermittent bouts of activity, need to be further explored so that minimal and optimal doses can be determined. Moreover, the parameters for initiating and maintaining these doses need to be determined.

Most physical activity assessment instruments are relatively insensitive to the lighter and more diverse forms of daily activities (e.g., walking, childcare) engaged in by many women. Recent studies of physical activity that have utilized more objective measures of participation in physical activity suggest that women may be more active than is typically reflected by current measurement instruments (Blair et al., 1989). Clearly, if knowledge is to be advanced in this area, more accurate and sensitive assessment instruments need to be developed.

Recent studies highlight the usefulness of process-oriented approaches to the understanding of the stages and processes applicable to individuals' decisions to consider, prepare for, initiate, and maintain increases in physical activity (B. H. Marcus, Eaton, et al., 1994; B. H. Marcus, Rossi, et al., 1992). Much more work is needed in this area, however, to formulate the most effective interventions for individuals at these different stages of participation. In particular, investigations of those in the precontemplation and contemplation stages of physical activity participation are scarce and are especially needed (Blair et al., 1993; B. H. Marcus, Banspach, et al., 1992; B. H. Marcus, Emmons, Simkin, Taylor, et al., 1994).

Similarly, the developmental stages and milestones that confront men and women throughout life present potential challenges for increasing and maintaining physical activity levels (King et al, 1991). Potentially important transitional periods that deserve further exploration include adolescence, entry into college or the workforce, pregnancy, parenthood, menopause, retirement, and family caregiving situations (King, 1991). Systematic investigation of how such milestones can enhance or inhibit physical activity participation is needed.

Although there is evidence for both behavioral and physiological synergy between physical activity and other health behaviors, such as cigarette smoking (B. H. Marcus, Emmons, Simkin, Albrecht, Honey, & Abrams, 1994) and dietary patterns (Wood, Stefanick, Williams, & Haskell, 1991), these three health behaviors typically have been studied in isolation. The evidence to date suggests that there is much to be gained by studying the ways in which systematically intervening in one health behavior can have positive consequences for another health behavior. For example, the planned introduction of a supervised exercise program as a component of a smoking cessation program for women has been shown to positively affect women's efforts to quit smoking and remain abstinent through a 12-month period (B. H. Marcus, Albrecht, Niaura, Abrams, & Thompson, 1991; B. H. Marcus, Albrecht, et al., 1995). Similarly, participation in any of three moderate-intensity physical activity programs was found to result in significant reductions in perceived stress levels among initially sedentary smokers (King et al., 1993), thereby reducing one frequently reported barrier to quitting smoking.

Finally, much more work needs to be conducted to address gaps in the literature on underserved and inadequately studied populations such as women, the elderly, members of minority groups, and individuals of lower socioeconomic status. A recent review of the literature (King et al., 1992) revealed that African-American women, the less educated, overweight individuals, and the elderly are consistently reported to be less active segments of the population. Future intervention research should therefore focus on these important subgroups.

REFERENCES

Abbott, M. W., & Raeburn, J. M. (1989). Superhealth: A community-based health promotion programme. *Mental Health in Australia, 2*, 25-35.

Alpert, B. S., Flood, N. L., Strong, S. B., Dover, E. V., DuRant, R. H., Montin, A. M., & Booker, D. L. (1982). Response to ergometer exercise in a healthy biracial population of children. *Journal of Pediatrics, 101*, 538-543.

American College of Sports Medicine. (1990). Position statement on the recommended quantity and quality of exercise for developing and maintaining cardiorespiratory and muscular fitness in healthy adults. *Medicine and Science in Sports and Exercise, 22*, 265-274.

Armstrong, C. A., Sallis, J. F., Hovell, M. F., & Hofstetter, C. R. (1993). Stages of change, self-efficacy and the adoption of vigorous exercise: A prospective analysis. *Journal of Sport and Exercise Psychology, 15*, 390-402.

Astrand, P. O. (1992). Why exercise? *Medicine and Science in Sports and Exercise, 24*, 153-162.

Ballard-Barbash, R., Schatzkin, A., Albanes, D., Schiffman, M. H., Kreger, B. E., Kannel, W. B., Anderson, K. M., & Helsel, W. E. (1990). Physical activity and risk of large bowel cancer in the Framingham Study. *Cancer Research, 50*, 3610-3613.

Bandura, A. (1977). Self-efficacy: Toward a unifying theory of behavioral change. *Psychological Review, 84*, 191-215.

Bandura, A. (1986). *Social foundations of thought and action: A social cognitive theory*. Englewood Cliffs, NJ: Prentice-Hall.

Barke, C. R., & Nicholas, D. R. (1990). Physical activity in older adults: The stages of change. *Journal of Applied Gerontology, 9*, 216-223.

Belisle, M., Roskies, E., & Levesque, J. (1987). Improving

adherence to physical activity. *Health Psychology*, *2*, 159-172.

Bernstein, L., Henderson, B. E., Hanisch, R., Sullivan-Halley, J., & Ross, R. K. (1994). Physical exercise and reduced risk of breast cancer in young women. *Journal of the National Cancer Institute*, *86*, 1403-1408.

Blair, S. N. (1984). How to assess exercise habits and physical fitness. In J. Matarazzo, S. Weiss, J. Herd, & N. Miller (Eds.), *Behavioral health: A handbook of health enhancement and disease prevention* (pp. 424-447). New York: Wiley.

Blair, S. N., Jacobs, D. R., & Powell, K. E. (1985). Relationships between exercise or physical activity and other health behaviors. *Public Health Reports*, *100*, 172-180.

Blair, S. N., Kohl, H. W., Paffenbarger, R. S., Clark, D. G., Cooper, K. H., & Gibbons, L. W. (1989). Physical fitness and all-cause mortality: A prospective study of healthy men and women. *Journal of the American Medical Association*, *262*, 2395-2401.

Blair, S. N., Piserchia, P. V., Wilbur, C. S., & Crowder, J. H. (1986). A public health intervention model for work-site health promotion. *Journal of the American Medical Association*, *225*, 921-926.

Blair, S. N., Powell, K. E., Bazzarre, T. L., Early, J. L., Epstein, L. H., Green, L. W., Harris, S. S., Haskell, W. L., King, A. C., Kaplan, J., Marcus, B., Paffenbarger, R. S., & Yeager, K. C. (1993). Physical inactivity: Workshop V. *Circulation*, *88*, 1402-1405.

Booth, M. L., Macaskill, P., Owen, N., Oldenburg, B., Marcus, B. H., & Baum, A. (1993). The descriptive epidemiology of stages of change in physical activity. *Health Education Quarterly*, *20*, 431-440.

Bovens, A. M., Van Baak, M. A., Vrencken, J. G., Wijnen, J. A., Saris, W. H., & Verstappen, F. T. (1993). Physical activity, fitness, and selected risk factors for CHD in active men and women. *Medicine and Science in Sports and Exercise*, *25*, 572-576.

Brill, P. A., Kohl, W. H., Rogers, T., Collingwood, T. R., Sterling, C. L., & Blair, S. N. (1991). Recruitment, retention and success in worksite health promotion: Association with demographic characteristics. *American Journal of Health Promotion*, *5*, 215-221.

Brownell, K. D., Stunkard, A. J., & Albaum, J. M. (1980). Evaluation and modification of exercise patterns in the natural environment. *American Journal of Psychiatry*, *137*, 1540-1545.

Calfas, K. J., Long, B. J., Sallis, J. F., Patrick, K., & Campbell, J. (1994). *The effect of counseling by primary care providers to increase physical activity: Project PACE*. Abstract presented at the annual meeting of the Society for Behavioral Medicine, Boston.

Caspersen, C. J., & DiPietro, L. (1991). National estimates of physical activity among older adults. *Medicine and Science in Sports and Exercise*, *23*(Suppl.), S106 (abstract).

Caspersen, C. J., Merritt, R. K., Heath, G. W., & Yeager, K. K. (1990). Physical activity patterns of adults aged 60 years and older. *Medicine and Science in Sports and Exercise*, *22*(Suppl.), S79.

Cohen, M. M., & MacWilliam, L. (1995). Measuring the health of the population. *Medical Care*, *33*, DS21-DS42.

Craighead, L. W., & Blum, M. D. (1989). Supervised exercise in behavioral treatment for moderate obesity. *Behavior Therapy*, *20*, 49-59.

Desharnais, R., Bouillon, J., & Godin, G. (1986). Self-efficacy and outcome expectations as determinants of exercise adherence. *Psychological Reports*, *59*, 1155-1159.

DiClemente, C. C., Prochaska, J. O., & Gibertini, M. (1985). Self-efficacy and the stages of self-change for smoking. *Cognitive Therapy and Research*, *9*, 181-200.

DiClemente, C. C., Prochaska, J. O., Velicer, W. F., Fairhurst, S., Rossi, J. S., & Velasquez, M. (1991). The process of smoking cessation: An analysis of precontemplation, contemplation and preparation stages of change. *Journal of Consulting and Clinical Psychology*, *59*, 295-304.

Dishman, R. K. (1982). Compliance/adherence in health-related exercise. *Health Psychology*, *1*, 237-267.

Dishman, R. K. (1990). Determinants of participation in physical activity. In C. Bouchard, R. J. Shephard, T. Stephens, J. R. Sutton, & B. D. McPherson (Eds.), *Exercise, fitness and health* (pp. 75-102). Champaign, IL: Human Kinetics.

Dishman, R. K. (1991). Increasing and maintaining physical activity and exercise. *Behavior Therapy*, *41*, 3-15.

Dishman, R. K., & Dunn, A. L. (1988). Exercise adherence in children and youth: Implications for adulthood. In R. K. Dishman (Ed.), *Exercise adherence* (pp. 155-200). Champaign, IL: Human Kinetics.

Dishman, R. K., Sallis, J. F., & Orenstein, D. R. (1985). The determinants of physical activity and exercise. *Public Health Reports*, *100*, 158-171.

Dubbert, P. M., Stetson, B., & Corrigan, S. A. (1991). *Predictors of exercise maintenance in community women*. Paper presented at the meeting of the American Psychological Association, San Francisco, CA, August.

Emmons, K. M., Marcus, B. H., Linnan, L., Rossi, J. S., & Abrams, D. B. (1994). The relationship between smoking, physical activity and nutrition behaviors among manufacturing workers. *Preventive Medicine*, *23*, 481-489.

Etkin, S. E. (1994). Reaching the hard to reach: Active living programs for low socioeconomic individuals. In H. A. Quinney, L. Gauvin, & A. E. T. Wall (Eds.), *Toward active living* (pp. 263-268). Champaign, IL: Human Kinetics.

Ewart, C. K., Stewart, K. J., Gillilan, R. E., & Kelemen, M. H. (1986). Self-efficacy mediates strength gains during circuit weight training in men with coronary artery disease. *Medicine and Science in Sports and Exercise*, *18*, 531-540.

Ewart, C. K., Taylor, C. B., Reese, L. B., & DeBusk, R. F. (1983). Effects of early postmyocardial infarction exercise testing on self-perception and subsequent physical activity. *American Journal of Cardiology*, *51*, 1076-1080.

Farquhar, J. W., Fortmann, S. P., Flora, J. A., Taylor, C. B., Heskell, W. L., Williams, P. T., Maccoby, N., & Wood, P. D.

(1990). Effects of community wide education on cardiovascular disease risk factors: The Stanford Five-City Project. *Journal of the American Medical Association, 264*, 359-365.

Feather, N. T. (1982). *Expectations and actions: Expectancy value models in psychology*. Hillsdale, NJ: Erlbaum.

Fiatarone, M. A., O'Neill, E. F., Ryan, N. D., Clements, K. M., Solares, G. R., Nelson, M. E., Roberts, S. B., Kehayias, J. J., Lipsitz, L. L., & Evans, W. J. (1994). Exercise training and nutritional supplementation for physical frailty in very elderly people. *New England Journal of Medicine, 330*, 1769-1775.

Fielding, J. E. (1984). Health promotion and disease prevention at the worksite. *Annual Review of Public Health, 5*, 237-265.

Fitness Profile in American youth. (1983). A report on 1981-1983 fitness tests involving more than 1 million boys and girls in over 10,000 schools. East Hanover, NJ: Nabisco Brands.

Folsom, A. R., Caspersen, C. J., Taylor, H. L., Jacobs, D. R., Luepker, R. V., Gomez-Marin, O., Gillum, R. F., & Blackburn, H. (1985). Leisure time physical activity and its relationship to coronary risk factors in a population-based survey. *American Journal of Epidemiology, 121*, 570-579.

Gartside, P. S., Khoury, P., & Glueck, C. J. (1984). Determinants of high-density lipoprotein cholesterol in blacks and whites: The Second National Health and Nutrition Examination Survey. *American Heart Journal, 108*, 641.

Godin, G., Desharnis, R., Jobin, J., & Cook, J. (1987). The impact of physical fitness and health-age appraisal upon exercise intentions and behavior. *Journal of Behavioral Medicine, 10*, 241-250.

Godin, G., & Shephard, R. J. (1990). An evaluation of the potential role of the physician in influencing community exercise behavior. *American Journal of Health Promotion, 4*, 255-259.

Goldstein, M. G., Marcus, B. H., Washburn, R., Jette, A. M., Rakowski, W., & Dubé, C. (1994). Medical office-based activity counseling of older adults. *National Institute on Aging* grant, Providence, RI.

Gomel, M., Oldenburg, B., Simpson, J., & Owen, N. (1993). Work-site cardiovascular risk reduction: A randomized trial of health risk assessment, education, counseling, and incentives. *American Journal of Public Health, 83*, 1231-1238.

Harris, S. S., Caspersen, C. J., DeFriese, G. H., & Estes, H. (1989). Physical activity counseling for healthy adults as a primary preventive intervention in the clinical setting. *Journal of the American Medical Association, 261*, 3590-3598.

Heiby, E. M., Onorato, V. A., & Sato, R. A. (1987). Cross-validation of the self-motivation inventory. *Journal of Sports Psychology, 9*, 394-399.

Hoyt, M. F., & Janis, I. L. (1975). Increasing adherence to a stressful decision via a motivational balance-sheet procedure: A field experiment. *Journal of Personality and Social Psychology, 31*, 833-839.

Hughes, J. R. (1984). Psychological effects of habitual aerobic exercise: A critical review. *Preventive Medicine, 13*, 66-78.

Iverson, D., Fielding, J., Crown, R., & Christenson, G. (1985). The promotion of physical activity in the United States population: The status of programs in medical, worksite, community, and school settings. *Public Health Reports, 100*, 212-224.

Janis, I. L., & Mann, L. (1977). *Decision making: A psychological analysis of conflict, choice and commitment*. New York: Free Press.

King, A. C. (1991). Community intervention for promotion of physical activity and fitness. *Exercise and Sport Science Reviews, 19*, 211-259.

King, A. C., Blair, S. N., Bild, D., Dubbert, P. M., Marcus, B. H., Oldridge, N. B., Paffenbarger, R. S., Powell, K. E., & Yeager, K. (1992). Determinants of physical activity and interventions in adults. *Medicine and Science in Sports and Exercise, 24*(Suppl.), S221-S236.

King, A. C., Carl, F., Birkel, L., & Haskell, W. L. (1988). Increasing exercise among blue-collar employees: The tailoring of worksite programs to meet specific needs. *Preventive Medicine, 17*, 357-365.

King, A. C., & Frederiksen, L. W. (1984). Low-cost strategies for increasing exercise behavior: Relapse preparation training and social support. *Behavior Modifications, 8*, 3-21.

King, A. C., Frey-Hewitt, B., Dreon, D. M., & Wood, P. D. (1989). Diet vs. exercise in weight maintenance: The effects of minimal intervention strategies on long-term outcomes in men. *Archives of Internal Medicine, 149*, 2741-2746.

King, A. C., Haskell, W. L., Taylor, C. B., Kraemer, H. C., & DeBusk, R. F. (1991). Group- vs. home-based exercise training in healthy older men and women. *Journal of the American Medical Association, 266*, 1535-1542.

King, A. C., Taylor, C. B., & Haskell, W. L. (1993). Effects of differing intensities and formats of 12 months of exercise training on psychological outcomes in older adults. *Health Psychology, 12*, 292-300.

Knapp, D. N. (1988). Behavioral management techniques and exercise promotion. In R. K. Dishman (Ed.), *Exercise adherence: Its impact on public health* (pp. 203-236). Champaign, IL: Human Kinetics.

Kohl, H. W., LaPorte, R. E., & Blair, S. N. (1988). Physical activity and cancer. *Sports Medicine, 6*, 222-237.

Kottke, T. E., Brekke, M. L., Solberg, L. I., & Hughes, J. R. (1989). A randomized trial to increase smoking intervention by physicians: Doctors helping smokers, Round 1. *Journal of the American Medical Association, 261*, 2101-2106.

Lee, C. (1993). Factors related to the adoption of exercise among older women. *Journal of Behavioral Medicine, 16*, 323-334.

Lewis, B. S., & Lynch, W. D. (1993). The effect of physician advice on exercise behavior. *Preventive Medicine, 22*, 110-121.

Lewis, C. E., Clancy, C., Leake, B., & Schwartz, J. S. (1991). The counseling practices of internists. *Annals of Internal Medicine, 114*, 54-58.

Lewis, C. E., Wells, K. B., & Ware, J. (1986). A model for predicting the counseling practices of physicians. *Journal of General Internal Medicine, 1*, 14-19.

Logsdon, D. N., Lazaro, C. M., & Meier, R. V. (1989). The feasibility of behavioral risk reduction in primary medical care. *American Journal of Preventive Medicine, 5*, 249-256.

Marcus, B. H., Albrecht, A. E., Niaura, R. S., Abrams, D. B., & Thompson, P. D. (1991). Usefulness of physical exercise for maintaining smoking cessation in women. *American Journal of Cardiology, 68*, 406-407.

Marcus, B. H., Albrecht, A. E., Niaura, R. S., Taylor, E. R., Simkin, L. R., Feder, S. I., Abrams, D. B., & Thompson, P. D. (1995). Exercise enhances the maintenance of smoking cessation in women. *Addictive Behaviors, 20*, 87-92.

Marcus, B. H., Banspach, S. W., Lefebvre, R. C., Rossi, J. S., Carleton, R. C., & Abrams, D. B. (1992). Using the stages of change model to increase the adoption of physical activity among community participants. *American Journal of Health Promotion, 6*, 424-429.

Marcus, B. H., Dubbert, P. M., King, A. C., & Pinto, B. M. (1995). Physical activity in women: Current status and future directions. In A. Stanton & S. Gallant (Eds.), *Women's health*. Washington, DC: American Psychological Association.

Marcus, B. H., Eaton, C. A., Rossi, J. S., & Harlow, L. L. (1994). Self-efficacy, decision making and stages of change: An integrative model of physical exercise. *Journal of Applied Social Psychology, 24*, 489-508.

Marcus, B. H., Emmons, K. M., Simkin, L. R., Albrecht, A. E., Stoney, C. M., Abrams, D. B. (1994), Women and smoking cessation: Current status and future directions. *Medicine, Exercise, Nutrition, and Health, 3*, 17-31.

Marcus, B. H., Emmons, K. M., Simkin, L. R., Taylor, E. R., Linnan, L., Rossi, J. S., & Abrams, D. B. (1994). Comparison of stage-matched versus standard care physical activity interventions at the workplace. *Annals of Behavioral Medicine, 16*, S035.

Marcus, B. H., & Owen, N. (1992). Motivational readiness, self-efficacy and decision-making for exercise. *Journal of Applied Social Psychology, 22*, 3-16.

Marcus, B. H., Pinto, B. M., Simkin, L. R., Audrain, J. E., & Taylor, E. R. (1994). Application of theoretical models to exercise behavior among employed women. *American Journal of Health Promotion, 9*, 49-55.

Marcus, B. H., Rakowski, W., & Rossi, J. S. (1992). Assessing motivational readiness and decision-making for exercise. *Health Psychology, 11*, 257-261.

Marcus, B. H., Rossi, J. S., Selby, V. C., Niaura, R. S., & Abrams, D. B. (1992). The stages of processes of exercise adoption and maintenance in a worksite sample. *Health Psychology, 11*, 386-395.

Marcus, B. H., Selby, V. C., Niaura, R. S., & Rossi, J. S. (1992). Self-efficacy and the stages of exercise behavior change. *Research Quarterly for Exercise and Sport, 63*, 60-66.

Marcus, B. H., & Simkin, L. R. (1993). The stages of exercise behavior. *Journal of Sports Medicine and Physical Fitness, 33*, 83-88.

Marcus, B. H., & Stanton, A. L. (1993). Evaluation of relapse prevention and reinforcement interventions to promote exercise adherence in sedentary females. *Research Quarterly for Exercise and Sport, 64*, 447-452.

Marcus, R., Drinkwater, B., Dalsky, G., Dufek, J., Raab, D., Slemenda, C., & Snow-Harter, C. (1992). Osteoporosis and exercise in women. *Medicine and Science in Sports and Exercise, 24*, S301-307.

Marlatt, G. A., & Gordon, J. R. (1985). *Relapse prevention: Maintenance strategies in addictive behavior change*. New York: Guilford Press.

Martin, J. E., & Dubbert, P. M. (1982). Exercise applications and promotion in behavioral medicine: Current status and future directions. *Journal of Consulting and Clinical Psychology, 30*, 1004-1017.

Martin, J. E., Dubbert, P. M., Katell, A. D., Thompson, J. K., Raczynski, J. R., Lake, M., Smith, P. O., Webster, J. S., Sikora, T., & Cohen, R. E. (1984). Behavioral control of exercise in sedentary adults: Studies 1 through 6. *Journal of Consulting and Clinical Psychology, 52*, 795-811.

Mayer, J., & Geller, E. S. (1982-1983). Motivating energy efficient travel: A community-based intervention for encouraging biking. *Journal of Environmental Systems, 12*, 99-112.

McMurray, R. G., Bradley, C. B., Harrell, J. S., Bernthal, P. R., Frauman, A. C., & Bangdiwala, S. I. (1993). Parental influences on childhood fitness and activity patterns. *Research Quarterly for Exercise and Sport, 64*, 249-255.

Oldridge, N. B., Donner, A. P., Buck, C. W., & Jones, N. L. (1983). Predictors of dropout from cardiac exercise rehabilitation. *American Journal of Cardiology, 51*, 70-74.

Oldridge, N. B., & Jones, N. L. (1983). Improving patient compliance in cardiac rehabilitation. Effects of written agreement and self-monitoring. *Journal of Cardiopulmonary Rehabilitation, 3*, 257-262.

Orleans, C. T., George, L. K., Houpt, J. L., & Brodie, K. H. (1985). Health promotion in primary care: A survey of U.S. family practitioners. *Preventive Medicine, 14*, 636-647.

Paffenbarger, R. S., Hyde, R. T., Wing, A. L., Lee, I. M., Jung, D. L., & Kambert, J. B. (1993). The association of changes in physical-activity level and other lifestyle characteristics with mortality among men. *New England Journal of Medicine, 328*, 538-545.

Pappas, G. P., Golin, S., & Meyer, D. L. (1990). Reducing symptoms of depression with exercise. *Psychosomatics, 31*, 112-113.

Pate, R. R., Pratt, M. ,Blair, S. N., Haskell, W. L., Macera, C. A., Bouchard, C., Buchner, D., Caspersen, C. J., Ettinger, W., Heath, G. W., King, A. C., Kriska, A., Leon, A. S., Marcus, B. H., Morris, J., Paffenbarger, R. S., Patrick, K., Pollock, M. L., Rippe, J. M., Sallis, J., & Wilmore, J. H. (1995). Physical activity and public health: A recommendation from the Centers for Disease Control and Prevention and the American College of Sports Medicine. *Journal of The American Medical Association*, *273*, 402-407.

Pinto, B. M., & Marcus, B. H. (1994). Physical activity, exercise and cancer in women. *Medicine, Exercise, Nutrition and Health*, *3*, 102-111.

Prochaska, J. O., & DiClemente, C. C. (1983). Stage and processes of self-change in smoking: Towards an integrative model of change. *Journal of Consulting and Clinical Psychology*, *51*, 390-395.

Prochaska, J. O., Velicer, W. F., DiClemente, C. C., & Fava, J. (1988). Measuring processes of change: Applications to the cessation of smoking. *Journal of Consulting and Clinical Psychology*, *56*, 520-528.

Raglin, J. S. (1990). Exercise and mental health: Beneficial and detrimental effects. *Sports Medicine*, *9*, 323-329.

Raglin, J. S., & Wallace, J. P. (1993). *Influence of spouse support, self-motivation and mood state on the adherence of married participants to a 12-month exercise program*. Paper presented at the annual meeting of the Society for Behavioral Medicine, San Francisco.

Reynolds, K. D., Killen, J. D., Bryson, S. W., Maron, D. J., Taylor, C. B., Maccoby, N., & Farquhar, J. W. (1990). Psychosocial predictors of physical activity in adolescents. *Preventive Medicine*, *19*, 541-551.

Rogers, R. L., Meyer, J. S., & Martel, K. F. (1990). After reaching retirement age, physical activity sustains cerebral perfusion and cognition. *Journal of the American Geriatric Society*, *38*, 123-128.

Rosen, M. A., Logsdon, D. N., & Demak, M. M. (1984). Prevention and health promotion in primary care: Baseline results on physicians from the INSURE project on lifestyle preventive health services. *Preventive Medicine*, *13*, 535-548.

Rowe, J. W., & Kahn, R. L. (1987). Human aging: Useful and successful. *Science*, *237*, 143-149.

Sallis, J. F., Haskell, W. L., Fortmann, S. P., Vranizan, K. M., Taylor, C. B., & Solomon, D. S. (1986). Predictors of adoption and maintenance of physical activity in a community sample. *Preventive Medicine*, *15*, 331-341.

Sallis, J. F., Hovell, M. F., & Hofstetter, C. R. (1992a). Predictors of adoption and maintenance of vigorous physical activity in men and women. *Preventive Medicine*, *21*, 237-251.

Sallis, J. F., Hovell, M. F., Hofstetter, C. R., Elder, J. P., Hackley, M., Caspersen, C. J., & Powell, K. E. (1990). Distance between homes and exercise facilities related to frequency of exercise among San Diego residents. *Public Health Reports*, *105*, 179-180.

Sallis, J. F., Hovell, M. F., Hofstetter, C. R., Faucher, P., Elder, J. P., Blanchard, J., Caspersen, C. J., Powell, K. E., & Christenson, G. M. (1989). A multivariate study of determinants of vigorous exercise in a community sample. *Preventive Medicine*, *18*, 20-34.

Sallis, J. F., Pinski, R. B., Patterson, T. L., & Nader, P. R. (1988). The development of self-efficacy scales for health-related diet and exercise behaviors. *Health Education Research*, *3*, 283-292.

Sallis, J. F., Simons-Morton, B. G., Stone, E. J., Corbin, L. B., Epstein, L. H., Faucette, N., Iannotti, R. J., Killen, J. D., Klesges, R. C., Petray, C. K., Rowland, T. W., & Taylor, W. C. (1992b). Determinants of physical activity and interventions in youth. *Medicine and Science in Sports and Exercise*, *24*, S248-S257.

Schoenborn, C. A. (1986). Health habits of U.S. adults: The "Alameda 7" revisited. *Public Health Reports*, *101*, 571-580.

Shephard, R. J. (1988). Exercise adherence in corporate settings: Personal traits and program barriers. In R. K. Dishman (Ed.), *Exercise adherence: Its impact on public health* (pp. 305-320). Champaign, IL: Human Kinetics.

Shephard, R. J. (1992). A critical analysis of work-site fitness programs and their postulated economic benefits. *Medicine and Science in Sports and Exercise*, *24*, 354-370.

Simons-Morton, B. G., O'Hara, N. M., & Simons-Morton, D. G. (1986). Promoting healthful diet and exercise behaviors in communities, schools and families. *Family and Community Health*, *9*, 1-13.

Somstroem, R. J. (1987). *Stage model of exercise adoption*. Paper presented at the meting of the American Psychological Association, August.

Study-Ropp, R. C., & DiLorenzo, T. M. (1993). Determinants of exercise in children. *Preventive Medicine*, *22*, 880-889.

Teufel, N. I. (1992). Diet and activity patterns of male and female co-workers: Should worksite health promotion programs assume homogeneity? *Women and Health*, *19*, 31-54.

Theberge, N. (1991). A content analysis of print media coverage of gender, women, and physical activity. *Journal of Applied Sport Psychology*, *3*, 36-48.

U.S. Centers for Disease Control and Prevention. (1993). Prevalence of sedentary lifestyle-behavioral risk factor surveillance system, United States, 1991. *Morbidity and Mortality Weekly Report*, *42*, 576-579.

U.S. Department of Health and Human Services. (1990). *The health consequences of smoking: Nicotine addiction. A report of the Surgeon General*. Rockville, MD: Office on Smoking and Health, Public Health Service.

U.S. Preventive Services Task Force. (1989). *Guide to clinical preventive services: An assessment of the effectiveness of 169 interventions* (pp. 297-304). Baltimore, MD: Williams & Wilkins.

Velicer, W. F., DiClemente, C. C., Prochaska, J., & Brandenburg, N. (1985). A decisional balance measure for assessing and predicting smoking status. *Journal of Personality and Social Psychology*, *48*, 1279-1289.

Verhoef, M. J., Hamm, R. D., & Love, E. J. (1993). Exercising at work: Barriers to women's participation. *American Association of Occupational Health Nurses*, *41*, 275-281.

Verhoef, M. J., & Love, E. J. (1992). Women's exercise participation: The relevance of social roles compared to non-role-related determinants. *Canadian Journal of Public Health*, *83*, 367-370.

Wallace, P. G., Brennan, P. J., & Haines, A. P. (1987). Are general practitioners doing enough to promote healthy lifestyle? Findings of the Medical Research Council's general practice research framework study on lifestyle and health. *British Medical Journal*, *294*, 940-942.

Wankel, L. M. (1984). Decision-making and social support strategies for increasing exercise involvement. *Journal of Cardiac Rehabilitation*, *4*, 124-135.

Wechsler, H., Levine, S., Idelson, R. K., Rohman, M., & Taylor, J. O. (1983). The physicians' role in health promotion—A survey of primary-care practitioners. *New England Journal of Medicine*, *308*, 97-100.

Wells, K. B., Lewis, C., Leake, B., Schleiter, M. K., & Brook, R. H. (1986). The practices of general and subspeciality internists in counseling about smoking and exercise. *American Journal of Public Health*, *76*, 1009-1013.

Wells, K. B., Lewis, C. E., Leake, B., & Ware, J. E., Jr. (1984). Do physicians preach what they practice? A study of physician's health habits and counseling practices. *Journal of the American Medical Association*, *252*, 2846-2848.

Weston, L. C., & Ruggiero, J. A. (1985-1986). The popular approach to women's health issues: A content analysis of women's magazines. *Women and Health*, *10*, 47-62.

Wiseman, C. V., Gray, J. J., Mosimann, J. E., & Ahrens, A. H. (1992). Cultural expectations of thinness in women: An update. *International Journal of Eating Disorders*, *11*, 85-89.

Wood, P. D., Stefanick, M. L., Williams, P. T., & Haskell, W. L. (1991). The effects on plasma lipoproteins of a prudent weight-reducing diet, with or without exercise, in overweight men and women. *New England Journal of Medicine*, *325*, 461-466.

Worsley, A. (1989). Perceived reliability of sources of health information. *Health Education Research*, *4*, 367-376.

Zakarian, J. M., Hovell, M. F., Hofstetter, C. R., Sallis, J. F., & Keating, K. J. (1994). Correlates of vigorous exercise in a predominantly low SES and minority school population. *Preventive Medicine*, *23*, 314-321.

19

Adherence to Smoking Cessation Regimens

Russell E. Glasgow and C. Tracy Orleans

INTRODUCTION AND SUMMARY OF EARLY APPROACHES

The field of smoking cessation is different from other topics discussed in this section. The ultimate goal is to stop doing something, rather than to follow a prescribed regimen directing how often to engage in a certain behavior. This goal contrasts with that of most other health behaviors, which is either to increase a baseline behavior or to adjust the rate or the conditions under which the behavior occurs. In the three decades after the first Surgeon General's Report on Smoking and Health in this country (U.S. Public Health Service [USPHS], 1964), there has also been a pronounced shift in the focus and goals of smoking cessation research, which differentiates it from most other areas of health behavior research.

Prior to the mid-1980s, the process of smoking cessation was largely conceptualized as a dichotomous outcome: A person either did or did not stop smoking. Also, most intervention approaches dealt with a relatively small percentage of smokers who were motivated to quit and who volunteered to participate in cessation programs. This early literature has been summarized in previous reviews (Schwartz, 1987; USPHS, 1993). Since the mid-1980s, the field has witnessed major changes, reflecting an increasing public health concern to reach more smokers, especially in high-risk and underserved populations. There has also been increasing interest in tailoring programs for particular kinds of smokers, rather than assuming that a single intervention will be effective for all smokers.

The purpose of this chapter is to summarize the literature of the last decade and describe current directions regarding adherence to stop smoking regimens both by smokers and by health care institutions, health professionals, and other change agents implementing cessation programs. These issues are discussed under two general categories: (1) reaching more smokers and (2) tailoring interventions. The chapter then concludes by discussing methodological and evaluation issues and important future directions.

Russell E. Glasgow • Oregon Research Institute, 1715 Franklin Boulevard, Eugene, Oregon 97403. **C. Tracy Orleans** • Fox Chase Cancer Center, 510 Township Line Road, Cheltenham, Pennsylvania 19012.

Handbook of Health Behavior Research II: Provider Determinants, edited by David S. Gochman. Plenum Press, New York, 1997.

It is essential to point out that smoking is determined by a variety of factors, including biological, biobehavioral, psychological, economic, and sociocultural influences. These factors have been the topic of recent reviews elsewhere (Orleans & Slade, 1993; U.S. Department of Health and Human Services [USDHHS], 1989). Since the mid-1980s, there has also been an increase in the percentage of interventions that address two or more of these factors (e.g., combining behavioral and pharmacological approaches; interventions tailored to take into account economic, cultural, and social factors affecting a given group of smokers), and the authors applaud this increasing sophistication.

Conceptually, there are three relevant types of adherence. From the perspective of the smoker, the end goal is permanent smoking cessation. For most smokers, however, this is not a straightforward, linear process. Instead, the change process usually involves *passing through a number of steps or stages of change* (Prochaska, DiClemente, & Norcross, 1992) and, for many persons, cycling many times through these different stages of readiness, action, and relapse.

A second type of smoker adherence concerns actions short of actually stopping smoking, but having to do with *participation in cessation activities*, sometimes including follow-through with program recommendations such as reading materials, attending a group, or watching a video.

Finally, a third type of adherence concerns *intervention by change agents*. As smoking cessation activities move further from programs conducted by staff whose primary function it is to deliver an intervention (e.g., graduate students or paid staff) to those involving implementation by personnel in settings devoted to other purposes (e.g., medical office staff, worksites), the extent to which intervention is delivered as intended becomes a relevant issue.

These three levels of adherence are invoked where relevant in the review that follows. There has been a great deal of research on factors related to the first category of adherence: stopping smoking. This research is summarized in the next section. There has been far less research on participation/follow-through and on adherence effected by change agents. The studies that have been conducted tend to have been conducted in one of the settings used to reach more smokers (e.g., worksites for participation, medical settings for change agent adherence) and will be discussed in those sections.

ADHERENCE TO STOP-SMOKING REGIMENS

On the basis of the 1986 Adult Use of Tobacco Survey, it is estimated that 17 million of America's 46 million smokers try to quit each year, but that only 1.3 million succeed in achieving permanent abstinence. The addictive nature of nicotine contributes to this high failure rate, with most relapse occurring in the first 2 weeks after quitting, at the time of most intense nicotine withdrawal (Kottke, Solberg, & Brekke, 1990). In addition, whether smokers quit on their own or in a formal intervention program, they are more likely to succeed if they possess certain motivations and expectations, employ certain self-change skills, and have certain social support and psychosocial resources available to them.

Table 1 summarizes the individual and smoking habit factors that have been found to predict quitting success in both self-quitting and treatment-assisted quitting (Orleans, 1993). Smoker characteristics that are especially important determinants of success in quitting include perceived severity of smoking-related illness/symptoms and measures of self-efficacy and readiness/intention to quit. In general, interventions have proven more efficacious with at-risk and high-risk populations (pregnant smokers, post-myocardial infarct [MI, heart attack] smokers) than with predominantly healthy populations. In two studies including inpatients and outpatients as subjects, the same brief intervention produced stronger treatment effects among *in*patients (Orleans, Rotberg, Quade, & Lees, 1990; Strecher, Becker, Kirscht, Eraker, & Graham-Tomasi, 1985). Like-

Table 1. Factors Associated with Successful Smoking Cessation

Motivational factors	Social support/psychosocial assets	Smoking habit factors	Effective quitting and maintenance skills/strategies
Desire to protect future health and overcome minor smoking-related symptoms (e.g., shortness of breath, coughing, loss of stamina)	Personal medical quit-smoking advice and follow-up	Lower smoking rate and nicotine intake (e.g., Fewer than 25 cigarettes/day, low-nicotine brand)	Using prequitting strategies, such as monitoring smoking rate, reviewing reasons for quitting, systematic brand switching to gradually reduce nicotine intake before quitting
Sense of personal vulnerability to smoking health risks	Support and encouragement from family, friends, and coworkers	Less dependence on smoking to regulate negative affect	Quitting abruptly on a target date
Desire for greater self-mastery, self-control, or self-esteem	Strong nonsmoking norms in one's immediate social environment	Shorter smoking history	Using a variety of methods to cope with withdrawal symptoms (e.g., deep breathing, positive thinking, concrete cigarette substitutes)
Confidence in ability to quit/quitting self-efficacy	Socioeconomic advantage (e.g., education, income, occupation, employment)	Past success quitting for six months or longer	Using a variety of methods to remain off cigarettes (e.g., avoiding temptations to smoke, finding alternative ways to relax and cope with stress such as hobbies or exercise, using substitute self-rewards to counteract sense of loss and prevent relapse)
One or more past quit attempts, especially in past year	Psychosocial assets (e.g., self-esteem, self-management skills, healthy coping skills, positive health habits, manageable life stress, freedom from other chemical dependencies, no past history of major depression)	Lower nicotine dependence (e.g., first cigarette at least 30 minutes after waking, few past difficulties with withdrawal after quitting)	Taking a long-range, problem-solving approach and making repeated attempts in a cumulative learning process
Expectation of many quitting benefits (e.g., health, social, psychological, cosmetic)			
Readiness to quit/stage of change			

wise, patients with greater quitting self-efficacy and readiness have been found more responsive to behavior change advice (Lichtenstein, Lando, & Nothwehr, 1994). A recent study by Ockene et al. (1992) of brief intervention for patients hospitalized for coronary angiography illustrates both effects. Long-term quit rates in that study were higher for patients hospitalized immediately post-MI or with at least two-vessel disease (65%) than for patients with less serious disease (46%). In addition, patients actively engaged in quitting at the time of intervention had a much higher long-term quit rate (43%) than those who said they wanted to quit in the next 6 months (24%) or those who expressed no intention to quit in the near future (11%).

The greatest theoretical advance in understanding patient adherence in smoking cessation is the transtheoretical model of behavior change (Prochaska et al., 1992). This model defines smoking cessation as a process involving progression through five motivational and behavior change stages:

1. Precontemplation—not thinking about quitting smoking.
2. Contemplation—seriously planning to quit in the next 6 months.
3. Preparation—planning to quit in the next month, with at least one quit attempt in the past year.
4. Action—active efforts to stop smoking and remain smoking-free.
5. Maintenance—beginning 6 months after quitting and involving efforts to resist relapse and remain permanently smoking-free.

Most smokers cycle (or recycle) through these stages several times before successfully "terminating" the behavior change sequence and achieving long-term smoking abstinence.

Cross-sectional and longitudinal research supporting the transtheoretical model has found that different motivational and behavioral self-change processes are important in different stages of quitting. The balance of perceived health risks of continuing versus the benefits of quitting and other decisional balance variables play an especially important role in early quitting, during shifts from precontemplation to contemplation and contemplation to action. Progress in the early stages involves shifts in the perceived "pros" and "cons" of smoking and the use of experiential change processes, including consciousness raising and a cognitive-emotional reevaluation of smoking behavior (e.g., fear arousal). In the transtheoretical model, health beliefs about smoking are related to stage of change, particularly for smokers in early stages of change. Quitting self-efficacy (Bandura, 1986) has been found important for smokers in all stages and increases linearly from precontemplation to maintenance. Besides improved self-efficacy, progress for quitters in the preparation, action, and maintenance stages involves the use of stage-appropriate active behavior change and cognitive coping strategies (e.g., see Table 1: using deep breathing to cope with withdrawal symptoms).

One major study found that smoking cessation treatments are most effective when they are targeted to the smoker's present stage of change (Prochaska, DiClemente, Velicer, & Rossi, 1993). For smokers in either the precontemplation or the contemplation stage, motivational interventions designed to alter the smoker's perceived pros and cons of quitting and to boost quitting self-efficacy seem most appropriate. For these smokers, action-oriented treatments may lead to failure and, over time, to demoralization—since smokers receiving them are not likely to quit or to advance toward greater quitting readiness. Smokers in the preparation, action, or maintenance stage, on the other hand, are more likely to benefit from the action stage-oriented treatments traditionally offered by change agents or smoking cessation programs.

NEWER RESEARCH DIRECTIONS: PUBLIC HEALTH EMPHASIS

The shift in smoking cessation research over the past decade has been characterized by a greatly increased emphasis on the public health goals of reaching more smokers (especially those who are underserved or at high risk) and producing population-wide (rather than individual) change. It is important to understand the profound changes involved in this switch before specific topics are discussed.

First, the settings in which intervention is delivered have changed from university smoking cessation clinics to "natural environments" such as worksites, physicians' offices, hospitals, churches, and other settings frequented by community members. Another key difference between clinical-individual and public health-population focused approaches involves the target audience. In smoking clinic-based approaches, one primarily sees motivated, often well-educated volunteers who have made the decision to stop smoking. In contrast, public health approaches are designed to reach a much larger, more heterogeneous and representative population—including persons who may not be considering smoking cessation. The key differences between public health and individual approaches are summarized in Table 2.

The intervention agents and interventions employed are also different, as can be seen in Table 2. Change agents in public health approaches are more likely to be either lay personnel or professionals (such as physicians or nurses) who are primarily performing other services rather than concentrating on smoking cessation. Public health interventions are brief, inexpensive, portable, and more focused on contextual and social-environmental factors such as smoking policies, taxes, and self-help materials. Individual-focused approaches are typically more intensive, expensive, and time-consuming, such as multisession group programs.

As might be expected from these differences, individual focused programs are usually more *efficacious* and produce higher short-term quit rates. Approximate figures for cessation rates from intensive, well-conducted smoking clinic interventions are 50-75% immediate cessation and 20-25% cessation at 1-year follow-up (Abrams, Emmons, Linnen, & Biener, 1994; Lando, 1993). Public health approaches usually produce lower cessation rates but are more likely to reach large numbers of smokers and to be more cost-effective. Abrams et al. (1994) have suggested use of the concept of *intervention impact*, which combines these factors to reflect the effect of an intervention on a defined population of smokers. Impact is defined as the reach of an intervention multiplied by its efficacy among those reached. These two approaches can be applied in concert, e.g., by using community-based public health approaches to identify individuals most appropriate for intensive, clinical intervention. However, the basic assumptions, focus, goals, and operations involved differ so markedly (Jeffery,

Table 2. Key Differences between Smoking Clinical/Individual-Based and Public Health/Population-Based Smoking Cessation Approaches

Factor	Smoking clinic/individual-based	Public health/population-based
Intervention setting	University or commercial stop-smoking clinic	Worksites, medical offices, churches, community settings
Target audience	Motivated, self-selected volunteers; interested in cessation	Large, heterogeneous, many not considering cessation
Intervention agent	Paid experts or research staff	Lay volunteers, or professionals primarily doing other activities
Intervention characteristics	Intensive, multisession; focus on personal characteristics, individual, proximal factors	Brief, inexpensive, focus on environmental, distal factors (policies, taxes)
Important outcomes	Efficacy; high cessation rates	Cost-effectiveness, reach, and dissemination

1989; Lichtenstein & Glasgow, 1992) that it is important to keep these differences in mind because the adherence issues and research findings also differ between these approaches.

REACHING MORE SMOKERS

Physician's Office and Hospital Interventions

The national shift to a public health model in tobacco control (see Table 2) and the emergence of nicotine replacement therapy as a standard part of treatment for nicotine addiction (e.g., Hughes, 1993) have provided a compelling rationale for using primary care and inpatient health care settings as smoking cessation treatment channels. Over two thirds of United States smokers see a physician on an annual basis, and most do so more than once. Glynn and Manley (1989) projected that if only *half* of United States physicians delivered even a brief quitting message to their patients who smoked and were successful with only 1 in 10, this effort would yield 1.75 million new ex-smokers every year—more than double the national annual quit rate. Furthermore, in all medical settings, nonphysician health care providers (e.g., nurses, physician assistants, respiratory therapists) have a critical role to play as change agents given physicians' limited time for preventive interventions.

Numerous controlled trials were conducted beginning in the mid-1980s to test the efficacy of so called "minimal-contact" office-based interventions using techniques that could be easily integrated into routine care and delivered on a population basis to *all* smokers in the practice, regardless of their interest in quitting. The emphasis was on brief physician counseling backed up by self-help quitting materials in combination with nicotine replacement therapy, if appropriate. Methodological advances included adequate controls for treatment contamination in designs randomizing patients and providers (versus practices) to interventions and greater similarities in intervention design and measurement strategies across studies to permit more meaningful meta-analyses.

The verdict was clear: Even brief interventions significantly improved quit rates. Glynn (1988), for instance, reviewed 28 physician-based trials and found that advice or counseling alone produced 6- to 12-month quit rates of approximately 5-10%, while more intensive physician-based interventions resulted in 20-25% quit rates. Similarly, five randomized, controlled clinical trials funded by the National Cancer Institute, involving over 30,000 patients and over 1000 providers, showed that patients in intervention conditions had long-term quit rates, 2-6 times higher than patients receiving usual care (Glynn & Manley, 1989). Kottke, Battista, DeFriese, and Brekke (1988) used meta-analysis to evaluate the findings of 39 controlled smoking intervention trials involving physicians and allied health care providers and found that minimal-contact interventions boosted quit rates an average of 6%.

The core elements of effective primary care interventions identified through this research include: a strong physician-delivered quit-smoking message; self-help materials presenting state-of-the-art motivational, behavioral, and relapse-prevention strategies; prescription of nicotine replacement, if appropriate; brief cessation counseling to include setting a quit date (usually provided not by the physician, but by an allied health professional); and follow-up support. Kottke et al. (1988) found that most effective interventions involved more than one modality (e.g., face-to-face advice/counseling, self-help materials, phone counseling, nicotine replacement therapy), involvement of both physician *and* nonphysician counselors, and a greater number of smoking-related contacts and follow-up visits. Nicotine gum has not consistently proven more effective than placebo control when provided with limited physician advice (e.g., Hughes, 1993). Both nicotine gum and transdermal nicotine, however, have proven to be effective adjuncts to more systematic minimal-contact treatments (e.g., Fiore, Smith, Jorneby, & Baker, 1994). Recent reviews of placebo-controlled trials indicate that transdermal nicotine doubles long-term quit rates, producing an effect size of approximately 9%.

Glynn and Manley (1989) distilled these core elements into a treatment equation that could be applied in a variety of health care settings by a variety of providers. The resulting algorithm has been widely applied—to physicians, nurses, respiratory care practitioners, and the oral health care team (dentists, hygienists)—and has been incorporated by the American Medical Association (AMA) (1993) in its recommended guidelines for the treatment of nicotine addiction. In summary form, the algorithm is:

1. Ask about smoking at every opportunity.
2. Advise all smokers to quit.
3. Assist smokers to quit, through use of self-help materials and nicotine replacement, when appropriate.
4. Arrange follow-up contacts or visits.

This model seems to apply equally well to *in*patient interventions (Orleans, Kristeller, & Gritz, 1993). Results of a handful of controlled studies suggest that a brief Ask-Advice-Assist-Arrange model to hospital patients can produce 20-25% long-term quit rates—rates that are, on average, 4-5% higher than for usual care, with intervention effects stronger among some high-risk medical inpatients (Orleans, Kristeller, & Gritz, 1993). A study by Stevens, Glasgow, Hollis, Lichtenstein, and Vogt (1993) documented a 13.5% quit rate (abstinent at both 3- and 12-month follow-ups) with *general hospital patients* who received brief nurse-delivered bedside quit-smoking counseling, a videotape presentation on behavioral quitting strategies, self-help materials, monthly follow-up mailings, and two proactive counseling calls—significantly higher than the usual care quit rate of 9.2%. A controlled study by Taylor, Houston-Miller, Killen, and DeBusk (1990) of a similar nurse-managed intervention for *post-MI inpatients* found significantly higher 12-month quit rates for intervention than for usual care subjects (62% versus 32%).

Health Care Provider Adherence

Nearly half of United States smokers still say they have never been advised by their physicians to quit smoking (e.g., Frank, Winkleby, Altman, Rockhill, & Fortmann, 1991). National physician surveys have shown that although physicians view smoking as a serious health risk and feel responsible for helping their patients quit, only about two thirds report routinely advising most of their smoking patients to quit, and fewer than one quarter report regularly offering or referring their patients for systematic treatment (e.g., Gottlieb, Mullen, & McAlister, 1987).

These same studies identified several common barriers to more systematic intervention: physician pessimism about their patients' abilities to quit smoking, a lack of time and training for quit-smoking counseling, coupled with a lack of confidence both in their own counseling skills and in the efficacy of outside treatments, and a lack of third-party reimbursement for treating nicotine dependence. Similar barriers have been reported by nurses (Goldstein, Hellier, Fitzgerald, Stegall, & Fischer, 1987). Inappropriate expectations about the outcomes of treatment undoubtedly also serve as a potent barrier to intervention by medical change agents. Even if a highly respectable 20% of smokers quit following a systematic intervention, the reality is that 8 in 10 smokers returning for care will *not* have quit. Correcting expectations about absolute quit rates, and helping physicians and other change agents to appreciate the public health importance of even low quit rates if achieved population-wide, and to view progress through the stages of change as a reasonable outcome, will help to overcome these barriers.

To address the lack of training in effective intervention techniques, most primary care trials reviewed (e.g., Glynn & Manley, 1989) included brief continuing medical education-type training protocols to teach intervention techniques and measures of provider adherence to recommended protocol, chiefly from exit and follow-up interviews with patients. These studies demonstrated that even brief physician training produces positive changes in a number of intervention activities, including increased time devoted to antismoking advice, increased use of chart stickers and reminders, greater frequency of setting quit dates, distributing self-help materials, using nicotine replacement therapy, more follow-up appointments, and referral to outside treatment (e.g., Cohen, Stookey, Katz, Drook, & Christen, 1989; Cummings, Emont, Jaen, & Sciandra, 1988). Booster sessions and performance feedback can help prolong training effects (Li, Coates, Ewart, & Kim, 1987).

Systemic barriers to medical office interventions on smoking cessation also are pervasive. America's health care system is organized chiefly to deliver care for acute and chronic illnesses rather than to deliver disease prevention or health promotion services (Orlandi, 1987). Accordingly, it is hardly surprising that providers are more likely to deliver advice to stop smoking to diseased and symptomatic patients than to healthy patients (e.g., Ockene et al., 1987). Efforts to institutionalize tobacco intervention must therefore introduce simple procedures to ensure that *all* patients who smoke are identified, monitored, and appropriately treated at every office visit.

Fiore (1991) recommended that smoking status be considered a vital sign and that practices flag patient records with a vital signs "stamp" as a reminder to obtain, along with blood pressure, pulse, respiratory rate, temperature, and weight, information about smoking status at every visit. Cohen and colleagues found that placing prominent reminder stickers on patient charts increases time spent counseling and the nature of counseling by both dentists and physicians (Cohen, Stookey, Katz, Drook, & Christen, 1989; Cohen, Stookey, Katz, Drook, & Smith, 1989). Likewise, the ready availability of patient materials and nicotine replacement samples in the office has improved provider adherence to recommended counseling strategies and the forcefulness of quitting advice (Cohen, Stookey, Katz, Drook, & Smith, 1989). Flow sheets outlining step-by-step protocols for nicotine dependence also have been used successfully (Glynn & Manley, 1989). Establishing such procedures usually requires selecting for the office a smoking cessation coordinator whose responsibilities include making the office tobacco-free and implementing ways to identify and monitor smokers and to remind health professionals to intervene (Glynn & Manley, 1989; Glynn, Manley, Solberg, & Slade, 1993).

In general, policy-related variables (e.g., smoking restrictions, treatment reimbursement policies) have not been examined as determinants of provider adherence. For instance, the Joint Commission on Accreditation of Health Care Organization's hospital smoking ban took effect so quickly that no studies were conducted to track pre- to postban changes in inpatient smoking cessation (Orleans, Kristeller, & Gritz, 1993). At present, most health insurance plans in the United States, public and private, exclude coverage for smoking cessation services. Little is known, either, about the impact of provider incentives to follow clinical practice guidelines with their patients who smoke, though promising results have been found giving physicians performance feedback about their compliance over time with quit-smoking advice protocols (Li et al., 1987). In mid-1996, the Agency for Health Care Policy Research released guidelines on smoking cessation counseling in medical settings, which will potentially impact clinical practice patterns (The Smoking Cessation Clinical Practice Guideline Panel and Staff, 1996).

Worksite Smoking Cessation Approaches

There have been substantial improvements in the contribution and methodological quality of worksite smoking cessation approaches since the mid-1980s (Abrams et al., 1994; Terborg & Glasgow, 1994). Smoking control activities represent one of the most prevalent worksite health promotion activities (USPHS, 1993). Early studies typically reported on only a small number of employees within one or two worksites who volunteered to participate in multisession group interventions. These early studies essentially used the worksite to recruit participants for individually focused, clinic-like interventions. In contrast, several recent studies have adopted more of an organizational or public health perspective and have randomly assigned several worksites to each treatment condition and have reported their impact on all employees or on representative samples.

Unfortunately, reported outcomes from these more recent studies have not been as positive (Glasgow, Terborg, Hollis, Severson, & Boles, 1995; Jeffery et al., 1993; Working Well Research Group, 1996). One finding has been that a relatively small percentage of smokers in the workforce will actively participate in cessation activities (see the review by Glasgow, McCaul, & Fisher, 1992). Studies in the mid-1990s also have shown large variability in outcomes across worksites within conditions (Glasgow et al., 1995; Jeffery et al., 1993). It remains to be seen whether these differences can be explained by worksite characteristics or whether there are certain types of programs that work better in some worksites than in others.

A 1990 meta-analysis of 20 well-controlled worksite smoking-intervention studies (Fisher, Glasgow, & Terborg, 1990) concluded that worksite interventions were significantly more effective than control conditions. The average long-term cessation rate was 13%. This figure may not seem high by absolute standards, but is encouraging given the reach of worksite programs and the fact that at least some of these studies included *all* smokers, rather than just those who actively participated in cessation activities. This meta-analysis also reported an interesting paradox regarding worksite size: There were far more smoking programs and studies in larger worksites, but intervention effect sizes and quit rates were higher in smaller worksites.

More recent studies have tended to emphasize greater involvement and ownership on the part of employees in the design and implementation of programs (e.g., Glasgow, Terborg, Strycker, Boles, & Hollis, in press; Sorensen et al., 1992; Working Well Research Group, 1996). Often this involvement is encouraged in the form of employee advisory boards (e.g., Sorensen et al., 1992). Although direct comparisons of worksite programs using such employee involvement approaches versus more standardized programs delivered by outside organizations have not yet been reported, most worksite researchers feel that such "buy-in" and tailoring to individual worksites are essential.

One interesting, large-scale project combined multiple intervention channels, conducting two separate studies of the effects of adding worksite group meetings (or, in the second study, group meetings and incentives) to a basic media and self-help intervention (Jason et al., 1987; Salina et al., 1994). Both studies also reported on the reach of the intervention among employees and used statistical procedures to address issues of intraclass correlation (nonindependent outcomes among employees within a given worksite) The first study (Jason et al, 1987) randomized 43 worksites and found that adding a series of peer-led support groups, held on work time, significantly increased cessation rates (41% versus 21% initial cessation, $p < 0.01$), but that this effect deteriorated over time. In the second study (Salina et al., 1994), which randomized 38 worksites, support groups and a $50 prize drawing were continued on a monthly basis over a 12-month period. This combined intervention was found to maintain differences between the support/incentives plus media/self-help worksites and the basic media/self-help worksites out to a 2-year follow-up (30% versus 19.5% cessation).

The most definitive data on worksite smoking cessation are from the National Cancer Institute's collaborative Working Well Trial (Sorensen et al., 1996), which targeted smoking, diet, and occupational exposures related to cancer. This study involved four research centers geographically dispersed across the United States and 114 worksites. Special features of this trial included: using the worksite as the unit of randomization and analysis, a theory-driven conceptual model that targeted both individual and organizational levels of change, and emphasis on both education and behavior change programs and on organizational practices and policies. Unfortunately, differences between intervention and control condition were significant in only one of the research centers.

In summary, worksite programs have focused on reaching and involving more employees, on tailoring interventions to meet the needs of different worksites, and on addressing other risk factors in addition to smoking. There have been considerable methodological advances in this area, but also an increased recognition that much remains to be learned. There are some promising results from studies combining intervention channels, but worksite smoking cessation, like other areas of worksite health promotion, does not appear to be the panacea declared by some. These issues are discussed in more detail in Abrams et al. (1994) and Terborg & Glasgow (1994).

Community-Wide Approaches

Interventions that target entire communities, or even whole states, in many ways epitomize the public health approach to cigarette smoking. Given logistical considerations and cost constraints, almost all community-based approaches have adopted social marketing approaches to reach diverse segments of the population. Several of these approaches have used mass media (Farquhar et al., 1990) to lay the groundwork for other intervention components.

Almost all community-based approaches also have two other characteristics. First, they attempt to maximize community participation through establishing voluntary community boards and task forces. Keys to success at this level seem to be the involvement of both (1) influential community members and stakeholders and (2) community members wiling to devote time and energy to implementing programs. Exactly how to achieve this optimum mix remains more art than science (Bracht, 1990).

The second key characteristic of community-wide approaches is that they involve multiple intervention channels. All community-based programs reported to date have included at least some focus on each of the following: media and public education, physician and medical setting interventions, worksite programs, involvement of community organizations (e.g., churches, voluntary health organizations), and widespread distribution of self-help materials and resources. Often the community board and task forces play a coordinating role in integrating the activities of different persons and organizations within and between channels.

The best-known and most completely reported community-wide intervention trials to date have been the three heart disease risk-factor modification trials funded by the National Heart, Lung, and Blood Institute (Farquhar et al., 1990; Lasater, Abrams, & Artz, 1984; Luepker et al., 1994). All of the trials addressed multiple risk factors (e.g., dietary behavior, exercise, blood pressure) in addition to cigarette smoking. Unfortunately, their smoking cessation outcomes are not encouraging. These interventions either have failed to increase cessation rates (or decrease prevalence rates) compared to comparison communities or have produced differences on only one of several measures (e.g., cohort but not cross-sectional findings, self-reported but not biochemically validated end points) for subgroups of the entire population.

It is not clear why these carefully developed and generally well-implemented, long-term interventions conducted with the collaboration and partnership of the intervention communities were not more successful. One possibility supported by the relatively high decreases in smoking among the *comparison* communities in these studies is that secular trends and the changing context around smoking overrode the effects of intervention (Luepker et al., 1994).

The initial results of the multifaceted "Proposition 99" statewide tobacco control program in the state of California (e.g., Pierce et al., 1993)—though it is essentially a demonstration project rather than a tightly controlled study—lend support to such an interpretation. Statewide efforts, funded in large part by a 25¢ increase per pack in the state cigarette tax, included aggressive television and radio antismoking ads and a variety of actions to promote nonsmoking policies and to reduce access to cigarettes, as well as prevention and quit-smoking activities. These efforts have produced a substantial statewide decrease in smoking prevalence statewide (Pierce et al., 1993). Time-series analyses suggest that the tax increase alone may have produced a 5-7% decline in cigarette consumption (Flewelling et al., 1992), and overall, California saw a 24% decrease from 1988 to 1992 in smoking prevalence among residents over age 18 (Pierce et al., 1993).

Initial results are available from the Community Intervention Trial for Smoking Cessation (COMMIT), which is the largest and best-controlled community-based smoking cessation trial ever conducted (COMMIT Research Group, 1995). Unlike the multiple-risk factor heart disease prevention studies discussed above, the National Cancer Institute-funded COMMIT trial focused solely on smoking. In COMMIT, 11 matched pairs of communities in North America were randomly assigned to intervention or comparison conditions. A 4-year intervention was conducted, involving the gamut of smoking intervention approaches discussed in this chapter, as well as others not considered here (e.g., media campaigns, school-based prevention). The COMMIT protocol emphasized the role of health care providers and worksites. Self-help materials were an important modality, and community-wide quitting contests were also prominently featured.

From a methodological perspective, COMMIT is noteworthy in that communities were both the unit of assignment and the unit of analysis. Quit rates in identified longitudinally tracked cohorts of 400 heavy smokers (25 or more cigarettes per day) in each community, and rates in a separate cohort of light to moderate smokers, were followed to assess the results of the intervention. The COMMIT intervention significantly increased the cessation rate among light to moderate smokers (30% for intervention communities versus 27% for comparison communities), but not among heavy smokers (18% for both conditions). It appears that some combination of earlier intervention, policy/taxation approaches, and more intensive intervention may be required to affect heavy smokers (COMMIT Research Group, 1995).

TAILORING INTERVENTIONS

Levels of Intervention and the Stepped-Care Approach

From a public health perspective, maximizing the reach and cost-effectiveness of smoking cessation services requires (1) tailoring treatments to match smokers' individual motivational characteristics, smoking habit factors, behavioral self-change skills, demographic/environmental characteristics, and medical needs and (2) introducing a stepped-care delivery model that offers the least intensive, least costly approaches to the largest number of smokers and reserves more costly and intensive treatments for those who do not succeed with minimal-contact approaches or who appear at the outset to require more intensive or specialized care. One such model is outlined in Figure 1 (Orleans, 1993).

The essential features of this model include the following:

1. It applies to *all* smokers, not just those smokers who are motivated to quit or to seek treatment.
2. It is based on the stages of change model, encompassing treatment for smokers in all stages of change from precontemplation to maintenance and recycling.
3. It incorporates an initial assessment to "triage" or match patients to the most appropriate type and intensity of treatment on

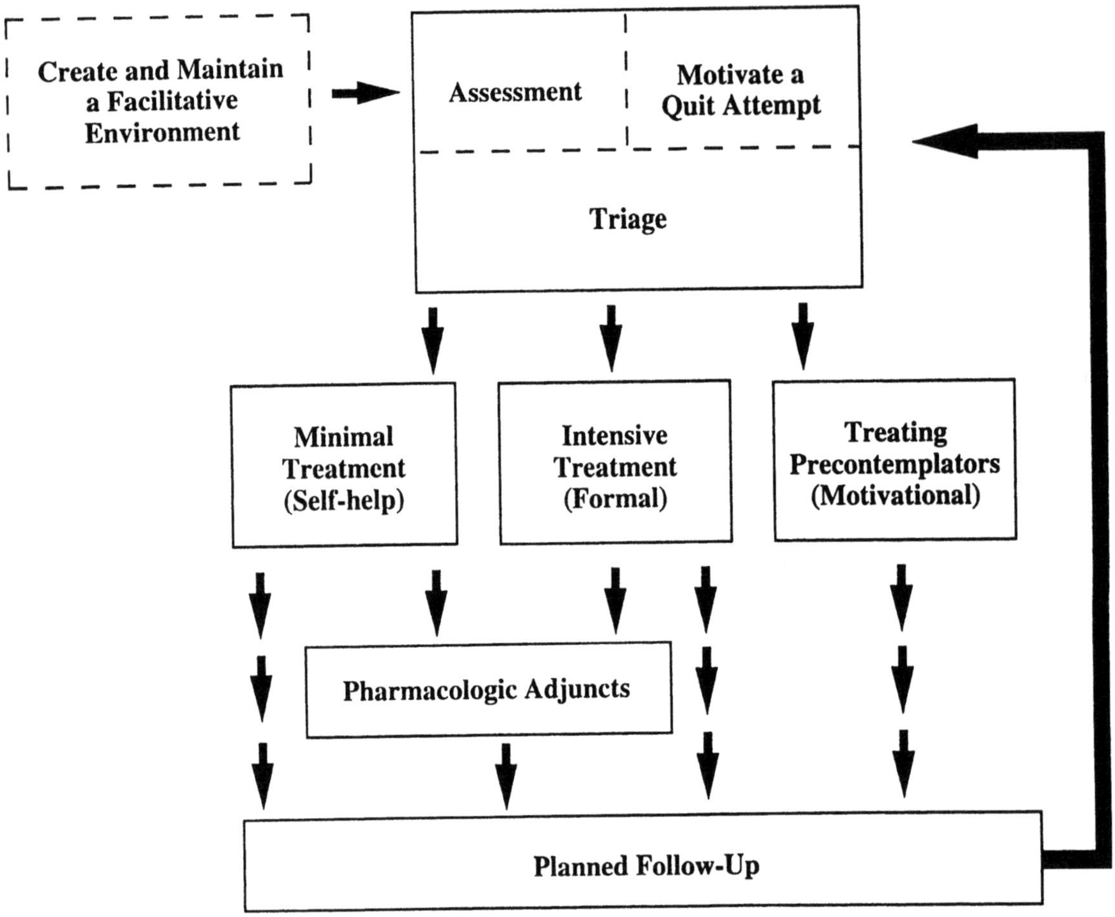

Figure 1. Treating nicotine addiction: A stepped-care, clinical treatment model.

the basis of their stage of change, existing nonsmoking skills, motivations and supports (e.g., Table 1), and level of nicotine dependence.

4. It is cyclical, offering smokers more specialized or intensive help as they progress through different stages of change and through repeated quit attempts.

Although stepped-care models have not been formally evaluated, there is good reason to believe that tailoring treatment through a stepped-care model such as this one will improve treatment adherence and efficacy. For instance, data supporting the stages of change model have shown improved treatment participation and completion rates and higher quit rates when treatments are matched to the smoker's current stage of change (Prochaska et al., 1993). Studies of strategies that personalize generic interventions to the individual smoker, e.g., via brief telephone counseling (Orleans et al., 1991) or computer-tailored messages (Prochaska et al., 1993; Strecher et al., 1994), have found improved use of self-change materials and treatment strategies and better outcomes. Similar benefits have been shown for programs tailored to specific demographic characteristics (e.g., age, ethnic/racial group) and medical status (e.g., pregnancy) (e.g., Perez-Stable, VanOss, Marin, & Marin, 1993; Rimer et al., 1994; Windsor et al., 1985).

This model can be applied in a variety of settings, including worksite, medical, and community. For instance, it fits well with the NCI's four-step Ask-Advise-Assist-Arrange treatment algorithm. Each part of the model is described briefly below, highlighting intervention, individual, and institutional features that bear on treatment adherence and outcomes.

Creating a Facilitative Environment. Glynn, Boyd, and Gruman (1990) define a facilitative environment as one in which "nonsmoking cues and cessation information are persistent and inescapable." Smoking restrictions, restrictions on tobacco advertising, new warning labels, and legislation to increase state and federal tobacco excise taxes or to improve reimbursement for cessation treatment are key tobacco control activities for motivating and supporting smokers in their individual behavior-change efforts. Similarly, state-level media and counteradvertising and health education campaigns (e.g., Pierce, Macaskill, & Hill, 1990), community-level or worksite quit-smoking contests, and community mass media cessation programs increase motivation, opportunity, and likelihood of quitting at a public health level (Glynn et al., 1990).

Assessment and Triage. Assessment and triage (tailoring treatment to patient characteristics and states) usually take place in a controlled treatment setting—a medical, worksite, or community setting in which quitting programs are offered or subsidized. The importance of having a system in place to identify all smokers has already been stressed (e.g., health risk appraisals in worksites, addition of smoking as a vital sign in medical settings). Inexpensive biomarkers of tobacco use may be used in some medical settings (e.g., low-cost urinary cotinine dipsticks are under development). There are many published samples of questionnaires used to diagnose nicotine dependence and collect the smoking history data required for triage (e.g., stage of change, level of nicotine dependence, past treatments and quitting barriers, medical comorbidity requiring special treatment) (Orleans, Glynn, Manley, & Slade, 1993). There are also examples of automated computer-based assessments developed to gather data and provide feedback on treatment recommendations for smokers and their health care providers (e.g., Orleans, Glynn, et al., 1993). These systems could be used in a controlled treatment setting or on a self-help mail correspondence basis.

The triage guidelines in Figure 1 recommend: (1) assigning precontemplators and contemplators to motivational treatments; (2) using self-help quitting programs as the starting point for most smokers, given their relative efficacy, cost, and availability and resulting population "impact"; (3) beginning with or moving to more intensive one-to-one and clinic treatments when the smoker expresses a preference for the structure or support a clinic, group, or counselor can provide or in the face of repeated self-quitting failures; and (4) introducing pharmacological treatment in conjunction with a minimal or formal treatment for regular smokers troubled by nicotine withdrawal in past quit attempts and without medical contraindications (Orleans, Glynn, et al., 1993). Treatment matching also includes choosing from a widening array of tailored self-help materials and programs (e.g., for women, older adults, Latino and African-American smokers).

The lack of research on stepped-care models leaves unanswered many questions about triage guidelines. For instance, when should relapsers be recycled through the *same* treatment and when should they be steered to more intensive or specialized care (Abrams, 1993)? Similarly, the role of patient preference in determining treatment adherence and outcome has not been systematically explored. Future research should give greater attention to these issues.

Motivational Interventions. One of the most basic goals of both population-based and individually focused smoking cessation initiatives is to heighten quitting motivation and self-efficacy (Glynn et al., 1990). A stage breakdown of the United States smoker population shows that the majority of smokers (70-80%) are in precontemplation and contemplation stages, not yet ready to benefit from cessation programs and activities (Prochaska et al., 1992). As noted, policy and environmental interventions can increase quitting motivation. A major adherence issue here centers around the need to enhance intrinsic versus extrinsic quitting motives. Curry and associates (1991) found that perceived social environmental pressure is related to high levels of extrinsic (versus intrinsic) motivation and a failure to quit or maintain abstinence.

Public education and counteradvertising media campaigns can effectively address these issues, helping smokers recognize and cope effectively with growing extrinsic pressures in a way that helps enhance intrinsic health, self-control, and self-esteem motives (cf. Table 1). At the individual treatment level, a number of promising motivational strategies for precontemplators and contemplators have been identified. In the stepped-care model (Figure 1), motivational interventions would be the major treatment used for smokers in the "precontemplation" stage. This is the area of tobacco intervention in which there has been the greatest innovation in the past decade.

Promising interventions include stage-based "motivational" manuals and feedback reports (Prochaska et al., 1993), personalized motivational feedback to enhance intrinsic quitting motives (Curry et al., 1991), "motivational interviewing" strategies originally developed to motivate problem drinkers to engage in self-change (Miller & Rollnick, 1991), and "biofeedback" (e.g., laboratory test results, genetic risk biomarkers) in combination with personal medical quitting advice to increase the salience and relevance of smoking-related health risks (Lerman, Orleans, & Engstrom, 1993). Several studies have shown that such feedback improves adherence to medical quit-smoking advice (Orleans, Glynn, et al., 1993). Risser and Belcher (1990), for instance, found that giving chronic disease outpatients feedback on spirometry and carbon monoxide breath test results along with quit-smoking advice and a medical review of pulmonary symptoms tripled 6-month quit rates compared to quit-smoking advice alone (34% versus 13%). The chief methodological requirement for further research in this area is the use of appropriate outcome measures—to detect both positive shifts in motivation and stages of change and potentially negative/iatrogenic shifts in anxiety level. Early research that gauged the efficacy of motivational interventions such as these primarily on the basis of whether they resulted in smoking abstinence underestimated their power to create change in *motivation*.

Self-Help Interventions. National survey data show that United States smokers strongly prefer minimal contact over more intensive programs (Curry, 1993; Fiore et al., 1990). These findings arc backed by research documenting low levels of participation in formal clinics and group treatments (patients not signing up, showing up, or finishing up), even among reportedly motivated and high-risk (e.g., post-MI, pregnant) smokers (Ockene et al., 1992; Taylor et al., 1990). Hence, for most smokers, self-help interventions represent a good starting point.

The greater reach and cost-effectiveness of self-help programs led the National Cancer Institute to fund seven large-scale controlled trials beginning in the mid-1980s to develop maximally effective self-help interventions. These trials reached over 200,000 smokers directly or indirectly in communities, worksites, hospitals, HMOs, and voluntary associations (Glynn et al., 1990). Results showed that smokers using self-help guides on their own achieved 14-15% long-term, biochemically verified, quit rates (Cohen, Lichtenstein, et al., 1989) and that several minimal-contact treatment adjuncts (e.g., brief follow-up counseling in person or by phone, personalized feedback concerning quitting strategies) could boost these rates by 50-100% to the 20-25% long-term quit rates achieved by most formal clinic programs (Curry, 1993; Glynn et al., 1990). "Reactive" (call-in) telephone "hot lines" showed some benefit, but less than expected because compliance with advice to use the hot lines was unexpectedly poor (Glasgow, Lando, Hollis, McRay, & LaChance, 1993; Ossip-Klein et al., 1991).

To date, surprisingly little is known about the relationship between smokers' use of self-help quit-smoking materials or the quitting strategies recommended therein and quitting outcomes (e.g., Curry, 1993). Only a handful of studies have collected data on the effects of varied treatment formats or adjuncts on smokers' use of self-help materials and suggested quitting methods (e.g., K. M. Cummings, Emont, Jaen, & Sciandra, 1988). In general, these studies have found a positive relationship between use of self-help materials/methods and improved outcomes. One study suggested that supplying smokers with repeated "cues to action" over time, by mail or phone, would itself have benefit (Ershoff, Mullen, & Quinn, 1989). Optimal "weaning" schedules for effective telephone counseling protocols have not been established, and more research is needed to explore stage by treatment (adjunct) interactions (e.g., does telephone counseling benefit smokers in preparation and action stages more than those in contemplation or maintenance?) (Curry, 1993; Rimer et al., 1994).

Intensive and Clinic Treatments. The core components of effective formal treatment programs were identified through programmatic clinical research conducted in the late 1970s and early 1980s to determine the optimal mix of educational, motivational, behavior change, and environmental elements. This research found that the most effective formal treatment programs have encompassed multiple cognitive-behavioral interventions, including strategies designed to prepare and motivate smokers to quit (e.g., self-monitoring, nicotine fading, stimulus control), to undermine the reinforcement value of smoking (e.g., aversive smoking, cognitive restructuring, covert sensitization), and to teach effective withdrawal coping skills and effective relapse prevention skills (e.g., Lando, 1993; Lichtenstein & Glasgow, 1992). Most formal treatments, even those offered by voluntary health organizations like the American Lung Association and the American Cancer Society, now incorporate these methods. In general, such programs produce 1-year quit rates of 20-25%, with some achieving results in the 40-50% range.

Compared to what has been learned over the past decade about effective self-help and pharmacological treatments, relatively little progress has been made in the formal treatment arena. In fact, in reviews of the literature on formal treatments, Lando (1993) and Shiffman (1993) called for significant innovation to advance the field. As Lichtenstein and Glasgow (1992) outlined, the answer probably will not lie in trying to combine *more* treatment elements into a single intervention. Past studies show diminishing returns from this approach. Better results are likely to come from programs that incorporate innovative motivational strategies, perhaps using biofeedback (Lerman et al., 1993) and motivational interviewing (Miller & Rollnick, 1991), and from more personalized interventions. A good example is work by Hall and colleagues showing that smokers with a history of major depressive disorder benefited from focused mood-management training in the context of a standard multicomponent treatment program (Hall, Munoz, Reus, & Sees, 1993). Even with more personalized programs, however, care must be taken not to overload the quitter. Poor results have emerged from programs that offer combined weight-control and cessation elements to quitters highly concerned about weight gain after quitting (e.g., Pirie et al., 1992).

Nicotine Replacement. Nicotine replacement therapy has proven an effective adjunct to medical setting treatment programs, doubling or even tripling quit rates, but it has little or no value over placebo when used on its own (Fiore et al., 1994; Hughes, 1993). The U.S. Food and Drug Administration currently mandates the use of nicotine replacement that includes smoking cessation treatment, and in 1996 approved nicotine gum and patches on an over-the-counter (rather than prescription-only) basis. To date, no other pharmacological interventions have proven as consistently effective as nicotine gum or transdermal nicotine. For these reasons, nicotine replacement therapy is indicated in the stepped-care model presented in Figure 1, but only as an adjunct to a minimal or formal treatment program.

Patient and provider adherence issues have proven key to the efficacy of nicotine replacement therapies. Patient adherence to recommended regimens for nicotine replacement therapy needs closer study. In general, compliance problems are greater with nicotine gum than with transdermal nicotine. Nicotine patches are easier to use, cause fewer side effects that might discourage or disrupt appropriate use, and produce higher blood nicotine levels and more stable nicotine replacement (e.g., Hughes, 1993). Moreover, dosing and weaning schedules are better defined and easier to follow for the patch. From the patient-adherence perspective, a major compliance issue for nicotine gum and transdermal nicotine is continued smoking, which may cause unsafe levels of nicotine intake and has been strongly associated with relapse to smoking (e.g., Orleans, Resch, Noll, et al., 1994). More research is needed to identify strategies that will boost the appropriate use of nicotine gum and patches (Fiore et al., 1994; Orleans, Resch, et al., 1994).

Instruction and support by health care providers also have been shown to play a major role in patient adherence (Killen, Fortmann, Newman, & Varady, 1990; Orleans, Jepson, Resch, & Rimer, 1994). A meta-analysis by Hughes (1993) found that nicotine gum had little value over placebo when combined with brief medical advice only, presumably because the protocol for appropriate gum use is relatively complex and requires time to teach (e.g., when to chew, how to chew, how long to chew, minimizing side effects, avoiding acidic beverages). Cummings, Hansen, Richard, Stein, and Coates (1988) in fact documented a number of common errors in internists' instructions about gum use, including lack of advice to stop smoking before using the gum. Provider instruction also appears very important to appropriate patch use. In a recent large-scale study of "real world" patch users, amount of provider advice was significantly related to higher quit rates and lower rates of concomitant smoking (Orleans, Resch, et al., 1994).

Tailoring for Special Populations

For any type of treatment covered by the stepped-care model (e.g., motivational, self-help, intensive, pharmacological), treatment tailoring is likely to improve reach, follow-through, and outcome. The dimensions on which treatment tailoring can occur include: sociodemographic and ethnic/cultural group membership, smoking habit factors and level of nicotine addiction, psychosocial variables including personal quitting motives and barriers, self-efficacy, stage of change and absence or presence of social support for quitting in the smoker's natural environment, and medical/psychiatric comorbidity. Examples are given below for several smoker subgroups.

Minority Smokers. High rates of smoking and smoking-caused disease within America's racial/ethnic minority groups, combined with poor access to mainstream quit-smoking programs and services, have made efforts to reach minority populations a national priority. To date, greatest progress has been made clarifying the smoking patterns and quitting needs of African-American and Hispanic smokers, with growing attention to the special needs of Native American and Asian-American smokers (Ramirez & Gallion, 1993). Though tailored treatments have not yet been systematically compared to "generic" treatments in any of these populations, formative research with African-American and Hispanic smokers has confirmed that culturally sensitive self-help quitting guides are more likely to be read and recalled, and are rated more highly, than "generic" guides—even when generic guides are multiracial (e.g., Perez-Stable et al., 1993). Research now under way will shed light on these issues and help to clarify the best channels for reaching smokers in varied United States racial/ethnic groups (Perez-Stable et al., 1993; Ramirez & Gallion, 1993).

Women Smokers. As the United States population has aged and tobacco industry advertising has helped to make smoking an equal opportunity killer, there are fewer and fewer differences in the smoking or quitting patterns of male and female smokers (Solomon & Flynn, 1993). There remain, however, important gender differences in the health consequences of smoking and in quitting motives and barriers. Women have therefore frequently been singled out as a high-risk group requiring tailored quit-smoking treatments.

Solomon and Flynn (1993) reviewed the literature on treating nicotine dependence in women and identified several salient concerns, including helping women to replace smoking as a coping technique, eliciting better social support for quitting, and coping better with fears of weight gain and with actual weight gain following quitting. Since depression is more common in women than in men, helping women cope with depression during and after quitting also may improve treatment effectiveness (Hall et al., 1993). To date, there are no studies comparing gender-tailored with generic treatment programs in women. Biofeedback techniques, however, including those related to monitoring children's exposure to parental environmental tobacco smoke (Emmons, Hammond, & Abrams, 1994), may help to increase the salience of smoking health harms for women (e.g., Lerman et al., 1993). Efforts to combine weight-management and smoking cessation treatments for weight-worried women have not proven beneficial, but the reason may be that they overburden the quitter with too many behavior change demands (Pirie et al., 1992). The area in which tailoring has proven effective for women quitters is during pregnancy. Windsor et al. (1985) found that pregnancy-tailored quitting guides were more effective than generic guides when used as part of a brief public health maternity clinic intervention to help pregnant smokers quit.

Older Smokers. Older smokers have been found to experience unique quitting motives and barriers. A reanalysis of the 1966 Adult Use of Tobacco Survey data found few differences in smoking pattern or level of nicotine dependence between older smokers and younger smokers (i.e., smokers 50–74 years of age versus 21–49 years of age). Older smokers, however, were found to underestimate significantly the "cons" of smoking, especially the personal and general health risks of smoking, and also to overestimate the "pros," perceiving smoking to be a more useful stress-control and weight-control tactic than younger smokers (Orleans, Jepsen, et al., 1994). The fact that today's cohort of older American smokers came of age in an era when smoking was widely promoted as safe and desirable helps to explain this age gap in awareness of health risks (Rimer, Orleans, Keintz, Cristinzio, & Fleisher, 1990).

These results and other characteristics of older adults have many implications for the best channels and contents of quit-smoking initiatives aimed at older smokers. The medical setting becomes an especially important treatment channel, given the need for clear and credible messages about smoking health harms and quitting benefits (e.g., "It's never too late to quit"). Other channels that reach older adults also can be exploited—preretirement seminars, community groups/activities, and media targeted at older adults. One program specifically developed for older smokers, the Clear Horizons program, was tailored to address the unique quitting benefits and barriers and to recommend quitting activities tailored to the capacities, resources, and lifestyles of older Americans. Results of a large clinical trial showed (1) higher than expected recruitment rates (a single short announcement in the magazine of the American Association of

Retired Persons elicited 10,000 inquiries), (2) greater use and more favorable ratings of the tailored Clear Horizons quitting guide compared to a comparable generic guide, and (3) better 3- and 12-month cessation rates (Rimer et al., 1994).

Adolescent Smokers. Smokers at the other end of the age continuum are equally likely to benefit from tailoring and from corrective messages about the perceived harms and benefits of smoking (e.g., "It's never too soon to quit"). Like older smokers, younger smokers have been found to possess a strong "optimistic bias" about the safety and benefits of smoking, as well as about the ease of quitting (e.g., Flay, 1993). Moreover, cultural sensitivity and appropriate "channel selection" is required in materials and programs targeted to younger smokers. The 1994 Surgeon General's Report (USDHHS, 1994) included the strong recommendation to develop and evaluate better youth-targeted programs and materials.

METHODOLOGICAL AND EVALUATION ISSUES

Smoking cessation researchers have contributed at least as much to the field of health behavior research from their methodological innovations as they have in terms of interventive or substantive developments. Smoking researchers have been leaders in moving toward population-based research; in developing standard measures of treatment outcome; in exploring the advantages and limitations of attempts to biochemically validate self-reports of behavior change; in developing and applying new analytic approaches, such as survival analysis and methods to account for clustering effects; and in conducting cost-effectiveness research. Each of these issues will be discussed in this section.

Over the past decade, smoking researchers have become bolder in the size of social units with which they intervene—and have learned to be more humble in what they claim. Research has moved from the study of small groups of volunteer participants to investigate the impact of cessation programs on entire populations of employees within one or more worksites, on representative members of health maintenance organizations (Curry et al., 1991; Hollis, Lichtenstein, Vogt, Stevens, & Biglan, 1993; Orleans et al., 1991), and on entire communities (COMMIT Research Group, 1995) and even multiple counties (Ossip-Klein et al., 1991) or states (Gruman & Lynn, 1993). The key to this research has been a focus on defined populations, i.e., known numbers of smokers living, working, or using the resources of a certain setting. This framework has also led to important research on participation and program reach (Glasgow et al., 1992; Koepsell et al., 1992) and to the realization that most programs attract only a small percentage of smokers in the population. This documentation, in turn, has contributed to the development of interventions and theoretical approaches applicable to the large percentage of persons who are not motivated to change their smoking at any given time (Abrams et al., 1994; Prochaska et al., 1992).

There has been a concerted effort by smoking cessation researchers to use comparable measures of treatment outcome to permit easier comparisons across studies. By the mid-1990s, almost all studies reported both short-term (e.g., post-treatment or 1- to 3-month follow-up) and a longer-term outcome measure (e.g., 12-month follow-up), and most used a standard item developed for a series of National Cancer Institute collaborative studies asking whether one "has smoked, even a single cigarette, in the past seven days" to define cessation. Although there is not as much consensus, more and more studies are also including a measure of continuous abstinence (e.g., reporting no smoking since end of treatment, or reporting abstinence at all follow-up assessments).

The field of smoking cessation research has undergone several swings in terms of biochemical verification procedures. It was recognized early on that self-reports of smoking cessation could be subject to demand characteristics. One of the oldest, easiest to collect, and least expensive biochemical confirmation procedures involves collecting breath samples, which are analyzed for carbon monoxide content (Hughes, Frederiksen, & Frazier, 1978). By the early 1980s, the prevailing choice had shifted to assays of serum or saliva thiocyanate, which has a longer half-life than does carbon monoxide and thus could potentially verify abstinence over a longer time period. Limitations with thiocyanate assays, involving collection of adequate samples for analysis, interference by certain dietary consumption patterns, and degree of specificity (Benowitz, 1983) led most investigators to switch to a new "gold standard" of cotinine. Being a by-product of nicotine metabolism, cotinine is a more direct and specific measure than either carbon monoxide or thiocyanate. It too has limitations, such as being elevated by nicotine patch or gum use, as well as by smokeless tobacco, but is now considered the biochemical assay of choice.

One controversy in the field concerns what to do in data analyses regarding subjects who do not provide saliva samples for biochemical confirmation. Previously, in smaller studies with volunteer samples in research settings where failure to provide such samples was usually minimal (less than 10%), the "conservative" standard of counting all subjects not providing samples as still smoking was developed. However, with the shift to more population-based studies in which the subjects do not volunteer for a research study, refusal or no-show rates are typically much higher—often around 50%. Simply considering all such subjects to be smoking, when in fact many do not participate for other reasons (e.g., invasion of privacy, fears of HIV testing or of insurance or employment ramifications), does not work so well in these settings and may not be "conservative." These issues and the conditions under which biochemical testing is most important (and least helpful) are discussed in Glasgow, Mullooly, et al. (1993) and Velicer, Prochaska, Rossi, and Snow (1992).

One of the conceptual reasons to intervene at the level of larger social units (e.g., worksites, doctors' offices, entire communities) is that it may be possible to change the culture (Steckler & Goodman, 1989) of these institutions and bring to bear prompts, incentives, and policies that will affect large numbers of employees, patients, or community residents. This likelihood that smokers within a given worksite or community will be more similar in their smoking behavior than those across such settings due to such common influences leads to data analysis complexities. Especially when combined with the common procedure of assigning entire worksites, medical offices, or communities (rather than individual smokers) to treatment conditions, this complexity leads to unit of analysis, clustering, or intraclass correlation issues that need to be taken into account when analyzing results. There are different methods of approaching this issue (Hedeker, Gibbons, & Flay, 1994; Koepsell et al., 1992), but the implication is that one must (1) study more units (e.g., worksites, communities) and subjects and (2) use more complex and conservative analysis procedures than would be the case if there were no clustering and one could simply use individuals as the unit of analysis. The later practice almost always inflates the significance level of treatment effects. An alternative, if one is able to repeat assessments over time but has a limited number of units (e.g., worksites, schools, communities) to study, is to employ multiple baseline or time-series designs.

FUTURE DIRECTIONS AND CONCLUSIONS

Dissemination

Since the mid-1980s, there has been an increase in the scope of health care institutions' efforts to disseminate research findings or to turn what has been learned into practice. Examples of three such efforts in different areas of smoking cessation research are briefly discussed below.

Lando, McGovern, and Sipfle (1989) joined forces with the American Lung Association to train community volunteers to implement their

8-week multicomponent cessation program. They demonstrated that the cessation rates resulting from this dissemination program are comparable to those obtained under more tightly controlled research evaluations (Lando et al., 1989).

In 1991, the National Cancer Institute embarked on a national "Train the Trainer" campaign with the goal of teaching 100,000 United States physicians and nurses the basic elements of the four-step Ask-Advise-Assist-Arrange protocol in a 3-hour course (Manley, Epps, Husten, Glynn, & Shopland, 1991).

Finally, the American Stop Smoking Intervention Trial for Cancer Prevention (ASSIST) exemplifies both broad-based dissemination efforts and the integration of policy and cessation approaches. ASSIST is a 5-year demonstration project (1993-1998) sponsored by the National Cancer Institute and the American Cancer Society in 17 states (Gruman & Lynn, 1993). Each participating state is forming broad-based coalitions, spearheaded by American Cancer Society offices and state and local health departments. Intervention will be based upon detailed assessments and tailored to the specific needs and conditions in each state. All states are using a common planning approach to develop a comprehensive initiative for each state that focuses on the integration of three different dimensions: (1) target groups (e.g., groups with high smoking rates, secondary risk factors), (2) major channels through which interventions will reach targeted groups (e.g., health care systems, worksites, community networks), and (3) intervention categories (e.g., media, policy, and program services).

Harnessing the Move to Managed Care

The move to managed care as the predominant model of medical care in the United States holds the promise of improving the infrastructure and incentives for preventive care, including smoking cessation programs and services. The creation of large regional health plans with more stable long-term enrollment should strengthen interest in the long-term savings and improved health outcomes associated with smoking cessation treatments. However, specifically mandating and reimbursing smoking cessation services as a component of the standard prevention benefits package will help realize this potential (Orleans, 1993). In fact, the 1994 Midcourse Revisions in the National Health Promotion and Disease Prevention Objectives for the Year 2000 include the objective of increasing to 100% the proportion of health plans offering treatment for nicotine addiction. Until this objective is a reality, however, regional managed care organizations will continue to compete for good prevention "report cards" based primarily on Health Plan Employer Data and Information Set (HEDIS) ratings. Expanding HEDIS prevention requirements (now limited to childhood immunization, cholesterol screening, mammography, and cervical cancer screening) to cover smoking cessation services could create unprecendented system-wide incentives to address smoking and tobacco use.

A restructured health care system involving health care plans and managed care organizations that provide care through integrated networks of providers will improve the integration of services provided across settings (hospital, pharmacy, clinic). Additionally, the growth in sophisticated information systems required to make this happen can be harnessed to prompt and direct the systematic treatment of tobacco use—removing critical systematic barriers to care. For instance, the computer-based system for cancer screening reminders/counseling developed by McPhee, Bird, Jenkins, and Fordham (1989) can be easily implemented to generate lists of smokers, to furnish computer-based screening and counseling reminders for every smoker at every visit, and to generate routine performance feedback ("report cards") to individual providers. Prescription plans used by a growing number of managed care organizations to administer and control costs of their pharmacy benefits can identify smokers using nicotine replacement therapies, supplying them automatically with timely and personalized advice on how to quit and how to use these therapies appropriately (Orleans, Resch, et al., 1994). Advanced information systems and technologies (including user-friendly patient interfaces) can be incorporated to facilitate patient and provider data collection and communication.

Conclusions

There have been substantial advances in the breadth and conceptualization of intervention approaches and in the methodological sophistication of evaluations in the smoking cessation area. There is far less emphasis on "horse race" studies or attempts to prove that "my approach is better than yours" (for all smokers) and more emphasis on multiple-channel interventions that are tailored to specific populations, subgroups, or even individual smokers. It has been recognized that smoking is multiply determined by a variety of biological, pharmacological, socioeconomic, institutional, cultural, and community factors, and that interventions must be similarly multifaceted. Perhaps the biggest shift over the past decade has been toward a public health approach that emphasizes extending the reach of interventions to encompass entire populations, and especially those persons at high risk and those who have historically been underserved by traditional approaches. With this shift in focus has also come increased appreciation that interventions on these multiple determinants are necessarily complex and that change in larger social units (e.g., worksites, medical organizations, and communities) usually occurs over a period of years rather than weeks or months.

ACKNOWLEDGMENTS. Preparation of this chapter was supported in part by Grant 1 R29 HL50181-01 to the first author and Grants 1 RO1 HL504-8902 and 5 PO1 CA5786-03 to the second author.

REFERENCES

Abrams, D. (1993). Treatment issues: Towards a stepped-care model. *Tobacco Control, 2*(Suppl.), S17-S29.

Abrams, D. B., Emmons, K. M., Linnan, L., & Biener, L. (1994). Smoking cessation at the workplace: Conceptual and practical considerations. In R. Richmond (Ed.), *Interventions for smokers: An international perspective* (pp. 137-169). Baltimore: Williams & Wilkins.

American Medical Association. (1993). *How to help patients stop smoking*. Chicago: American Medical Association.

Bandura, A. (1986). *Social foundations of thought and action: A social cognitive theory*. Englewood Cliffs, NJ: Prentice-Hall.

Benowitz, N. L. (1983). The use of biologic fluid samples in assessing tobacco smoke consumption. In J. Grabowski & C. S. Bell (Eds.), *Measurement in the analysis and treatment of smoking behavior*. NIDA Research Monograph 48, DHHS Publication No. ADM 83-1285. Washington, DC: U.S. Government Printing Office.

Bracht, N. (1990). *Health promotion at the community level*. Newbury Park, CA: Sage.

Cohen, S., Lichtenstein, E., Prochaska, J. O., Rossi, J. S. Gritz, E. R., Carr, C. R., Orleans, C. T., Schoenbach, V. J., Biener, L., Abrams, D., DiClemente, C., Curry, S., Marlatt, G. A., Cummings, K. M., Emont, S. L., Giovino, G., & Ossip-Klein, D. (1989). Debunking myths about self-quitting: Evidence from 10 prospective studies of persons quitting smoking by themselves. *American Psychologist, 44*, 1355-1365.

Cohen, S. J., Stookey, G. K., Katz, B. P., Drook, C. A., & Christen, A. G. (1989). Helping smokers quit: A randomized controlled trial with private practice dentists. *Journal of the American Dental Association, 118*, 41-45.

Cohen, S. J., Stookey, G. K., Katz, B. P., Drook, C. A., & Smith, D. M. (1989). Encouraging primary care physicians to help smokers quit. *Annals of Internal Medicine, 110*, 648-652.

COMMIT Research Group. (1995). Community Intervention Trial for Smoking Cessation (COMMIT). I. Cohort results from a four-year community intervention. *American Journal of Public Health, 85*, 183-192.

Cummings, K. M., Emont, S. L., Jaen, C. K., & Sciandra, R. (1988). Format and quitting instructions as factors influencing the impact of a self-administered quit smoking program. *Health Education Quarterly, 15*, 199-216.

Cummings, S. R., Hansen, B., Richard, R. J., Stein, M. J., & Coates, T. J. (1988). Internists and nicotine gum. *Journal of the American Medical Association, 260*, 1565-1569.

Curry, S. J. (1993). Self-help interventions for smoking cessation. *Journal of Consulting and Clinical Psychology, 61*, 790-803.

Curry, S. J., Wagner, E. H., & Grothaus, L. C. (1991). Evaluation of intrinsic and extrinsic motivation interventions with a self-help smoking cessation program. *Journal of Consulting and Clinical Psychology, 59*, 318-324.

Emmons, K. M., Hammond, K., & Abrams, D. (1994). Smoking at home: The impact of smoking cessation on nonsmokers' exposure to environmental tobacco smoke. *Health Psychology, 13*, 496-507.

Ershoff, D. H., Mullen, P. D., & Quinn, V. P. (1989). A randomized trial of a serialized self-help smoking cessation program for pregnant women in a public health setting. *American Journal of Public Health*, *79*, 182-187.

Farquhar, J. W., Fortmann, S. P., Flora, J. A., Taylor, C. B., Haskel, W. L., Williams, P., Maccoby, N., & Wood, P. D. (1990). Effects of community-wide education on cardiovascular disease risk factors: The Stanford Five-City Project. *Journal of the American Medical Association*, *264*, 359-365.

Fiore, M. C. (1991). The new vital sign. Assessing and documenting smoking status [commentary]. *Journal of the American Medical Association*, *266*, 3183-3184.

Fiore, M. C., Novotny, T. E., Pierce, J. P., Giovino, G. A., Hatziandreu, E. J., Newcomb, P. A., Surawicz, T. S., & Davis, R. M. (1990). Methods used to quit smoking in the United States: Do cessation programs help? *Journal of the American Medical Association*, *263*, 2760-2765.

Fiore, M. C., Smith, S. S., Jorneby, D. E., & Baker, T. B. (1994). The effectiveness of the nicotine patch for smoking cessation: A meta-analysis. *Journal of the American Medical Association*, *271*, 1940-1947.

Fisher, K. J., Glasgow, R. E., & Terborg, J. R. (1990). Worksite smoking cessation: A meta-analysis of controlled studies. *Journal of Occupational Medicine*, *32*, 429-439.

Flay, B. R. (1993). Youth tobacco use: Risks, patterns, and control. In C. T. Orleans & J. Slade (Eds.), *Nicotine addiction: Principles and management* (pp. 365-384). New York: Oxford University Press.

Flewelling, R. L., Kenney, E., Elder, J. P., Pierce, J., Johnson, M., & Bal, D. G. (1992). First-year impact of the 1989 California cigarette tax increase on cigarette consumption. *American Journal of Public Health*, *82*, 867-869.

Frank, E., Winkleby, M. A., Altman, D. G., Rockhill, B., & Fortmann, S. P. (1991). Predictors of physician's cessation advice. *Journal of the American Medical Association*, *266*, 3139-3144.

Glasgow, R. E., Lando, H., Hollis, J., McRae, S. G., & LaChance, P. (1993). A stop-smoking telephone helpline that nobody called. *American Journal of Public Health*, *83*, 252-253.

Glasgow, R. E., McCaul, K. D., & Fisher, K. J. (1992). Participation in worksite health promotion: A critique of the literature and recommendations for future practice. *Health Education Quarterly*, *20*, 391-408.

Glasgow, R. E., Mullooly, J. P., Vogt, T. M., Stevens, V. J., Lichtenstein, E., Hollis, J. F., Lando, H. A., Severson, H. H., Pearson, K. A., & Vogt, M. R. (1993). Biochemical validation of smoking status in public health settings: Pros, cons, and data from four low-intensity intervention trials. *Addictive Behaviors*, *18*, 511-527.

Glasgow, R. E., Terborg, J. R., Hollis, J. F., Severson, H. H., & Boles, S. M. (1995). Take Heart: Results from the initial phase of a worksite wellness program. *American Journal of Public Health*, *85*, 209-216.

Glasgow, R. E., Terborg, J. R., Strycker, L. A., Boles, S. M., & Hollis, J. F. (in press). Take Heart II: Replication of a worksite health promotion trial. *Journal of Behavioral Medicine*.

Glynn, T. J. (1988). Relative effectiveness of physician-initiated smoking cessation programs. *Cancer Bulletin*, *40*, 359-364.

Glynn, T. J., Boyd, G. M., & Gruman, J. C. (1990). Essential elements of self-help/minimal intervention strategies for smoking cessation. *Health Education Quarterly*, *17*, 329-345.

Glynn, T. J., & Manley, M. W. (1989). Physicians, cancer control and the treatment of nicotine dependence: Defining success. *Health Education Research*, *4*, 479-487.

Glynn, T. J., Manley, M. W., Solberg, L. I., & Slade, J. (1993). Creating and maintaining an optimal medical practice environment for the treatment of nicotine addiction. In C. T. Orleans & J. Slade (Eds.), *Nicotine addiction: Principles and management* (pp. 162-180). New York: Oxford University Press.

Goldstein, A. O., Hellier, A., Fitzgerald, S., Stegall, T. S., & Fischer, P. M. (1987). Hospital nurse counseling of patients who smoke. *American Journal of Public Health*, *77*, 1333-1334.

Gottlieb, N. H., Mullen, P. D., & McAlister, A. L. (1987). Patients' substance abuse and the primary care physician: Patterns of practice. *Addictive Behaviors*, *12*, 23-31.

Gruman, J., & Lynn, W. (1993). Worksite and community intervention for tobacco control. In C. T. Orleans & J. S. Slade (Eds.), *Nicotine addiction: Principles and management* (pp. 396-411). New York: Oxford University Press.

Hall, S. M., Munoz, R. F., Reus, V. I., & Sees, K. I. (1993). Nicotine, negative affect and depression. *Journal of Consulting and Clinical Psychology*, *61*, 761-767.

Hedeker, D., Gibbons, R. D., & Flay, B. R. (1994). Random-effects regression models for clustered data: With an example from smoking prevention research. *Journal of Consulting and Clinical Psychology*, *62*, 757-764.

Hollis, J. F., Lichtenstein, E., Vogt, T. M., Stevens, V. J., & Biglan, A. (1993). Nurse-assisted counseling for smokers in primary care. *Annals of Internal Medicine*, *118*, 521-525.

Hughes, J. R. (1993). Pharmacotherapy for smoking cessation: Unvalidated assumptions, anomalies and suggestions for future research. *Journal of Consulting and Clinical Psychology*, *61*, 751-760.

Hughes, J. R., Frederiksen, L. W., & Frazier, M. (1978). A carbon monoxide analyzer for measurement of smoking behavior. *Behavior Therapist*, *9*, 293-296.

Jason, L. A., Gruder, C. L., Buckenberger, L., Lesowitz, T., Belgredan, J., Flay, B. R., & Warnecke, R. B. (1987). A 12-month follow-up of a worksite smoking cessation intervention. *Health Education Research*, *2*, 185-194.

Jeffery, R. W. (1989). Risk behaviors and health: Contrasting individual and population perspectives. *American Psychologist*, *44*, 1194-1202.

Jeffery, R. W., Forster, J. L., French, S. A., Kelder, S. H., Lando, H. A., McGovern, P. G., Jacobs, D. R., Jr., & Baxter, J. E.

(1993). The Healthy Worker Project: A work-site intervention for weight control and smoking cessation. *American Journal of Public Health, 83*, 395-401.

Killen, J. D., Fortmann, S. P., Newman, B., & Varady, A. (1990). Evaluation of a treatment approach combining nicotine gum with self-guided behavioral treatments for smoking relapse prevention. *Journal of Consulting and Clinical Psychology, 58*, 85-92.

Koepsell, T. D., Wagner, E. H., Cheadle, A. C., Patrick, D. L., Martin, D. C., Diehr, P. M., Perins, E. B., Kristall, A. R., Allan-Andrilla, C. H., & Dey, L. J. (1992). Selected methodological issues in evaluating community-based health promotion and disease prevention programs. *Annual Review of Public Health, 13*, 31-57.

Kottke, T. E., Battista, R. N., DeFriese, G. H., & Brekke, M. L. (1988). Attributes of successful smoking cessation interventions in medical practice: A meta-analysis of 39 controlled trials. *Journal of the American Medical Association, 259*, 2883-2889.

Kottke, T. E., Solberg, L. I., & Brekke, M. L. (1990). Initiation and maintenance of patient behavioral change: What is the role of the physician? *Journal of General and Internal Medicine, 5*(Suppl.), S26-S67.

Lando, H. A. (1993). Formal quit smoking treatments. In C. T. Orleans & J. Slade (Eds.), *Nicotine addiction: Principles and management* (pp. 221-244). New York: Oxford University Press.

Lando, H. A., McGovern, P. G., & Sipfle, C. L. (1989). Public service application of an effective clinic approach to smoking cessation. *Health Education Research, 4*, 103-109.

Lasater, T., Abrams, D., & Artz, L. (1984). Lay volunteer delivery of a community-based cardiovascular risk factor change program: The Pawtucket experiment. In J. H. Matarazzo, S. M. Weiss, & J. A. Herd (Eds.), *Behavioral health: A handbook of health enhancement and disease prevention*. New York: Wiley.

Lerman, C. L., Orleans, C. T., & Engstrom, P. F. (1993). Biological markers in smoking cessation treatment. *Seminars in Oncology, 20*, 359-367.

Li, V. C., Coates, T. J., Ewart, C. K., & Kim, Y. J. (1987). The effectiveness of smoking cessation advice given during routine medical care: Physicians can make a difference. *American Journal of Preventive Medicine, 3*, 81-86.

Lichtenstein, E., & Glasgow, R. E. (1992). Smoking cessation: What have we learned over the past decade? *Journal of Consulting and Clinical Psychology, 60*, 518-527.

Lichtenstein, E., Lando, H. A., & Nothwehr, R. (1994). Readiness to quit as a predictor of smoking changes in the Minnesota Heart Health Program. *Health Psychology, 5*, 393-396.

Luepker, R. V., Murray, D. M., Jacobs, D. R., Jr., Mittelmark, M. B., Bracht, N., Carlaw, R., Crow, R., Elmer, P., Finnegan, J., Folsom, A. R., Grimm, R., Hannan, P. J., Jeffery, R., Lando, H., McGovern, P., Mullis, R., Perry, C. L., Pechacek, T., Pirie, P., Sprafka, J. M., Weisbrod, R., & Blackburn, H. (1994). Community education for cardiovascular disease prevention: Risk factor changes in the Minnesota Heart Health Program. *American Journal of Public Health, 84*, 1383-1393.

Manley, M., Epps, R., Husten, C., Glynn, T., & Shopland, D. (1991). Clinical interventions in tobacco control: A National Cancer Institute training program for physicians. *Journal of the American Medical Association, 266*, 3172-3173.

McPhee, S. J., Bird, J. A., Jenkins, C. N. H., & Fordham, D. (1989). Promoting cancer screening: A randomized controlled trial of three interventions. *Archives of Internal Medicine, 149*, 1866-1872.

Miller, W. R., & Rollnick, S. (1991). *Motivational interviewing: Preparing people to change addictive behavior*. New York: Guilford Press.

Ockene, J., Kristeller, J., Goldberg, R., Ockene, I., Merriam, P., Barret, S., Pekow, P., Hosmer, D., & Gianelly, R. (1992). Smoking cessation and severity of disease: The coronary artery smoking intervention study. *Health Psychology, 11*, 119-126.

Ockene, J. K., Hosmer, D. W., Williams, J. W., & Goldberg, R. J. (1987). The relationship of patient characteristics to physician delivery of advice to stop smoking. *Journal of General and Internal Medicine, 2*, 117-340.

Orlandi, M. A. (1987). Promoting health and preventing disease in health care settings: An analysis of barriers. *Preventive Medicine, 16*, 119-130.

Orleans, C. T. (1993). Treating nicotine dependence in medical settings: A stepped-care model. In C. T. Orleans & J. Slade (Eds.), *Nicotine addiction: Principles and management* (pp. 145-162). New York: Oxford University Press.

Orleans, C. T., Glynn, T. M., Manley, M. W., & Slade, J. (1993). Minimal-contact quit smoking strategies for medical settings. In C. T. Orleans & J. Slade (Eds.), *Nicotine addiction: Principles and management* (pp. 181-221). New York: Oxford University Press.

Orleans, C. T., Jepson, C., Resch, N., & Rimer, B. K. (1994). Quitting motives and barriers among older smokers: The 1986 Adult Use of Tobacco Survey revisited. *Cancer, 74*, 2055-2061.

Orleans, C. T., Kristeller, J. L., & Gritz, E. R. (1993). Helping hospitalized smokers quit: New directions for treatment and research *Journal of Consulting and Clinical Psychology, 61*, 778-789.

Orleans, C. T., Resch, N., Noll, E., Keintz, M. K., Rimer, B. K., Brown, T. V., & Snedden, T. M. (1994). Use of transdermal nicotine in a state-level prescription plan for the elderly. *Journal of the American Medical Association, 271*, 601-607.

Orleans, C. T., Rotberg, H., Quade, D., & Lees, P. (1990). A hospital quit-smoking consult service: Clinical report and intervention guidelines. *Preventive Medicine, 19*, 198-212.

Orleans, C. T., Schoenbach, V. J., Quade, D., Salmon, M. A., Pearson, D. C., Fiedler, J., Porter, C. Q., & Kaplan, B. H.

(1991). Self-help quit smoking interventions: Effects of self-help materials, social support instructions, and telephone counseling. *Journal of Consulting and Clinical Psychology, 59*, 439-448.

Orleans, C. T., & Slade, J. (Eds.). (1993). *Nicotine addiction: Principles and management*. New York: Oxford University Press.

Ossip-Klein, D. J., Giovino, G. A., Megahed, N., Black, P. M., Emont, S. L., Stiggins, J., Shulman, E., & Moore, L. (1991). Effects of a smokers' hotline: Results of a 10-county self-help trial. *Journal of Consulting and Clinical Psychology, 59*, 325-332.

Perez-Stable, E. J., VanOss, T., Marin, B., & Marin, G. (1993). A comprehensive smoking cessation program for the San Francisco Bay Area Latino community: Programa Latino Para Dejar de Fumar. *American Journal of Health Promotion, 51*, 390-395.

Pierce, J., Farkas, A., Evans, N., Berry, C., Chio, W., Rosbrook, B., Johnson, M., & Bal, D. G. (1993). *Tobacco use in California: A focus on preventing uptake in adolescents*. Sacramento: California Department of Health Services.

Pierce, J. P., Macaskill, P., & Hill, D. (1990). Long-term effectiveness of mass media led antismoking campaigns in Australia. *America Journal of Public Health, 80*, 565-569.

Pirie, P. L., McBride, C. M., Hellerstedt, W., Jeffery, R. W., Hatsukami, D., Allen, S., & Lando, H. (1992). Smoking cessation in women concerned about weight. *American Journal of Public Health, 82*, 1238-1243.

Prochaska, J. O. (1991). Assessing how people change. *Cancer, 67*(Suppl.), S805-S807.

Prochaska, J. O., DiClemente, C. C., & Norcross, J. C. (1992). In search of how people change: Applications to addictive behavior. *American Psychologist, 47*, 1102-1114.

Prochaska, J. O., DiClemente, C. C., Velicer, W. F., & Rossi, J. S. (1993). Standardized, individualized, interactive and personalized self-help programs for smoking cessation. *Health Psychology, 12*, 399-405.

Ramirez, A. G., & Gallion, K. J. (1993). Nicotine dependence among blacks and Hispanics. In C. T. Orleans & J. Slade (Eds.), *Nicotine addiction: Principles and management* (pp. 349-364). New York: Oxford University Press.

Rimer, B. K., Orleans, C. T., Fleisher, L., Cristinzio, S., Resch, N., Telepchak, J., & Keintz, M. K. (1994). Does tailoring mater? The impact of a tailored guide on ratings and short-term smoking-related outcomes for older smokers. *Health Education Research, 9*, 69-84.

Rimer, B. K., Orleans, C. T., Keintz, M. K., Cristinzio, S., & Fleisher, L. K. (1990). The older smoker: Status, challenges and opportunities for intervention. *Chest, 97*, 547-553.

Risser, N. L., & Belcher, D. W. (1990). Adding spirometry, carbon monoxide feedback and pulmonary symptom results to smoking cessation counseling. *Journal of General and Internal Medicine, 97*, 547-553.

Salina, D., Jason, L. A., Hedeker, D., Kaufman, J., Lesondak, L., McMahon, S. C., Taylor, S., & Kimball, P. (1994). A follow-up of a media-based worksite smoking cessation program. *American Journal of Community Psychology, 22*, 257-271.

Schwartz, J. L. (1987). *Review and evaluation of smoking cessation methods: The United States and Canada, 1978-1985*. NIH Publication No. 87-2940. Bethesda, MD: Division of Cancer Prevention and Control, National Cancer Institute, U.S. Department of Health and Human Services.

Shiffman, S. (1993). Smoking cessation treatment: Any progress? *Journal of Consulting and Clinical Psychology, 61*, 718-722.

Solomon, L. J., & Flynn, B. S. (1993). Women who smoke. In C. T. Orleans & J. Slade (Eds.), *Nicotine addiction: Principles and management* (pp. 339-349). New York: Oxford University Press.

Sorensen, G., Hsieh, J. Hunt, M. K., Morris, D. H., Harris, D. R., & Fitzgerald, G. (1992). Employee advisory boards as a vehicle for organizing worksite health promotion programs. *American Journal of Health Promotion, 6*, 443-450.

Sorensen, G., Thompson, B., Glanz, K., Feng, Z., Kinne, S., DiClemente, C., Emmons, K., Heimendinger, J., Probart, C., & Lichtenstein, E. (for the Working Well Trial). (1996). Worksite-based cancer prevention: Primary results from the Working Well trial. *American Journal of Public Health, 86*, 939-947.

Steckler, A., & Goodman, R. M. (1989). How to institutionalize health promotion programs. *American Journal of Health Promotion, 3*, 34-44.

Stevens, V. J., Glasgow, R. E., Hollis, J. F., Lichtenstein, E., & Vogt, T. M. (1993). A smoking-cessation intervention for hospital patients. *Medical Care, 31*, 65-72.

Strecher, V. J., Becker, M. H., Kirscht, J. P., Eraker, S. A., & Graham-Tomasi, R. P. (1985). Evaluation of a minimal-contact smoking cessation program in a health care setting. *Patient Education and Counseling, 7*, 395-407.

Strecher, V. J., Kreuter, M., Den Boer, D., Kobrin, S., Hospers, H. J., & Skinner, C. S. (1994). The effects of computer-tailored smoking cessation messages in family practice settings. *Journal of Family Practice, 39*, 262-268.

Taylor, C. B., Houston-Miller, N., Killen, J. D., & DeBusk, R. F. (1990). Smoking cessation after acute myocardial infarction: Effects of a nurse-managed intervention. *Annals of Internal Medicine, 113*, 118-123.

Terborg, J. R., & Glasgow, R. E. (1994). Worksite interventions: A brief review of health promotion programs at work. In A. Baum, C. McManus, S. Newman, J. Weinman, & R. West (Eds.), *Cambridge handbook of psychology, health and medicine*. London: Cambridge University Press.

The Smoking Cessation Clinical Practice Guideline Panel and Staff. (1996). Consensus Statement: The Agency for Health Care Policy and Research Smoking Cessation Clinical Practice Guideline. *Journal of the American Medical Association, 275*, 1270-1280.

U.S. Department of Health and Human Services. (1989). *Reducing the health consequences of smoking: A report of the Surgeon General*. DHHS Publication No. CDC 89-8411. Washington, DC: U.S. Government Printing Office.

U.S. Department of Health and Human Services. (1994). *Preventing tobacco use among young people: A report of the Surgeon General*. Washington, DC: U.S. Government Printing Office.

U.S. Public Health Service. (1964). *Smoking and health: Report of the Advisory Committee to the Surgeon General of the Public Health Service*. PHS Publication No. 1103. Atlanta, GA: Centers for Disease Control, U.S. Public Health Service, U.S. Department of Health, Education and Welfare.

U.S. Public Health Service. (1993). 1992 National Survey of Worksite Health Promotion Activities: Summary. *American Journal of Health Promotion*, 7, 452-464.

Velicer, W. F., Prochaska, J. O., Rossi, J. S., & Snow, M. G. (1992). Assessing outcome in smoking cessation studies. *Psychological Bulletin*, *111*, 23-41.

Windsor, R. A., Cutter, G., Moris, J., Reese, Y., Manzella, B., Bartlett, E. E., Samuelson, C., & Spanos, D. (1985). The effectiveness of smoking cessation methods for smokers in public health maternity clinics: A randomized trial. *American Journal of Public Health*, *75*, 1389-1392.

Working Well Research Group. (in press). Cancer control at the workplace: The Working Well Trial. *Preventive Medicine*.

20

Accepting Occupational Safety and Health Regimens

Alexander Cohen and Michael J. Colligan

INTRODUCTION

In October 1991, the National Institute of Mental Health (NIMH) sponsored a workshop the aim of which was to identify the major parameters of behavioral influence. It was expected that the end product would serve as a general paradigm or set of guidelines for designing behavioral interventions related to the prevention of AIDS. The participants were well-recognized figures in behavioral science and related fields.[1] Following three days of discussion, eight variables were identified as the primary determinants of behavior: (1) ability, (2) intention, (3) environmental constraints, (4) anticipated outcomes, (5) norms, (6) self-standards, (7) emotion, and (8) self-efficacy.

The first three variables were viewed as necessary and sufficient causes of action. If a person is to follow a prescribed routine reliably (e.g., to practice safe sex), the person must be capable of performing that act, want to or intend to perform that act, and not be constrained from performing that act. Behavior is therefore best understood as the product of ability, motivation, and opportunity.

The remaining five variables were viewed as factors that influence the intentional or motivational component of behavioral influence, in terms of both strength and direction. Thus, even though an individual may be knowledgeable and competent in a particular area (i.e., well trained), the person's actual level of performance depends on such motivational considerations as the anticipated costs and rewards, self-esteem, confidence, and conformity pressures toward internal and external standards.

For individuals responsible for workplace safety management, the model outlined above serves as a humbling reminder that the develop-

[1]Invited attendees were Drs. Albert Bandura, Marshall Becker, Anita Eichler, Martin Fishbein, Frederick Kanfer, Susan E. Middlestadt, and Harry C. Triandis. The workshop proceedings are summarized in a 1992 report titled "Factors Influencing Behavior and Behavior Change," which is available from the National Institute of Mental Health, Rockville, Maryland.

Alexander Cohen • Consultant—Occupational Human Factors, 6752 East Farmacres Drive, Cincinnati, Ohio 45237. **Michael J. Colligan** • Education and Information Division, National Institute for Occupational Safety and Health, Cincinnati, Ohio 45226.

Handbook of Health Behavior Research II: Provider Determinants, edited by David S. Gochman. Plenum Press, New York, 1997.

ment and maintenance of safe behaviors is an arduous and continuous task. Simplistic safety campaigns that rely solely on poster displays, lost-time accident graphics, and packaged training videos to establish safe work practices and other prescribed risk-reducing behaviors are doomed to fail. Yet occupational injury and illness remain serious threats to public health. According to Bureau of Labor Statistics reports, 3 million workers were disabled by work injuries and more than 6000 fatally injured in 1992 (*Safety Compliance Letter*, 1994). These figures do not include workers debilitated by occupation-related illness and disease.

Traditional attempts to reduce or abate workplace hazards have involved a number of approaches including the application of engineering or physical controls, the use of monitoring systems, the promotion of safe work practices, and the use of personal protective equipment. Machines designed or retrofitted with built-in safety features, substitution of less hazardous materials, closed (containment) ventilation systems, and automation of hazardous operations are examples of engineering or physical techniques to attain hazard control and risk reduction.

Monitoring systems furnish information about whether industrial processes or operating equipment are in fact functioning normally, i.e., are under control. If there is a process control breakdown or malfunction, signals can be communicated, including worker alerts to take evasive action. Safe work practices are procedures or behavioral sequences that employees are expected to follow in order to reduce exposures to harmful agents or to minimize the probability of injury. Protective equipment consists of devices or materials (e.g., respirators, hearing protectors, hard hats, safety goggles) that employees wear to reduce exposure to potentially harmful conditions.

Eliminating known dangers in industrial processes through engineering controls is the preferred strategy, in large part because physical or process controls "engineer out" the hazard at the source with little or no apparent worker involvement. Adherence to safe procedures and the wearing of protective equipment, in comparison, require much more active worker participation and are therefore viewed as less reliable control strategies due to human variance. In addition, labor unions fear that management, given the choice, will endorse behavioral interventions over more costly engineering controls, thereby shifting the burden and responsibility for safety to the individual worker.

In actuality, workers' actions and behaviors are important components of any workplace hazard control program. Even the most automated engineering controls are ineffective if workers do not use them properly. Ventilatory systems do not work if individuals do not turn them on or do not change filters and perform routine maintenance. Machine guards are useless if they are dismantled, and pressure-sensitive switches, monitoring systems, and alarms can be overridden to make them inoperable. It simply isn't possible to eliminate the "human element" from the safety formula. A. Cohen (1987) has previously stressed this point in commenting on a report by Conard (1983) that listed the following eight broad categories of behaviors that affect safety performance in the workplace:

1. Proper use and operation of the hazard control systems in place, thus realizing their maximum protective benefits. To illustrate, spray painting in ventilated booths with spray mist arrestors is one means of reducing hazards in spray painting. Without prescribed employee actions, however, such as activating the booth ventilation system, spraying within the capture range of the ventilation, and ensuring that the mist arrestors are not saturated, these control measures would have little effect.

2. Work habits in performing job tasks that could include acts that unnecessarily increase the risk of injury or illness. Employees have under their control many behavioral options that can influence exposure to hazards. H. H. Cohen and Jensen (1984) found in observing driver behaviors in forklift truck operations that the drivers frequently failed to signal or yield to coworkers

at intersections, a factor implicated in accidents involving their equipment.

3. An increased awareness and recognition of workplace hazards. Recognition of hazards is a necessary first step to avoiding them. Educational and informational techniques for this purpose may include the use of labels, information posters, safety pamphlets, pocket cards, and safety data sheets, all of which may be coupled with regular training activities in which the avoidance actions themselves are expected to be addressed.

4. Acceptance and use of personal protective equipment. Respirators and hearing protectors are the best-known protective devices, but present particular difficulties in terms of effective fit, encumbrance, and general discomfort (Acton, 1977; Morgan, 1983).

5. Observance of housekeeping and maintenance measures to keep work areas clear of agents that could pose additional risks of illness or injury. Hopkins (1981) observed that simply failing to replace lids on trash contains of styrene-coated scraps in laminated plastics manufacturing processes increased the concentration of the toxic styrene material in the work environment.

6. Following good personal hygiene practices, such as regularly washing, showering, changing, and laundering work clothes, and not eating in processing and production areas. Failure to follow these practices can nullify other modes of contact or exacerbate retention of toxic materials that could amplify their hazard potential.

7. Proper responses to emergency situations. Proper employee responses are critical if there is a chemical spill, fire, control equipment failure, explosion, or machine malfunction. Employees must be informed, trained, and rehearsed in procedures that will enable them to cope effectively with the apparent danger.

8. Self-monitoring and early recognition of any signs or symptoms of hazardous exposures. Instructing workers in early symptom recognition can help to avoid more serious problems.

It is clear from these examples that worker involvement and cooperation are essential in reducing workplace injury and illness. Accordingly, it is the intent of this chapter to address issues of worker acceptance of occupational safety and health regimens. The approach to be taken will be to first analyze and examine impediments to workers' behaving safely—i.e., adopting and complying with safe, healthful workplace practices—and then to identify strategies for overcoming these obstacles. The treatment throughout is organized around the three general factors identified by the NIMH workshop as being critical behavioral determinants: (1) ability factors, (2) intentional and motivational factors, and (3) environmental factors.

IMPEDIMENTS TO SAFE BEHAVIOR

It is tempting to assume that if workers are given enough information about an occupational or environmental hazard and instruction on how to avoid or control it, they will automatically adopt recommended safe work practices. This assumption is consistent with beliefs that safety and self-protection are basic human motives (e.g., Maslow, 1954). The challenge for the safety manager, then, would be to develop training programs and health communications designed to apprise employees of work-related risks and their respective safeguards. In fact, recent "right to know" regulations at both the local and the national level already require employers to inform workers about job-specific hazards as part of the work contract. The federal Hazard Communications Standard (Code of Federal Regulations 1910.120), for example mandates that employers establish comprehensive hazard communication programs that include container labeling and other forms of warning, material safety data sheets, and employee training.

The intent of these regulations is admirable, and they are a necessary step in promoting worker safety and well-being. As noted by Atkin and Wallach (1990), however, information alone does not lead to prevention, and there are nu-

perceptual biases, which predispose one to see safe behavior as the other party's responsibility, may diminish one's willingness or capacity to understand the nature of the hazard and the importance of self-protection.

It should be apparent that training and health risk communication are extremely important components of any hazard control program. Furthermore, these efforts have to be tailored to the specific information needs of the workforce. Perceptual sets, attribution biases, heuristics, and similar cognitive processes may interfere with workers' ability to objectively interpret the material as presented and respond to it in the prescribed manner. Considerations for designing occupational health risk communications have been discussed elsewhere (e.g., A. Cohen, Colligan, & Berger, 1985). Specific suggestions for improving occupational safety and health training programs are detailed later in this chapter.

Intentional and Motivational Factors

Unfortunately, compliance with safe behavior practices often imposes on the worker a variety of costs that must be overcome. These costs can take on many forms involving added time, effort, discomfort, cognitive or attentional demands, and social or interpersonal penalties. For example, OSHA-mandated procedures require a worker to go through a series of elaborate and time-consuming (though vitally necessary) steps before working in a confined space. Among others, the steps involved are: (1) isolating the space prior to entry; (2) taking air samples in the space to identify any atmospheric hazards; (3) purging, flushing, or ventilating the space to eliminate any such hazards detected; (4) securing and donning necessary protective equipment; (5) establishing a communication link between those entering the space and posted observers; and (6) setting up the equipment and identifying standby personnel in the event of an emergency requiring rescue (Code of Federal Regulations 1910.147). Each of these steps, in turn, involves a separate set of actions that are to be followed. As can be seen, proper entry into a confined space can be a burdensome chore for a hurried worker under pressure to make a repair as quickly as possible.

In order to ensure compliance, the individual not only must be properly trained but also highly motivated such that the benefits of behaving safely are perceived as outweighing the costs (e.g., Rosenstock, 1974). Benefits of safe behavior can be intrinsic, such as the satisfaction of a "job well done" or the avoidance of anxiety from knowing that one has taken the necessary precautions to protect one's health. The benefits can also be extrinsic, such as recognition and appreciation of others, improved performance ratings, material rewards, or similar outcomes. Costs can likewise be intrinsic or extrinsic, can vary from worker to worker, and to some extent are situationally specific. Workers' reasons for not wearing hearing protection in a foundry will differ from their reasons for not following mandated procedures for a confined-space entry at a construction site. Nevertheless, it is important to understand, at least generically, the types of motivational impediments to safe behavior. Failure to recognize and address these obstacles in a safety-management program will nullify the effects of even the best-laid training programs.

Perhaps one way to understand at least some of the impediments to safe behavior is to examine the reasons for worker resistance to the use of personal protective equipment. In situations in which engineering controls (e.g., ventilation, material substitution) are not feasible, workers must rely upon protective apparel such as gloves, safety glasses, respirators, and impermeable garments to protect themselves against workplace hazards. Often this equipment is either inconvenient, uncomfortable, or even hazardous to the workers who use it. Latex gloves, worn as a protection against bloodborne pathogens, have been associated with a variety of dermatological problems. Heat stress is a frequent complaint of hazardous waste workers who must wear encapsulated suits when working at cleanup sites. Plastic safety goggles may fog in hot or humid environments, resulting in impaired vision. Morgan

(1983), for example, has presented a wide range of complaints associated with respirator usage including tunnel vision, restricted communication, labored breathing, impaired performance, and personal discomfort.

Such problems are immediate and salient to the worker, whereas the hazards the equipment is designed to combat may be remote and imperceptible. It is not surprising that under these circumstances, workers are inclined to ignore the safety equipment. One solution available to the safety manager is to reduce worker burden by such means as selecting equipment that has been engineered to be user-friendly and as comfortable as possible. Invoking such a solution, however, is not as easy as it appears. In the first place, not all costs involve physical discomfort. White, Baker, Larson, and Wolford (1988) surveyed a sample of painters regarding their beliefs about the protective benefits of respirators as well as usage patterns. While personal discomfort and inconvenience were the most frequently cited reasons for not wearing respirators, other factors such as concerns about appearing foolish, feeling entrapped, and being unable to smoke were also significantly related to intended usage. The authors conclude that the most effective strategy to increase worker acceptance of respirators would have to be multidimensional in nature due to the range of cognitive, emotional, and physical factors that affect usage.

In the second place, it must be recognized that behaving safely will always involve some cost or added burden; to expect otherwise is unrealistic. To the extent that workers are inconvenienced, they are likely to examine their share of the safety burden relative to other segments of the work environment. If they feel that their costs are disproportionate, the resulting resentment may interfere with their willingness to follow recommended practices. Requiring workers to wear a respirator or hearing protection when they believe that low-cost engineering controls are available for abating workplace hazards produces a state that Brehm (1966) has referred to as "reactance." Individuals who feel that their behavior is being manipulated or unfairly coerced will react defiantly as a means of establishing their independence and restoring their sense of control. Such defiance can occur when management relies upon punitive tactics such as reprimands or threats to enforce safety policy or when workers perceive that they are bearing the brunt of the responsibility for the safety function. Consequently, workers may behave safely in the presence of their managers but resort to shortcuts and risky actions in the absence of supervision. Unfortunately, the resulting "illusion of safety" may serve to convince management that it has done its job.

Finally, it must be noted that reactance can also be generated by safety programs that emphasize positive incentives or reinforcements. If workers feel that management is using a reward system insincerely or unilaterally in an attempt to avoid its own responsibilities in the safety effort, hostility and noncompliance are likely to occur. This possibility indicates the importance of organizational climate and managerial style in promoting behavioral safety.

Environmental Factors

No matter how well trained and highly motivated, individuals cannot perform safely on the job without the necessary resources and organizational support. Feeney (1986), for example, has listed some of the conditions that must be met before workers can be expected to effectively use protective equipment: (1) They must be aware of the hazard that surrounds them; (2) the protective equipment must be easily and conveniently accessible; (3) workers must understand how the equipment works in protecting them against the hazard and how to use it properly; and (4) there must be no other factors present that will interfere with workers carrying out their jobs productively while using the equipment. Even a cursory examination of these conditions indicates that management must be heavily involved in creating the proper climate.

Smith, Cohen, Cohen, and Cleveland (1978),

in an attempt to describe the influence of organizational factors on accident rates, conducted on-site surveys of seven matched pairs of high- versus low-frequency accident rate plants. The plants with low accident rates were characterized by high efficiency, good human resource practices and policies (i.e., the presence of affirmative action, counseling, and career development programs), good supervisor-employee relations in terms of both frequency and quality, low turnover, and low absenteeism.

Similar findings were described in an earlier study by Simonds and Shafai-Sahrai (1977), who compared 11 pairs of high- and low-accident worksites. Again, low accident rates were associated with involvement of top management in safety promotion, better injury record-keeping systems, roomy and clean workspace, the existence of employee recreational programs, and good supervisor-employee relations.

Interestingly, neither study found a relationship between the quality and quantity of safety rules and accident rate. The absence of such a relationship is not surprising if one accepts the idea that the informal climate or culture of an organization may have an impact on safety practices greater than that of formal policy. In making this distinction, Pidgeon (1991) argues that the development of a safety culture is contingent, not on the formulation of explicit rules and procedures, but on the cultivation of a set of shared beliefs, attitudes, roles, and norms regarding the importance of worker safety to the organization. Cues that workers use to gauge the underlying commitment of management to safety will be discussed later.

Summary

The preceding sections elaborated on various impediments to workers' adopting safe work practices and behaviors for reducing risk of occupational disease and injury. As presented, the various obstacles touched on ability/knowledge, intentional/motivational, and situational/organizational concerns and were so classified. To summarize the more troubling issues:

- In the ability/knowledge area, the discussion noted perceptual and cognitive biases that have the effect of distorting one's knowledge or appreciation of actual risk levels and one's attribution processes in ways that can undercut needs for self-protection.
- In the intentional/motivational area, mention was made of the added time, effort, discomfort, and penalties imposed by adhering to safety regimens, especially in the absence of any apparent benefit or sense of shared responsibility.
- In the situational/organizational area, there were implicit questions of whether the workplace climate, as determined by management's policies, actions, and allocation of resources, fully supported appropriate, safe behaviors among those at risk.

STRATEGIES FOR OVERCOMING PROBLEMATIC FACTORS

This section will address strategies to overcome these problems. In doing so, it is important to acknowledge that the behavioral science and occupational safety and health literature documents many ideas in dealing with skill or knowledge problems bearing on ability issues, feedback/incentive approaches to bolster intention or motivation, and organizational changes to relieve constraints or create an environment more supportive of the behavior goals in question. The section first offers a brief summary of this literature, acknowledging elements that have implications for addressing the particular problems noted. Subsequently, two studies illustrating certain applications in more detail are described.

Training to Enhance Ability and Knowledge

One's ability to function effectively in various tasks is in large measure dependent on the knowledge, skill, and attitudes one has acquired through proper training and practice. While many worksite studies report training successes in effecting safe work practices and other actions aimed at reducing exposure to workplace hazards, these successes seem to be the products of efforts guided by individual researchers and not the norm. Indeed, current training activities for industry as a whole appear suspect, especially since lack of compliance with OSHA training rules is among the most frequently reported violations (communication with OSHA Office of Data Management). Part of the problem is that OSHA training rules appear as a mix of fragmented statements in different standards and give no sense of the need for an orderly plan.

Recognizing this shortcoming, OSHA (1988) has issued guidelines for developing a training plan in more systematic fashion, mirroring steps found effective in general job training (Campbell, 1988; A. Cohen & Colligan, 1995). The guidelines are to assure that (1) a problem is solvable by training, (2) the training objectives are clearly defined, (3) the learning material and activities appropriately stress the particular needs and active participation of the trainees, and (4) evaluations are performed to determine whether objectives are met or revisions are in order. A. Cohen and Colligan (1995), in their review of workplace safety training, offer excerpts from the literature pointing out the merits of these guidelines.

Emergent too are program efforts not only to instruct workers in safety fundamentals, but also to give them skills in problem solving and teamwork to identify and solve job hazards, and even to learn how to effect actions aimed at creating a safer workplace through networking, committee processes, and contract negotiations (Office of Technology Assessment, 1985). These developments are viewed as positive in respecting the fact that today's workers are on the whole better educated, seek greater involvement in decisions affecting their jobs, and have greater expectations about their job roles. The changes also recognize the subtler nature of today's workplace hazards, given shifts from heavy industry to "high-tech" work environments, more varied and complex forms of human-equipment interactions, and a much faster pace of work.

Feedback and Incentives as Intentional and Motivational Factors

Sulzer-Azaroff, Harris, and McCann (1994) charted over 40 workplace studies that make a strong case for showing how feedback, goal setting, and incentive/reward strategies can shape safe, protective behaviors among workers at risk. The greatest number of these citations reflect how goal setting and feedback techniques, by giving knowledge of results, can motivate the learning of safe behaviors during training. Even more dramatic results for these treatments are seen posttraining or in the actual job situation. In many of these studies, in fact, the training seems incidental, merely taking the form of workers viewing right and wrong ways of performing various tasks, usually in one session. The main emphasis is on monitoring of worker compliance with the safe acts when at the job site and varying the nature of information feedback to the workers who may have set up safe performance goals to further spur compliance behavior. The overwhelming results from these studies prompted the conclusion that training by itself did not account for improvements in worker safety and health, but rather that the improvements derived from feedback indicating compliance or progress in meeting performance goals. To quote Sulzer-Azaroff et al. (1994, p. 336): "Training alone might have promoted [behavioral] change, but often this change tended to dissipate unless it was coupled with specific, timely, frequent feedback with goal setting and/or positive consequences."

The literature on performance feedback and use of incentives as a means of altering behavior in general and workplace safety in particular was reviewed by Lindell (1994) and McAfee and Winn (1989). Conditions that favor consistently positive results are those in which the feedback includes a tangible reward, is administered by a supervisor, and occurs at least biweekly. Private versus public feedback and individual versus group performance feedback appear to be about equally effective. Lindell (1994) explains how workers respond to feedback and incentive programs in different ways depending upon their expectations regarding the outcomes of their actions and the values they see in the rewards offered. He notes that individualized rewards such as T-shirts, jackets, and caps may offer the best reminders of the safe actions that achieved them, yet may be viewed as least rewarding to those who would prefer cash or gift certificates offering more options to fit their wants. Group awards may decrease the size of individual awards but provide for peer pressure to maintain safe performance.

Organizational and Environmental Factors

It is contended that a company's safety climate, as defined by the workers' shared perceptions of management's attitude toward safety and its importance in everyday operations, can guide and direct appropriate task behaviors (Zohar, 1980). By their direct involvement in safety matters, by giving priority to safety issues in company meetings and planning decisions, and by affording stature to the safety officer's role and holding supervisors accountable for the safety performance of their units, top management can send a strong message about how the subject of safety is to be viewed by the workforce as a whole. So too can its sanction of program practices that emphasize (1) instruction in hazard identification and control as part of early employee indoctrination and follow-up training and (2) close contact and interaction among workers, supervisors, and management, enabling free, open communications on all job issues including safety. The value of these measures appears well substantiated; studies show that companies with these program practices have exemplary safety records or better safety performance than those with poorer performance (A. Cohen, 1977).

A specific strategy that encompasses these considerations of management style, safety awareness, and communications is one accenting a worker-participatory approach. Benefits that high-level interactions among managers, supervisors, and workers can achieve include these:

1. Greater involvement and sustained interest of all parties in safety issues, and related activities.
2. Broadened problem-defining and problem-solving capabilities.
3. Improved coordination among different groups and greater knowledge of company operations.

Worker participation in industrial management practices is growing as a result of two developments. One is that the need to remain competitive in today's markets has caused companies to downsize and restructure their operations. In so doing, they have removed layers of middle management or supervision to save on costs and have given work units at lower levels more autonomy in directing operations, including those concerned with workplace safety and health (LeBar, 1993). Greater worker involvement is seen as the key to success in making this change. The second development is the acceptance of total quality management (TQM) principles, which empower workers to solve problems, help improve processes, and foster teamwork to ensure quality efforts at each stage of producing a product or delivering a service (Millar, 1993). Safety and health objectives can be readily folded into TQM programs in which work-related injury and illness cases are treated as defects in the quality of the work process. Signs of unsafe conditions, poor work practices, and risky worker behaviors are targets for joint worker-management actions aimed at eliminating them.

Worker-participation successes have been reported in two types of job hazard control activities (see the review in Gjessing, Schoenborn, & Cohen, 1994): (1) enhancing the detection of previously unrecognized physical hazards by having workers play a more direct role in hazard surveillance and (2) having workers serve on ergonomics work teams with the aim of modifying work environments and processes that place workers at risk of strain or wear-and-tear musculoskeletal injuries, or otherwise complicate safe work behaviors. At the same time, these cases point up certain requirements to make the strategy work. For example, both workers and management involved in the joint effort will need added training not only in the technical skills of hazard control but also in learning how to communicate with each other. Indeed, workers will need instruction in how to interact in groups, supervisors in how to listen and in feedback skills. Related to the latter requirement, precautions also have to be taken to prevent supervisors and managers on a team from intimidating worker members or dominating discussions. Further, the first problems chosen for study should be relatively easy ones to solve and offer promise of quick implementation; to begin by tackling more difficult problems or those requiring proposed changes that will not be immediately realizable can have demoralizing effects on the group's efforts. These and other issues concerned with worker participation in occupational safety and health are discussed in Gjessing et al. (1994).

Applications to the Problems at Hand

How do these training, motivational, and organizational considerations help to resolve the problems discussed earlier? Foremost should be the thought that any effective strategy must take account of all three factors; total reliance on any one will not prove worthwhile. Two studies (Zohar, Cohen, & Azar, 1980; Zohar & Fussfeld, 1981) in effecting greater use of ear protectors for reducing noise hazards to hearing are illustrative. One study setting was the metal fabrication plant and the other a textile factory, in both of which workers were exposed to noise levels that posed a risk of permanent hearing loss. In both plants, earplugs were provided and efforts were made to enhance use of the plugs through presentation of hearing conservation lectures, poster campaigns, talks by safety officials, and even threats to remove nonusers from the production line. Despite these efforts, use rates were merely 35%. The prevailing view among workers and supervisors alike was that earplugs were uncomfortable and hindered the monitoring of machine operations. Managers also feared that the disciplinary threats to remove nonusers would be too disruptive of operations.

Overcoming the earplug-use problem at the two plants involved different approaches. The one used in the metal fabrication plant recognized that noise-induced hearing loss is an insidious disorder. Daily noise exposure in itself does not cause readily perceptible signs that would alert workers to impending ear damage, which typically results from cumulative years of exposure. To make workers aware of this reality, the metal fabrication plant introduced an intervention program in which, in addition to instructions on hearing conservation and use of earplugs, workers were given hearing tests before and after their workshifts on days during which they did wear and did not wear the earplugs. The intent was to show workers how their hearing was being affected by measuring temporary threshold changes in their ears' response to sound from each day's noise insult and how these changes would be minimized by use of the protectors. Brief exposure to noise levels that will cause permanent hearing damage after long-term exposure invariably produces temporary changes that subside after a period of quiet, reflecting the ear's recovery from the overstimulation (Kryter, 1970). In this case, the temporary changes were used as an early warning indicator of the risk of permanent hearing loss. To further reinforce this idea, the audiograms of workers who regularly wore protection and of those who did not were also posted, the latter showing substantial permanent loss.

Following this program, earplug use rose to near 90% and remained there even though there was a significant turnover of personnel in this plant and new hires were present who had not gone through the threshold testing. The sustaining effect of this behavioral change was explained as due to two factors. First, the acceptance of earplugs by such a large number of workers in effect created new norms and behavior standards favoring their use. Second, managerial standards were also changed. Seeing the success of the intervention, managers became more insistent about the use of ear protection.

The second approach, used in the textile factory, utilized a token reinforcement plan developed jointly by workers and department managers. Inputs from both were used to determine the values of tokens to be issued to workers found to be wearing earplugs during tours of work areas taken at random times, appealing products for which the tokens could be exchanged, and details on how managers would monitor the overall effort. Recognizing that workers require some time to adapt to wearing earplugs, the joint worker-manager group defined time bands of increasing length for token-dispensing tours at the outset of the program and agreed that the program would be in effect for no more than 2 months.

The results of this effort were similar to those noted in the metal fabrication plant. The level of earplug use jumped to nearly 90% shortly after the start of the token-dispensing program and remained there long after the program was terminated. As in the metal fabrication plant, this result was explained by noting that the upsurge in earplug use marking the success of the token strategy caused a change in managers' behavior. Given this outcome, their initial skepticism changed, and having been involved in the planning, application, and monitoring stages of the program, they continued to reinforce the heightened level of earplug use through greater oversight and example.

The reader will recognize in these studies elements of the problems summarized earlier and the dependence on training, motivational, and organizational factors in efforts to overcome them. For example, on the matter of perceptual bias hindering one's appreciation of true risk levels, adding a special form of feedback to a conventional training effort was seen as enhancing workers' awareness of a hazard that would otherwise go unheeded, and in ways that showed personal vulnerability. As a result, through demonstration of its effectiveness in reducing risk, use of protective equipment, though uncomfortable and burdensome, became more acceptable. This finding is in accord with the health belief model, which posits that people's likelihood of complying with a safety regimen is a joint function of (1) the extent to which they believe themselves susceptible to a particular health threat, (2) whether they believe the outcome is serious, and (3) whether they believe the preventive action would be effective (Rosenstock, 1974). Other examples in which surrogate indicators have been used to make workplace hazard exposures and risk more personally salient are to be found in the literature. They include use of "near-miss" incidents to heighten attention to would-be accident risks and use of certain biological measures as early warning indicators of exposure to toxic materials (Maples, Jacoby, Johnson, Ter Haar, & Buckingham, 1982; A. Cohen & Colligan, 1995). In each instance, these approaches prompted increased self-protective actions.

In the absence of these kinds of displays, and reflecting motivational approaches, offering rewards as an incentive also overcame the resistance to burdensome protective measures. Moreover, making workers party to the plan, including rewards that had appeal to them, and allowing time for them to accommodate to wearing the protective equipment added to the positive effect. Similarly, management's participation with workers in mounting the program and its apparent success caused both workers' and managers' behaviors to change. Their later actions to sustain the benefits of the program once the reward phase ended meant more organizational support for the protective measures taken. In respect to these observations, Zohar and Nussfeld (1981) suggest that maintaining safe work regimens need not require continued use of the reward/incentive practices used to establish them. Rather, concurrent changes in the organizational environment can provide the needed reinforcement.

The reader may ask whether any thought was given to an engineering solution to the problem in these two workplaces, which would have relieved the workers of the burden of wearing ear protection. While not noted in either report, noise control technology for the operations in question would have been prohibitively expensive and the expected suppression still not substantial enough to eliminate the hazard. The studies do not mention whether this point was included in justifying earplug use to the workers, but perhaps it should have been if it was not. Doing so could have helped counter any worker sentiment that management was not doing its share in hazard control, one of the concerns raised earlier in analyzing impediments to workers' acceptance of safety regimens.

FURTHER RESEARCH ISSUES

Problem-defining and problem-solving aspects of worker acceptance of safety regimens raise a number of issues requiring follow-on work. This last section mentions a few such needs in the training, motivational, and organizational factor areas that were focal points for the review.

Training Issues

Scheduling Training. Defensible recommendations as to the frequency and length of instruction needed to sustain safe and healthful workplace behaviors are in order. Current schedules for refresher training of this nature appear arbitrary, and their importance in maintaining performance in critical skill or emergency situations cannot be stressed enough. Some research data on retention of job skill training over time (Sitterley, Pietan, & Metaftin, 1974) suggest that lacking practice or task activity, job skills requiring high levels of performance can deteriorate much sooner than anticipated (e.g., between 1 and 4 months for piloting aircraft or firefighting). Also, different skills degrade at different rates; losses in performance of more complex, procedural tasks are greater than those for simpler or straightforward manual operations. In terms of retraining, the same studies found methods that offered dynamic, pictorial representations of the task situation (i.e., movies, videotapes) to be as effective as hands-on practice, although the combination of representation and practice resulted in the greatest recovery.

The implications of these findings for retraining issues in occupational safety and health are obvious. For example, they suggest that priority candidates for more frequent safety and health refreshment training would be those procedures that are rarely used but are nevertheless critical when situations that demand appropriate action arise. Emergency events would fit this category and would therefore justify frequent practice and drills to offset any deterioration in the knowledge and performance of actions to be taken in such occurrences. Cole et al. (1988) discussed this need in connection with evaluating miner skills in donning the self-contained self-rescuer breathing device used in cases of mine fire or explosion. Similar needs for frequent drill may also exist for prescribed safety and health practices that run counter to natural behaviors or that add extra steps to task performance, especially when the hazard risks are not that apparent. Procedures to ensure safe performance in confined-space work and rescue actions as needed would appear to fall in this category.

For other situations, the basis for establishing training and retraining schedules is less clear. Presumably, criteria for determining such scheduling would take account of the complexity of the hazard control measures to be taught, the degree to which they are integrated into everyday work routines (and thus afford opportunities for practice), and local and industry-wide injury and disease incident data for the work in question, among other considerations. It would seem worthwhile to develop a decision logic for occupational safety and health training that would dictate selective scheduling of training and retraining when appropriate, not sooner or later or more or less frequent than required. As part of this exercise, it would also be important to determine the kinds of retraining or refresher experience that could best sustain the desired outcome.

Underserved Groups. Minority and illiterate workers frequently fill the dirtiest menial jobs where there are major occupational safety and health hazards and where knowledge and use of protective measures are imperative. Strategies to train these workers in safety actions and promote adherence to them need to be formulated. Involving minority professionals in leadership roles in this program and engaging respected workers in such groups to help package and present materials in ways that can reach this audience would appear to have merit. There is a need for documentation of experiences in applying these or other approaches in eliminating obstacles and facilitating learning.

Motivational and Promotional Issues

Alternative Reinforcers. That rewards and incentives of various types can shape and reinforce safe behaviors and promote their transfer to the workplace has been well demonstrated. Alternatives to these ideas need to be sought if opportunities for effective use of these techniques prove problematic for reasons already noted. Techniques used for other behavior-management purposes may have some utility, and Ford and Fisher (1994) suggest three different methods used in health promotion programs, in which lifestyle behaviors are the major concern. One is a "buddy system" approach successfully used in smoking reduction, which pairs trainees, each reinforcing the other's need to maintain learning, offer advice, and be alert for signs of relapse in self or buddy. A second is use of "booster sessions," which as an extension of training require periodic face-to-face contact between trainee and trainer. In weight-control studies, inclusion of booster sessions at 2-, 3-, and 5-week intervals induced a greater percentage of maintained weight loss than did the absence of such sessions. The third is a relapse-prevention method that has been used in treating addictive behaviors. In this method, trainees are exposed to situations that pose obstacles to their trained skills and are led through exercises that prepare them to cope with these difficulties.

Research to show how these techniques can support safety behaviors in a workplace subject to a variety of factors that can both enhance and inhibit their expression deserves consideration. Since many worksites are also settings for health promotion programs as well as hazard control activities, real possibilities for integrating the two efforts exist. A. Cohen and Murphy (1989) discuss the benefits of an integrated approach in realizing behavioral outcomes that meet both improved job safety and healthier lifestyle objectives.

Generalization of Effect. As evident in earlier discussions, feedback/incentive programs work best in situations in which the safety behaviors in question are well defined and can be readily observed. Use of protective equipment and compliance with prescribed safe work methods meet these conditions, and the near-uniform success of such interventions in promoting positive results is impressive. One can question, however, whether the effect of reinforcing these specific behaviors is being internalized so as to create a more general, heightened state of safety consciousness. If it is not, what supplemental treatment could help to realize this outcome?

Organizational Issues

Studies analyzing the program practices in companies that display exemplary safety performance have served to define key factors in their success. But using these results to generate a blueprint or model for effective programs is limited for at least two reasons. First, the database does not permit an assessment that would enable one to rank-order the different program factors in terms of their importance. While there is reason to believe that management commitment is controlling, it is not clear how much other considerations such as open communications, extent of training, workforce career growth, and other attributes of successful programs contribute to the end result.

Second, the studies themselves are focused almost entirely on manufacturing and mining companies; the movement to a service-type economy over the past decade brings the relevancy of the findings into question. Along these lines, high-technology jobs and shifts from heavy manual work to mental labor are presenting a new array of potential workplace problems. Job stress and strain, both physical and mental, are more prominent, and each poses added challenges in finding effective solutions. On the basis of consultations with managers of "healthy companies," Rosen (1991) places much weight on a people-oriented culture, defined as one in which (1) there is a strong partnership between employees and managers; (2) individual differences are respected, as is an appreciation of flexibility in doing one's job; (3) high priority is given to the health and well-being of the workforce; and (4) a commitment is made to their self-development. Operational definitions of these ideas and suitable tests to verify their importance are in order.

REFERENCES

Acton, W. I. (1977). Problems associated with the use of hearing protection. *Annals of Occupational Hygiene, 20*, 387-395.

Atkin, C., & Wallach, L. (Eds.) (1990). *Mass communication and public health*. Newbury Park, CA: Sage.

Brehm, J. (1966). *A theory of psychological reactance*. New York: Academic Press.

Campbell, J. P. (1988). Training design and performance improvement. In J. P. Campbell & R. J. Campbell (Eds.), *Productivity in organizations: New perspectives from industrial and organizational psychology* (pp. 117-215). San Francisco: Jossey-Bass.

Cohen, A. (1977). Factors in successful occupational safety programs. *Journal of Safety Research, 9*, 168-178.

Cohen, A. (1987). Perspectives on protective behaviors in the workplace. In N. Weinstein (Ed.), *Taking care: Understanding and encouraging self-protective behavior* (pp. 298-322). New York: Cambridge University Press.

Cohen, A., & Colligan, M. J. (1995). *Assessing occupational safety and health training: A literature review. Final report* Cincinnati: National Institute for Occupational Safety and Health.

Cohen, A., Colligan, M. J., & Berger, P. (1985). Psychology in health risk messages to workers. *Journal of Occupational Medicine, 27*, 543-551.

Cohen, A., & Murphy, L. (1989). Indications of health promotion behaviors at the workplace. In: S. B. Kar (Ed.), *Health promotion indicators and actions* (pp. 249-270). New York: Springer-Verlag.

Cohen, H. H., & Jensen, R. C. (1984). Measuring the effectiveness of an industrial lift truck operator safety training program. *Journal of Safety Research, 15*, 125-135.

Cole, H. P., Mallett, L. G., Haley, J. V., Berger, P. K., Lacefield, W. E., Waslielewski, R. D., Lineberry, G. T., & Wala, A. M. (1988). A new SCSR donning procedure. In *Research and evaluation methods for measuring non-routine mine health and safety skills: Vol. I* (pp. 120-165). Lexington: University of Kentucky.

Conard, R. J. (1983). *Employee work practices*. NIOSH Contract Report 81-2905. Cincinnati: National Institute for Occupational Safety and Health.

DeJoy, D. (1985). Attributional processes and hazard control management in industry. *Journal of Safety Research, 16*, 61-71.

DeJoy, D. (1989). The optimism bias and traffic accident risk perception. *Accident Analysis and Prevention, 21*(4), 333-340.

Edwards, D. S., & Hahn, C. P. (1980). A chance to happen. *Journal of Safety Research, 12*, 59-67.

Feeney, R. J. (1986). Why is there resistance to wearing protective equipment at work? Possible strategies for overcoming this. *Journal of Occupational Accidents, 8*, 207-213.

Ford, J. K., & Fisher, S. (1994). The transfer of training in work organizations: A systems perspective to continuous learning. In M. J. Colligan (Ed.), *Occupational safety and health training* (pp. 241-260). Philadelphia: Hanley & Befus.

Gjessing, C. C., Schoenborn, T. F., & Cohen, A. (1994). *Participatory ergonomic interventions in meatpacking plants*. DHHS (NIOSH) Publication No 94-124. Cincinnati: National Institute for Occupational Safety and Health.

Hopkins, B. L. (1981). *Behavioral procedures for reducing worker exposure to carcinogens*. NIOSH Contract Report 210-77-0042. Lawrence: University of Kansas.

Kryter, K. D. (1970). *Effects of noise on man*. New York: Academic Press.

LeBar, G. (1993). Safety management in tight times. *Occupational Hazards, 6*, 27-30.

Lindell, M. K. (1994) Motivational and organizational factors affecting implementation of worker safety training. In M. J. Colligan (Ed.), *Occupational safety and health training* (pp. 211-240). Philadelphia: Hanley & Befus.

Manwaring, J. C., & Conroy, C. (1990). Occupational confined space-related fatalities: Surveillance and prevention. *Journal of Safety Research, 21*, 157-164.

Maples, T. W., Jacoby, J. A., Johnson D. E., Ter Haar, G. L., & Buckingham, F. M. (1982). Effectiveness of employee training and motivation programs in reducing exposure to inorganic lead and lead alkyls. *American Industrial Hygiene Association Journal*, *43*, 692-694.

Maslow, A. H. (1954). *Motivation and personality*. New York: Harper.

McAfee, R. B., & Winn, A. R. (1989). The use of incentives/feedback to enhance workplace safety: A critique of the literature. *Journal of Safety Research*, *20*, 7-19.

Millar, J. D. (1993). Valuing, empowering employees vital to health and safety management. *Occupational Safety and Health*, *9*, 100-101.

Morgan, W. P. (1983). Psychological problems associated with the wearing of industrial respirators: A review. *American Industrial Hygiene Association Journal*, *44*, 671-676.

Occupational Safety and Health Administration. (1988). Training requirements. In *OSHA standards and training guidelines*. (pp. 3-8). OSHA Report No. 2254. Washington, DC: U.S. Department of Labor.

Office of Technology Assessment. (1985). Training and education for preventing work-related injury and illness. In *Preventing illness and injury in the workplace* (pp. 189-202). Report OTA-H-256. Washington, DC: U.S. Congress.

Pidgeon, N. F. (1991). Safety culture and risk management in organizations. *Journal of Cross-Cultural Psychology*, *22* (1), 129-140.

Rosen, R. H. (1991). *The healthy company: Eight strategies to develop people, productivity, and profits* (pp. 9-17). Los Angeles: Jeremy P. Tarcher.

Rosenstock, I. M. (1974). The health belief model: Origins and correlates. *Health Education Monographs*, *2*, 336-353.

Safety Compliance Letter with OSHA Highlights. (1994). No. 2217 Sept. 10. Waterford, CT: Bureau of Business Practice.

Simonds, R. H., & Shafai-Sahrai, Y. (1977). Factors apparently affecting injury frequency in eleven matched pairs of companies. *Journal of Safety Research*, *9*, 120-127.

Sitterley, T. E., Pietan, O. D., & Metaftin, W. E. (1974). *Firefighter skills study: Effectiveness of training and retraining methods*. Seattle, WA: Boeing Aerospace Company.

Slovic, P. (1978). The psychology of protective behavior. *Journal of Safety Research*, *10*, 58-68.

Smith, M. J., Cohen, H. H., Cohen, A., & Cleveland, R. J. (1978). Characteristics of successful safety programs. *Journal of Safety Research*, *10*, 5-15.

Sulzer-Azaroff, B., Harris, T. C., & McCann, K. B. (1944). Beyond training: Oganizational performance management techniques. In M. J. Colligan (Ed.), *Occupational safety and health training* (pp. 321-340) Philadelphia: Hanley & Befus.

White, M. C., Baker, E. L., Larson, M. B., & Wolford, R. (1988). The roles of personal beliefs and social influences as determinants of respirator use among construction painters. *Scandinavian Journal of Work, Environment, and Health*, *14*, 239-245.

Wichman, H., & Ball, J. (1983). Locus of control, self-serving biases, and attitudes toward safety in general aviation pilots. *Aviation, Space, and Environmental Medicine*, *54*, 507-510.

Zohar, D. (1980). Safety climate in industrial organizations: Theoretical and applied implications. *Journal of Applied Psychology*, *65*, 96-102.

Zohar, D., Cohen, A., & Azar, N. (1980). Promoting increased use of ear protectors in noise through information feedback. *Human Factors*, *22*, 69-79.

Zohar, D., & Fussfeld, N. (1981). Modifying earplug wearing behavior by behavior modification techniques: An empirical evaluation. *Journal of Organizational Behavior Management*, *3*, 41-52.

IV

INTEGRATION

21

Provider Determinants of Health Behavior

An Integration

David S. Gochman

This chapter integrates major points and findings presented in Volume II. Although its contents primarily reflect the contributions to this volume, rather than the larger body of scholarship about how providers—health care professionals and institutions—affect health behavior, they are consistent with this knowledge. The section on future directions is the major exception to this principle, and includes additional perspectives. The chapter's organizing framework is a "work in progress" and is intended to become the foundation for a future synthesis and integration of this larger body of knowledge.

Complementing the contributions in Volume I, which deal primarily with specific levels of personal or social determinants, the chapters in this volume focus on selected aspects of health providers as personal, interpersonal, social, or institutional systems, and on the effects of these aspects on adherence to a range of health-related regimens. In a fashion similar to that of the integrating chapter in Volume I, a major part of this chapter is organized around four of the six categories of health behaviors. These categories are presented with some modest reframing and in a different order, to reflect the major thrusts of the volume: adherence to disease-focused regimens (which is a rephrasing, more appropriate for this volume, of the more general category "responses to illness"); preventive, protective, and safety behaviors; lifestyle behaviors; and care seeking. Risk behaviors and health cognitions emerged rarely in their own right in the chapters, and are not included as separate behavior categories. However, findings involving risk behaviors and perceptions of professionals, especially related to satisfaction with care, are included in relation to these four categories.

Each of these categories of health behavior is examined in terms of the relevant personal, interpersonal, and social processes within health institutions, as well as in terms of the personal and social determinants examined in Volume I. These determinants are: interactional, including

David S. Gochman • Kent School of Social Work, University of Louisville, Louisville, Kentucky 40292.

Handbook of Health Behavior Research II: Provider Determinants, edited by David S. Gochman. Plenum Press, New York, 1997.

information sharing and communication, and role and power issues; structural, including interventions and programs, and organization and location; personal; family; social; nonhealth institutional and community; and cultural. The major emphasis of this volume, however, is adherence to or acceptance of disease-focused regimens, and the largest part of this section naturally involves analyses of the determinants of such adherence. The chapter continues with an analysis of some common themes and concludes with some directions for future research.

SELECTED HEALTH BEHAVIORS

Adherence to Disease-Focused Regimens (Responses to Illness)

Interactional Determinants

Communication. Inadequate or inappropriate communication or instruction is a primary barrier to adherence to a range of regimens. DiMatteo (Chapter 1) emphasizes the role of communication in providing information necessary for successful adherence. The blockage of successful communication may impede the patient's expression of preferences in relation to treatment and, ultimately the patient's decision not to adhere. Poor communication leads to avoidance of discussion of expectations and ultimately to poor adherence. DiMatteo also notes that adherence is greater when communications lead to greater trust in the provider.

Creer and Levstek (Chapter 7) similarly note that inadequate instruction impedes adherence to asthma regimens and underscore how important it is that the provider use clear, understandable vocabulary; provide opportunity for active questioning by the patient; negotiate, contract, and arrive at joint treatment goals with the patient; instruct the patient in monitoring skills; and track the patient's behavior.

The importance of physician and patient agreement on treatment goals is further emphasized in relation to adherence to adult diabetes regimens along with evidence that patients and physicians differ in their judgments and perceptions about such adherence (Fisher et al., Chapter 10). As Fisher et al. note, health professionals tend to view nonadherence as a patient problem and to believe that the patient is not able to adhere. However, when health professionals recognized the difficulties in adherence in their "demands" or expectations, and were thus more realistic, their patients were more truthful about reporting glucose monitoring than were patients of physicians whose expectations were unrealistically high.

Fisher et al. (Chapter 10) further emphasize that the patient is the primary provider of 90–99% of care. The patient needs to understand all aspects of the regimen, and the goals and objectives of the management plan should reflect collaboration and a convergence between provider expectations and what the patient can actually do.

The role of provider-patient interaction is also stressed by Clark (Chapter 8) in terms of advice and counseling about heart disease relative to health status. Clark notes that interaction and communication can be impeded when patients are demographically dissimilar to the provider. Physicians tend to provide less instruction for these patients. Clark also points out critical incongruities: Physicians often do not perceive patients as wanting advice, yet most patients do want it, and although patients with hypertension perceived the physician as less empathetic than did patients with other conditions, they attributed greater importance to physician discussions than these other patients.

The importance of interaction and communication is seen in the linkage between adherence to regimens in seizure disorders and physician monitoring activities and the provision of support from health care providers (Di Iorio, Chapter 11). Di Iorio also notes that adherence was linked to positive patient attitudes toward providers. Christensen, Benotsch, and Smith (Chapter 12) note that adherence to the dietary components of renal dialysis regimens is related to the fit between patient and physician preferences about the level of patient involvement in the treatment process.

Negative interactions with providers by persons with tuberculosis generated negative attitudes toward providers, which resulted in the greater likelihood that patients would terminate treatment prematurely (Morisky & Cabrera, Chapter 14). On the other hand, perceptions of sincere provider encouragement, possibly taking the form of asking about the patient's fears and beliefs about tuberculosis, and expressions of belief in the patient's skills necessary to complete treatment, are thought to improve communication and the relationship and thus increase adherence. When patients enjoy good relationships with a clinic staff, they are more likely to appear for appointments and to complete the tuberculosis treatment. Physicians' perceptions of "sufficient" communication are often inappropriate; some define it simply in terms of spending additional time with patients; others overestimate the amount of time they spend. Such inappropriate perceptions impede adherence.

The importance of instruction about symptoms, of providing feedback, and of any reasonable educational intervention in increasing adherence to a plaque control/flossing regimen is noted by McCaul (Chapter 16). McCaul also points out the importance of maintaining patient contact in increasing the likelihood that the patient will return for treatment.

Role and Power. Changes in professional-patient roles and in the physician's professional power also have implications for adherence to a range of regimens (Haug, Chapter 3; Salloway, Hafferty, & Vissing, Chapter 4). The power of the physician role is clearly linked to political and economic power (Trostle, Chapter 6). Di Matteo (Chapter 1) notes that nonadherence itself may be an active coping strategy to restore the patient's lost sense of control.

The degree of physician expertise, or the ability to enact the physician role appropriately, is linked to adherence to asthmatic regimens (Creer & Levstek, Chapter 7). Specialists' ability to provide more complete or adequate information has implications for an instructional role for physicians and an active questioning role for the patient.

Creer and Levstek also note that a collaborative role relationship between physician and patient in deciding on treatment goals is associated with increased patient commitment to perform self-regulatory skills and establishes expectancies that drive patient efforts and performance. Providers' skill in shaping and modeling of appropriate inhalation behaviors is an additional factor in adherence. Pharmacists and physicians may lack appropriate expertise in doing this. Providing patients with a written summary of the regimen and giving them reinforcement and support also underlie adherence. Physician ignorance may be the most serious impediment to adherence in asthmatic regimens.

Clark (Chapter 8) observes that while patients want their education and counseling to come from physicians, evidence suggests that no category of provider—physicians, physician assistants, dieticians, nurses, counselors—demonstrated superiority in educational and counseling skills. The active patient role also is related to the success of educational and counseling interventions in heart disease.

Physicians who themselves are poor compliers with regimens for tuberculosis may be less enthused about assuring compliance by their own tuberculosis patients (Morisky & Cabrera, Chapter 4). Finally, McCaul (Chapter 16) stresses the importance of the dentist or direct service provider's role as a health educator/health promoter.

Structural Determinants

Interventions and Programs. The complexity of regimens is a major barrier to adherence, particularly in asthmatic regimens (Creer & Levstek, Chapter 7) and seizure disorders (Di Iorio, Chapter 11). Tailoring interventions to specific population needs, beliefs, and perceptions of risk improves adherence and increases acceptance of tuberculosis screenings, as do telephone reminders (Morisky & Cabrera, Chapter 14). The importance of provider support, including feedback and monitoring, and of the accessibility and availability of staff was also identified as a critical factor in adherence in adults with diabetes (Fisher et al., Chapter 10).

Organizational Issues. The control of academic research on "adherence" or compliance by medical interests that have an interest in maintaining physician power and authority is emphasized by Trostle (Chapter 6), who demonstrates that for decades such research has been framed from the physician's perspective. Trostle views "compliance" as a problematic concept, transforming physicians' theories about appropriate patient behavior into a series of research strategies that appear to legitimate physician power and control.

The conflicts between the multiple physician roles of provider, bureaucrat, and researcher also have implications for satisfaction with care and thus for adherence, remaining in care, and appropriate use of services (Ben-Sira, Chapter 2). In addition, medical education fails to stress the sociobehavioral components of health care and the need to involve patients in their own treatment plans for cardiac rehabilitation (Clark, Chapter 8).

The "crumbling infrastructure of public health programs adversely affects efforts of tuberculosis control and management" (Morisky & Cabrera, Chapter 14) and can have a negative impact on perceptions of availability and accessibility. Such infrastructure problems include compromised quality of care—failures to provide follow-up services, including missed appointments and monthly checking for signs and symptoms; incomplete or unavailable charts; personnel changes that result in lower satisfaction with the provider; affordability; distance; transportation; waiting times; inflexible clinic hours; lack of bilingual and bicultural staff; policies targeting undocumented immigrants; deficiencies in provider skills; and inadequate or delayed testing and misinterpretation of test results (Morisky & Cabrera). Shifts in tuberculosis care from public to private practice physicians with minimal training in tuberculosis also reduce adherence. There is also poor supporting infrastructure in social and health-related agencies that deal with other health problems. Morisky and Cabrera affirm that deficiencies in organizational decision-making generate many of the clinic-related problems.

Other organizational barriers within health institutions include some capitation programs that exclude diabetes and the lack of inclusion of patient education in standards of care (Fisher et al., Chapter 10). Fisher et al. point out that the type of emotional and social support that sustains adherence is considered "soft" within the health care culture. The lack of patient education that emphasizes behavioral change as an integral part of the social and cultural health care environment is a barrier to adherence to adult diabetes regimens.

Personal Determinants

A wide range of personal and demographic characteristics have been examined in relation to diverse components of adherence and acceptance, and patterns of adherence itself vary considerably. Ben-Sira (Chapter 2) notes the importance of patient affective needs—particularly needs for emotional support and reduction of anxiety—in the overall treatment process. When these needs are not met satisfactorily, the patient will be less satisfied and presumably less likely to adhere to regimens. Patient anxiety and emotional upset may also impede communication, with negative implications for adherence (DiMatteo, Chapter 1).

Creer and Levstek (Chapter 7), for example, indicate that patients vary along a continuum ranging from obsessive-compulsive self-regulation to total nonacceptance. Patients tend to balance the costs or side effects with the benefits of adherence to treatment.

There are no consistent demographic or personal characteristics related to acceptance of heart disease regimens (Clark, Chapter 8). Older patients seem more receptive to patient education than younger patients, but not consistently so. Some linkages exist between patients' perceptions about susceptibility and seriousness, costs and benefits, and adherence but again, they are not appreciable. Self-efficacy and outcome expectations, however, were important beliefs related to adherence. Higher levels of knowledge are also sometimes predictors of adherence. Clark notes that the impact of patient beliefs seems to be in their influence on what recommendations patients receive from their physicians. Time-management skills, adaptation to illness, and "laziness" were found to be linked to adherence to the exercise components of heart disease self-regulation. Older persons following rehabilitation regimens reported issues in many areas, among them differentiating changes due to aging from changes due to their conditions, setting priorities and making choices, maintaining independence, managing the burden of caring for others, and dealing with fears and anxieties.

Di Iorio (Chapter 11) also reports no consistent linkage between demographic characteristics or health status or perceived health status characteristics, emotional adjustment, or costs, on one hand, and adherence to seizure disorder regimens, on the other, although she does observe some predictive value for educational level and age. Lower perceptions of financial distress were also predictive of greater adherence. Persons with higher levels of life responsibilities also showed more adherence. Adherence was not linked to locus of control, although uncertainty about illness was related to lower adherence. Fear of seizures, however, did seem to be related to adherence.

On the other hand, Di Iorio notes that attempts at self-management could be related to lower "compliance" by medical standards, since patients developed their own regimens. Compliers, moreover, were more likely to have had a seizure while off medication. Parents of "compliant" children showed more information seeking and higher levels of belief in their children's susceptibility to seizures, and felt that treatment was beneficial. Adult compliers also showed more information seeking, had higher levels of perceived susceptibility and perceived benefits, and had more positive attitudes toward taking medication. Noncompliant patients were more likely to be undecided about the benefits of the treatment. Moreover, among adults, those with *more complex* regimens and with *greater concerns* about side effects were *more likely* to comply. Di Iorio also found self-efficacy, measured by the Epilepsy Self-Managment Scale, to be positively related to self-management practices.

In renal dialysis regimens, no consistent demographic or personal characteristics were found to be related to adherence, other than some positive linkages with age (Christensen et al., Chapter 12). Little support was found for health belief model variables, which may be due to the difficulty in executing the behaviors. Self-efficacy was observed to have some predictive value, but not locus of control. Perceived health competence may have predictive value in conjunction with health locus of control. These observations suggest that perceived ability to manage health effectively is related to adherence only when the patient believes that positive health outcomes are contingent upon following the advice and actions of health care providers. The possible linkage between differences in learned resourcefulness and fluid intake may be mediated by self-efficacy.

The five-factor theory of personality had limited usefulness in predicting adherence to renal dialysis (Christensen et al., Chapter 12). Conscientiousness was found to be linked to medical compliance, but not to other components of the regimen. The information vigilance factor was related to adherence for patients with high needs for self-monitoring and self-care, but this factor was inversely related to adherence for patients for whom no opportunity for self-care exists. Fluid-intake adherence was best for persons using planful problem solving for solvable problems.

But in dealing with less controllable stressors, adherence was related only to emotional self-control. Overall, self-efficacy is a modest predictor.

Increased understanding of tuberculosis as a condition increases the likelihood that therapy will be completed (Morisky & Cabrera, Chapter 14). Belief in its curability (benefits of treatment) also increases the likelihood that appointments will be kept. Other health belief model variables were not that valuable in predicting adherence to tuberculosis regimens. Attitudes toward the provider are related to adherence, as are the experiences of symptoms; as symptoms disappear, compliance decreases. Patients' fears of the stigma attached to tuberculosis are reflected in systematic avoidance of their use of the term *tuberculosis*. Perceptions of support from physician are related to adherence.

Confusion over the changing nature of treatment is a factor that has a negative effect on adherence to diabetes regimens (Fisher et al., Chapter 10). There is no "diabetic" personality. Perceived severity and perceived benefits increase adherence to regimens in adults with diabetes.

Family Determinants

A family's failure to obtain medications, apathy, the social stigma attached to a condition, and parental perceptions, and understandings of a disease, i.e., whether it is "physical" or "psychosomatic," may be barriers to adherence to asthmatic regimens by children (Creer & Levstek, Chapter 7). Clark (Chapter 8) notes the importance of spousal support in adherence to heart disease regimens and also observes that family members may have interests that are different from the patient's interests and therefore may not support adherence to the regimen.

The family is considered to be the basic component of adherence to diabetes in children (Wysocki & Greco, Chapter 9). Adherence is increased to the degree that parents maintain a developmentally appropriate balance of parent-child responsibilities, involving problem-solving skills, communication about diabetes management, and expression of emotional adjustment. Wysocki and Greco suggest that adherence is more likely when parents encourage the development of appropriate skills in children relevant to obtaining social support, foster appropriate interactions between the child and professionals, and advocate for the child at school and in the community. The family's likelihood of engaging in these supportive behaviors is itself mediated by socioeconomic status (SES), ethnicity, the family's level of functioning/dysfunctioning, and the family's structure and organization.

Parental worrying seems to reduce the degree of a child's adherence to seizure disorder regimens (Di Iorio, Chapter 11). Families who worried more also placed more restrictions on children, a practice that in turn was linked to lower levels of adherence. Family support was positively related to adherence to seizure disorder regimens. Parents of compliant children were more likely to seek information and do special things to keep the child healthy, were less likely to run out of medication or miss a dose, and were more likely to believe their child was at risk for a seizure than were parents of noncompliant children. None of the parental health belief model variables presumed to be related to threat reduction were associated with the child's compliance. Parents of compliers noted more difficulty in affording medications (barriers) and were less likely to be on government assistance. They also reported fewer weeks since the last clinic visit. Parents of noncompliers, on the other hand, had higher goals for their children.

Families perceived as more supportive, i.e., showing greater cohesion and expressiveness, and having less conflict, were associated with greater adherence to the fluid-intake component in renal dialysis regimens, but not to adherence to the dietary component (Christensen et al., Chapter 12). Better marital adjustment was also related to adherence in fluid intake.

Openness of feelings in families, as opposed to criticality, was linked to adherence in adults with diabetes (Fisher et al., Chapter 10). On the other hand, family attempts at support sometimes ended up being detrimental. Living alone was also linked to good adherence.

Social Determinants

Social support is also a critical factor in adherence to a range of regimens. Clark (Chapter 8) provides evidence that social support in the form of providing information and advice, appraisal, emotional support, and availability was related to adherence to heart disease regimens, especially when the social support was more family-centered and came from a "dense" network, i.e., one made up of more close members. Moreover, patients from families that participated in social support training were more likely to keep medical appointments and to achieve weight and blood pressure control.

Di Iorio (Chapter 11) found, to the contrary, that social support had mixed effects on adherence to epilepsy regimens. Although there was evidence that adult compliers had more supportive social networks than noncompliers, some data indicated that social support in the form of reminders to take medication increased the patients' negative views about the medicaton, with possible negative impacts on adherence. Di Iorio further noted that the linkage between social support and self-managment may be mediated by self-efficacy beliefs and by being epilepsy-specific.

Instrumental support from friends or families (e.g., transportation, child care) appears to be related to keeping follow-up appointment in tuberculosis management. Emotional support is also likely to improve adherence (Morisky & Cabrera, Chapter 14). Fisher et al. (Chapter 10) note a number of linkages between social support and adherence in adult diabetes; they also note that social support is the only factor not related to control of overeating. On the other hand, social support does not appear to be related to components of renal dialysis adherence (Christensen et al., Chapter 12).

Fisher et al. (Chapter 10) also observed a social role effect in the form of gender differences: Social support is related to adherence in men, but not in women. At the same time, they note that such support has value for women in terms of their morale levels, even if it does not affect levels of adherence or control. The finding that although women were as adherent to heart disease regimens as men, they were observed to drop out of cardiac rehabilitation programs more and to attend less, is another gender effect (Clark, Chapter 8).

Institutional and Community Determinants

The linkage between the framing of research questions about compliance or adherence and physician power and control needs to be viewed in terms of community and larger system political and economic issues. Trostle (Chapter 6) demonstrates how such larger system factors, e.g., the economic interests of pharmaceutical and food and nutritional companies and the "interests" of the academic research community within medicine and related social sciences, become "medicalized" and transformed into issues of the physician–patient relationship, physician power and authority, and information and product control, and ultimately are rephrased in terms of "patient compliance."

Lack of community input to promote a sense of ownership is a barrier to adherence to tuberculosis regimens, as is the community's perception that tuberculosis has disappeared as a problem (Morisky & Cabrera, Chapter 14). Any legislation that isolates undocumented immigrants increases their isolation and facilitates perceptions of stigma about tuberculosis. Such legislation also damages the trust in the provider that is necessary for successful adherence.

The importance of organizational factors is further emphasized by Fisher et al. (Chapter 10), who note that organizational culture, size, and structure can have implications for adherence to diabetes regimens. Larger organizations seem more likely to have resources to invest in employee health (benefits, cafeterias with wider menu choices), but may at the same time be less accommodating of individuals. Large companies are often less aware of whether an employee has diabetes. Work schedules allowing for flexible mealtimes and breaks can also increase adherence. Community- and worksite-based programs are also envisioned as involving peers as agents of change (Fisher et al.). In the context of identifying possible community interventions, Di Iorio (Chapter 11) mentions the role of community myths and stigma about epilepsy as barriers to adherence.

Cultural Determinants

Cultural beliefs about drugs and treatments can transcend the physician-patient relationship and take precedence over the medically dictated regimen (Trostle, Chapter 6). Moreover, the concept of "health culture" is emphasized by Morisky and Cabrera (Chapter 14) to refer to patients with coherent alternative views of health and disease, who may not understand or accept the rationale for tuberculosis treatment and thus vary in their responses to the results of tests and their decisions to continue in care. Cultural beliefs about tuberculosis may not consider it either as communicable or as a health threat. Cultural stigmatization also varies; Spanish-speaking Latinos stigmatize tuberculosis to a greater degree than do English-speaking Latinos. Tuberculosis may also invoke beliefs about sorcery. Similar barriers exist for adherence to adult diabetes regimens in the form of cultural norms for eating, body image, and beliefs about fatalism and activism (Fisher et al., Chapter 10).

Preventive, Protective, and Safety Behaviors

Interactional Determinants

The importance of physician communications about mammograms is noted by Champion and Miller (Chapter 13). The absence of a physician's recommendation is a critical barrier to participation in a mammogram screening program; physicians' recommendations increase the likelihood of women's participating in such screening. Physicians with greater knowledge are more likely to make recommendations for mammograms (Champion & Miller).

Structural Determinants

Interventions and Programs. Tailoring interventions to specific populations needs, beliefs, and perceptions of risk improves adherence and increases acceptance of mammography (Champion & Miller, Chapter 13). Use of individualized telephone counseling and automated and computerized reminder systems, specifically tailored letters to African-American and lower income populations, door-to-door canvassing and outreach, and in-home education by lay health workers all increased patricipation in screenings. Breast self-examination (BSE) improved with demonstrations of corrective feedback from professionals (Champion & Miller). Rimer et al. (Chapter 15) further affirm the importance of provider initiatives in relation to screening for cervical, colorectal, skin, and prostate cancer.

Organizational Issues. Medical specializations affect recommendations to have a mammography; gynecologists are more likely to make such recommendations than internists, internists more likely than family practitioners (Champion & Miller, Chapter 13). Physicians with greater knowledgeability are also more likely to make such recommendations. Institutional accessibility and availability also influence participation. HMO membership is likely to increase mammography (Champion & Miller), although the effect of Medicare coverage is unclear, depending in part on physician recommendations to elderly women. Continuing medical education activities were also related to increasing the likelihood of physicians' making such recommendations. Rimer et al. (Chapter 15) note that clinics often miss opportunities to make recommendations about cancer screening and that increasing convenience increases participation in skin cancer screening.

Personal Determinants

Age is inversely related to acceptance of mammography, and perceived susceptibility and benefits—but not perceived severity—are positively related to it (Champion & Miller, Chapter 13). Primary barriers are costs and not having a physician recommend mammography. Most studies show some predictive value for health belief model (HBM) variables. Perceptions of benefits were consistently related to acceptance of mammography. The value of HBM variables also interacted with stages of adoption. Perceived benefits, for example, along with subjective norms derived from the theory of reasoned action, had the most positive value at the maintenance stage compared to both precontemplative and contemplative stages. There were fewer perceptions of barriers for women at the maintenance stage. Moreover, a group that relapsed (did not continue to participate) had higher negative decisional balance levels.

Locus of control variables were not related to predictions of BSE, but HBM variables seemed to show some modest predictive values in many studies, with perceived barriers having the most consistent value as a predictor, and perceived seriousness the least value, probably because there is little if any variability about the perceptions of the seriousness of cancer. In some research, self-efficacy appeared to be the strongest predictor of BSE.

Personal embarrassment or discomfort about Pap tests, colorectal screening, and other cancer prevention procedures has a negative impact on participation (Rimer et al., Chapter 15). On the other hand, personal experiences with people who have had cancer, and beliefs that cancer is curable, increase the likelihood of participation in cancer screenings. Having signs of possible skin cancer or, holding beliefs that one is at risk for it increases the likelihood of skin cancer screenings. Low SES, on the other hand, reduces the likelihood of skin cancer screening. Race has an impact on acceptance of screening for prostate cancer, whites being more likely to participate than nonwhites. Lack of knowledge appears to be a major factor in not seeking testicular cancer screening.

Self-efficacy and outcome expectancy appear to be major predictors of adherence to dental flossing regimens (McCaul, Chapter 16). Persons with a history of flossing or who had greater levels of flossing skills were more likely to adhere and less likely to relapse. Worry about gum disease seems to be a possible predictor. Persons who relapsed had lower intentions to floss and lower levels of self-efficacy. Readiness to change was also related to adherence.

Cohen and Colligan (Chapter 20) note the importance of perceived ability and perceptual factors in adherence to occupational safety regimens. Younger and less experienced workers often are more at risk because of lack of training in safety skills and practices. Lack of safety information together with the perceived remoteness of threat and the disproportionate emphasis on machine-related (as opposed to behaviorally related) causes of accidents decreases acceptance of safety regimens. There is an optimistic bias present in workers' estimates of their own competence that results in their discounting safety and risk-related information. Even when workers recognize threat, they may attribute responsibility for it elsewhere, e.g., to supervisors. Safety behaviors involve costs and interpersonal penalties. Equipment use is often inconvenient; wearing rubber gloves can result in dermatological problems, for example, and encapsulated suits may result in heat stress.

Institutional and Community Determinants

Champion and Miller (Chapter 13) point out from community-focused studies that participation rates for mammograms increased as a result of outreach programs involving community advisory and gospel groups among African-American women and health and beauty programs for Hispanic-American women.

Lack of training and lack of risk information within the worksite are cited as barriers to acceptance of safety regimens; on the other hand, selection of equipment that is least inconveniencing can increase acceptance (Cohen & Colligan, Chapter 20). Management has the responsibility for assuring that protective equipment is readily and conveniently available. "Safe" work organizations seem to be those with high efficiency, good human resources practices and policies (such as affirmative action, counseling, career development), good supervisor-supervisee relationships, low turnover, and low absenteeism. It is not necessary to have a lot of safety rules. There is no relationship between quality or quantity of safety rules and accident rates, but organizations should have safety training programs, should provide feedback and incentives, and should increase employee participation (increase worker "ownership") in the development of safety programs.

Cultural Determinants

Champion and Miller (Chapter 13) note some ethnic differences in adherence; Hispanic women who have poor English language skills are less likely to participate in mammography screenings.

Lifestyle

Interactional Determinants

Communication. The role of communication in lifestyle change is underscored by Chrisler's observations (Chapter 17) that low provider expectations are associated with low adherence to weight loss and nutritional regimens. Adherence to such regimens is also associated with physician communication that is high in affectivity and information and expressive of empathy, helps the patient to acquire consumer skills as well as the skills necessary for adherence, and provides relapse training.

Marcus et al. (Chapter 18) emphasize the importance of professional recommendations and counseling in adherence to and acceptance of an exercise regimen, as well as the role of relapse-prevention efforts. Professional advice and information about treatment are also identified by Glasgow and Orleans (Chapter 19) as important factors in adherence to and acceptance of smoking cessation regimens, while physicians' and nurses' pessimistic perceptions about patients' ability to quit, the professionals' own lack of time, their lack of training for smoking cessation counseling, their lack of confidence in their own counseling skills, and their inappropriate expectations about change outcomes are barriers to adherence and acceptance.

Roles and Power. Type of specialization is also a factor in increasing adherence to weight loss and nutritional programs; patients under the care of an endocrinologist were more likely to adhere than those under other types of care, possibly because conditions under endocrinological treatment are perceived by the patient as more serious than those being treated by other types of medical practitioners (Chrisler, Chapter 17).

Structural Determinants

Interventions and Programs. Tailoring interventions to the needs and beliefs of specific populations increases acceptance of and improves adherence to weight loss and nutritional programs (Chrisler, Chapter 17) and exercise programs (Marcus et al., Chapter 18). Treating smoking status as a "vital sign" and then routinely flagging this sign on patient charts increases time spent by physicians in counseling patients about smoking cessation (Glasgow & Orleans, Chapter 19). Glasgow and Orleans point out that interventions to alter decisional balance and self-efficacy were most effective during precontemplation or contemplation stages. Action-oriented interventions, in contrast, were more appropriate in preparation, action, and maintenance stages.

Organizational Issues. Since the health system is focused on delivering care for illness rather than on disease prevention, physicians and other providers often lack the ability to advise patients about lifestyle change. Marcus et al. (Chapter 18) point out that physicians do not believe they have the ability to provide counseling about exercise and that there is often no organizational support for their doing so. Training physicians to discuss exercise would increase their perceptions that they have the ability to provide counseling for it (Marcus et al.). Training physicians and other providers to advise patients to quit smoking (Glasgow & Orleans, Chapter 19) and to recognize persons at risk for relapse or nonadherence to flossing regimens (McCaul, Chapter 16) would be likely to increase adherence.

The availability of smoking literature in waiting rooms can also increase participation in smoking cessation programs (Glasgow & Orleans, Chapter 19). On the other hand, there is little support from insurance companies in the form of coverage for attendance at smoking cessation clinics.

Personal Determinants

Chrisler (Chapter 17) introduces the idea that some persons may be biologically wired for calorie-dense foods because evolutionarily, before culture supervened, the sweetest foods available were also high in vitamins and fibers. Moreover, she points out, the developmental changes in food needs are often not recognized or appreciated. Medical conditions and health status tend to predict adherence to a weight loss or nutritional regime; persons who are asymptomatic, however, manifest lower adherence. People with greater control over food selection and preparation are more likely to adhere to regimens; when food preparation is expensive or difficult, adherence is less likely. Pessimism, stress, social isolation, depression, high external locus of control, and low frustration tolerance are all linked to lower levels of adherence, while persons who perceive themselves to have potentially shorter life spans are more adherent.

Demographic characteristics do seem to have some consistent linkage to acceptance of exercise regimens (Marcus et al., Chapter 18). African-Americans, persons with less education, and persons who are overweight, elderly, or have negative health status tend to be more inactive. Self-efficacy, self-motivation, beliefs in benefits, and enjoyment of exercise seem to predict adherence.

Glasgow and Orleans (Chapter 19) clearly identify the interactions between stages of change and the impact of selected beliefs on acceptance of a smoking cessation program. Perceived severity of smoking-related illness or symptoms interacts with readiness to change and self-efficacy. Perceived risks of smoking in relation to the perceived benefits of quitting and other decisional balance variables are most important during shifts from precontemplation to contemplation, and from contemplation to action. Self-efficacy is an important predictor at all stages, however, increasing in value from precontemplation to maintenance.

Family Determinants

Family interactions may make it difficult to change eating habits (Chrisler, Chapter 17). A family's understanding is necessary for a child to adhere to a diet. Attitudes and behaviors of family members and the importance of adherence to significant others are all related to adherence. When families are supportive, understanding, and organized, adherence is increased. Families have the potential for rewarding a person for successful adherence and can provide appropriate feedback.

Family and spousal support is important in women's maintenance of an exercise regimen

(Marcus et al., Chapter 18). Family participation also increases adherence to an exercsie regimen. On the other hand, family responsibilties are likely to decrease participation by women in exercise regimens.

Social Determinants

Social supports affect adherence to nutritional and weight regimens (Chrisler, Chapter 17). Peer pressures are important components in adherence to dietary and nutritional regimens in adolescents, as are gender issues. Some foods, for example, are more likely to be seen as women's fare than as men's; other foods are likely to be viewed oppositely.

Social expectations that women and the elderly will be less active may have implications for the participation of these population segments in exercise regimens (Marcus et al., Chapter 18). On the other hand, peer role models may increase participation in exercise programs.

Institutional and Community Determinants

The convenience of facilities and the flexibility or rigidity of child and occupational schedules have an impact on acceptance and adherence to exercise regimens, this effect being greater for women and low-income persons (Marcus et al., Chapter 18). Availability of exercise facilities such as bicycle trails, swimming pools, tennis courts, playing fields, and recreation centers, and worksite programs, are important community determinants of adherence to exercise regimens. Moreover, signs posted near escalators promoting stair climbing can be an important institutional determinant of exercise behavior. On the other hand, certain types of "fitness" institutions may create an atmosphere in which persons without the money to buy fashionable attire may feel out of place. Workplace programs offering a diversity of programs maximizing convenience, use of company time, flexible schedules, and employee involvement in program development can increase the likelihood of participation in and adherence to exercise programs (Marcus et al.).

The importance of worksite programs for increasing acceptance of and adherence to smoking cessation programs is noted by Glasgow and Orleans (Chapter 19). Although data are not available, there is a sense that participant "ownership" of programs increases their success. Tax increases and community-level statutes and legislation against smoking may also contribute to adherence to smoking cessation regimens. Finally, the availability of fresh food and dietary choices for weight control and nutritional regimens may be linked to such characteristics of a community as its rural or urban nature (Chrisler, Chapter 17).

Cultural Determinants

Cultural barriers to weight loss and nutritional adherence may also be found in some religious dictates or in religious celebrations. Observation of certain holidays, such as Lent, Passover, Ramadan, or Kwanzaa, during which certain eating behaviors are either mandated or proscribed, may impede adherence.

Care Seeking

Interactional Determinants

Patterns of care seeking are linked to the communication process by both DiMatteo (Chapter 1) and Ben-Sira (Chapter 2). Affective responses and skilled communication on the part of the provider are viewed as critical in determining appropriate care seeking and utilization of services. Good communication, involving both information and affect, can decrease inappropriate use of services and inappropriate care, i.e., more risky and instrusive procedures, and increase use of appropriate, i.e., less risky services and procedures. Ben-Sira's concept of lay-intelligible cues posits that those actions on the part of the physician that increase the patient's understanding of a condition and its treatments and that serve as a basis for evaluation of the physician's treatment and competence are linked to decisions to remain in care and to selection of physicians, as well as to appropriate use of services.

Structural Determinants

The degree to which health care reflects corporate versus public interests is a predictor of its use (Scarpaci & Kearns, Chapter 5). Locational attributes, such as proximity, centrality, and convenience, are also important determinants and interact with economic, personal, social, and cultural factors (Scarpaci & Kearns). Scarpaci and Kearns point out that market forces may determine the location of physician's offices, but market forces are not directly linked to care seeking.

Institutional and Community Determinants

Land use and population density contribute to care-seeking behavior, as do communities' characteristics, such as the degree to which they are rural or urban (Scarpaci & Kearns, Chapter 5). Concentration of therapeutic and diagnostic practitioners and procedures in highly urban areas permits increased access to these in urban areas. Communities with larger and denser populations offer a wider range of provider services and thus increased accessibility and use of care.

Cultural Determinants

Scarpaci and Kearns (Chapter 5) show that culture determines what physician behaviors will be valued. In Britain, touching by physicians was not valued; in Chile, among lower-income patients, it was. Although this behavior is a "health cognition" rather than care seeking as such, perceptions of satisfaction with care are important factors in care-seeking behavior.

COMMON THEMES

Five themes underlying a number of aspects of health behavior research dimensions appear regularly throughout this volume: conceptual issues, methodological issues, professional versus phenomenological perspectives, the role of affect, and the size of the focal system.

Conceptual Issues

Understandably, this volume focuses less on specific theories or conceptual models than Volume I, several chapters of which are devoted to particular conceptual frameworks. At the mid-1990s, there is less interest in demonstrating the superiority of one theory over another, as Glasgow and Orleans (Chapter 19) note, than in using diverse theories to tailor interventions and programs to specific behaviors and populations. Important conceptual issues in this volume can be organized under three headings: conceptual content, conceptual integration, and a reconceptualization of "compliance."

Conceptual Content

The major conceptual frameworks deal with relationships between persons, patients, or clients, on one hand, and health professionals, settings and treatments, interventions, and programs, on the other. The models are thus interactional—involving communication, roles and role relationships, and power and control—as well as predictive.

Communication, roles, and role relationships between individuals and professionals are viewed as evolving and dynamic in nature and as moving increasingly away from a strict paternalistic model toward a model that more closely resembles a partnership (Haug, Chapter 3; Salloway et al., Chapter 4; Trostle, Chapter 6). Physicians and professionals have traditionally been conceptualized as having the sole authority to define illness, provide treatment, and mandate patient behaviors (Salloway et al.). As Haug observes, this physician-professional dominance was based in large measure on a monopoly of knowledge and was enhanced by age, gender, race, and practice style; physicians who spent too much time listening were at risk for having their power diminished. Social forces and changes in societal norms have expanded the physician's traditional responsibilities to include other roles, including that of health educator in the community as well as in the clinic, and of health advocate, with resulting role confusion and role strain (Salloway et al.).

Conflicts between physicians and patients are often reflected in the encounter between them. Haug notes that physicians and patients do not necessarily have the same goals, and DiMatteo (Chapter 1) notes that the encounter and provision of information can be viewed as a "micropolitical process" that reinforces social status and power relationships that parallel those in the larger society, in which physicians have social dominance.

Self-management (or self-regulation, or self-care) represents a major framework for several chapters on adherence, especially in relation to heart disease and hypertension (Clark, Chapter 8), childhood diabetes (Wysocki & Greco, Chapter 9), and epilepsy (Di Iorio, Chapter 11). Di Iorio notes that the terms "self-management," "self-regulation," and "self-care" are often used interchangeably. A self-management perspective moves the locus of responsibility for adherence away from the physician and onto the patient. It reflects the totality of actions a person takes to deal with a condition (Di Iorio) or, alternatively, a way of activating patients: the mechanism through which health behavior change is effected (Clark). Within a self-management framework, taking of medications as prescribed is only one of a constellation of behaviors necessary for living successfully with the condition. Other components would include initiating and maintaining non-medication actions such as dietary, fluid-reduction, exercise, risk avoidance, or stress-reduction practices. Self-management emphasizes the mobilization of resources, both personal and external, and the acquisition of skills to reach certain objectives. There is thus interaction between patients and role models, health professionals, and social support systems. Self-management denotes conscious manipulation of situations toward the enhancement of daily life and the reduction of the impact of disease on the activities of daily living. The concept of self-efficacy, the belief that one has the skills to perform a specific behavior or adhere to a regimen, is a core element of self-management models, along with outcome expectancy, the perceived value of the consequence of a specific behavior.

Two unusual concepts that merit special attention in relation to adherence behaviors are "smoking status as a vital sign" (Glasgow & Orleans, Chapter 19), and "availability bias" (Cohen & Colligan, Chapter 20). Glasgow and Orleans recommend that smoking status be considered a vital sign, to be routinely assessed or queried by physicians. It is presumed that this practice would increase physician recommendations for a smoking cessation program. "Availability bias" refers to the inclination of a person to be inordinately influenced by dramatic events that have low probabilities of happening, but that are vivid in memory and easily recalled. Persons may thus be preoccupied with the improbable and be less inclined to engage in safety behaviors for more likely events.

Conceptual Integration

The several cognitive models—health belief, locus of control, protection motivation, and behavioral intention—dealt with in individual chapters in Volume I, together with stages of change models, all have relevance for prediction of some aspects of adherence regimens (already discussed in the sections on determinants of adherence). Research and interventions for improving adherence often combine elements of more than one model. For example, Fisher et al. (Chapter 10) point out that there are benefits to combining the health belief and stages of change models, since these models have differential predictive value for different components of an adult diabetes regimen. Glasgow and Orleans (Chapter 19) note the interactions between stage models and selected cognitive models; Champion and Miller (Chapter 13), the interactions between health belief and stage models; and Marcus et al. (Chapter 18), the interactions between stage and decisional balance models.

Reconceptualizing "Compliance"

There is broad consensus that "compliance" or "adherence" needs to be reconceptualized or redefined. It is clearly something more than obeying a physician's dictates; it is complex and multidimensional (Di Iorio, Chapter 11), it involves a wide range of determinants beyond the physician's dictates (Trostle, Chapter 6), and it must be understood in "systemic" terms. For example, adherence to a tuberculosis regimen must be viewed in terms of the social context in which the disease occurs and the context of the person's possible daily problems with housing, substance abuse, domestic violence, alienation from the system, and basic survival needs (Morisky & Cabrera, Chapter 14).

Nonadherence can be viewed as a reflection of poor interactions with providers and professionals, underscored by inadequate communication (Di Matteo, Chapter 1). It can also be viewed as a corollary of attempts to be self-managing or self-regulating, in which departures from the medically dictated regimens represent conscious efforts to achieve better control or to determine whether medication was still needed (Di Iorio). It can be viewed as a way of reacting to the stigma that society attaches to a condition such as tuberculosis (Morisky and Cabrera). It can also reflect the lack of fit between a prescribed medicine-taking schedule and the demands and rigidities of community institutions (Fisher et al., Chapter 10).

The increasing questioning of the linkage between compliant behavior and physiological indexes such as levels of blood glucose (Fisher et al.) or antiepileptic drugs (Di Iorio) also raises doubts about the criticality of strict adherence for health status. Adherence is clearly no longer considered to be solely a medical issue, and there is no longer any legitimacy, if ever there was, in thinking of the nonadhering, nonaccepting patient or layperson as the problem, or as a defaulter, or as behaving in an inappropriate, unacceptable way.

Methodological Issues

The methodological issues presented in this volume can be dealt with using the same broad categories used in the integrating chapter for Volume I: measurement, sampling, and procedure. Again, in many instances these are "boilerplate" concerns—criticisms that can be made for nearly any corpus of research.

Measurement

There is little consensus on how relevant health behaviors are to be measured or on what is being measured (Champion & Miller, Chapter 13; Chrisler, Chapter 17; Glasgow & Orleans, Chapter 19). A lack of agreement on what is meant by adherence or compliance translates into lack of consensus on measuring it, what behaviors it represents, and the time frame in which to observe it (Champion & Miller; Di Iorio, Chapter 11). This lack of agreement is also reflected in lack of consensus on what success means and how it is measured. Does success refer to a physiological outcome or to some aspect of social and personal functioning related to quality of life (Clark, Chapter 8)? The diversity of measures makes it difficult if not impossible to compare the findings of different investigations (e.g., Chrisler). Even when using the same theoretical framework, researchers use different scales to measure the same variables (Champion & Miller). Pervasive problems in reliability and validity problems have been noted (e.g., Champion & Miller; Chrisler), even in physiological measures such as saliva (e.g., Glasgow & Orleans). Finally, components of measures of adherence may not be correlated with one another, as Champion and Miller note in their observations that frequency of BSE does not correlate with proficiency in its practice.

The Epilepsy Self-Management Scale (Di Iorio) represents one attempt to resolve a number of measurement issues. Data indicate that it is internally consistent and offers promise of being a productive research tool, and it could become a standardized measure in relation to epilepsy. Glasgow and Orleans suggest that a single item developed from a series of National Cancer Institute studies—asking if one "has smoked even a single cigarette in the past seven days"—be incorporated into all measures of adherence to smoking cessation programs. The specification of a time frame for adherence remains unresolved, with little attention paid to long-term behavior change or continuous abstinence (Glasgow & Orleans; McCaul, Chapter 16).

Sampling

As is true of much behavioral research, the data base for studies on the impact of health institutions on health behavior is made up largely of white males, with a disproportionately small number of studies on nonwhites. A major sampling issue is thus the underrepresentation of a number of ethnic and cultural groups, particularly African-American and Hispanic women in relation to mammography and BSE (e.g., Champion & Miller, Chapter 13) and women in general, and the aging, in relation to exercise (Marcus et al., Chapter 18). Moreover, little is known about the adherence behaviors of persons who do not appear for regular clinic visits (Morisky & Cabrera, Chapter 14) or who do not attend smoking programs (Glasgow & Orleans, Chapter 19).

Procedure

Since intervention research is such a large contributor to understanding how health behaviors are influenced by health care institutions, several procedural issues related to such interventions must be mentioned. Paradoxically, the interventions themselves are often hard to define (e.g., Fisher et al., Chapter 10).

There is consensus across several chapters that interventions must be multilevel or multidimensional (e.g., Rimer et al., Chapter 15), that they must involve not only the patient but also family members, social networks, and community resources as well as health institutions and providers. Moreover, they must deal with a range of lifestyle activities beyond medically prescribed actions.

Successful interventions are those that seem to be especially designed for and tailored to fit particular problems in identified populations (e.g., Fisher et al., Rimer et al.). Provider initiatives are emphasized throughout the volume. The importance of the cultural acceptability of an intervention cannot be overestimated (e.g., Champion & Miller, Chapter 13; Morisky & Cabrera, Chapter 14). Characteristics of successful programs include providing feedback and reinforcement, individualized learning, skill instruction, access to resources, efforts to address patient needs continuously, active patients, and social support (e.g., Clark, Chapter 8). Moreover, there is often a need to train staff members to carry out the interventions (e.g., Fisher et al.; Morisky & Cabrera).

Professional versus Phenomenological Perspectives

While Trostle (Chapter 6) points out that historically the literature on compliance research has largely dealt with physician power and control and has been written largely by physicians about themselves, the discussions in this volume of adherence and other health behaviors indicate that the research questions are being reframed. The traditional model of physician power based on a monopoly of knowledge is diminishing, and patient and layperson perspectives are increasingly incorporated into research and practice.

Shared decision making (e.g., DiMatteo, Chapter 1; Haug, Chapter 3) involving questioning and challenging by patients, together with negotiations, is being seen as a model for physician-patient interaction, rather than the model of physician determination. The consumerist movement has led to a contrasting conception of purchaser's "rights" and seller's "obligations" (Haug). The HMO movement (prior to its becoming increasingly corporate for-profit) also encouraged patients to demand services. Physician power is also being eroded by other professions (Haug; Salloway et al., Chapter 4), such as nurse-practitioners and nurse midwives, and by the bureaucratization and corporatization of the medical system (Haug; Salloway et al.). Finally, the increasing awareness that a good part of medical practice was based less on empiricism than on ideology (Trostle), and an accumulation of dubious medical results such as the thalidomide scandal (Haug), make consumers reluctant to accept medicine in an uncritical way.

The Role of Affect

Complementing the conceptualization of adherence and other health behaviors in terms of rational, conscious self-management are the affective components of interactions between laypersons and health care providers and institutions. Both DiMatteo (Chapter 1) and Ben-Sira (Chapter 2) emphasize the emotional side of such interactions. Ben-Sira notes that patients bring anxiety about illness into their encounters with physicians; that physicians, by training and by the structure of institutional rewards, tend to be unwilling or unable to deal with such anxiety; and that the gap between technological medicine and the patient's emotional needs has an impact on satisfaction with care, on utilization of services, and on adherence. DiMatteo notes that communication between physicians and patients is impeded by anxiety and by the patient's emotional state. Such impaired communication has negative implications for the success of treatment and for adherence to regimens.

A further "nonrational" issue is the "vividness" of memories for improbable but dramatic events. Cohen and Colligan (Chapter 20) note that workers' memories for unlikely but vivid events can be obstacles to their engaging in appropriate safety behaviors. This phenomenon is parallel to the "optimistic bias" discussed in several chapters in Volume I.

Size of the Focal System

There is consensus in this volume that adherence and other health behaviors are best understood and improved when multiple levels of personal and social systems are included, and that more traditional models that focus only on the patient, or that assume that only the physician can or should dictate regimens, are inappropriate (e.g., Morisky & Cabrera, Chapter 14). While there may be appropriate focus on a single system, such as the family in relation to adherence to juvenile diabetes regimens (Wysocki & Greco, Chapter 9), the family is simultaneously in interaction not only with the young patient, but also with the caregiver, the care institutions, and the community.

Social and societal values also play a role in the changing patterns of role relationships (Salloway et al., Chapter 4) and in the power of physicians (Haug, Chapter 3). Finally, Trostle (Chapter 6) provides a cogent argument, in addition, that larger political and economic systems must be considered. He provides compelling evidence of the interlocking commercial interests—of physicians, of pharmaceutical suppliers, and of food manufacturers—that contribute to making compliance a medical issue.

FUTURE RESEARCH DIRECTIONS

Methodological Directions: The "Boilerplate"

A discussion of future directions for health behavior research would be remiss if it did not include a restatement of "boilerplate" themes, although many of these themes are the mirror images of the dicussion of methodological issues earlier in this chapter. Future research on institutional determinants (as on any of the dimensions of social or behavioral science) must be increasingly longitudinal; must embrace more diverse samples, including African-Americans, Hispanics, and women, cross-cultural comparisons, illiterate workers performing the dirtiest industrial tasks where knowledge of use of protective measures is imperative, care providers and children, nonusers of services and nonparticipants in programs; must use more appropriate, valid, and reliable measures; must employ agreed-upon identical or comparable measures across diverse studies; must eliminate errors of subject recall; and must avoid uncritical acceptance of medical perspectives.

Conceptual Models

Future research related to conceptual models must use existing theory more effectively in developing interventions and developing research in a way that will yield more robust theoretical explanations (Clark, Chapter 8). There is also a need for detailed theoretical development and empirical examination of communication between professionals and patients, linking this communication to improving the process of shared decision making (DiMatteo, Chapter 1).

Lines of research related to specific conceptual models include increasing understanding of the transtheoretical/stages of change models through applying them systematically to the design of interventions (Marcus et al., chapter 18). Of particular interest are the precontemplative and contemplative stages of change. The role of developmental milestones or transitions that have the potential to increase and maintain behaviors, such as exercise and physical activity, should be explored, and there should be increased investigation of relapse-prevention, social, and cognitive learning models (Marcus et al.).

Research on Institutional Factors and Interventions

Important topics suggested for future research include the impact on adherence, prevention, and patient satisfaction of such institutional and structural factors as changing power relationships (Haug, Chapter 3), corporate medicine (Haug; Scarpaci & Kearns, Chapter 5), and managed care (Glasgow & Orleans, Chapter 9; Salloway et al., Chapter 4). Future intervention programs should be based on what is already known about behavior change (e.g., Clark, Chapter 8), and research on these programs should focus on improving their fit with specific problems and populations, i.e., their specific tailoring (Rimer et al., Chapter 15); examining the impact on adherence of manipulations of mediating factors such as social support and coping skills (Christensen et al., Chapter 12); and use of culturally appropriate educational materials (Morisky & Cabrera, Chapter 14).

As an alternative to specifying an endless list of theories and concepts and their interactions, questions for future research can be framed in terms of bald empiricism: "What makes for ...?" "What constitutes the most effective ...?" For example, as Clark suggests, there is need for research on determining the elements of successful programs; on what processes and methods best engender self-management and on whether these measures are best directed at individuals, groups, or combinations thereof; and on what external factors, such as organizational arrangements and community resources, contribute to program success. Similarly, Wysocki and Greco (Chapter 9) suggest that research is needed to determine what factors create higher levels of skill in self-management, what types of parents are most likely to benefit from (or fare poorly in) skills building, and how parental involvement can be maintained. More specifically Christensen et al. (Chapter 12) encourage research that attempts to increase patient self-management or problem-solving skills in dialysis treatments involving greater patient control and to increase emotional regulation or cognitive change for patients whose dialysis is less controllable. Marcus et al. (Chapter 18) suggest research into the determinants of acceptance of exercise in older persons. They also encourage thinking beyond the traditional types of programs to consider examining exercise in terms of lighter physical activity engaged in by women, such as walking and child care, and to examine the effects that changing one health behavior has on other health behaviors.

What is the impact of worksite interventions on acceptance of mammography (Champion & Miller, Chapter 13) and other programs? What organizational structures lend themselves to more effective worksite programs? What types of companies are "healthy," i.e., have good safety behavior records (Cohen & Colligan, Chapter 20)? What are the reinforcers of adherent behavior in the workplace? What role is played, for example, by the buddy system, by booster sessions, or by relapse-prevention programs?

Timing and scheduling issues are also thought to be important directions for future research. DiMatteo (Chapter 1) raises the question of the timing of providing information; Cohen and Colligan (Chapter 20) raise the question of scheduling of training to increase workplace safety behaviors. Finally, the entire research time frame must be expanded to include more longitudinal investigation of long-term adherence rather than one-time or interval study (Champion & Miller; McCaul, Chapter 16).

Major barriers to future legitimate and uncompromised health behavior research may be found in the degree to which managed care engulfs the delivery of health services. Salloway et al. (Chapter 4), noting the extent to which managed care is driven by corporate economic interests, raise the questions of whether findings emerging from institutions under managed care will be too company-specific, whether they will be considered the property of the corporate ownership, and whether the research agenda will be set by private, corporate funding sources and not by public interest.

The Search for Meaning

Meaning of Illness

The role of the meaning of illness is amplified in Ben-Sira's discussion (Chapter 2) of "lay-intelligible explanations" and of the importance of relief from the illness-generated anxiety as an objective in the patient's interactions with a health care practitioner. Stimson and Webb (1975, p. 2) also point out how patients attempt to make sense out of what has happened to them.

Meaning of Treatment

In the context of their analysis of how pressures for reputation in persons and institutions lead to increased technological interventions, Fox and Swazey (1978) raise critical questions about the meaning of treatment and about whether treatment must be employed simply because it is available. Fox and Swazey (1978, p. 379) ask: "Is it medically and morally proper to dialyze or transplant *all* these patients because monies are available, whether or not they will benefit from treatment?"

Similarly, Elinson (1985) raises the question of the meaning of treatment by pointing to the potential conflict between therapeutic goals aimed at increasing the quality of life and those aimed at increasing its quantity. Such conflicts are likely to increase in older populations, whose values may not always be deferent to medical technology, and whose concern for quality of life may transcend acceptance of "good" medical care, particularly when evidence is accumulating that an acceptable quality of life can be maintained even during the terminal stages of illness (Morris, Suissa, Sherwood, Wright, & Greer, 1986). Compliance studies are increasingly identifying what the medication means to the patient. Conrad (1985), for example, has shown that compliance can be a reminder that the patient has a stigmatized condition (e.g., epilepsy).

Furthermore, as DiMatteo (Chapter 1) and Ben-Sira (Chapter 2) make clear, the affective components of treatment—what the treatment means in terms of the feelings and emotional needs of the patient—in contrast to the instrumental or technical components, are increasingly important areas for systematic future research.

The meaning of treatment in these contexts is juxtaposed with the question of the quality of life. Thus, the meaning of treatment in relation to personal needs, values, and conceptions of what constitutes quality of life appears to be an important factor in reconsidering definitions of "compliance," "adherence," or "acceptance" of treatment, and is thus a promising area for future health behavior research.

Meaning of Environment

Whitehead, Fusillo, and Kaplan (1988) urged that the way in which laypersons—patients, clients, consumers—attempt to make sense out of their physical environments be investigated systematically. Specifically, they note the importance of movement, contours, bulk, and simplicity as determinants of ability to remember a location; the role of graphic displays in making settings comprehensible and thus maximally useful; and some hypothesized relationships between these physical dimensions of the environment and the degree to which clients feel that the environment is manageable and predictable and that they are being treated as responsible persons.

The manner in which more general aspects of space and time generate meanings also has subtle implications for health behavior. In the context of analyzing social constructions of space and time, Armstrong (1985) examined changes in the spatial and temporal arrangements of British medical practice and how these changes have modified conceptions about the meaning of the treatment process and about how professionals and patients relate to one another. According to Armstrong, the traditional British "surgery" was part of the physician's "smoke room" and was not partitioned or separated from it in any way. Thus, medical space was not divorced from domestic space. The traditional British surgery did not have distinct areas for specialized medical functions, i.e., testing, diagnosis, and treatment. Medical space, however, eventually became differentiated from domestic space, at first through the establishment of a separate surgery, possibly with its own entrance, and later through the establishment of clinics and health centers as sites for primary care practice. As a consequence of such physical separation, it became less common for physicians to visit patients at home, solidifying the separation of medical and domestic spaces. Such changes are interpreted as having powerful implications for divorcing medical problems, issues, and practices from the total life of the patient and the community. Further spatial separation of functions in modern clinics and practice settings is seen to be related to the fragmentation of the treatment process.

Parallel with and related to spatial changes were changes in the social construction of the temporal aspects of practice. Armstrong notes that the separation of the medical from the domestic established and strengthened the boundaries between the physician's own personal life and professional activities. Physicians could now have "off-duty time" that they previously lacked. It also led to setting appointments and to other forms of "time management" that are related to fragmentation of the interactions between physicians and patients.

Scarpaci and Kearns (Chapter 5) enlarge on the concept of the "sense of place" and reveal that while the social constructions of the meanings of space and time have received little attention, they present an important area for future health behavior research.

SUMMARY

Historically, research on health institutions as determinants of health behavior has focused largely on "compliance"—or, more broadly, on adherence to disease-focused and lifestyle regimens—and on care seeking. By the mid-1990s, research had moved away from a professionally defined conception of medical compliance and toward a more multidimensional conception of adherence or acceptance that increasingly focuses on self-regulation or self-maintenance, with the patient interacting continuously and dynamically with health providers, family members, social networks, community resources, organizational structures, and institutions beyond the health care system.

The single institutional factor that appears to have the greatest impact on health behaviors is communication. Good communication within the medical encounter is likely to reduce patient anxiety, bringing a corollary increase in patient satisfaction with care, remaining in care, and appropriate care-seeking behavior. Good communication will improve patients' understanding of treatment regimens, with a resulting improvement of adherence. Furthermore, within the broad context of communication, provider initiatives, i.e., health professionals' taking on the responsibility for making suggestions or recommendations, will increase the likelihood of patients' participating in a range of preventive screening programs

Much research is needed to increase the generalizability of existing findings, including increasing the reliability and validity of measurements, standardizing instrumentation, and expanding the range of data bases. Finally, there is a great need for research on the phenomenology of illness, on the meanings of conditions and treatments and the settings that deal with them.

REFERENCES

Armstrong, D. (1985). Space and time in British general practice. *Social Science and Medicine, 20,* 659-666.

Conrad, P. (1985). The meaning of medications: Another look at compliance. *Social Science and Medicine, 20,* 29-37.

Elinson, J. (1985). The end of medicine and the end of medical sociology. *Journal of Health and Social Behavior, 26,* 268-275.

Fox, R. C., & Swazey, J. P. (1978). *The courage to fail: A social view of organ transplants and dialysis* (2nd ed., rev ed.). Chicago: University of Chicago Press.

Morris, J. N., Suissa, S., Sherwood, S., Wright, S. M., & Greer, D. (1986). Last days: A study of the quality of life of terminally ill cancer patients. *Journal of Chronic Diseases, 39,* 47-62.

Stimson, G., & Webb, B. (1975). *Going to see the doctor: The consultation process in general practice.* London: Routledge & Kegan Paul.

Whitehead, B. A., Fusillo, A. E., & Kaplan, S. (1988). The design of physical environments and health behavior. In D. S. Gochman (Ed.), *Health Behavior: Emerging research perspectives* (pp. 231-241). New York: Plenum Press.

Concepts and Definitions

A Glossary for Health Behavior Research

With few exceptions, the definitions in this Glossary are either taken verbatim, paraphrased, or abstracted from this *Handbook*. Specific chapters and, where appropriate, sources cited herein are identified. Italicized terms within a definition denote additional Glossary entries.

Consistent with the focus of this *Handbook* on health *behavior*, the Glossary does not routinely define diseases or medical treatments. Space limitations preclude defining every "named" intervention or program, or every social or behavioral science model that is not especially focused on health behavior. A number of these programs and models, however, are listed in the Index.

acceptance See *adherence; compliance*.

access framework A conceptual refinement of the *health services utilization model* that predicts the use of and satisfaction with health care; basic components are health policy, the organizational and accessibility characteristics of the delivery system, and *predisposing*, *enabling*, and *need factors* (Aday & Andersen, 1974, in Aday & Awe, I, 8). See *utilization framework*.

action stage In the *transtheoretical model*, the phase in which persons have modified their behavior and are participating in the appropriate health practice (Prohaska & Clark, III, 2).

active coping In health contexts, a tendency or motivation to exercise personal control, reflecting preference for decision making in health care, preference for behavioral involvement, and low expectations that health care professionals can control one's health (Christensen, Benotsch, & Smith, II, 12).

active patient orientation See *mutual participation model*.

active prevention See *prevention, active*.

activities of daily living (ADL) Instrumental and basic behaviors necessary for everyday life (Prohaska & Clark, III, 2).

adherence Practice of following health care provider recommendations (Clark, II, 8; Chrisler, II, 17); "an interdependent network of regimen behaviors rather than a single behavior" (Wysocki & Greco, II, 9); following recommended screening procedures (Rimer, Demark-Wahnefried, & Egert, II, 15); congruence between patient behaviors and advice or instructions provided by health care providers; medical adherence: how closely a patient's medication-taking behaviors match instructions prescribed by a physician (Creer & Levstek, II, 7). The concept embraces total adherence and acceptance, as well as degrees thereof; in relation to smoking, it includes not only total cessation, but also participation in cessation activities, as well as the actions of change agents (Glasgow & Orleans, II, 19). It connotes active, voluntary behavior designed to produce a therapeutic effect (Chrisler, II, 17). See *compliance*.

ADL See *activities of daily living*.

affective behavior, physician's Comprises acts aimed at establishing a relationship with patients in which the physician accepts the patient as a human being whose anxiety-arousing problems cannot be alleviated by technical procedures; it involves the physician attributing therapeutic importance to, and engaging in warm, open relations with the patient; being attentive to problems that may not be related to disease; gathering information about personal and family problems and social relations; and explaining the rationale of the diagnosis and treatment (Ben-Sira, II, 2).

AIDS Acquired immunodeficiency syndrome: a condition in which exposure to the *HIV* (human immunodeficiency virus) leads to the destruction of the body's natural defenses against infection (Thomason & Campos, III, 8).

analytical framework for the study of child survival A conceptual model designed to understand morbidity and mortality in children in developing countries; basic components are maternal factors, environmental contamination, nutrient deficiency, and injury and personal illness control (Mosley & Chen, 1984, in Coreil, III, 9).

anthropology of medicine See *medical anthropology*.

appropriate interventions/care Lists of indications for use of procedures consensually generated by nationally recognized experts (Rand Corporation/McGlynn, Kosecoff, & Brook, 1990, in DiMatteo, II, 1). Compare *inappropriate/unnecessary care*.

attributable risk Amount of disease (disability or mortality) in a population group that could be eliminated if a risk factor were eliminated (Prohaska & Clark, III, 2).

authority, physician The physician's power over others (Haug, II, 3).

autonomy, physician The physician's power or ability to resist or withstand being compelled by others (Haug, II, 3).

autonomy, principle of A moral standard stressing the obligation to respect rights to self-determination (Nilstun, IV, 11).

autonomy, self-care See *self-care autonomy*.

availability bias A concept that explains safety and risk avoidance behaviors, denoting the inclination to be inordinately influenced by dramatic events that have low probabilities of happening but are vivid in memory; ease of recall being a function of saliency, recency, and emotional impact (Slovic, 1978, in Cohen & Colligan, II, 20).

behavioral epidemiology The study of the relationships between lifestyles and mortality and morbidity patterns in a population (Rakowski, III, 5).

behavioral model See *health services utilization model*.

beneficence, principle of A moral standard stressing the obligation to benefit others, especially not to harm them (Nilstun, IV, 11).

bruxism Spasmodic grinding of the teeth in other than chewing movements (Gift & White, IV, 7).

caregiver, informal Layperson who provides personal care to an older, ill family member or close friend (Wright, III, 13).

care-seeking behavior, theory of A conceptual framework in nursing, incorporating components of the *health belief model*, *theory of reasoned action*, and Triandis's theory of interpersonal behavior; designed to predict preventive rather than illness-related behaviors; basic components are affective arousal, perceived utility, *social norms*, and habits (Lauver, 1992a, in Blue & Brooks, IV, 5).

central place theory A conceptual framework based on land economics that is used to relate a hierarchy of levels of health care services to concentrations of population and distances (Scarpaci & Kearns, II, 5).

children's health belief model A conceptual framework for understanding children's health behaviors, incorporating components of the *health belief model*, environmental variables, and readiness factors (O'Brien & Bush, III, 3).

chronic Referring to an illness or condition that is incurable and lasts through a person's lifetime (Gallagher & Stratton, III, 11).

cognitive appraisal The process of intellectually evaluating and deciding on available options to engage in a particular behavior (Cowell & Marks, III, 4).

cognitive developmental theory A conceptual framework for understanding the development of children's thinking; assumes that children take an active rather than a passive role in constructing their own knowledge and understanding of health and illness and that they move through universally recognized sequences in doing so (O'Brien & Bush, III, 3).

cognitive representations Personal images or schemata of illness, disease, and being healthy, and the meanings attached to these images; persons develop their own individualized images or schemata in relation to symptoms and illness that are often different from the representations of physicians and the medical community (Lau, I, 3).

coming out Disclosure of nonheterosexual identity by a lesbian or a gay man (VanScoy, III, 7); can also mean self-recognition of such identity.

commonsense representation of illness The images or schemata of illness, disease, or symptoms held by a layperson; the images include an identity, a set of consequences, a time-line, a cause, and a cure or control (Lau, I, 3).

communication Exchange of meaning, either verbally or nonverbally, between people to establish a commonality of thought, attitude, feeling, and ideas (DiMatteo, II, 1).

communication campaign Use of mass media on a health topic, typically involving television, radio, newspaper, magazines, and other channels to convey health information or to provide motivation for health actions (Swinehart, IV, 18).

community A social entity or system made up of individuals together with formal organizations, such as local government, businesses, and educational institutions, and voluntary organizations, such as religious, fraternal, or service groups; informal social networks; and families. Critical to the concept is the premise that various components are related to each other and have the potential for being mobilized in relation to health promotion programs (Schooler & Flora, IV, 15).

community health promotion Interventions for effecting change in communities that involve social planning, social action, and locality development (Rothman, 1979, in Schooler & Flora, IV, 15).

community organization An intervention strategy designed to empower a community and to enhance its competence and problem-solving ability; of particular importance for increasing the success of a *health promotion* program (Schooler & Flora, IV, 15).

compadrazgo A system of selecting *comadres* (female friends) and *copadres* (male friends) for one's children; levels of perceived support from these friends are related to health status and health behavior (Dressler & Oths, I, 17).

competence gap The difference in health-related knowledge and skill between physicians and other health professionals and their patients or clients (Haug, II, 3).

compliance Degree of correspondence between the physician's prescription and the patient's behavior (Sackett & Haynes, 1976, in DiIorio, II, 11; Morisky & Cabrera, II, 14); congruence between medical recommendations and the degree to which a patient takes medicine, follows a diet, or changes lifestyle behaviors (Trostle, II, 6); an ideology that transforms a physician's theories about patients' behavior into research strategies and potentially coercive interventions that strengthen physicians' authority (Trostle, II, 6). See also *adherence*.

conscientiousness factor A theoretical personality dimension reflecting "will to achieve," "dependability," and "self-control" thought to be related to medication adherence in renal dialysis patients (Christensen et al., II, 12).

consciousness raising A component of the *transtheoretical model*, denoting a process by which people move from not being ready to initiate a behavior to being ready to initiate it (Rakowski, III, 5).

consumerism A framework for viewing physician–patient interactions that argues for patient autonomy and sole decision making as essential in combating physician paternalism (DiMatteo, II, 1), or in which an "activist" patient approaches health care as a problem-solving endeavor that requires active coping (Pratt, 1978, in Wiese & Gallagher, IV, 4).

contemplation In the *transtheoretical model*, the stage in which people are aware that a problem exists and are seriously thinking about overcoming it (Prohaska & Clark, III, 2).

contracting Use of a written document, resulting from the negotiation of a treatment plan between a patient and medical personnel, that identifies the reinforcements the patient will receive contingent on performing the behaviors stipulated in the treatment plan (Creer & Levstek, II, 7).

control beliefs See *locus of control*.

control demand model A conceptual framework developed to understand how workplace characteristics are related to health behaviors such as smoking, alcohol use, exercise, and self-protective behavior; basic components are levels of control over work, psychological demands, and social support (Eakin, I, 16).

control, perceived behavioral See *perceived behavioral control*.

convergence hypothesis A proposition that suggests that as gender roles become more similar, gender differences in health behavior decrease or disappear (Waldron, I, 15).

conversation model A conceptual framework for viewing physician–patient interactions in which the patient continually provides the physician information about values, preferences, and constraints and the physician engages in "thinking out loud" about possible courses of action, recommended interventions, and their implications, using language that is understood by the patient (DiMatteo, II, 1).

coping appraisal Evaluation of adaptive responses to threat; a component of the *protection motivation theory* (Rogers & Prentice-Dunn, I, 6).

coping mode Way of responding to threat messages (Rogers & Prentice-Dunn, I, 6). See *protection motivation theory*.

cue to action A stimulus, either internal or external, that can trigger health-related cognitive processes or health actions (Strecher, Champion, & Rosenstock, I, 4).

cultural consensus model A conceptual framework to assess the degree to which a body of information is shared within a social group; provides an estimate of shared beliefs related to health and illness (Dressler & Oths, I, 17).

culture A set of interlocking cognitive schemata that literally construct much of what people do on a daily basis; the manner in which a social group stores and transmits information; a system of symbols or abstract elements that are learned and patterned socially (Dressler & Oths, I, 17).

damaging cycle A chain of events in which a somatic disturbance leads to a detrimental appraisal of health, which then precipitates stress, which then increases the risk of further somatic disturbance (Ben-Sira, II, 2).

decisional balance theory A conceptual framework for understanding how persons make specific choices, based on comparisons of perceived positive and negative aspects of a behavior, and including gains and losses to self and others and approval or disapproval of self and others (Janis & Mann, 1977, in Marcus, Bock, & Pinto, II, 18).

demography, health See *health demography*.

deskilling Transference of work functions once controlled exclusively by physicians or nurses to positions lower down on the occupational hierarchy (Salloway, Hafferty, & Vissing, II, 4).

developing country A designation based on economic, demographic, and social/health indicators, given to a nation that is relatively poor, with a relatively young and fertile population and relatively scarce health and social resources (Coreil, III, 9).

developmental model of diabetes self-management A conceptual framework for understanding the responsibilities that patients and families can assume in monitoring, evaluating, and adjusting treatment for insulin-dependent diabetes mellitus; basic components include demographic factors, family functioning, psychological stress, and interactions with providers to acquire necessary skills (Wysocki & Greco, II, 9). See *self-management, childhood diabetes*; *self-regulation/self-regulatory skills*.

diagnosis Naming of a condition by medical professionals; represents the interplay of social, institutional, and cultural factors together with personal symptoms through which time and location at which medical professionals and other parties determine the existence and legitimacy of a condition (Brown, 1995, in Gochman, IV, 20).

diagnosis related group/diagnostic related group (DRG) One of 438 groupings of patient conditions that have been the basis for federal reimbursements to hospitals for Medicare patients since 1983 (Daugherty, IV, 10); hospitals are paid a fixed amount for a given DRG regardless of length of stay and services provided.

disease A biological/organic abnormality; not identical to illness (Lau, I, 3); the measurable deviation of an organic system from some independently defined optimum (Dressler & Oths, I, 17).

doctrine of specific etiology See *specific etiology, doctrine of*.

DRG See *diagnosis related group*.

drinking culture Group norms, particularly within work settings, that encourage and support consumption of alcohol; closely related to *occupational culture* (Eakin, I, 16).

ecological model A conceptual framework that integrates five levels of personal and social systems: intrapersonal, interpersonal, organizational, community, and public policy in public health efforts (Buchanan, IV, 9).

edentulous Without teeth; toothless (Gift & White, IV, 7).

effectiveness Benefits of medical care measured by improvements in health (Aday & Awe, I, 8).

efficiency A relationship between improvements in health and the resources required to produce them (Aday & Awe, I, 8).

elaboration likelihood model A conceptual framework to predict attitude change; persuasion is proposed to be a function of the audience's active involvement in processing a message and the importance of the message's topic to the audience (Petty &

Cacioppo, 1986, in Rogers & Prentice-Dunn, I, 6; Wiese & Gallagher, IV, 4).

emic Denotes a way of knowing reflecting an internal or cultural "insider" perspective (Weidman, 1988, in Gochman, I, Part V); emic behavior is behavior that a person believes to be related to health, regardless of whether it is externally validated (Eakin, I, 16). Compare *etic*.

empowerment Enabling individuals, families, and communities to take control over their lives and their environment (e.g., Rappaport, 1984, in Schooler & Flora, IV, 15).

enabling factor A resource characteristic, such as family income or community availability, that predicts use of health services; a component of the *health services utilization model* (Aday & Awe, I, 8).

energized family A conceptual framework for understanding the family as a social system; basic components are regularity of interaction among members, contacts with the larger community, working together to advance members' interests, and coping with and mastering their lives. Energized families tend to encourage autonomy, rather than use "autocratic" parenting, and to socialization methods, resulting in children with better levels of health behaviors (Pratt, 1976, in Gochman, I, 10; Tinsley, I, 11).

epidemiology "Study of the distribution and determinants of diseases and injuries in human populations" (Inhorn, 1995, in Gochman, IV, 20).

epidemiology, behavioral See *behavioral epidemiology*.

epidemiology, psychosocial See *psychosocial epidemiology*.

equity The degree to which the benefits and burdens of medical care are fairly distributed in a population (Aday & Awe, I, 8); the degree to which participants (either patients or professionals) believe that the ratio of benefits received to their efforts and resources expended is equal or skewed in their favor (Daugherty, IV, 10).

etic Denotes a way of knowing reflecting an external or cultural "outsider" perspective (Weidman, 1988, in Gochman, I, Part V). Etic behavior is behavior that external observers believe to be related to health, independent of the behaving individual's beliefs (Eakin, I, 16). Compare *emic*.

eudaimonistic health A state of exuberant well-being (Lau, I, 3).

exercise Physical activity of moderate intensity (Marcus et al., II, 18).

explanatory model A cognitive framework of health processes based on both cultural knowledge and idiosyncratic experience that is used to understand health status, illness, and sickness; basic components include etiology, timing of onset of symptoms, pathophysiology, course of sickness, and treatment. Explanatory models exist at both lay and professional levels (Kleinman, 1980, & Kleinman, Eisenberg, & Good, 1978, in Dressler & Oths, I, 17).

facilitative environment An environment in which "nonsmoking cues and cessation information are persistent and inescapable" (Glynn, Boyd, & Gruman, 1990, in Glasgow & Orleans, II, 19).

familism Importance of family and relatives in a person's live, particularly in relation to care-seeking behavior (Geertsen, I, 13).

family aggregation A concept denoting intrafamilial similarities in health variables compared to nonfamilial similarities (Sallis & Nader, 1988, in Gochman, I, 10).

family code A system of norms for a family's behavior, including core assumptions, beliefs, family stories, myths, and rituals (Tinsley, I, 11).

family concordance Degree to which members of a family exhibit similarity in a specified health behavior (Baranowski, I, 9).

family, energized See *energized family*.

family health culture The unique combination of family experiences, beliefs, perceptions of symptoms, and reactions to the perceptions that influences the way in which families seek care or treatment (Black, 1986, in Gochman, I, 10).

fighting the illness A posture of gritty defiance as a way of dealing with a chronic illness (Gallagher & Stratton, III, 11).

fixed role hypothesis A proposition suggesting that men's more structured role obligations, compared with women's, may make it more difficult for men to engage in care-seeking behavior and thus accounts for women's greater use of health services (Marcus & Siegel, 1982, in Gochman, I, Part IV).

Flexner Report An analysis and recommendations relevant to United States medical education, prepared by Abraham Flexner in 1910, that became the basis for the reform of and standardization of medical training; remains a critical foundation for late 20th-century medical education (Weise & Gallagher, IV, 4).

folk illness A shared interpretation of a cluster of symptoms within a social group that is at variance with a biomedical framework (Dressler & Oths, I, 17).

framework of relationships model A conceptual scheme for understanding compliance behavior, especially for epilepsy; basic components are the ***health services utilization model***, the ***health belief model***, and health education, with an emphasis on adequate financial and community resources (Di Iorio, II, 11).

gay Without a gender qualifier, refers to a homosexual, a person who engages or desires to engage in sexual behavior with a person of the same gender (Kauth & Prejean, III, 6).

gay man A male who engages or desires to engage in sexual behavior with another male; a homosexual (Kauth & Prejean, III, 6).

gender role The social roles, behaviors, attitudes, and psychological characteristics that are more common, more expected, and more accepted for one sex or the other; includes a group of interrelated behaviors, attitudes, and psychological characteristics that influence a variety of risk and risk-taking behaviors as well as care-seeking behaviors (Waldron, I, 15).

GOBI Acronym for *G*rowth monitoring, *O*ral rehydration, *B*reast-feeding and *I*mmunization, the four cornerstone child survival interventions in developing countries (Coreil, III, 9).

grazing Snacking throughout the day (O'Brien & Bush, III, 3).

group ties See *social ties*.

habit A behavior that does not require conscious effort but is set in motion by situational cues (Schneider & Shiffrin, 1977, in Maddux & DuCharme, I, 7) and is less under the control of conscious cognitive processes and deliberate decisions.

healing The social processes and actions brought to bear to deal with a condition of disease or illess (Fabrega, I, 2).

healing culture The totality of institutions involved in treatment of disease, including biomedical and alternative approaches and the range of choices available, and the culture of medicine and its rituals and stresses (e.g., Foster & Anderson, 1978, in Gochman, IV, 20).

healmeme A unit of symbolic cultural information that gives meaning to the domain of health, well-being, sickness, and healing; underlies and constitutes a society's health-related beliefs and behaviors (Fabrega, I, 2).

health A state of being, almost impossible to define satisfactorily; includes components of physiological, psychological, and social functioning (Gochman I, 1; Lau, I, 3). What is considered to be health is appreciably determined by societal and cultural factors (Fabrega, I, 2). A continuous variable reflecting a capacity or ability to perform, as well as the use of that capacity to achieve expectations and to negotiate the demands of the social and physical environment (Tarlov, 1992, in Reed, Moore-West, Jernstedt, & O'Donell, IV, 2); "an individual or group capacity relative to potential to function fully in the social and physical environment" (Tarlov, 1992, in Flipse, IV, 3).

health behavior, formal Actions taken for the prevention or treatment of a condition or for the maintenance or enhancement of health that involve the use of institutionalized services such as physicians and hospitals (Pol & Thomas, III, 1).

health behavior, informal Actions taken for the prevention or treatment of a condition or for the maintenance or enhancement of health that do not involve the use of institutionalized services such as physicians and hospitals; these actions include self-care, tooth brushing, and use of over-the-counter medications (Pol & Thomas, III, 1).

health belief model A conceptual framework designed to predict preventive actions and eventually used to predict illness and sick role behaviors; basic components of the model are perceived susceptibility to some illness, perceived severity or seriousness of that condition, perceived benefits of taking a specified action, and perceived barriers to taking such action (Strecher, Champion, & Rosenstock, I, 4).

health care management See ***management, health care***.

health care manager See ***manager, health care***.

health culture A society's repertoire of patterns for cognition, affect, and behavior in relation to health, sickness, and well-being (Weidman, 1988, in Gochman, I, Part V).

health demography Application of the content and methods of demography to the study of health-related phenomena; analyzes the influence of demographic factors such as age, marital status, and income on the health status and health behavior of poplations and the differential impact of health-related phenomena on demographic groupings; focuses on the implications of population change for health care (Pol & Thomas, III, 1). See ***behavioral epidemiology***; ***psychosocial epidemiology***.

health education Efforts to change behavior in order to improve health (Glanz & Oldenburg, IV, 8); "any combination of learning experiences designed to facilitate voluntary adaptations of behavior conducive to health" (Green, Kreuter, Deeds, & Partridge, 1980, p. 7, in Glanz & Oldenburg, IV, 8).

health input–output model See *input-output model, health.*

health maintenance organization (HMO) A prepaid group practice for delivering comprehensive health care from a specific set of providers. See *managed care.*

health policy Aggregate of federal, state, and local laws, rules, and regulations that govern the financing, regulation, and organization of health care (Aday & Awe, I, 8).

health-promoting self-care system model A conceptual framework for nursing, integrating self-care deficit nursing theory, the *interaction model of client health behavior*, and the *health promotion model of nursing*, designed to predict individual autonomy and responsibility for health-promoting behaviors (Simmons, 1990a, in Blue & Brooks, IV, 5).

health promotion "any combination of health education and related organizational, economic, and environmental supports for behavior of individuals, groups, or communities conducive to health" (Green & Kreuter, 1991, in Glanz & Oldenburg, IV, 8); "the science and art of helping people change their lifestyle to move toward a state of optimal health ... by a combination of efforts to enhance awareness, change behavior, and create environments that support good health practices" (O'Donnell, 1989, in Glanz & Oldenburg, IV, 8); "the process of enabling people to increase control over, and to improve, their health ... a commitment to dealing with the challenges of reducing inequities, extending the scope of prevention, and helping people to cope with their circumstances ... creating environments conducive to health, in which people are better able to take care of themselves" (Epp, 1986, in Glanz & Oldenburg, IV, 8). The term was seldom used prior to 1980.

health promotion model, nursing A conceptual framework for nursing, similar to the *health belief model*, used to predict engaging in behaviors that maintain or improve well-being, rather than prevent disease; basic components are importance of health, perceived control of health, perceived *self-efficacy*, definition of health, perceived health status, *perceived benefits* of health-promoting behaviors, and *perceived barriers* to health-promoting behaviors (Pender, 1982, in Blue & Brooks, IV, 5).

health psychology "The aggregate of the specific educational, scientific, and professional contributions of the discipline of psychology to the promotion and maintenance of health, the prevention and treatment of illness, the identification of etiologic and diagnostic correlates of health, illness and related dysfunction" (Matarazzo, 1980, p. 815, in Gochman, IV, 20); "any aspect of psychology that bears upon the experience of health and illness, and the behavior that affects health status" (Rodin & Stone, 1987, pp. 15–16, in Gochman, IV, 20).

health-seeking process model A conceptual framework for understanding people's experiences with sickness holistically as natural histories of illness; basic components are symptom definition, illness-related shifts in role behavior, lay referral, treatment actions, and adherence (Chrisman, 1977, in Dressler & Oths, I, 17).

health service system Arrangements for the potential rendering of care to consumers, including the volume and distribution of services and their accessibility and organization (Aday & Awe, I, 8). See *health services utilization model.*

health services utilization model A conceptual framework designed to predict use of health care, such as visits to physicians and dentists and use of medications and clinical facilities; basic components are *predisposing*, *enabling*, and *need factors* (Aday & Awe, I, 8); sometimes referred to as the *behavioral model.*

heterosexism An assumption, especially among health providers and institutions, that heterosexuality, or male–female sexual expression, is normative and superior to others (VanScoy, III, 7).

HIV See *AIDS.*

HMO Acronym for *health maintenance organization* (Daugherty, IV, 10). See *managed care.*

homeless assistance act, Stewart B. McKinney A 1987 federal law that extended the National Health Care for the Homeless Initiative to a total of 109 cities (Wright & Joyner, III, 10).

homeless, literally Persons who spend their nights either in outdoor locations, in temporary overnight shelters, or in other places not intended for human habitation (Wright & Joyner, III, 10).

homelessness No agreed-upon definition (Wright & Joyner, III, 10). See *homeless, literally*; *housed, marginally.*

homophobia An irrational fear of homosexuality (Eliason, Donelan, & Rundall, 1992, in Vanscoy, III, 7).

housed, marginally Persons with a claim to some minimal housing, but who are at high risk of being *homeless* (Wright & Joyner, III, 10).

illness The subjective experience of some biological/organic/social/emotional abnormality; not identical to disease (e.g., Lau, I, 3); the social and psychological concomitants of putative physiological problems (Conrad, 1990, in Gochman, I, 1); incapacity for role performance (Gerhardt, 1989a, in Gochman, I, 1); motivated deviance (Segall, I, 14); the individual experience of suffering or distress, or disvalued states of being and functioning (Dressler & Oths, I, 17).

illusion of safety Workers' practicing of safe behavior under supervision but of unsafe behavior, such as taking shortcuts and engaging in risky actions, in the absence of supervision; convinces management that it has done its job and that safety regimens are being followed when in reality they are not (Cohen & Colligan, II, 20).

image theory A conceptual framework for decision making based on the fit between alternative choices and an individual's images, plans, or principles (Mitchell & Beach, 1990, in Rogers & Prentice-Dunn, I, 6).

inappropriate/unnecessary care A medical intervention with risks that exceed the potential benefit to the patient (DiMatteo, II, 1). Compare *appropriate intervention/care*.

informal caregiver See *caregiver, informal*.

information seeking A generic process that underlies behavior change and comprises a cluster of behaviors including but not limited to reading articles about health, attending to media programs on health, and reading food package labels (Rakowski, III, 5; Swinehart, IV, 18).

information vigilance factor A tendency or motivation to attend actively to threat-relevant information and sensory experiences related to health and treatment, reflecting *information seeking*, internal health *locus of control*, and monitoring of sensory information (Christensen et al., II, 12).

inoculation theory A conceptual framework suggesting that providing persons in advance with information and counterarguments enables them to resist persuasive and pressuring appeals to engage in risk behaviors; sometimes termed "social inoculation theory" (McGuire, 1968, in Kelder et al., IV, 14; Bruhn, IV, 1).

input–output model, health A framework combining external factors such as the physical and community environments and the macrosocial structure with internal biological-genetic-psychic factors as predictors of role fulfillment and well-being (Tarlov, 1992, in Flipse, IV, 3).

inreach Directing health promotion and prevention strategies at persons already in the health care system (Rimer et al., II, 15).

intention, behavioral A person's subjective probability or prediction of performing a specified behavior; a basic component of the *theory of reasoned action*/theory of planned behavior. It has been inaccurately defined as what a person intends or plans to do and the degree to which a person has developed conscious plans to enact some behavior in the future (Maddux & DuCharme, I, 7). See *self-prediction*.

interaction model of client health behavior A conceptual framework in nursing to explain and predict a range of health behaviors; basic components are elements of client singularity, such as background, motivation, cognitive appraisal, and affective responses, and elements of client-professional interactions, such as affective support, health information, decisional control, and professional competence (Cox, 1982, in Blue & Brooks, IV, 5).

interfamilial consensus A concept denoting the degree of similarity in illness-related conceptions in randomly selected pairs of persons (Susman et al., 1982, in Gochman, I, 10).

intrafamilial transmission A concept denoting the degree of similarity in illness-related conceptions found in parent-child pairs (Susman et al., 1982, in Gochman, I, 10).

justice as fairness A conceptual framework applied to health issues that stipulates that each person has an equal right to liberty, that persons with similar abilities and skills should have equal access to services, and that social and economic institutions should be arranged to benefit maximally the least well off (Nilstun, IV, 11).

justice, principle of A moral standard stressing the obligation to act fairly in the distribution of burdens and benefits, especially not to discriminate against anyone (Nilstun, IV, 11).

KAP (acronym for *K*nowledge, *A*ttitudes, and *P*ractices) A standardized measure to assess knowledge of disease risk factors, use of a health service, and perceptions of therapeutic efficacy; used extensively in *developing countries* (Coreil, III, 9).

landscape, therapeutic A combination of physical and humanly imposed environmental characteristics of treatment settings that facilitate the healing process (Gesler, 1992, in Gochman, IV, 20).

language of distress Terminology as well as nonverbal cues that patients use to present their conditions to health professionals (Helman, 1991, in Gochman, IV, 20).

lay-intelligible cues An action on the part of the physician that serves as a basis for the patient's understanding of a condition and its treatment and for the patient's evaluation of the physician's treatment and competence (Ben-Sira, II, 2).

lay referral system The informal network of family members, friends, and community contacts who provide information and advice about the care-seeking process prior to use of a professional (Geertsen, I, 13).

learned resourcefulness Tendency to apply self-control skills in solving behavioral problems, e.g., use of strategies to delay gratification or tolerate frustration (Rosenbaum, 1980, in Christensen et al., II, 12).

lesbian A woman who engages or desires to engage in sexual behavior with another female; the preferred term is "lesbian identity," denoting a woman whose identity is defined by other women (VanScoy, III, 7).

lesbian epistemology A way of knowing the world that reflects a lesbian's own identity and constructions of reality, including of health and illness, in contrast to patriarchal, heterosexist constructions (VanScoy, III, 7).

lesbian invisibility The degree to which lesbian health issues or lesbian identity are hidden or ignored in health services and in the lesbian's interactions with the health care system (VanScoy, III, 7).

libertarianism A conceptual framework applied to health issues that emphasizes the liberty of all individuals to do what they please with themselves and their property, provided they do not interfere with the like liberty of others (Nilstun, IV, 11).

lifespan A framework for individual development that includes chronological age as well as biological and social role transitions (Prohaska & Clark, III, 2).

lifestyle Utilitarian social practices and ways of living adopted by an individual that reflect personal, group, and socioeconomic identities. A health lifestyle involves decisions to live or not to live healthfully; decisions about food, exercise, coping with stress, smoking, alcohol and drug use, risk of accidents, and physical appearance; and reflects social norms and values (Cockerham, I, 12).

lifestyle changes Modifications of behavior resulting from negotiated agreements rather than physician's orders (Chrisler, II, 17).

locality development A cooperative, broadly based approach to community health promotion interventions involving wide discussion and joint problem solving among many diverse groups (Rothman, 1979, in Schooler & Flora, IV, 15).

locational attributes Proximity, centrality, and convenience of health care facilities (Scarpaci & Kearns, II, 5).

locus of control, internal Beliefs that things that happen are a result of one's own ability to influence events as opposed to being the result of chance or fate or of powerful other forces; has been used to predict varied health behaviors (Reich, Zautra, & Erdal, I, 5).

managed care A form of delivering health services in which an organization assumes total responsibility and financial risk for its participants' health, providing all needed services and treatments on a prepaid, capitation basis; an outgrowth of *health maintenance organizations (HMOs)* (Daughtery, IV, 10).

management, health care Tasks of planning, organizing, directing, communicating, coordinating, and monitoring organizational functions in health settings by persons specifically designated and empowered to do so; execution of these tasks through an orderly institutional process carried out by persons designated as managers, regardless of their specific titles (Daugherty, IV, 10).

manager, health care An administrator, executive, director, or chief; anyone who has, or shares in, the legal authority and responsibility for the functions, direction, and achievements of a health organization (Daugherty, IV, 10).

media advocacy Use of mass media to advance a social or public policy objective (Pertschuk, 1988, in Schooler & Flora, IV, 15).

medical anthropology The study of cultural factors related to disease and its explanations, and to healing, treatment, responses to illness and interactions between healers and persons who are sick (Gochman, IV, 20).

medical geography The study of physical, climatic, and locational factors related to disease and its explanations and to healing, treatment, responses to illness, and interactions between healers and persons who are sick (Barrett, 1993, in Gochman, IV, 20).

medical model A framework for looking at illness that is based largely on the 19th-century linkages of germ theory and acute diseases and that accords physicians and medical institutions primacy in diagnosis and treatment; an overdependence on medical metaphors in dealing with behavioral variability and problems in living.

medical pluralism Existence of a multiplicity of medical systems, usually biomedical plus varied indigenous ones, within a society; alternatively, a multiplicity of healing techniques, rather than of medical systems (Durkin-Longley, 1984, in Gochman, I, Part V; Stoner, 1986, in Gochman, IV, 20).

medical sociology The study of social and societal factors related to disease and its explanations and to healing, treatment, responses to illness, and interactions between healers and persons who are sick (Gochman, IV, 20).

medicalization Expansion of the jurisdiction of the profession of medicine to include many problems not previously defined as medical entities (Gabe & Calnan, 1989, in Gochman, I, Part IV).

medication event monitor system A device attached to a medication bottle that records the date and time of every opening, for use in studying adherence (Di Iorio, II, 11).

medicocentrism Practice of viewing health- and illness-related phenomena solely from the point of view of the physician, particularly in reference to *sick role* (Segall, I, 14).

meme A unit of symbolic cultural information (Fabrega, I, 2). See *healmeme*.

mental illness, severe (SMI) A diagnosis in the family of schizophrenic or any other psychotic disorders, or any bipolar disorder, as well as any other medical disorder that is of at least 2 years' duration and disables the patient in at least two major areas of life (Hawley, III, 12).

mutual participation model A framework for physician-patient interaction in which the patient takes an active role in care and both parties share the goal of the patient's well-being (Szasz & Hollender, 1956, in DiMatteo, II, 1).

narrative representation Presentation of materials in the context of a story about someone doing something, for some purpose, that results in specific consequences; used in interventions to increase safety and reduce injury (Cole, IV, 17).

narrative thinking Translation of personal experiences into stories that integrate facts, perceptions, emotions, intentions, actions, and consequences into coherent meaning; involves knowing through stories lived and stories heard and told; contrasted with *paradigmatic thinking* (Howard, 1991, in Cole, IV, 17).

National Health Care for the Homeless An initiative take in 1984 by the Robert Wood Johnson Foundation and the Pew Charitable Trusts to establish health care clinics for the homeless in 19 United States cities (Wright & Joyner, III, 10).

need factor A characteristic such as health status or illness that predicts use of health services; a component of the *health services utilization model* (Aday & Awe, I, 8).

negotiating An intervention to increase adherence that involves medical personnel and the patient jointly discussing and agreeing upon the treatment plan (Creer & Levstek, II, 7).

negotiating model of decision making A framework for physician-patient interaction in which physician and patient belief systems and expectations are given equal value (Reed et al., IV, 2).

occupational culture Group norms and practices within work settings that often shape the discourse on health, including how workers define situations of threat and danger, and influence risk behaviors such as smoking and alcohol use (Eakin, I, 16).

operational research model A way of conducting investigations that begins with a practical, problem-focused question rather than with a conceptual framework; characteristic of research in international health (Coreil, III, 9).

oral rehydration therapy (ORT) An intervention to treat diarrheal conditions in *developing countries* (Coreil, III, 9).

organizational barrier A structural problem within the health care system that hampers a patient's perceptions of availability and accessibility of care; organizational barriers may include compromised quality of care, patient's perceptions of inhospitable facilities, distance and transportation problems, waiting time, inflexible hours, dearth or lack of bilingual or bicultural staff, and exclusionary policies (Morisky & Cabrera, II, 14).

organizational culture See *occupational culture.*

outcome expectancy A person's beliefs about the consequences of some behavior (e.g., Maddux & DuCharme, I, 7; Baranowski, I, 9); perceived value of the consequence of a given behavior (Di Iorio, II, 11).

pain A multifaceted noxious experience involving sensory, cognitive, and emotional dimensions (Gift & White, IV, 7).

paradigmatic thinking Cognitive processes concerned with the construction of context-free and abstract formal concepts and principles; both the goal and method of science, logic, and mathematics, in contrast to *narrative thinking* (Cole, IV, 17).

parochialism/cosmopolitanism A conceptual framework for understanding social ties within families and families' relationships to the larger community. Parochial families are presumed to demonstrate strong commitment to family (usually paternal) tradition and authority and to have enduring friendships primarily with persons whose backgrounds are similar to their own; cosmopolitan families demonstrate less commitment to family authority and expand their friendships over time, including persons with diverse backgrounds. This typology has guided some research into use of health services and attitudes toward health professionals, but its value has been limited (Suchman, 1965, in Geertsen, I, 13).

passive prevention See *prevention, passive.*

paternalism Characterizing an act by a person or a group, *P*, intended to avert some harm or promote some good for a person or a group, *Q*, where *P* has no reason to believe that the act agrees with the current preferences, desires, or dispositions of *Q*, and *P*'s act is a limitation of *Q*'s right to self-determination (Nilstun, IV, 11).

patient role The component of the sick role that involves interaction with health professionals and/or the formal health care system, in contrast to *self-care* and informal care behaviors (Segall, I, 14).

perceived barriers A person's belief that a specified health action has negative value, particularly in terms of impediments or costs; a component of the *health belief model* (Strecher et al., I, 4).

perceived behavioral control A person's belief in the relative ease or difficulty of performing a specified health action; importance increases as volitional control decreases (Maddux & DuCharme, I, 7); similar to *self-efficacy.*

perceived benefits A person's belief that a specified health action has positive value, particularly in reducing the threat of an illness or health condition; a component of the *health belief model* (Strecher et al., I, 4).

perceived health competence Belief in one's ability to influence one's personal health outcomes effectively (Christensen et al., II, 12).

perceived severity/seriousness A person's belief that an illness or health condition would have negative consequences; a component of the *health belief model* (Strecher et al., I, 4).

perceived social norm A person's belief about how other people view and evaluate a behavior (e.g., Maddux & DuCharme, I, 7).

perceived susceptibility A person's belief about risk for an illness or health condition; a component of the *health belief model* (Strecher et al., I, 4).

perceived threat A function of perceived susceptibility and perceived seriousness providing an impetus for taking some action; a component of the *health belief model* (Strecher et al., I, 4); also a component of *protection motivation theory.*

physician authority See *authority, physician.*

physician autonomy See *autonomy, physician.*

poverty An exceptionally low standard of living officially defined by the U.S. Bureau of the Census, based ultimately on cost of food and adjusted annually for inflation (Wright & Joyner, III, 10).

power, patient The degree to which patients exert control over encounters with physicians and other health care professionals; basic factors are the patient's age, gender, race, education and knowledge, and health status (Haug, II, 3).

power, physician Dominance of and control by the physician over patients and other health professionals; basic factors are the physician's age, gender, race, practice style, and social status (Haug, II, 3).

precaution adoption process model A conceptual framework to predict protective or risk-reducing behavior; identifies five basic stages—unaware, aware but not personally engaged, engaged but deciding on a course of action, planning to act but not yet doing so, and acting—plus a maintenance stage (Weinstein & Sandman, 1992, in Gochman, I, Part II). See *transtheoretical model.*

PRECEDE Acronym for part of a conceptual framework for developing and evaluating health education programs, denoting the basic terms: *P*redisposing, *R*einforcing, and *E*nabling *C*auses in *E*ducational *D*iagnosis and *E*valuation (Green, Kreuter, Deeds, & Partridge, 1980, in Glanz & Oldenberg, IV, 8). See *PROCEED*.

precontemplation In the *transtheoretical model*, the stage at which there is no apparent intention to change behavior (Prohaska & Clark, III, 2).

predisposing factor A characteristic such as a health belief, family composition, or social position of family that predicts use of health services; a component of the *health services utilization model* (Aday & Awe, I, 8).

preparation In the *transtheoretical model*, the stage at which a person has taken small steps to engage in some behavior but has not yet taken effective action (Prohaska & Clark, III, 2).

PREPARED™ Acronymic name of a system of improving provider–patient communication and patient self-efficacy and satisfaction; denotes the basic components: recommended *P*rocedure, *R*eason for it, patient's *E*xpectations, *P*robability of achieving them, *A*lternative treatments, *R*isks, *E*xpenses, prior to making a *D*ecision (DiMatteo, II, 1).

prevention, active Individual actions to eliminate or reduce the likelihood of a negative health outcome, in contrast to *passive prevention* (Gauff & Miller, 1986, in Gochman, I, 1).

prevention, passive Societal, institutional, or governmental activities to eliminate or reduce the likelihood of a negative health outcome, in contrast to *active prevention* (Gauff & Miller, 1986, in Gochman, I, 1).

prevention/preventive behavior Any activity (medically recommended or not) undertaken to eliminate or reduce the likelihood of contracting a disease or incurring a negative health outcome, or of detecting a disease at an early, asymptomatic stage (Gochman, I, 1).

prevention, primary Reduction or elimination of risk factors (Last, 1987, in Buchanan, IV, 9).

prevention, secondary Asymptomatic detection of a disease in its early stages (Gochman, I, 1).

principle of justice See *justice, principle of*.

problem-based learning An approach to professional education in which curricular materials resemble problems that students will face as practitioners (Bruhn, IV, 1).

PROCEED Acronym for part of a conceptual framework for developing and evaluating health education programs, denoting the basic terms: *P*olicy, *R*egulatory, and *O*rganizational *C*onstructs for *E*ducational and *E*nvironmental *D*evelopment (Green et al., 1980, in Glanz & Oldenburg, IV, 8). See *PRECEDE*.

professional role See *role, physician/provider*.

protection motivation theory A conceptual framework to determine the effects of threatening health information on attitude and behavior change; basic components are internal and external sources of information, cognitive mediating processes of *threat appraisal* and *coping appraisal*, and adaptive or maladaptive coping modes (Rogers & Prentice-Dunn, I, 6).

psychosocial epidemiology Application of epidemiological methods to determine health-related personal and social characteristics in a population, e.g., people's perceptions of social support, religiosity, and health (Rakowski, III, 5).

public health Collective actions of society to assure the conditions for people to be healthy (Institute of Medicine, 1988, in Buchanan, IV, 9).

reactance Workers' tendency to be defiant about safety and risk behaviors as a way of maintaining their control when they believe their behavior is being manipulated (Cohen & Colligan, II, 20). See *illusion of safety*.

reciprocal determinism A concept expressing the constant interaction between a person, the person's behavior, and the person's family and social environment in the development and maintenance of health behaviors (Baranowski, I, 9; Baranowski & Hearn, IV, 16).

relapse In the *transtheoretical model*, the movement from one stage to a previous stage (Prohaska & Clark, III, 2); in the context of regimens of dental flossing and brushing for plaque removal, defined as *adherence* at less than 43% (McCaul, II, 16).

relapse prevention model A conceptual framework, derived from *social learning theory*, for understanding how and why people backslide from a path of behavior change (Marlatt & Gordon, 1985, in Marcus et al., II, 18).

relative risk Ratio of adverse health consequences of a specified behavior accruing to groups who do and do not perform that behavior (Prohaska & Clark, III, 2).

resource model of preventive health behavior A conceptual framework in nursing to predict health actions; basic components are health resources, including perceived health status, energy level, concern about health, feelings about taking care of one's health; and social resources, such as educational level and income (Kulbok, 1985, in Blue & Brooks, IV, 5).

response efficacy Belief that adopting a behavior will reduce some threat (Strecher et al., I, 4).

risk behavior, sexual Any behavior that increases the likelihood of a sexually transmitted disease (STD), including *AIDS*; such behaviors include sexual intercourse without latex protection, actions that expose open sores or cuts to infected bodily fluids, and sharing intravenous drug use apparatus (Thomason & Campos, III, 8).

risk, relative See *relative risk*.

role, physician/provider A set of normative expectations for the full-time professional activity of caring for the sick, involving the development of technical proficiency, affective neutrality, and objectivity and placing the welfare of the patient above that of the professional's personal interests (Parsons, 1951, 1975, in Salloway et al., II, 4).

role, sick See *patient role*; *sick role*.

safe sex Sexual behavior in which there is no chance of direct bloodstream access to infected blood, blood products, seminal fluid, vaginal fluid, or breast milk (Thomason & Campos, III, 8).

safer sex Sexual behavior that reduces the likelihood of exchange of bodily fluids (Thomason & Campos, III, 8).

secular trend Health behavioral changes in a community that are not attributable to health education or health promotion intervention (Glanz & Oldenburg, IV, 8).

selective survival Changes in the composition of a population due to the higher mortality rates at advancing age of individuals participating in risk behaviors (Prohaska & Clark, III, 2).

self-care A process whereby laypersons can function effectively on their own behalf in health promotion and prevention and in detecting and treating disease (Levin, 1976, in Gochman, I, Part IV); often used interchangeably with *self-management*, *self-regulation* (Di Iorio, II, 11). See *self health management*.

self-care agency An individual's capacity to gather information, make decisions, and perform skillfully the behaviors necessary to assume personal control in health promotion and maintenance as well as in the prevention and treatment of illness (e.g., Orem, 1985, in Blue & Brooks, IV, 5).

self-care autonomy Demonstrating the ability and skills necessary to self-manage a condition (Wysocki & Greco, II, 9).

self-care autonomy, appropriate Expecting a child to have the requisite ability and skills to manage a condition at a level appropriate to the child's maturity (Wysocki & Greco, II, 9).

self-care autonomy, constrained Expecting a child to have the requisite ability and skills to manage a condition at a level less than appropriate to the child's maturity (Wysocki & Greco, II, 9).

self-care autonomy, excessive Expecting a child to have the requisite ability and skills to manage a condition at a level greater than appropriate to the child's maturity (Wysocki, II, 9).

self-efficacy Belief or judgment about one's ability to execute some action successfully (Strecher et al., I, 4; Maddux & DuCharme, I, 7); confidence in one's ability to perform a particular behavior (Baranowski, I, 9). See *health belief model*; *perceived behavioral control*; *protection motivation theory*; *theory of reasoned action*.

self health management Undertaking of lay activities to promote health, to prevent illness, and to detect and treat illness when it occurs; includes a range of behaviors such as: health maintenance activities, illness prevention, symptom evaluation, self-treatment, and use of a variety of health resources such as lay network members as well as diverse health professionals (Segall, I, 14).

self-management, childhood diabetes Assumption of responsibility by a patient and the patient's family for monitoring, evaluating, and adjusting treatment; basic components include demographic factors, family functioning, psychological stress, and interactions with providers to acquire necessary skills (Wysocki & Greco, II, 9). See *self-regulation/self-regulatory skills*.

self-management, epilepsy Sum total of steps a person takes to control seizures and to control the effects of having a seizure disorder; common practices include taking medications at prescribed times, avoiding factors that trigger seizures, following safety precautions such as not driving when seizures are not under control, avoiding running out of medications, consulting with professionals about treatment or unexpected problems, and monitoring seizure frequency; often used interchangeably with *self-care*, *self-regulation* (Di Iorio, II, 11).

self-prediction What one states one will do in contrast to *behavioral intention*: what one predicts one will do (Maddux & DuCharme, I, 7). See *intention, behavioral; theory of reasoned action.*

self-regulation/self-regulatory skills Ability to control or change one's health behavior, including goal setting, monitoring movement toward goals, exerting effort and skill to reach goals, and rewarding self for attaining goals (Baranowski, I, 9); used interchangeably with *self-care, self-management* (Di Iorio, II, 11); a conceptual framework designed to understand behavior change, particularly in relation to disease management; basic components include *self-efficacy, outcome expectancy,* monitoring feedback, role modeling, social support, and learning of necessary skills (Clark, II, 8).

sense of place Personal and social meanings or particular significance that people attach to physical locations or settings, as distinct from the objective or physical space dimensions (Tuan, 1974, in Scarpaci & Kearns, II, 5; Gochman, IV, 20).

setting The conventional "bricks and mortar" facilities in which health care takes place as well as the psychosocial implications of such places for provider-patient encounters (Scarpaci & Kearns, II, 5).

sex, safe See *safe sex.*

sexism In health care, a focus primarily on male health issues and on health roles for women that are subordinate to those of men (Elder, Humphreys, & Lakowski, 1988, in VanScoy, III, 7).

shared decision making model A framework for physician-patient interaction in which the physician is obliged to present the patient with all available information without filtering it, and without giving advice, in order for the patient to be able to make the most informed decision about care (Wennberg, 1990, in Reed et al., IV, 2).

sick call The processing of health complaints in correctional facilities, which requires that inmates sign up, have their requests reviewed and triaged, and then be seen by a provider; inmates have no choice of providers or of appointment time (Anno, III, 14).

sick role A conceptual framework developed by Parsons (1951, in Segall, I, 14) for analyzing the behavior of a person who has been diagnosed as ill; basic components are the person's rights to be exempt from responsibility for the incapacity and from normal role and task obligations and the person's duties to seek professional care and to abide by professional advice and recover (Segall, I, 14).

sick role, alternative Elaboration of the Parsonian *sick role* model, adding the person's rights to make decisions about health care and to be dependent on lay others for care and social support and the person's duties to maintain health and overcome illness and to engage in routine self-management; assumes that members of the person's social network are prepared to take on added responsibilities and to function as caregivers as needed (Segall, I, 14).

sickness A departure from being healthy, often defined through a combination of symptoms experienced, not feeling "right" or "normal," and consequences such as restricted activity (Lau, I, 3); the social side of illness (Gochman, I, 1); the social construction of an episode of illness, the way illness is dealt with in society (Fabrega, I, 2); a form of deviance (Segall, I, 14); the contextualized definition of dysfunction, a process by which signs and symptoms are given socially recognizable meanings (Dressler & Oths, I, 17).

social action An approach to community health promotion interventions involving advocacy or conflict strategy that entails mass mobilization of low-power components and use of political pressure (Rothman, 1979, in Schooler & Flora, IV, 15).

social cognitive theory A general social psychological conceptual framework adapted to understand the acquisition or health behaviors; basic components are *outcome expectancy, self-efficacy,* skills, and social evaluation of and feedback on behavior (Baranowski, I, 9; Di Iorio, II, 11; Marcus et al., II, 18).

social epidemiology See *psychosocial epidemiology.*

social learning theory A conceptual framework for understanding the acquisition of health behaviors; basic components are observation, modeling, and reinforcement in interpersonal contexts (Tinsley, I, 11; Marcus et al., II, 18).

social marketing Use of merchandising and advertising techniques to increase the effectiveness of health-related campaigns, e.g., for immunizations and family planning; basic components are lowering the price; responding to market demands, such as needs; emphasizing relative advantages of the service or product; making the service or product accessible to the population; and using a full range of mass media to promote the service or product (Buchanan, IV, 9).

social network A broad conceptual framework for examining social ties and social support; includes dimensions of structure (e.g., number and density of linkages, interaction (e.g., nature and quality), and function (e.g., provision of information, resources, and emotional support). Not identical to *social support*; networks may be unsupportive (Ritter, 1988, in Gochman, I, Part IV).

social norms Generally held beliefs about the appropriateness or desirability of some behavior.

social planning A technical approach to community health promotion interventions using rational empirical processes of data accumulation, and persuasion involving experts (Rothman, 1979, in Schooler & Flora, IV, 15).

social structure The organization or patterning of social ties; regularities in interpersonal linkages. *Parochialism/cosmpolitanism* has been a major typology of social structure relevant to health behavior research (Geertsen, I, 13).

social support Aggregate of social ties involving interpersonal relationships that protect people from negative experiences, including both structural (e.g., living arrangements, participation in social activities) and functional (e.g., emotional support, encouraging expression of feelings, provision of advice) dimensions (e.g., Ritter, 1988, in Gochman, I, Part IV); a range of interpersonal exchanges that include not only the provision of physical, social, and emotional assistance, but also the subjective consequences of making individuals feel that they are the subject of enduring concern by others (Pilisuk & Parks, 1981, in Morisky & Cabrera, II, 14).

social support, directive Assumption by others of responsibility for tasks or decisions in relation to *adherence* (Fisher et al., II, 10).

social support, nondirective Participation by others in cooperating, sharing, and expressing understanding of feelings in relation to *adherence* without attempts to control or alter tasks or decisions (Fisher et al., II, 10).

social ties Interpersonal linkages, including those with household members, relatives, and friends (Geertsen, I, 13).

sociology of medicine See *medical sociology*.

specific etiology, doctrine of An essentially mechanistic medical model that specified that for each illness there was a single, necessary, and sufficient causal agent or pathogen (Pasteur, 1873 [cited in Hamann, 1994], in Wiese & Gallagher, IV, 4).

stage models of adoption See *transtheoretical model*.

stages of change models See *transtheoretical model*.

stepped-care model A conceptual framework for increasing smoking cessation that matches intensity of treatment to stages of change (Glasglow & Orleans, II, 19).

stereotyping Physician's categorization of a patient as bad or undesirable, using the patient's behavior as a clue indicative of potential challenge to the physician's authority (Ben-Sira, II, 2).

support-mobilizing hypothesis A conceptual framework for understanding caregiver behavior, based on the assumption that stress will motivate the caregiver to elicit support (Bass, Tausig, & Noelker, 1988/1989, in Wright, III, 13).

t'ai chi An ancient Chinese system of exercise and meditation being introduced in selected religious communities as a health behavior intervention (Duckro, Magaletta, & Wolf, III, 15).

theory of planned behavior See *theory of reasoned action*.

theory of reasoned action A conceptual framework designed to predict intentions to engage in or change specified health behaviors (Maddux & DuCharme, I, 7); basic components are a person's attitudes toward a specified behavior and a person's perceptions of the social norms regarding the behavior. See *intention, behavioral*; *self-prediction*.

therapeutic landscape See *landscape, therapeutic*.

threat appraisal Evaluation of maladaptive responses (Rogers & Prentice-Dunn, I, 6). See *protection motivation theory*.

transtheoretical model A conceptual framework for predicting behavior change that assumes a progression of stages from *precontemplation* of change through *contemplation*, *preparation*, *action*, maintenance, and *relapse*, with different intervention approaches appropriate for each stage (Prohaska & Di Clemente, 1992, in Gochman, I, Part II; Rimer et al., II, 15; Glasgow & Orleans, II, 19); incorporates behavioral intentions, *decisional balance theory*, *self-efficacy*, and individual processes of behavioral change (Marcus et al., II, 18).

utilitarianism A conceptual framework applied to health issues that emphasizes the maximization of some desired state (Nilstun, IV, 11).

utilization framework A refinement of the *health services utilization model* designed to predict type and purpose of health care use; basic components are societal determinants such as technology and social norms, health service system resources and organizations, and *predisposing*, *enabling*, and *need factors* (Andersen & Newman, 1973, in Aday & Awe, I, 8).

value-based learning An approach to professional education that places values, ethics, and moral issues at the curricular core (Bruhn, IV, 1).

wellness Realization of the optimum health potential of an individual, family, or community; achieved by enhancing physical, psychological, and sociological well-being through activities aimed at the promotion of health (Blue & Brooks, IV, 5).

window of vulnerability A period in the family life cycle when the strength of the family's influence on health behaviors has the potential for diminishing (Lau, Quadrel, & Hartman, 1990, in Gochman, I, 10).

worksite program One or more health promotion activities conducted in an occupational setting (Schooler & Flora, IV, 15).

Contents of Volumes I–IV

VOLUME II. PROVIDER DETERMINANTS

VOLUME III. DEMOGRAPHY, DEVELOPMENT, AND DIVERSITY

VOLUME IV. RELEVANCE FOR PROFESSIONALS AND ISSUES FOR THE FUTURE

Index to Volumes I–IV

In addition to the entries in this Index, the reader is encouraged to look at the Contents of each volume and the Contents of Volumes I–IV that appears at the end of each volume, as well as at the Glossary contained in each volume. Space limitations precluded listing *every* intervention or program, government document, or disease or condition identified in the chapters. Similarly, passages dealing *solely* with etiologies, morbidity, mortality, and demographic correlates of diseases with no relevance for health behavior were not indexed.

MIX
Papier aus verantwortungsvollen Quellen
Paper from responsible sources
FSC® C105338

If you have any concerns about our products,
you can contact us on
ProductSafety@springernature.com

In case Publisher is established outside the EU,
the EU authorized representative is:
Springer Nature Customer Service Center GmbH
Europaplatz 3, 69115 Heidelberg, Germany

Printed by Libri Plureos GmbH
in Hamburg, Germany